Health and Humanity

*A History of the Johns Hopkins Bloomberg School
of Public Health, 1935–1985*

KAREN KRUSE THOMAS

Johns Hopkins University Press
Baltimore

Johns Hopkins University Press
2715 North Charles Street
Baltimore, Maryland 21218-4363
www.press.jhu.edu

Library of Congress Cataloging-in-Publication Data

Names: Thomas, Karen Kruse, author.
Title: Health and humanity : a history of the Johns Hopkins Bloomberg School
of Public Health, 1935–1985 / Karen Kruse Thomas.
Description: Baltimore : Johns Hopkins University Press, 2016. | Includes
bibliographical references and index.
Identifiers: LCCN 2016005169 | ISBN 9781421421087 (hardcover : alk. paper) |
ISBN 1421421089 (hardcover : alk. paper) | ISBN 9781421421094 (electronic) |
ISBN 1421421097 (electronic)
Subjects: | MESH: Johns Hopkins University. School of Hygiene and Public Health. |
Schools, Public Health   history | Education, Public Health Professional   history |
History, 20th Century | Baltimore
Classification: LCC R747.H722 | NLM WA 19 AM3 | DDC 610.71/17526— dc23 LC
record available at http://lccn.loc.gov/2016005169

A catalog record for this book is available from the British Library.

*Special discounts are available for bulk purchases of this book. For more information,
please contact Special Sales at 410-516-6936 or specialsales@press.jhu.edu.*

To three people whose support was essential in writing this book but who did not live to see it finished.

My postdoctoral adviser, Harry M. Marks (1946–2011)

My father, H. William Kruse (1926–2012)

My guide and encourager at the School of Public Health, Timothy D. Baker (1925–2013)

CONTENTS

Epilogue   392

In 2008, I began a postdoctoral fellowship at the Institute of the History of Medicine at the Johns Hopkins School of Medicine. This fellowship, which would profoundly and happily change my life, resulted from the foresight of Michael J. Klag, dean of the Johns Hopkins Bloomberg School of Public Health. Soon after becoming dean in 2005, he began planning for the school's centennial in 2016, and at the top of his list was commissioning a follow-up volume to Elizabeth Fee's history of the school's founding and early years, *Disease and Discovery: A History of the Johns Hopkins School of Hygiene and Public Health, 1916–1939*. Fee's insightful volume is among the most widely cited sources on the twentieth-century history of public health; it set high expectations for the sequel. Before I even interviewed for the fellowship, I cold-called Elizabeth from the Baltimore–Washington airport and asked for her advice. She very graciously gave it to me and would subsequently share her abundant trove of research materials.

Many people guided me in conceptualizing, gathering widely scattered sources, and writing the narrative for this ambitious project. For nearly eight years, Mike Klag has shown an enduring commitment to the success of the book and the Bloomberg School Centennial celebration for which it was written; I could not ask for a more supportive dean in my corner. At the Institute of the History of Medicine, I was privileged to work with Harry M. Marks, who urged me to explore the complex roots of the vast intellectual networks of mid-twentieth-century public health. Randall M. Packard, director of the institute, and faculty member Graham Mooney also provided expert guidance. Participants in the institute's renowned colloquium offered their very helpful suggestions on an earlier draft of chapter 7, and I also thank those who offered feedback on other parts of the book presented to the American Association for the History of Medicine, the National Institutes of Health Office of History, the *Journal of Policy History* Conference, and the Bloomberg School's Centennial Lunch and Learn Lecture Series.

The records of the School of Hygiene and Public Health (JHSPH) are held in the Alan Mason Chesney Archives of the Johns Hopkins Medical Institutions, where I spent four fun and fascinating years researching this book. I could not have written it without the Chesney's knowledgeable staff, including its director, Nancy McCall, and staff members Phoebe Letocha, Tim Wisniewski, Andy Harrison, and Marjorie Kehoe. With their able guidance, I had the privilege of being the first to delve into the many unprocessed JHSPH collections, which represent one of the world's most comprehensive and in-depth resources on the history of public health, spanning the areas of public policy, practice, education, research, philanthropy, and international development. JHSPH faculty served as consultants to every major organization engaged in domestic and international public health, including federal and military agencies such as the US Public Health Service, US Armed Forces Epidemiology Board, Atomic Energy Commission, Tennessee Valley Authority, National Institutes of Health, and US Agency for International Development; state and local health departments (in 1960, JHSPH alumni headed 21 of the nation's 50 state health departments); voluntary health organizations such as the National Foundation for Infantile Paralysis, American Cancer Society, American Heart Association, and American Red Cross; philanthropies such as the Rockefeller, Ford, and Commonwealth foundations; international health agencies such as the World Health Organization, UNICEF, and Pan American Health Organization; professional groups such as the American Public Health Association and Association of Schools of Public Health; and a wide variety of schools of medicine and public health in the United States and abroad. One of this project's many collateral benefits has been to expand the Chesney's public health collections and make them more accessible to researchers. I am also grateful to James Stimpert, archivist at the Johns Hopkins University Special Collections, and the staff of the National Archives at College Park.

I am truly blessed to have astonishingly supportive colleagues in the Bloomberg School Office of External Affairs, who have gamely listened, offered consolation when necessary, and shared my excitement about this project throughout the four years I have served on staff. In particular, Heath Elliott, Susan Sperry, Josh Else, Barb Verrier, Brian Simpson, Robert Ollinger, Konrad Crispino, and Kyle Rudgers have coached me along (and lit a fire under me on occasion) to ensure that this book and everything else we have worked so hard on together for the centennial actually happened. I also want to thank my longsuffering children, Phoebe and Fletcher, who have patiently endured having a parent who is obsessed with writing a book on the history of public health. My father, Bill Kruse, and sister, Carolyn Freedell, provided wonderful encouragement, as they always have. And last but not least, I want to thank the many Bloomberg School faculty, staff, and alumni who were interviewed for the book, read drafts, or otherwise contributed to making this a more interesting and accurate history. Professor Tim Baker was an amazing resource on the history of the school and provided invaluable guidance on what questions to ask and to whom. Kelley Squazzo and Elizabeth Demers at Johns Hopkins University Press were indispensable to the success of the book.

This book was incredibly difficult to write, for several reasons. First, during the writing phase, I experienced in quick succession the death of my postdoctoral adviser, a divorce, the death of a parent, and a family member's severe illness. Second, I had to balance many competing agendas and goals for what this book would be: a scholarly, objective, well-footnoted work in the history of medicine and public health; a compelling—and marketable—story about personalities and politics that would reach a general audience; and a homage to the trials and accomplishments of the men and women who have built one of the world's oldest and most recognized schools of public health. Third, public health is so diverse, and the school's reach is so extensive, that it was agonizing to decide what to include and what to leave out. My hope is that the resulting book is comprehensive enough to be a valuable resource for historians and other scholars of public health, compelling enough to appeal to readers who are unaffiliated with the Bloomberg School, and humane enough to adequately recognize the heroic yet flawed individuals who are the heart of the story. Some readers will doubtless question my decisions on which people, departments, and topics to feature most prominently, but please bear in mind that my hand was forced in some cases by the absence of archival documents on otherwise worthy figures, or simply the difficulty of fitting disparate parts into the flow of the narrative.

Throughout the text, Johns Hopkins School of Hygiene and Public Health alumni are denoted at first mention by their degree and graduation year in parentheses. The school is referred to interchangeably as JHSPH, the School of Hygiene, or Hygiene, and the Johns Hopkins School of Medicine is called the School of Medicine, the medical school, or Medicine.

I am deeply grateful to the Johns Hopkins Bloomberg School of Public Health for making this book possible. I am, however, solely responsible for its contents, which do not represent the official views of the Bloomberg School.

ACGs	adjusted clinical groups
AFDC	Aid to Families with Dependent Children
AFEB	Armed Forces Epidemiological Board
AMA	American Medical Association
ANA	American Nursing Association
APHA	American Public Health Association
ASPH	Association of Schools of Public Health
BCG	bacillus Calmette–Guérin vaccine against tuberculosis
BCHD	Baltimore City Health Department
CDC	Communicable Disease Center of the US Public Health Service (renamed Center for Disease Control in 1970, Centers for Disease Control in 1980, and Centers for Disease Control and Prevention in 1992)
DrPH	Doctor of Public Health
EHD	Eastern Health District
EHS	Department of Environmental Health Sciences
EIS	Epidemic Intelligence Service of the Communicable Disease Center
EPA	US Environmental Protection Agency
FDA	US Food and Drug Administration
GEB	Rockefeller General Education Board
GIS	geographic information systems
HEW	US Department of Health, Education and Welfare (established as cabinet-level agency in 1953)
HHS	US Department of Health and Human Services (successor to HEW in 1979)
Homewood	arts and sciences campus of Johns Hopkins University
HPM	Department of Health Policy and Management
ICA	US International Cooperation Administration
ICD	International Classification of Diseases

ICDDR,B	International Centre for Diarrheal Disease Research, Bangladesh
IHD	Rockefeller Foundation International Health Division
IRB	institutional review board
IUD	intrauterine device
JHMI	Johns Hopkins Medical Institutions (the Johns Hopkins Hospital, School of Medicine, School of Hygiene and Public Health, and, after 1984, School of Nursing)
JHSPH	Johns Hopkins School of Hygiene and Public Health
JHU	Johns Hopkins University
MCH	Department of Maternal and Child Health
MHS	Master of Health Science
MPH	Master of Public Health
MSc	Master of Science in Hygiene
NAACP	National Association for the Advancement of Colored People
NAMRU	US Naval Medical Research Unit
NATO	North Atlantic Treaty Organization
NCHS	CDC National Center for Health Statistics
NCI	National Cancer Institute
NGO	nongovernmental organization
NHI	National Heart Institute (to reflect its broadened mission, NHI was renamed the National Heart and Lung Institute in 1969 and the National Heart, Lung and Blood Institute in 1976)
NIAAA	National Institute on Alcohol Abuse and Alcoholism
NIAID	National Institute of Allergy and Infectious Diseases
NICHD	National Institute of Child Health and Human Development
NIDA	National Institute on Drug Abuse
NIEHS	National Institute of Environmental Health Sciences
NIH	National Institutes of Health
NIMH	National Institute of Mental Health
NRC	National Research Council
ORO	US Army Operations Research Office, headquartered at Johns Hopkins
OSHA	US Occupational Safety and Health Administration
PAHO	Pan American Health Organization (before 1959, Pan American Sanitary Bureau)
PHA	Department of Public Health Administration
PhD	Doctor of Philosophy

PHS	US Public Health Service
P.L. 480	Public Law 480, the Agricultural Trade Development and Assistance Act of 1954
ScD	Doctor of Science in Hygiene
SEATO	Southeast Asia Treaty Organization
SS	Social Security Act of 1935
TB	tuberculosis
TPI	*Treponema pallidum* immobilization test for syphilis
UNICEF	United Nations Children's Fund
USAID	US Agency for International Development
VA	Veterans Administration
VD	venereal disease
WEPREC	West Pakistan Population Research and Evaluation Center
WHO	World Health Organization
WIC	Women, Infants and Children

Health and Humanity

Prologue

Through the prism of the oldest and largest independent graduate school of public health, this book surveys the growth of academic public health in the mid-twentieth-century United States. The Johns Hopkins School of Hygiene and Public Health (JHSPH) was established in 1916 to carry out the mandate of its founding dean, William Henry Welch, to "cultivate the science of hygiene." Welch and the Rockefeller Foundation promoted a new model of scientific training that wove the laboratory mind-set together with the methods of public health administration and epidemiological fieldwork. By developing and transmitting that model, JHSPH was a catalyst for exponential growth in the evidence base for public health. Its faculty and alumni would launch public health agencies and schools around the world.

Origins of US Graduate Public Health Education

At the turn of the twentieth century, death was a familiar event to most Americans, rich and poor. Respiratory infections killed 1 in 250 people each year, and waterborne diseases killed 1 in 500. Women averaged eight births during their reproductive lives (not including miscarriages), and without access to contraceptives or prenatal care, near-constant childbearing frequently ended tragically for mothers, their infants, or both. Malnutrition, parasitic infections, and serious injuries were accepted as facts of life, and nearly 20 percent of infants died before their first birthdays. From the federal to the local levels, governments exercised little authority to protect consumers or the environment.

During the Progressive Era, crusading reformers such as Upton Sinclair, Jane Addams, and Lewis Hine had employed muckraking journalism and the rising influence of scientific experts to push for government regulation and other changes to safeguard the most vulnerable members of society, especially children. A central thrust of Progressivism was to establish public health as a basic responsibility of state and local governments. By 1920, most large cities provided the standard "basic six" services: vital statistics, environmental sanitation (including ensuring food, milk, and water purity), communicable disease control, maternal and child health, health education, and public health laboratory services. Yet many less-populated areas remained without full-time health departments until after World War II, particularly in the rural South and West.[1]

As the gospels of germs and social reform advanced together, the common goal of conquering infectious disease united public health and medicine. Their relationship was mapped out along two axes: prevention/cure and population/individual. Traditionally, public health was defined by its broad-gauged preventive approach to protecting the health of whole populations, while clinical medicine focused on curing acute disease in the individual patient. The single largest patron of public health and medicine, in the United States and abroad, was the Rockefeller Foundation. Created with the spoils of John D. Rockefeller's Standard Oil empire, the foundation employed a multipronged strategy of research, training programs, and practical demonstration projects. By funding major scientific initiatives and endowing modern schools of medicine and public health, Rockefeller played a key role in establishing the basis for biomedical research as well as health-oriented philanthropy. The foundation would also provide the funding, leadership, and institutional prototypes necessary to establish the Johns Hopkins School of Hygiene and Public Health.[2]

At the Johns Hopkins University in Baltimore, Quaker banker Johns Hopkins had endowed the School of Medicine and the Johns Hopkins Hospital as the first American medical institutions dedicated to scientific clinical investigation and instruction. William Henry Welch, the medical school's founding dean from 1893 to 1898, was a key Rockefeller adviser. In 1901, he helped organize the Rockefeller Institute for Medical Research, the nation's first biomedical research institute. Welch was president of the board of trustees, and his former student Simon Flexner was the institute's first director.[3]

As a young pathologist in the 1880s, Welch had visited the German institutes of hygiene, particularly Max von Pettenkofer's institute in Munich, and he longed to bring the model of laboratory-driven health reform back to the United States. According to science historian Robert E. Kohler, the Johns Hopkins School of Medicine "deliberately pushed to the limit the idea that basic science was the engine of medical progress." But Welch knew that the science of hygiene could accomplish even more than it had at the School of Medicine and the Rockefeller Institute. The whole structure of medical education and research centered on the acutely ill hospital patient, yet treating disease in its advanced stages often proved futile, particularly in the pre-antibiotic era. In the 1910s and 1920s, Welch and other Rockefeller leaders extended the foundation's scope of activity to develop the first effective disease control programs in the American South and Latin America.[4]

The first of these programs was the Rockefeller Sanitary Commission for the Eradication of Hookworm Disease, established in 1909. Hookworm was not a deadly disease, but it caused stunted growth and lethargy, earning it the moniker, "the germ of laziness." Hookworm disease was especially common in young children, since it was contracted by walking barefoot in soil fertilized with infested human waste. The Sanitary Commission's director in North Carolina, John Ferrell, rhapsodized about hookworm as a disease that "affords the opportunity for the eternal demonstration." Diphtheria and malaria were too sporadic, and typhoid fever and tuberculosis were too resistant to treatment. Hookworm, the South's most prevalent disease, was available "every day of the year in every community. It has a causative agent discernible to the naked eye, is both preventable and curable by methods the simplicity of which appeals to everyone. The results following treatment are so prompt and emphatic that they have been aptly compared with the miracles of the New Testament."[5]

The Sanitary Commission cooperated with the Public Health Service (PHS) Hygienic Laboratory to conduct extensive testing in the southeastern United States that established a hookworm infection prevalence rate of approximately 40 percent of the population. Health workers provided the vermifugal drug thymol to those whose stool samples revealed evidence of infection, and the campaign also built sanitary privies and conducted extensive health education to reinforce preventive methods, especially wearing shoes. By 1915, nearly a million southern children in 600 counties had been examined, even though some southern residents and doctors regarded the Rockefeller agents and PHS officers as meddling outsiders.

The hookworm campaign helped generate the political will and government funding to establish and strengthen public health departments across the South. In the long term, hookworm proved difficult to control, much less eradicate. But, as the first disease control program to combine modern scientific methods of screening, data collection, mass communication, and treatment, the hookworm campaign set the stage for everything that followed in public health.[6]

After Rockefeller officials voted in 1915 to disband the Sanitary Commission, its director, Wickliffe Rose, convinced the foundation to create a permanent International Health Division (IHD) to carry on the methods developed against hookworm to fight it and other diseases in foreign countries. (The division underwent several name changes during its 36-year existence, but for the sake of simplicity, it will be referred to as the IHD.) The division's first order of business was to establish an independent school of public health (for a comprehensive account of this process, see Elizabeth Fee's *Disease and Discovery: A History of the Johns Hopkins School of Hygiene and Public Health, 1916–1939*, on which this volume builds). In 1915, Welch and Rose submitted a report to the Rockefeller General Education Board (GEB) that described public health training opportunities as well as laboratories of hygiene at existing institutions as "woefully lacking"; the quality of instruction was "all inadequate and unsatisfactory." Welch and Rose proclaimed that correcting these deficiencies was "at present the most urgent [need] in medical education and in public health work, and is recognized on all sides."[7]

This allegedly sorry state of affairs must be understood in proper context as a funding appeal to the Rockefeller Foundation. In response to Abraham Flexner's 1910 report on medical education in the United States and Canada, the GEB had already begun to award grants to medical schools that Flexner deemed worthy of investment. By 1915, seven universities granted graduate degrees in hygiene and public health (table 1), and the GEB could have funded the expansion of some or all of them. Instead, Rockefeller first chose to put all its eggs in one basket to establish an entirely new school at Johns Hopkins.[8]

This decision was based less on the inadequacy of existing programs than on the substantial agreement of early public health leaders on two key points. First, public health was an interdisciplinary field that extended far beyond the laboratory—and the medical school—to encompass a powerful set of methodological tools for systematically examining the host of factors that shaped the health of populations. The second point followed from the first: public health degree programs should ideally be housed in independent units that were co-equal with medical schools, not controlled by them, as most programs then were. Welch and Rose proposed that the new school should (1) cultivate hygiene as a science, (2) have access to a first-class medical school and hospital yet remain fully independent of them, and (3) train public health leaders, scientists, and university faculty.[9]

With the proclamation that "public health work constitutes a distinct profession," the Welch–Rose Report was a Declaration of Independence for public

TABLE I
US Graduate Degrees Awarded in Hygiene or Public Health, 1909–1923

Institution and Year First Awarded	Division	Degree Name	Years to Complete
University of Pennsylvania[1]			
1909	Medicine	Certified Sanitarian[2]	1
1911	Medicine	Doctor of Public Hygiene	1
University of Wisconsin[3]			
1912	Graduate	Doctor of Public Health	2
1915	Graduate	Master of Public Health	1
Harvard University/ Massachusetts Institute of Technology			
1914	Medicine, Science, Engineering	Certificate of Public Health	1
Tulane University			
1914	Medicine	Certificate of Public Health	1
Yale University			
1915	Medicine	Doctor of Public Health	2
1915	Graduate	Certificate of Public Health	1
University of Michigan[4]			
1915	Medicine	Master of Science in Public Health	1
1916	Medicine	Doctor of Public Health	2
Harvard University			
1918	Medicine	Doctor of Public Health	2
Massachusetts Institute of Technology			
1918	Graduate	Master of Science in Biology and Public Health[2]	1
New York University/ Bellevue Hospital			
1918	Medicine	Doctor of Public Health	1
University of California, Berkeley			
1918	Graduate	Graduate in Public Health[2]	2
Johns Hopkins University			
1919	Hygiene and Public Health	Doctor of Public Health	2
1919	Hygiene and Public Health	Doctor of Science in Hygiene[2]	3
1922	Hygiene and Public Health	Certificate of Public Health[5]	1

(*continued*)

TABLE I (*continued*)

Institution and Year First Awarded	Division	Degree Name	Years to Complete
DeLamar Institute of Public Health at Columbia College of Physicians and Surgeons 1923	Medicine	Master of Science in Public Health	1

[1] Public health program discontinued after 1929.
[2] Denotes degree for individuals who do not hold MD degrees.
[3] Public health program discontinued after 1916.
[4] Public health program was expanded and transferred from the medical school to the graduate school in 1921.
[5] Renamed the Master of Public Health in 1939, and all Certificate of Public Health degrees were retroactively converted to Master of Public Health degrees.

health. Fee calls public health education's independence from both medical schools and government health agencies "the most remarkable single fact" about its development in America. By contrast, public health education in Europe was subsumed under government bureaucracies, and in Great Britain, it remained under control of the medical profession. From the beginning, Rockefeller officials urged JHSPH to exercise leadership in preventive medicine and public health administration and to beware of subordinating itself to the medical school. The foundation's 1917 annual report noted, "The School of Hygiene and Public Health will have its own quarters, its own faculty, its own problems and purposes, its own distinct body of students, and will develop from the outset a corporate individuality and a professional spirit." After JHSPH opened in October 1918, Rockefeller officials called it "A West Point for Health Officers," which underlined the school's mission to prepare high-level administrators and scientific researchers.[10]

JHSPH offered degrees in hygiene to train nonphysicians for research careers and in public health for physicians who wanted to prepare for leadership positions in government, academics, and private foundations (table 2). Ferrell, who had served as Rose's second-in-command, enrolled in the first DrPH class, even though he had more public health experience than some of the instructors. As associate director of the IHD from 1914 to 1944, Ferrell remained a close adviser to the school, guiding the growth of research and training programs at Johns Hopkins and brokering its relationships with many other institutions. Ferrell saw the big picture beyond the immediate effort to rid the South of hookworm. "In a long and profitable experience with petroleum," he wrote, "Rockefeller had learned that the byproducts of his industry rival in impor-

TABLE 2
Degrees at the Johns Hopkins School of Hygiene and Public Health before 1960

Degree Track	Degree Name	Description
Professional leadership (primarily physicians). Mix of foreign and US students.	Certificate of Public Health	Renamed Master of Public Health in 1939. One year of coursework, no exam or thesis.
	Doctor of Public Health	Two years of coursework and an individual study on a subject in public health or hygiene.
Scientific research (nonphysicians).	Master of Science in Hygiene	Two years of coursework and a written exam in a special field. Must produce an original thesis. Highest number of female students. Most ScM degrees are awarded in laboratory sciences, biostatistics, and epidemiology.
	Doctor of Science in Hygiene	Three years of coursework and a written exam in a special field. Must produce a work of rigorous original research. Most students are from United States. Most ScDs are awarded in parasitology, bacteriology, and physiological hygiene.

tance the refined oil." Not eradication but the disease's eternal presence and dramatically demonstrable disappearance made hookworm the perfect entering wedge for public health. And such an enormous task demanded a vast, dedicated labor force.[11]

Grants from Rockefeller and other private philanthropies established a growing number of independent schools of public health in the United States and abroad (table 3). But in the post–Flexner Report era, a degree from a Flexner-approved medical school would nearly guarantee entry into a lucrative private practice, whereas an additional year or more of advanced study to qualify as a health officer would likely reduce a doctor's earnings. Schools of public health now proposed to recruit from a smaller pool of better-qualified physicians and distill them still further into Renaissance men with a command of basic science, epidemiology, vital statistics, sanitary engineering, and public health administration.[12]

Herein lay a financial conundrum that would dog schools of public health throughout the twentieth century. The Rockefeller model of public health training was expensive. It required high-quality applicants who were willing to sacrifice future earnings in the name of science and humanity to work

TABLE 3
Early Schools of Public Health Established with Philanthropic Grants[1]

Year	Name	Location
1916	Johns Hopkins School of Hygiene and Public Health (opened 1918)	Baltimore, Maryland, USA
	Institute of Hygiene[2]	São Paulo, Brazil
1918	School of Hygiene	Warsaw, Poland
1921	University of Michigan Division of Hygiene and Public Health[3]	Ann Arbor, Michigan, USA
1921	State Institute of Public Health (opened 1925)	Prague, Czechoslovakia
1922	Harvard School of Public Health	Cambridge, Massachusetts, USA
1922	Columbia College of Physicians and Surgeons DeLamar Institute of Public Health	New York, New York, USA
1924	London School of Hygiene and Tropical Medicine[4]	London, England
1924	University of Toronto School of Hygiene	Toronto, Canada
1924	Central Hygiene Institute	Belgrade, Yugoslavia (now Serbia)
1929	University of Manila School of Hygiene and Public Health	Manila, Philippines
1932	All India Institute of Hygiene and Public Health	Calcutta, India

[1] The DeLamar Institute was founded with a bequest from Joseph DeLamar; all other schools listed were established with Rockefeller Foundation grants.

[2] Became the University of São Paulo School of Public Health and Hygiene in 1945.

[3] The public health program was expanded and transferred from the medical to the graduate school in 1921.

[4] The London School of Tropical Medicine was founded in 1899 and renamed when the Rockefeller Foundation awarded a grant to expand the school's capacity in public health.

wherever disease was rampant. These students would need scholarships to lure them into public health and sustain them through full-time studies without employment. Second, Rockefeller prescribed administrative (and budgetary) independence from medical schools. Without their financial support and without wealthy alumni or grateful patients, schools of public health were almost entirely dependent on private philanthropy. This kept the number of graduates small and left schools vulnerable to economic downturns, when endowment income decreased. Dependence on a single source of income could spell doom if a school's patron either withdrew support or ran into financial trouble.

Johns Hopkins, the first school of public health founded with a Rockefeller endowment, would later lead academic public health's crusade to replace private funding with federal grants. But first, JHSPH leaders had to decide what constituted essential knowledge for the health officer.

Public Health Problem Solving

The Rockefeller Foundation's 1924 annual report noted, "The idea that an ordinary medical education fits a doctor to be a health officer is a serious error which does much harm." Instead, public health professionals needed training "under expert guidance in the practical work of the public health laboratory, the bureau of vital statistics, the health-center, baby welfare station, the house-to-house service of the sanitary inspector, the public health nurse, etc."[13] To provide a sense of how closely Johns Hopkins aligned itself with public health practice, table 4 compares the development of special sections in the American Public Health Association (APHA) with the founding of corresponding departments at JHSPH.

The school's departments of immunology and virology were the first of their kind in the world. By establishing basic science departments, the school recognized the early importance of hygienic laboratories in public health practice, in keeping with Welch's experience as a member of the advisory board of the PHS Hygienic Laboratory and as president of the Maryland State Board of Health from 1900 to 1922. Public health scientists explored the immunology

TABLE 4
American Public Health Association Sections and Corresponding JHSPH Departments

APHA Sections, with Year Established		JHSPH Departments, with Year Established	
Laboratory Section	1899	Bacteriology	1917
		Immunology	1917
		Medical Zoology	1917
		Filterable Viruses	1925
		Helminthology	1927
		Biology	1930
Health Officers	1908	Public Health Administration	1917
Vital Statistics	1908	Biometry and Vital Statistics[1]	1917
Engineering	1911	Sanitary Engineering	1937
Industrial Hygiene	1914	Physiological Hygiene[2]	1917
Food and Nutrition	1917	Chemical Hygiene[3]	1917
Maternal and Child Health	1921	Maternal and Child Hygiene[4]	1947
Public Health Education	1922	Public Health Education	1974
Public Health Nursing	1923	Public Health Nursing[5]	1950
Epidemiology	1929	Epidemiology	1917
Mental Health	1955	Mental Hygiene[6]	1941

[1] Renamed Biostatistics in 1930.
[2] Renamed Environmental Medicine in 1950.
[3] Renamed Biochemistry in 1932.
[4] Established as a division of Public Health Administration in 1947, became an independent department in 1961.
[5] Established as a division of Public Health Administration in 1950.
[6] Established as a division of Public Health Administration in 1941, became an independent department in 1961.

of antigen–antibody relationships to develop vaccines, antitoxins, and diagnostic tests for communicable diseases. In municipal laboratories, technicians analyzed samples of food, water, and soil for pathogens. Out in the field, health officers needed to know not only how the relationship between hosts, parasites, and environmental conditions promoted the spread of disease in humans but also the regulations, standards, and sanitary procedures to ensure the quality and purity of food, water, meat, and drugs; metabolic and bacterial analysis of blood, urine, and excreta; and the identification of essential vitamins and minerals and the corresponding diseases caused by nutritional deficiencies. These topics comprised the core of public health instruction in bacteriology, biochemistry, parasitology, and sanitary engineering. Johns Hopkins was the only school of public health that required bacteriology or offered graduate science degrees to train nonphysician researchers until 1946, when Harvard instituted ScM and ScD degrees. Some schools of public health did not even offer science as an elective.[14]

Laboratory discoveries could be applied in mass screening and vaccination programs, whose success depended on effective public health administrative methods, including management, communication, and popular education. The health officer also used epidemiology and biostatistics to survey the forest of human disease and discover how it spread. By collecting data on rates of morbidity and mortality in a population and then carefully observing and comparing the potential causative role of social, environmental, and behavioral factors, the epidemiologist could unlock the modes of disease transmission and prevention. JHSPH roughly paralleled the APHA in establishing departments in public health administration, biometry and vital statistics, physiological hygiene, and chemical hygiene (dedicated to the biochemistry of nutrition). The school was significantly ahead of the APHA in the physician-dominated fields of epidemiology and mental hygiene. Since JHSPH neglected nonphysician occupational categories, it lagged behind other schools and the APHA in establishing departments of sanitary engineering, health education, maternal and child hygiene, and public health nursing. These would prove to be major growth areas that would constitute the majority of the public health workforce.

In the 1910s, health departments began to experiment with decentralized administration schemes for delivering basic sanitation and disease prevention services more efficiently, and by 1930, over 1,500 neighborhood health centers operated across the country. In 1932, the Baltimore City Health Department (BCHD) and the Rockefeller International Health Division signed an agreement with JHSPH to establish the Eastern Health District (EHD), which became the engine of the school's work in applied public health. As the first of eight local health districts to be established in Baltimore, the EHD was designed to provide a full range of health services to a delimited population from a strategically located health center, a model also promoted heavily abroad by the Rockefeller Foundation. The EHD was conceived as a national model for public health research, training, and administration, as stipulated in the grant agreements with the PHS, Rockefeller Foundation, and later the Milbank Memorial Fund and Commonwealth Fund. Just as the Johns Hopkins Hospital provided the clinical bedside for medical education and research, JHSPH leaders envisioned the EHD as a population laboratory, demonstration area, and field training site for JHSPH faculty and students as well as for BCHD personnel.[15]

The EHD occupied a 1-square-mile area surrounding JHSPH with a mostly working-class population of 60,000. The district was enlarged in 1938 to encompass nearly 110,000 residents, of whom approximately one-quarter were African American, with many Eastern European Jews and other ethnic minorities among the remaining "white" population. As the keystone of JHSPH's multidisciplinary approach to public health research and teaching, the EHD hosted clinics for mental hygiene, prenatal care, and screening for syphilis and tuberculosis (TB), as well as research projects on key issues such as infant nutrition, diphtheria inoculation, and the prevalence of chronic diseases. These activities significantly involved both medical and public health faculty and provided clinical training to students at both schools as well as to Johns Hopkins Hospital residents and graduate nurses. New health department employees received training in the EHD, and the BCHD experimented with new administrative procedures for controlling communicable diseases, including the initiation of school health programs in cooperation with Baltimore City public schools.[16]

Under the guidance of Lowell J. Reed, the EHD played a critical role in efforts to develop sophisticated methods for demographic research and statistical sampling. Reed's early work with Raymond Pearl, founding chair of Biometry and Vital Statistics, developed his lifelong interest in the statistical analysis of population growth. Their partnership provided an excellent foundation for building further collaborations with the medical school, where Pearl held a joint appointment as professor of biology and headed the Institute for Biological Research. Reed succeeded Pearl in 1925 as both chair of Biometry and Vital Statistics and editor of the respected scientific journal *Human Biology*, which Pearl founded. In 1930, Reed renamed the department, coining the term *biostatistics* to indicate the broad applications for statistics across biomedicine and the life sciences.[17]

Reed, trained as a mathematician, remains the only nonphysician to serve as JHSPH dean, from 1937 to 1946, as well as the only public health faculty member to serve as president of Johns Hopkins University, from 1953 to 1956.

Reed emulated Welch's broad-minded leadership and was elected president of the APHA, American Statistical Association, and Population Association of America and later served as the nation's leading public health statesman on the President's Commission on the Health Needs of the Nation and the National Health Advisory Council.[18]

In his history of the Johns Hopkins Medical Institutions, Thomas Turner called the EHD "a new and exciting approach to public health, especially in the hitherto statistical jungle of large urban centers." Whether in the American South or in developing countries abroad, an almost total lack of reliable vital statistics abetted government officials in ignoring health problems or denying their existence, particularly among remote populations who had little political power or contact with physicians and public health workers. Through the first half of the twentieth century, the quality of vital statistics varied widely, since compliance with PHS and US Census Bureau guidelines varied according to local and state codes and different levels of funding and personnel to enforce them. Until well into the 1920s, southern health departments failed to verify that at least 90 percent of annual births or deaths had been accurately reported using a standardized certificate, and, therefore, the first southern state was not admitted to the US Census death registration area until 1916 nor the birth registration area until 1921. Similar conditions obtained in the developing world for much of the twentieth century, and disease-fighting efforts in these countries suffered from inadequate morbidity and mortality data to guide health policy.[19]

Reed's Department of Biostatistics collaborated with statisticians in the Census Bureau, who collected local statistics on births and deaths, and in the PHS, who tracked morbidity for reportable communicable diseases. These activities were facilitated by the school's proximity to the offices of the Social Security Administration in downtown Baltimore's Candler Building, minutes from campus, as well as to the PHS headquarters in Washington, DC, about 40 miles away. JHSPH faculty and students also collaborated with Baltimore physicians, hospital administrators, and health department officials to develop workable statistical methods, such as improved sampling, uniform coding practices for causes of death, and a standard medical certification form. The EHD studies used what was then cutting-edge computing technology, punchcard tabulating machines, which the school purchased and loaned to the Maryland State Health Department. The punchcards represented the first step in the school's development of the critical public health discipline of biomedical computing, without which there would be no modern public health as we know it today.[20]

After statistical surveys had mapped out a community's size and demographic characteristics, epidemiologists could then measure the prevalence of specific diseases and employ these data to zero in on the most important targets for prevention and control measures. EHD studies analyzed the distribution and spread of both communicable and mental illness as well as the reproductive characteristics of the population. JHSPH's research on the social and economic determinants of both disease and population dynamics directly relied on "the unusual and valuable nature of the family files of the Eastern Health District [which] result in its being one of the few places in the world where scientific answers to some of these relationships can be found." The family files and survey reports formed "a backdrop of considerable expanse against which may be painted the individual portraits of particular health problems under study in a way to give deeper significance than could otherwise be possible." Out of the school's research in the EHD grew many of JHSPH's signature strengths, including the social epidemiology of the family, the life-course approach to disease in populations, advanced methods of biostatistics and demography, communicable disease control (especially syphilis, diphtheria, TB, and influenza), and some of the earliest epidemiological studies of developmental disability and chronic diseases.[21]

Reed, Wade Hampton Frost, and Allen Weir Freeman, the chairs of Biostatistics, Epidemiology, and Public Health Administration, respectively, were the primary developers of the EHD alongside Baltimore Health Commissioner Huntington Williams (DrPH 1921). The three professors trained Hygiene faculty and students to painstakingly collect and analyze data on EHD residents' age, sex, race, occupation, living conditions, economic status, and family size. They checked this baseline information against patient records from local hospitals, physicians, and EHD clinics, using a unique identifying number for each individual, most of whom were treated as either inpatients or outpatients at Johns Hopkins Hospital. Biostatistics faculty members Carroll E. Palmer and Edwin Crosby designed the hospital's top-notch medical records system and provided aggregated patient data for analysis. This cross-checking technique, called record linkage, enables records from multiple data sets to be matched to a common identifier, and it would become an invaluable tool for epidemiological investigations and population research. Halbert L. Dunn, chief of the PHS National Office of Vital Statistics, published the first article on record linkage in the *American Journal of Public Health* in 1946, and the concept has since become influential in information management across a variety of disciplines (the school's work in developing record linkage is discussed in chapters 4 and 11).[22]

The introductory courses in biostatistics and epidemiology required students to analyze real-life raw data and case studies from the EHD, and JHSPH alumni cited them as the best and most relevant courses in the curriculum. Biostatistics students learned the mathematical theory and methods of statistical analysis, as well as its public health applications such as sampling techniques, population changes, life tables, and variables determining morbidity and mortality. Reed and Frost guided their students to go beyond merely isolating the infectious agent to seek the broader causes of disease among large numbers of cases in a population, under a wide spectrum of environmental conditions. Students learned "shoe-leather epidemiology," which emphasized the value of fieldwork and extensive interaction with the community to gather data and make observations. Such firsthand knowledge was essential for recognizing and responding effectively to changes in the relationships between disease-causing agents, hosts, and environments. Biostatistics and epidemiology were also required courses for the MD at Johns Hopkins, and by 1938, the Department of Biostatistics taught as many students from outside as within JHSPH in courses that were open to students and staff from the medical school, hospital, and science departments. Lydia Edwards, a postdoctoral fellow in preventive medicine, called Reed "one of the most brilliant teachers I ever had." Reed's students learned that "just as x-rays had permitted us to see what was going on inside the human body, so statistics enabled me to see what was occurring within a population."[23]

Students gained practical experience by working alongside BCHD nurses on the four EHD census surveys conducted in 1933, 1936, 1939, and 1947. The 1936 survey was part of the National Health Survey conducted by the PHS, the largest morbidity survey to date. W. Thurber Fales (ScD 1924), who was appointed director of the BCHD Bureau of Vital Statistics in 1934, was a critical collaborator for EHD research and its application to address national statistical standards. He worked closely with Reed and the US Census Bureau to revise the International List of Causes of Death and coauthored many of the articles published from the EHD studies. Fales also consulted with the Bureau of Old-Age and Survivors Insurance of the Social Security Administration to develop a uniform national system of recording death certificates for beneficiaries.[24]

The EHD studies helped secure Reed's selection to chair both the US Committee on Joint Causes of Death and the World Health Organization (WHO) International Committee on Vital and Health Statistics. Together, these committees oversaw the modernization and international adoption of standard classifications for diseases, injuries, and causes of death. This framework is known today as the International Classification of Diseases (ICD), the standard diagnostic tool for epidemiology, health management, and clinical medicine. The achievement would merit a Lasker Foundation Award, public health's highest honor, in 1947.[25]

The universal adoption of the *Manual of the International Statistical Classification of Diseases, Injuries and Causes of Death* also redounded to the benefit of US state and local health departments. Dunn, Reed's collaborator at the PHS National Office of Vital Statistics, observed that "it would have been almost impossible to obtain the use of a single classification for morbidity within the United States, even within the states and cities, if this world-wide International Statistical Classification had not emerged." Indeed, the WHO International Committee on Vital and Health Statistics urged national committees to "study the problems of producing health statistics which are related to the family structure and to the social-economic and occupational background of the individual," a direct reference to the EHD Family Studies that formed an influential template for subsequent research in demography and population health.[26]

Federal Funds for Public Health Training

After the first group of schools was established, the movement to professionalize public health made further headway in 1932, when the APHA created the Committee on Professional Education to establish minimum hiring standards and develop guidelines for university degree programs and in-service training. Among state and local health workers, most sanitary officers, half of physicians, and one-third of nurses had no public health training. Public health reformers in the APHA, PHS, and Association of State and Territorial Health Officers aimed to extend public health services nationwide while also upgrading the quality of the public health workforce. A major goal of public health reform was to replace unqualified political appointees with properly trained, full-time health officers. Proposed qualifications included an MD, at least one year's internship at an approved hospital, a year of public health graduate instruction, and an initial period of supervised field experience in a health department.[27]

As the Great Depression intensified community health needs, health departments had few resources to implement the APHA's recommendations. The economic crisis eroded state budgets for public universities and deflated the endowment income of private schools and the Rockefeller Foundation itself. At Hopkins, endowment income furnished about 80 percent of the School of Hygiene operating budget, and administrators were forced to consolidate departments, cut faculty salaries, and abolish vacant positions. After cutting the budget for 1935–1936 by over 10 percent from the previous year, school administrators warned the Board of Trustees that any further reduction would do "serious and permanent damage to the work of the School." This was the first of what would become cyclical financial downturns besetting the school every 20 years or so.[28]

Relief for schools of public health and support for the APHA's professional standards came through the 1935 Social Security Act. Title V aided maternal and child health programs and Title VI strengthened state and local health departments, including the first federal training grants for public health personnel. Social Security's Title VI had been proposed by members of President Franklin D. Roosevelt's Science Advisory Board, which included New York State Health Commissioner Thomas Parran. He credited Social Security's public health programs as "the first large scale effort to shorten the lag between what we know and what we do." After Roosevelt appointed Parran as surgeon general in 1936, he built the prestige of the Public Health Service and expanded its scope. Echoing Welch, Parran championed public health as "a dynamic science" that was advancing modern disease control methods so rapidly that past sickness and death rates were "inadequate yardsticks for the present and are utterly useless as goals for the future." Parran would figure prominently in the midcentury development of JHSPH.[29]

Social Security and other federal programs underwrote new health department positions in maternal and child health, environmental sanitation, VD control, and general health services. The legislation required states to establish minimum hiring criteria, including a recommended one year of coursework in an approved public health degree program. Enrollments surged, and by 1938, more than 4,000 public health workers nationwide had received training (including short courses lasting from a few weeks to six months).[30]

In 1939, the Rockefeller Foundation requested Parran and Livingston Farrand, the noted public health reformer and just-retired president of Cornell University, to analyze the state of public health education and assess the future need for trained public health professionals. Commonly known as the Parran–Farrand Report, the *Report to the Rockefeller Foundation on the Education of Public Health Personnel* relied on the estimate of Rockefeller officer John Ferrell (DrPH 1919) that the nation's federal, state, and local public health agencies would need to train 1,500 physicians, 6,000 nurses, 750 sanitary engineers, and 500 other types of technical workers over the next ten years to reach adequate staffing levels to provide full-time public health services to all US residents. Yet only nine universities in the United States and Canada conferred graduate public health degrees, about half by Johns Hopkins, followed distantly by University of Toronto, Harvard, and University of Michigan.[31]

Both the Flexner Report and its public health analog, the Parran–Farrand Report, were based on site visits to every school in the United States and Canada. Parran and Farrand made three central recommendations to schools of public health: facilitate the interdisciplinary training of public health professionals from a variety of backgrounds in a single degree program, include opportunities for field study and practical experience, and improve undergraduate teaching of preventive medicine to medical students. The Rockefeller Foundation had already endowed the schools of public health at Harvard,

Johns Hopkins, and the University of Toronto, and Parran and Farrand designated them as "national and international" level schools worthy of increased support to expand the production of graduates.[32]

The guidelines for training public health professionals set forth in the Social Security Act and the Parran–Farrand Report challenged private, research-oriented schools such as Hopkins and Harvard to increase their emphasis on pedagogy and applying public health knowledge. Since the 1920s, the Rockefeller Foundation had sponsored 25 fellows at JHSPH annually, but beginning in 1936, Social Security supported about 50 new students each fall, which increased the numbers of municipal and state health personnel at the school. By 1939, the Social Security training program had more than tripled JHSPH's annual output of MPH graduates. In keeping with the southern focus of JHSPH and the PHS, nearly half of these graduates were southerners.[33]

Social Security training funds expanded enrollments at existing schools and spurred state legislatures to establish new ones. North Carolina, with its record of progressive leadership in higher education and its key role in the hookworm campaign, was a logical choice for the first state university to found a school of public health. In December 1935, just four months after President Franklin D. Roosevelt signed the Social Security Act into law, the PHS and the state of North Carolina allotted funds to establish a Division of Public Health at the University of North Carolina (UNC) Medical School in Chapel Hill. In 1940, the division became an independent school.[34]

The UNC School of Public Health was shaped by three public health luminaries. Its first head from 1936 to 1946 was the august Milton J. Rosenau, founding chair of preventive medicine at Harvard and director of the Harvard–MIT School for Health Officers. Rosenau was assisted in developing the school at UNC by Ferrell, who had retired from the Rockefeller Foundation and returned to his home state to serve as the first executive director of the North Carolina Medical Care Commission. Third was Carl V. Reynolds, North Carolina's state health officer and a national leader in venereal disease (VD) control. Rose's first draft of the 1915 Welch–Rose Report had envisioned a practice-oriented school aligned with both a medical school and a state health department, a plan finally realized in the cooperative founding agreement between UNC, the PHS, and the North Carolina State Board of Health. The schools of public health founded at the state universities of Michigan (1941), California–Berkeley (1943), and Minnesota (1944) were organized along similar lines.[35]

Under Rosenau, Ferrell, and Reynolds's influence, UNC's new school conformed to the models of public health education and research put forth by Johns Hopkins and Harvard, yet also represented a challenge to their hegemony. Johns Hopkins hosted a PHS venereal disease research laboratory and the training center for public health workers in PHS Sanitary District 2, which included West Virginia and the seven Atlantic coast states from Florida to Delaware. But since Chapel Hill was more centrally located 300 miles south of Baltimore, Rosenau and Reynolds influenced Parran in 1936 to relocate the lab and training center to UNC.[36]

Public health deans at the more established schools viewed the unprecedented expansion of public health graduates with alarm. Leaders at Hopkins and Harvard worried that their "high-quality" programs might be "undermined" by schools that awarded certificates in public health to "persons with only a bachelor's degree who have taken a few special courses in public health." Harvard already called its nine-month program the Master of Public Health (MPH), and in 1939, JHSPH applied Harvard's title to rename the Certificate of Public Health, to ensure that it was recognized as a graduate degree. The enormous personnel needs of military and defense agencies stimulated the expansion of both enrollments and curricula for the MPH, which shifted the balance of enrollment at JHSPH from doctoral to master's students and promoted a more even balance between research and practice.[37]

E. B. Wilson, chair of Vital Statistics at the Harvard School of Public Health, wrote to Reed in December 1941 about the implications of the proliferation of new schools for Hopkins and Harvard. The previous April, Reed had convened the deans of seven schools at Hopkins, who elected him the first president of the Association of Schools of Public Health (ASPH). Wilson worried that Hopkins and Harvard might lose their autonomy to set professional and educational standards. "Indeed," he commented, "if we take in not only North Carolina but Minnesota and MIT and a number of other of the weaker schools we shall probably be under pressure to lower our requirements or at any rate to give basic definitions for the whole profession which will be somewhat lower than we should ourselves wish to maintain."[38]

Reed was less worried than Wilson about the new schools usurping the leadership of the older, privately endowed schools. As a member of the APHA Committee on Professional Education, Reed worked to implement the Parran–Farrand Report's recommendations and cheerfully advised institutions that were planning to establish new public health schools or degree programs. He stressed to the new schools that the MPH degree should, with few exceptions, be reserved for physicians training to be health officers and should not be awarded to students who entered with only a bachelor's degree. During the 1940s, public health deans would be primarily concerned with maintaining the quality of their degree programs during a period of rapid expansion. The ASPH collaborated with the PHS and APHA Committee on Professional Education to outline standards for degree programs, minimum facilities for graduate public health education, and professional qualifications for public health workers in a variety of fields.[39]

Conclusion

The Rockefeller campaign against hookworm created a southern health nexus of philanthropy, academic research, and public health agencies that would give birth to the first independent school of public health at Johns Hopkins and shape the course of regional, national, and international public health throughout the twentieth century. JHSPH was the first in a series of institutions to receive Rockefeller grants to establish new schools of public health that carried out the Welch–Rose Report's recommendations on a global scale under the strong influence of IHD officials (table 3). The school's early success in propagating the Welch–Rose model is indicated by the large number of alumni who founded or led schools of public health, served as senior officials in national and international government health agencies, and led military, philanthropic, and voluntary health organizations. Yet from the beginning, financial stability and independence from medical schools posed challenges for fledgling schools of public health.

CHAPTER ONE

The Southern Roots of Public Health at Johns Hopkins

[William Henry] Welch had turned the Hopkins model into a force. He and colleagues at . . . a handful of other schools had in effect first formed an elite group of senior officers of an army; then, in an amazingly brief time, they had revolutionized American medicine, created and expanded the officer corps, and begun training their army, an army of scientists and scientifically grounded physicians. . . . The army Welch had created was designed to attack, to seek out particular targets, if only targets of opportunity, and kill them.

—John M. Barry, *The Great Influenza:*
The Story of the Deadliest Pandemic in History, pp. 86–87

The language of public health is rife with military terms, and wars have always strengthened the mandate for public health. Troops mustered from disparate environments are vulnerable to disease outbreaks that can be the deciding factor in an army's defeat. Even among civilians, health officers launch campaigns against disease by conducting surveillance, mapping out the best targets, and deploying magic bullets to kill enemy pathogens. The US Public Health Service, since its establishment in 1798 as the Marine Hospital Service, has functioned as a quasi-military organization with a hierarchical chain of command and uniformed commissioned officers. Public health is a game of risk, in more than one sense: it involves complex calculations to determine the health risks of behaviors or substances, but it also resembles the military strategy board game in its marshalling of limited resources to achieve practical aims.

Historically, wartime measures to protect health have not usually outlasted the conflict, but World War II proved to be exceptional, triggering a sea change in the practice of public health in the United States and abroad. The 1944 Public Health Service Act consolidated the agency's reorganization during World War II on a permanent basis. Even after demobilization, the PHS retained its 16,000 employees, double the number who had served in 1940; the full-time staff would more than double again by 1950. In June 1945, President Harry S. Truman issued Executive Order 9575, designating the Commissioned Corps of the PHS as members of the armed forces "with full military rights and obligations." The order remained in effect until 1956, when Congress passed legislation naming the PHS and the National Oceanic and Atmospheric Administration as the two civilian commissioned corps that, along with the five branches of the armed forces, today constitute the uniformed services of the United States.[1]

From the 1940s through the 1960s, World War II and the Cold War profoundly shaped the development of the Johns Hopkins School of Hygiene and Public Health as well as public health practice and graduate education. National defense and foreign policy considerations suffused not only the nomenclature but also the methods and objectives of American public health. In an era of extreme anxiety about the potential for another world war, national defense was a politically potent justification for expanding the scope of public health, particularly training and research programs. But by harnessing public health to the engine of the military–industrial complex, the field's leaders risked losing sight of its humanitarian ethos: to improve and protect health for its own sake, because all human life is precious, not only the lives of one's countrymen. However, by making population-wide health improvements a key facet of "winning hearts and minds" (and lives), public health professionals gained the opportunity to humanize and ennoble the American enterprise abroad, with important and often unforeseen consequences for domestic public health programs.

Although this book deals substantially with the origins and evolution of international health, careful attention is paid to the continuities and contrasts between JHSPH's domestic and international programs, especially the reasons that it was in many ways more difficult for the school to make a significant impact on the health of the people at its own doorstep in East Baltimore than on the populations of Brazil, India, and Turkey. Academic public health leaders repeatedly made the case that founding new schools of public health and increasing the supply of graduates were crucial steps toward solving the nation's most pressing health problems. But since schools of public health were a hybrid of graduate and professional education, faculty often placed top priority on publishing cutting-edge scientific research rather than preparing frontline health officers, especially at research-oriented schools such as JHSPH and Harvard. As schools of public health proliferated after the war, mainly at state universities, they established degree programs across the gamut of public health occupations and disciplines. Johns Hopkins, by contrast, remained focused on its traditional constituencies, the physician and elite research scientist.

In the realm of public health policy and practice, the way forward was often perilous and unclear. In the United States, unlike Europe and Latin America, national policymakers did not integrate social security programs for wage earners with government-sponsored medical care services. From 1935 to 1985, American health reformers unsuccessfully pursued national comprehensive health insurance whenever the political climate seemed propitious, and meanwhile enacted a series of categorical health programs (that is, focused on a specific disease, such as cancer, or system of the body, such as the heart and lungs) that were incremental but easier to pass. This siloed approach to providing health services to different population groups according to type of disease, age, military service, economic status, or other such criteria was reflected in and reinforced by vertically organized public health programs such as those for maternal and child health or sexually transmitted disease control. The history of the Johns Hopkins School of Hygiene and Public Health is in many important respects an ongoing debate over the wisdom of vertical versus horizontal methods of planning and implementing public health interventions.[2]

Closely related to the debates over health reform, funding sources were another key factor that determined the parameters of growth at JHSPH and all schools of public health. Although Johns Hopkins and most other early schools had been founded with endowments at private universities, endowment and tuition income could support teaching and research only on a small scale. During the 1950s, Rockefeller and the other philanthropies that had launched the first wave of schools stopped awarding open-ended, unrestricted grants. Competition for funding intensified as both public health and medical schools attempted to expand their enrollments and research programs as well as to rebuild their neglected campuses after more than a decade of depression and war. Johns Hopkins was at the forefront of both precipitating and capitalizing on the midcentury shift toward federal sponsorship of public health and medical education. By 1970, federal grants accounted for 85 percent of the JHSPH budget, which resulted in rapid but chaotic growth.

During the 1970s, Johns Hopkins, like all schools of public health and universities generally, faced severe budgetary constraints posed by inflation and vacillating support for federal research and education programs, including those in health. Yet by forcing academic public health to reinvent itself, the erosion of national defense as a basis for funding would ultimately be the "best worst thing" to ever happen to JHSPH.

This chapter sketches the school's transition under Lowell J. Reed's deanship from 1937 to 1946 in two settings: first, tropical disease research in the United States and global South, and then community health in Baltimore. These layers of activity coalesced in the school's new venereal disease control program that made Baltimore the "best place in the world to study syphilis" and redrew the boundaries for the MPH degree. The VD control program aptly illustrates the impact of the war as well as civil rights concerns on educational programs at JHSPH. Chapter 2 examines the growth triggered by national defense priorities and funding, which generated a series of specialized master's programs that branched out from public health's traditional focus on infectious diseases into areas such as environmental medicine and mental hygiene.

Disease Hunting in Dixie

Isaiah Bowman, president of Johns Hopkins University, noted ruefully in 1938 that William H. Welch had "lived in another period when it was possible to make spectacular investigations and win public support. Advances in bacteriology today only rarely have spectacular features. The work in that field is a tough slugging process."[3] Bowman's pessimism would be dispelled once the School of Hygiene stepped onto the national and international stages by participating in the war effort and the campaigns against syphilis, polio, and malaria. Reed and his successor, Ernest L. Stebbins, solidified the school's primacy in international health, clinical trials, and vaccine development, and both deans were instrumental in helping to found new schools of public health in the United States and abroad.[4]

When Reed became dean, all 10 of the school's departments were still headed by members of the original faculty, including Reed himself (see appendix A). From 1937 to 1939, Reed recruited three dynamic new chairs who would help chart the school's direction for the next 20 years. His first appointment was Abel Wolman, chair of Sanitary Engineering from 1937 to 1961. Wolman had co-developed the chlorination formula used to protect public water supplies against waterborne diseases, once a scourge in his childhood neighborhood of East Baltimore. Just as important, he had traveled across the country, using his considerable skills at persuasion to convince local officials to adopt chlorination. When the Johns Hopkins School of Engineering recruited him to chair the Department of Sanitary Engineering, Wolman insisted on a joint appointment as chair of the department's analog in the School of Hygiene, so that engineers would be exposed to public health methodology and public health students would understand the importance of environmental health. He thought this would be a deal-breaker, but Johns Hopkins administrators were eager to lure Wolman and agreed. By the end of his career, Wolman had helped plan the national water and sewer systems in more than 50 countries. He was consultant to the PHS and myriad other organizations and chaired the sanitary engineering committees of the National Research Council (NRC), federal Office of Foreign Relief and Rehabilitation Operations, and Pan American Health Organization (PAHO).[5]

Reed's second hire was Kenneth F. Maxcy (DrPH 1921), chair of Bacteriology from 1937 to 1939. Maxcy's mentor at JHSPH had been Wade Hampton Frost, founding chair of Epidemiology. Like Frost, Maxcy was a master of observation and comparison who adored John Snow, the British epidemiologist famous for tracing the source of the 1854 London cholera epidemic to the Broad Street pump. Frost and Maxcy's combined influence ensured that *Snow on Cholera* was widely taught in schools of public health. After Frost's death in 1939, Maxcy succeeded him as chair of Epidemiology, making him the only person ever to lead more than one JHSPH department, excluding interim chairs.[6]

Thomas B. Turner, who came to JHSPH in 1936 to head the new VD control training program, was tapped as chair of Bacteriology. Reed, Wolman, Maxcy, and Turner were all on close terms with President Franklin D. Roosevelt's new surgeon general, Thomas Parran, who helmed the PHS from 1936 to 1948. Turner and Parran both hailed from Calvert County in rural southern Maryland, and Turner was married to Parran's cousin, Anne Parran Somervell. Wolman had grown up as the son of Jewish Polish immigrants in East Baltimore, and Maxcy was raised in Washington, DC, a large but still segregated city. The only nonsoutherner among them was Reed, a quiet, genial mathematician from New Hampshire.[7]

This new group of leaders piloted the school through a critical decade of depression and war, during which Reed, Wolman, and Parran all served as president of the American Public Health Association. In their leadership of American public health, the five men took bold and sometimes controversial stands that injected politics into public health, especially in their efforts to align medicine and public health to improve access to health care for all citizens.

Geography was destiny for the school, which had grown out of Baltimore's unique context as a port city and leading East Coast railhead that sat at the intersection of southern agriculture, northern manufacturing, and international commerce. During JHSPH's first 25 years, from 1916 to 1941, its priorities had mirrored those of its primary patron, the Rockefeller Foundation: fighting the tropical diseases that accompanied poverty in the American South, the Caribbean, and Latin America. Johns Hopkins University, apart from its internationally renowned medical school, was still transforming from a regional into a national institution. The university's home state of Maryland was poor and overwhelmingly rural, bearing more resemblance to its southern neighbors than to other more prosperous mid-Atlantic states.

Compared to the rest of the United States, the South's population was poorer, younger, and more rural; had higher fertility and lower standards of living; posted shorter life expectancy and higher rates of illiteracy, morbidity, and mortality; and was more isolated, with a much smaller supply of doctors and hospital beds. In short, the South was still part of the developing world. Yet because Parran considered the region "the number one health problem of the Nation," he made it the PHS's public health laboratory.

The South was an ideal field for public health work for two related reasons: its economy and ecology fostered the types of communicable epidemic disease that responded most dramatically to public health initiatives, and its relatively underdeveloped private health system was less a source of competition than in the North, where fee-for-service hospital-based practice, well-established academic medical centers, organized medicine, and group payment plans all flourished. Under the guidance of Parran and other likeminded reformers, a flurry of government reports, academic journal articles, and dispatches in the popular press trumpeted the South's abysmal health status and identified it as a crucial target of federal intervention that would both end the Depression and build an effective labor force during peace and war.[8]

Many diseases were endemic in both the American and the global south, including typhus, malaria, and hookworm. JHSPH faculty and alumni used their disease-hunting experiences in Dixie to guide wartime vector-control campaigns against pathogen-carrying insects, worms, and snails. Maxcy was the ideal candidate to lead public health expeditions into the southern wilds. As a young man, he had spent his summers as a federal surveyor with the US Forestry Service and the Bureau of Indian Affairs, exploring the American West by camping and mountain climbing. Maxcy's biographer noted, "The knowledge he gained of the great variety of terrain and wildlife of his own country later proved invaluable to him as an epidemiologist." He personified epidemiology's close alliance with the disciplines of bacteriology, ecology, parasitology, and sanitary engineering.[9]

As a PHS officer in the 1920s, Maxcy had hunted down the vectors of malaria and other diseases spread by intermediate hosts. Slogging through the canebrakes of the Southeast, Maxcy made a critical discovery that shaped his career and established him as an expert in rickettsial diseases, caused by a family of tiny bacteria that had only recently been discovered and distinguished from viruses.[10]

At the time, the only known vector of typhus fever was the human body louse, which spread epidemic typhus in crowded, extremely unsanitary conditions, such as refugee camps and jails. Based on field surveys in Savannah,

Georgia, and Montgomery, Alabama, Maxcy discovered a new, milder, endemic form of typhus among scattered rural residents and hypothesized that wild rodents were the natural reservoir that incidentally infected humans through fleas. In studies at the PHS Hygienic Laboratory in Washington, DC, he confirmed that guinea pigs inoculated with the blood of patients with this type of typhus became infected with the disease, which he named "murine typhus" after its rodent vector. This greatly aided subsequent research, since murine typhus had previously been denoted by a confusing mix of names, including Brill's disease and endemic, sporadic, or Mexican typhus, for which there was no confirmation yet of biological distinctions. During World War II, Maxcy would prove that a third strain of typhus, endemic in the South Pacific, was spread by yet another insect vector, mites. This knowledge would help control "scrub typhus," or tsutsugamushi disease, among thousands of Allied troops in the South Pacific. Because there was no effective treatment or vaccine available for the disease, identifying the correct vector for intervention was the only hope for preventing outbreaks.[11]

On the eve of the war, malaria still plagued the Atlantic and Gulf coastal areas from the Carolinas to Alabama, and rates were highest in the Mississippi Delta cotton-growing regions. Maxcy observed, "The Mississippi Delta . . . is particularly favorable to heavy production of *Anopheles quadrimaculatus*. The flat 'river bottom' land is everywhere traversed by sluggish streams, with dendritic bayou connections forming innumerable cypress and sweet-gum swamps." The greatest risk of malaria exposure was on the "great cotton plantations worked by thousands upon thousands of negro families living under conditions of maximum exposure to mosquito bites."[12]

Public health researchers took careful note of racial differences in death and disease rates, which might illuminate the underlying causes of epidemics or, perhaps, reveal weaknesses in the statistics themselves. Splenomegaly (enlarged spleen), a sign of malaria, was twice as prevalent among black Mississippi schoolchildren as their white counterparts. The growing racial disparities in malaria were evidence of the plummeting economic status of black sharecroppers as cotton prices slid after the end of World War I. Studies conducted between 1912 and 1930 by Maxcy and other researchers showed a black infection rate ranging from 20 to 54 percent. Throughout the 1920s and 1930s, approximately 10 times as many blacks as whites died of malaria, although the total number of deaths declined for both races during that period.[13]

Maxcy and his two coauthors had concluded that a high proportion of black deaths classified as caused by malaria were unattended by a physician. In the two South Carolina counties with the highest recorded US malaria death rates, only 4 of 95 deaths had been certified by a doctor. Frost and Reed's student, Ruth Rice Puffer (ScM 1938), built on this work in a 1937 paper that examined the validity of African-American mortality statistics and compared the results across 12 southern states. A startling percentage of nonwhite death certificates listed the cause of death as ill-defined or unknown (at this juncture, nearly all individuals in the South classified as "nonwhite" were of African ancestry, albeit many with European and Native American heritage as well). The problem was particularly acute among nonwhites under age 1, for whom the cause of death was unknown in nearly one in four cases; this figure was as high as 49 percent in Mississippi. As Puffer noted, "This large percentage of deaths from unknown causes invalidates any discussion of colored death rates from specific causes." Puffer's work highlighted the ways that race, poverty, and geography skewed birth and death statistics, which paved the way for both the field of health disparities research and the strategic use of a scientific evidence base to inform health policy.[14]

Alongside Maxcy and Puffer's work, Justin M. Andrews (ScD 1926) was instrumental in planning and executing efforts to eradicate malaria in the American South. Andrews served on the JHSPH Protozoology and Medical Entomology faculty from 1926 to 1938, where he studied host–parasite relations in zoonotic and human disease, including malaria. He mentored numerous future public health leaders, particularly in the field of malaria control, and according to his student and colleague Lloyd Rozeboom, no student ever missed his lectures. Rozeboom described Andrews as "exud[ing] an aura of considerable self-respect. With his erect bearing, clipped mustache, and magnificent mane of wavy red hair he was indeed an impressive figure. He was also a lot of fun." In 1938, Andrews left to apply his skills in the Georgia Department of Public Health as director of the Malaria and Hookworm Service, where he instituted training programs and publicized the problems and solutions for these diseases through health education materials in print and radio broadcasts. During World War II, the southern antimalaria campaign culminated in the PHS Malaria Control in War Areas program around southern military bases. These experiences informed Andrews when he, Joseph Mountin, and others within the PHS reorganized the wartime malaria program on a permanent basis as the Communicable Disease Center (CDC) in 1946.[15]

The war was also the impetus for expanding malaria control efforts worldwide, since malaria struck an estimated 300 million people each year and killed roughly 3 million. While Andrews was still teaching at Hopkins, the Rockefeller International Health Division sent Fred L. Soper (DrPH 1925) to Brazil. By 1935, he had conducted the first successful vector eradication campaign against yellow fever, spread by *Aedes aegypti*. He then turned his attention to the *Anopheles gambiae*, an African mosquito that had brought malaria to rural Brazil, and eradicated both the species and the disease in only nine months. In both campaigns, Soper and his team of 40,000 workers had employed the same expensive, labor-intensive methods that the PHS used in the southeastern United States. They treated breeding sites in standing water with oil or the highly toxic insecticide powder Paris green (copper(II) acetate triarsenite) and fumigated houses and buildings with pyrethrum, a newly available, low-toxicity insecticide that today remains the most common home and garden insecticide in the United States.[16]

Soper was aided by some of the world's best medical entomologists at JHSPH, including Andrews and Ottis R. Causey (ScD 1931). Causey's team of researchers painstakingly secured the eggs of identified female anophelines during more than 50,000 isolated ovipositions (egg-layings). After the larvae were reared to adults, they were used to identify the precise correlation of egg, larval, and adult female characteristics used in species recognition as well as the structural differences in male genitalia that best aided anopheline speciation. Causey published his detailed descriptions of more than 30 mosquito species in the book *Studies on Brazilian Anophelines from Northeast and Amazon Regions*. While still in Brazil, Causey married Soper's classmate, JHSPH bacteriologist Calista Eliot (ScD 1925), by proxy in Baltimore so that she could join her new husband and Soper at the IHD field office. The Causeys published extensively on mosquitoes, malaria, and arboviruses in Brazil and Africa.[17]

During the war, Andrews, Soper, and many other JHSPH parasitologists helped to forge both of the primary weapons against malaria, prophylactic drugs in humans and powerful new vector control methods that killed mosquitoes or prevented them from reproducing. In order for Allied soldiers to fight the Axis powers in the European, North African, and Pacific theaters, US Army medical officers first had to learn how to protect troops against tiny, deadly enemies: worms and insects. The US military hired consultants from the Rockefeller Foundation and JHSPH who had extensive experience in controlling malaria and hookworm. Andrews served as the chief malariologist for the US Army in North Africa, and Soper advised the Rockefeller Foundation and the Army. Beginning in 1941, malaria-carrying mosquitoes had invaded the upper delta of the Egyptian Nile, which had the same favorable breeding conditions as the Mississippi and Amazon deltas. One mosquito species was causing trouble in both Brazil and Egypt: *A. gambiae*, which carried the deadlier *P. falciparum* strain of malaria (named by William Welch in 1897). By late 1942, hundreds of thousands of Allied troops had gathered along the Nile's lower delta for the final battle for Egypt and the Suez, and Andrews predicted that half of the Allied armies would be sickened with malaria at the time of the planned offensive. He convinced his superiors to deploy twice the number of soldiers as originally planned, and in the spring of 1943, Allied forces routed Nazi General Erwin Rommel's Afrika Korps, which retreated into Tunisia before surrendering in May. The Army awarded Andrews the Legion of Merit and promptly sent him to oversee malaria control in the Pacific theater.[18]

Meanwhile, the US Department of Agriculture Division of Insecticide Investigations was developing and testing a potent long-acting insecticide, DDT (dichlorodiphenyltrichloroethane), at two main sites in Orlando, Florida, and Beltsville, Maryland, just outside Baltimore. News quickly spread of the spectacular results and scope of the new substance, which newspapers dubbed one of the war's top scientific developments. DDT killed lice, flies, bedbugs, and both adult and larval mosquitoes, and it was far cheaper to manufacture and apply than existing insecticides, since it could be sprayed aerially. Soper, working with the Rockefeller Foundation Health Commission, eagerly seized the opportunity to test DDT's effectiveness in curbing an epidemic of typhus in Naples, Italy, during the winter of 1943–1944. By conducting a mass delousing campaign among the city's inhabitants, the participating military and civilian organizations were able to achieve a remarkable feat: aborting the spread of disease just as the epidemic curve of cases was reaching its peak. The campaign used public delousing stations in jails, refugee camps, air-raid shelters, and public squares, where squads of workers equipped with hand-pumped cans and mechanical air-compressed guns blew DDT powder beneath each individual's clothes and over the neck and scalp. After the war, Soper made DDT the centerpiece of global vector campaigns against malaria and other insect-borne diseases. He served as director of PAHO from 1947 to 1959, presiding over the successful malaria eradication campaign in Latin America and advising the World Health Organization on its antimalaria campaigns in Asia and Africa. Like Soper, many JHSPH experts in tropical disease gravitated to PAHO.[19]

Andrews, however, was both humbler and more cautious than Soper about the potential for new technology to eradicate malaria. Andrews attributed the 1936 resurgence of malaria in the American South to the Great Depression. In 1947, he summarized the emerging expert consensus that, in many parts of the South, malaria eradication had resulted from overall socioeconomic improvements and better standards of living, since rates of malaria infection had begun to taper off in some areas even before large-scale programs had been implemented to drain swamps and apply insecticides to reduce mosquito populations. After the war, Andrews and other CDC malariologists worried that a postwar depression might trigger another outbreak.

Andrews and Soper represented different poles of the debates about whether economic underdevelopment was the cause or the result of environmental vector diseases such as malaria and hookworm, both of which were blamed for diminishing labor productivity in endemic areas. But if, as Andrews posited, poverty and low living standards created conditions ripe for the spread of epidemic disease, including malnutrition and poor sanitation, then these problems could not be solved solely with Soper's technocentric philosophy, which traced its roots directly back to the Rockefeller Sanitary Commission for the Eradication of Hookworm Disease. Notwithstanding John Ferrell's excitement about their miraculous properties, thymol and sanitary privies had reduced but not eliminated hookworm. Latter-day malariologists who once more plotted to eradicate a disease would run up against the limits of DDT as well.[20]

The school's participation in the war effort triggered the long-term development of international health and scientific research programs under the federal sponsorship of military and civilian agencies. Andrews and Soper both had studied under Robert W. Hegner, chair of the Department of Protozoology and Medical Entomology. Hegner's department played an important role in identifying and testing synthetic antimalarial drugs, a top military priority. His studies of mosquito physiology complemented his colleagues' research on the physiology and immune systems of birds, mammals, and humans. JHSPH investigators had experimented with several types of bird species and avian malaria strains to develop and perfect some of the most widely used models to study malaria. Since none of the strains of the *Plasmodium* parasite that caused human malaria could be cultured either in vitro or in a nonhuman living host, Hegner's lab helped to identify the best match of malaria parasite and bird species to support studying the physiological interaction of host and agent.[21]

As early as 1927, one student wrote a dissertation on the infectivity of bird malaria parasites in mosquitoes and how mosquitoes developed immunity. This was exceptionally sophisticated research at a time when most parasitologists were still focused on the taxonomy and life cycle of various organisms. Not until the 1940s did the field see intensive studies to address problems of parasite physiology, metabolism, immunology, and host reactions. After the war, parasitology research would explore the connection between parasite metabolism and chemotherapy. The understanding of host immunity to malaria and helminths would be applied to developing control methods against malaria and hookworm disease.[22]

The bird model of malaria perfected at JHSPH and other research centers served as a system to test the effectiveness of chemical agents that might also kill malaria in humans. After the supply of quinine, the traditional antimalarial, was cut off by the Japanese offensive in Southeast Asia in 1942, finding new synthetic drugs to protect troops against malaria was the top priority of the NRC Committee on Chemotherapy. William Mansfield Clark, professor of physiological chemistry in the Johns Hopkins School of Medicine, oversaw the NRC Office for the Survey of Antimalarial Drugs from 1942 to 1946. Hegner's student, Ernest Hartman (ScD 1926), developed the *Plasmodium cathemerium* model, one of the most productive models of avian malaria, since its wide variety of behavior closely mimicked the human parasite. Since young Peking ducklings were highly susceptible to malaria and could be easily inoculated, this species was chosen to host another model of malaria infection, the *P. lophurae* model, designed to evaluate structure–activity relationships in therapeutic compounds. The survey office was based in the Welch Medical Library, and across the street in the School of Hygiene, the entire sixth floor was commandeered to house the ducklings for the evaluations.

Scientists in the schools of Medicine and Hygiene conducted testing that yielded precise pharmacological and toxicological data on over 14,000 drugs, roughly 10 a day for four years. The malaria research program proved to be the largest biomedical undertaking to date in the United States, and it served as a model for postwar scientific medical research. It also proved essential for developing and testing two main antimalarial drugs, atabrine and chloroquine. Although the military's heavy prophylactic use of atabrine saved lives and reduced soldiers' risk of contracting malaria, they hated taking the bitter yellow pills and their unpleasant side effects. The malaria drug survey decisively identified chloroquine, more effective and less toxic than atabrine, as the drug of choice for malaria after the war.[23]

The Naval Research Laboratory (reorganized by Congress as the Office of Naval Research in August 1946) was another example of a wartime JHSPH research collaboration that built on southern antecedents. Several current and former JHSPH parasitologists were deployed in the Pacific at the US Naval Medical Research Unit No. 2 (NAMRU-2) on Guam, established with the resources and expertise of the Rockefeller Foundation to study infectious diseases of military significance in Asia. Colonel Thomas M. Rivers, the peacetime director of the Rockefeller Institute Hospital in New York, was the commanding officer of NAMRU-2. In January 1945, Norman R. Stoll (ScD 1923) arrived to direct the parasitology lab, where he conducted parasitic disease surveys among the island's residents and the US Marines who had been transferred there from the Philippines.[24]

While on the JHSPH Helminthology faculty in the mid-1920s, Stoll had invented the dilution egg-counting method, a quantitative tool for estimating hookworm infection in population groups. With E. H. Loughlin on Guam, Stoll used the dilution egg-counting method to demonstrate an important new mode of hookworm transmission: contact with soiled sheets. The Marines had been infected while handling hospital bedding that, after remaining unwashed and damp for over a week, had fostered the growth of enormous numbers of hookworm larvae. In the high temperatures and humidity, fecally soiled bedding had also resulted in outbreaks of severe and sometimes fatal hookworm disease in native infants and young children. Rivers called the work on treating and preventing this source of hookworm transmission the most important wartime contribution of NAMRU-2.[25]

After Hegner's death, the JHSPH Department of Helminthology merged with the Department of Protozoology and Medical Entomology to form Parasitology in 1942. The department's chair, William W. Cort, was elected president of the American Society of Parasitology and the American Academy of Tropical Medicine and also advised the NRC Division of Biology and Agriculture on the potential danger posed by snails as intermediate hosts of human parasitic diseases in the South Pacific. The Parasitology faculty's Pacific Theater experiences enlivened helminthology courses on hookworm and other widespread, debilitating tropical diseases such as filariasis, caused by thread-like roundworms and their larvae, and schistosomiasis, caused by trematodes (or flukes, a species of flatworm). Cort brought jars of helminths back from around the world to use in teaching parasitology classes, and JHSPH students today can still view the liver flukes that Cort collected in China in 1917. The etiologies of these diseases are often quite complex, moving through multiple intermediate hosts and life stages of the parasite. Filariasis, for example, is caused by infected mosquitoes depositing the parasitic worm larvae into a human host through a blood meal, followed by the larvae developing into adult worms in the lymphatic vessels, causing severe damage and swelling. In its late stage, the disease causes elephantiasis—painful, disfiguring swelling of the legs and genitals.[26]

It is difficult to overestimate the public health significance of parasitic worm diseases, which Stoll memorably assayed in a landmark 1947 paper in the *Journal of Parasitology*, aptly titled "This Wormy World." Stoll estimated that 25 different helminth species produced 2.3 billion infections distributed among 2.2 billion people alive at the time (since some people were infected by more than one species). Stoll, as a member of the WHO expert panel on parasitology for two decades, conducted the first major survey of hookworm infection in West Africa in 1961. By 2012, there were still 4.2 billion helminth infections among the world's 7 billion people, but parasitic worms had become much more concentrated among the world's poorest billion inhabitants, especially in sub-Saharan Africa and tropical Asia.[27]

The wartime exploits of JHSPH faculty and alumni energized the curriculum and flooded the admissions office with applications. No other JHSPH department produced more publications or graduates, with 112 ScD degrees between 1923 and 1953. Parasitology faculty authored six of the seven JHSPH-authored articles published in the journal *Science* through 1945. Of all the school's departments, Parasitology most effectively married its research to the teaching and practical application of public health methods.[28]

Women were also among the JHSPH alumni whose early careers in southern settings helped them to shape postwar international health. Ruth Rice Puffer had served before the war as chief statistician for the Tennessee Department of Public Health, and from 1953 to 1970, she directed the health statistics division of PAHO. During the 1960s, she oversaw the Inter-American Investigation of Mortality in adults and children, an international collaborative project including 12 large cities—1 English, 1 American, and 10 Latin American. Puffer was determined to obtain the most complete and comparable death data possible to find out whether the differences in mortality patterns in published statistics were real or resulted from inferior data.

As she had in her earlier studies of southern state death statistics, she paid close attention to unregistered and misclassified deaths, which were most common in infants and young children, whether in the rural United States or in Latin America. Measles was the most common cause of death among children aged 1 to 4 in Brazil, and more than 60 percent of these deaths were associated with malnutrition. Armed with these statistics before the study was even completed, Puffer convinced the Brazilian Ministry of Health to start a measles vaccination program and used the alarming new data on malnutrition to encourage the Brazilian government to create the National Institute of Food and

TABLE 1.1
Selected Baltimore City Statistics, 1939

	Black		White		Total	
Population	173,482 (20%)		695,508 (80%)		868,990	
Births/1,000 population		19.1		13.2		14.4
	Rank	Rate	Rank	Rate	Rank	Rate
Deaths/1,000 population		14.3		11.4		12.0
Heart disease	1	2.5	1	3.5	1	3.4
Cancer	7	1.0	2	1.5	2	1.4
Nephritis	4	1.3	3	1.1	3	1.2
Cerebral hemorrhage	6	1.1	4	0.9	4	0.9
Tuberculosis	2	1.9	7	0.5	5	0.8
Pneumonia	3	1.4	5	0.6	6	0.8
Accidents	—	—	6	0.6	7	0.6
Syphilis	5	1.3				
Deaths/1,000 live births						
Infant		63.1		32.1		40.8
Maternal		5.1		3.0		3.6

Source: City of Baltimore 125th Annual Report of the Department of Health, 1939.

Nutrition, which instituted food assistance programs for children. Puffer's achievements in improving the quality and quantity of vital statistics in Brazil led directly to the creation in 1975 of the Information System on Mortality and the Information System on Live Births, which implemented the International Classification of Diseases standards for morbidity and mortality data.[29]

The southern landscape from Baltimore to Brazil had fostered the school's prewar work on hookworm and malaria. In the 1920s and 1930s, service in the Rockefeller Foundation and PHS was a formative experience for many future public health leaders. This generation was likely to follow the career path of Maxcy, Andrews, Soper, Rivers, Stoll, Cort, and Puffer: they entered wartime military service and/or consulting with federal agencies and then played pioneering roles in the postwar global health campaigns. The school's southern roots continued to nourish its research, education, and practice programs as they blossomed in the fertile postwar environment for international cooperation in public health.

Baltimore Confronts the Color Bar

The School of Hygiene's southern context shaped its efforts to conquer urban maladies as well as tropical plagues. Baltimore's health problems were a unique product of its industrial economy and large international port, a growing population squeezed into an aging housing stock, and the injustices and inefficiencies of racial segregation. All these factors featured prominently in the work of the Eastern Health District.

The Rockefeller IHD agreed in 1942 to increase its support for the EHD by splitting the budget evenly with the school, since Parran and Farrand had praised the EHD as "particularly useful as a study area" and deemed its long-term stability "of the highest importance." The additional funding enabled the JHSPH Department of Public Health Administration (PHA) to collaborate with the EHD to offer new courses in infant hygiene, maternal hygiene, public health education, and public health nursing. In the innovative public health nursing course, nurses learned in groups by sharing responsibility for cases referred to the mental hygiene clinic and discussing them together with an EHD social worker at family case study conferences. JHSPH researchers also partnered with EHD staff to conduct whooping cough vaccine trials, comparing the secondary attack rates and severity of disease in vaccinated versus unvaccinated children in families with reported cases of whooping cough.[30]

As JHSPH leaders embraced the lofty goals of improving health in Baltimore and beyond, they upheld Maryland's racial segregation laws. From its inception, the school had admitted a multiethnic student body that included physicians from Latin America, Europe, and East and South Asia. A significant number of the school's early alumni were Jewish, of whom the most prominent were Harry Eagle (ScM 1929), Morton L. Levin (MPH 1933), Margaret Gene Arnstein (MPH 1934), Morton D. Kramer (ScD 1939), and Abraham Horwitz (MPH 1944) (all were American but Horwitz, who was from Chile, and all are profiled in the following chapters). But Johns Hopkins University remained firmly closed to African Americans, who could only attend segregated colleges with inferior funding, libraries, and research facilities. Isaiah Bowman, president of Johns Hopkins from 1935 to 1948, was openly segregationist and anti-Semitic (despite his first name, he was not Jewish and resented that assumption). Although Bowman was a Canadian, he had no inclination to challenge longstanding discriminatory policies. Black Marylanders had to leave the state to earn graduate or professional degrees.[31]

At JHSPH, the two deans who preceded Reed were sons of the Old South. Wade Hampton Frost, dean from 1931 to 1934, was named after Wade Hampton, the Confederate brigadier general under whom Frost's father had served in the Civil War. During Reconstruction, Hampton had been elected governor of South Carolina with the violent assistance of the Red Shirts, a paramilitary group formed to help the Democratic Party wrest the state from Republican control by disrupting elections and brutally intimidating black voters, sometimes by resorting to murder. Allen Freeman, dean from 1934 to 1937, was the son of General Walker Burford Freeman, the honorary commander-in-chief of the United Confederate Veterans; Freeman's brother, Douglas Southall Freeman, edited the Richmond *News Leader* and authored the definitive multivolume biography of Robert E. Lee. Bowman, Frost, and Freeman, therefore, were disinclined to challenge Johns Hopkins' whites-only admissions policy for US students. Black applicants always received the same rebuff from the school's Advisory Board: the university received an annual payment from the Maryland General Assembly and was therefore a *state-supported institution* obliged to follow segregation laws.[32]

In April 1938, Bowman met with B. M. Rhetta, a local black physician who was president of the Monumental City Medical Society and chairman of the Baltimore Interracial Commission. Rhetta had been applying unsuccessfully to JHSPH since 1922, but this time, he saw glimmers of hope on the horizon. The University of Michigan had recently become the first US school of public health to admit a black student, Paul Cornely, who earned a DrPH in 1934 (he went on to become the first black president of the APHA in 1968). Closer to home, the National Association for the Advancement of Colored People (NAACP) Legal Defense Fund, led by Maryland's own Thurgood Marshall, had won in *Murray v. Maryland* (1936), which forced the University of Maryland Law School to admit the black plaintiff. Marshall and the NAACP would continue to push for the integration of the School of Nursing and other professional schools at University of Maryland's Baltimore campus.[33]

Rhetta informed Bowman that the Harvard School of Public Health had just accepted a black Baltimore physician, H. Maceo Williams, and that therefore Johns Hopkins should consider admitting qualified black physicians to the one-year Certificate of Public Health (CPH) program. Postgraduate education was extremely difficult to obtain for Baltimore's black health professionals, who could not work or train in hospitals that cared for white patients, even facilities with separate "Jim Crow" wards, such as Johns Hopkins Hospital. But under the slogan "germs know no color line," southern health departments, including the Baltimore City Health Department, began to enlist black doctors, nurses, and laypeople to extend public health programs into the black community. City Health Commissioner Huntington Williams, who had written Maceo Williams's recommendation letter for Harvard, pledged his support for four more black physicians to apply to the Hopkins CPH program, but the JHSPH Advisory Board was unmoved.[34]

Private universities such as Johns Hopkins were free to discriminate because they were not bound by the Constitution's "equal protection" clause, which only applied to government-supported institutions. By claiming to be a government-supported institution, Hopkins was actually setting itself up for an antidiscrimination lawsuit. In November 1938, the US Supreme Court ruled in *Missouri v. Gaines* that the constitutionality of segregation laws rested "wholly upon the equality of the privileges which the laws give to the separated groups within the State." If none of a state's public universities agreed to admit blacks to graduate and professional programs offered to whites, then the state government would be obliged to build new separate schools for blacks that were demonstrably equal to those for whites.[35]

The *Gaines* decision prompted one member of Johns Hopkins' all-white faculty to mount a public critique of the university's segregationist admissions policy. Broadus Mitchell, a political science professor, charged that by excluding black students, Johns Hopkins was "turning our backs on the part of the population that needs us most," citing the racial disparity in Baltimore's mortality rates. Mitchell took aim at the School of Hygiene's international reputation to reinforce his point. "The Caroline Islands have our solicitude before Caroline Street Baltimore," he declared, "and the Dutch East Indies before Druid Hill Avenue."[36]

After Maceo Williams graduated from Harvard, he returned to Baltimore and became the first African-American doctor to join the BCHD staff on a full-time basis. From 1939 to 1966, he served as the founding director of the Druid Hill Health Center in West Baltimore, the city's first neighborhood clinic for black patients. Among his first tasks was to assist JHSPH with obtaining the cooperation of black residents of the EHD for the second major survey in 1939, which used 45 BCHD nurses. The move to bring Maceo Williams on the BCHD staff was part of a larger movement by health departments to address black health needs in response to the growing influence of the medical civil rights movement, but the BCHD still would not allow a black physician to treat white patients. When the PHS attempted to assign its first black commissioned officer to Baltimore during the war, Commissioner Williams bowed to local pressure, explaining that local whites would refuse to be served by a black physician in uniform. The expansion of public health and sanitation services for black residents was also motivated by white employers' desire for a healthy labor force, business interests who feared that high disease rates would drive away economic and population growth, and white residents who feared the spread of illness from black into white neighborhoods.[37]

When Hopkins officials met in December 1938 with Commissioner Williams and Mayor Howard W. Jackson to discuss a new EHD building, they were hoping to solve both the school's space crunch and its need to expand field training opportunities. Since the EHD's original Rockefeller grant was about to expire, the university offered to donate the land for the building and asked the city to take over the full EHD budget as well as provide $350,000 for construction and $5,500 for annual maintenance. The original proposal was for a grand structure with six floors of 4,000 square feet each, featuring clinics for syphilis, tuberculosis (TB), maternal and child hygiene, and dentistry; nursing and administrative offices; and one floor each for teaching and research activities.[38]

Baltimore's mayor and city council deemed improving black health a higher priority than helping Johns Hopkins expand its School of Hygiene. Instead of moving forward with the university's proposal to build a new EHD building on land owned by Johns Hopkins, the city government decided to construct a second black neighborhood clinic in East Baltimore at Central and Orleans Avenues, a few blocks from JHSPH. Commissioner Williams had named the opening of the Druid Hill Health Center "the most important health event of 1939," and he likewise praised the Somerset Health Center as "one of the most important City Health Department new developments associated with the Johns Hopkins School of Hygiene and Public Health."[39]

The Best Place in the World to Study Syphilis

Venereal disease control was the main catalyst for founding the Somerset Health Center, and several faculty members in the Department of Venereal Diseases spoke at the opening ceremony in 1944. Syphilis ranked fifth as a cause of black mortality in Baltimore, but the disease also destroyed lives in myriad ways before it ended them. Neurosyphilis was the leading diagnosis for admissions to state mental hospitals, since patients exhibited cognitive decline, paranoia, hallucinations, and other features consistent with general paresis, an acronym coined to catalog the changes in personality, affect, reflexes, eyes, senses, intellect, and speech. Syphilis also caused a range of other complications ranging from weakening of the heart muscle to severe skin problems. Nowhere was the impact of local attitudes and conditions more evident than in Baltimore's venereal disease control program, the impetus for record growth and far-reaching changes in the school's research and teaching missions.[40]

After he became surgeon general, Parran called on medical and public health leaders to contribute "the best professional thinking" to create a new health system that coordinated the government, business, and nonprofit sectors. He claimed that physicians and the public had already accepted the essential connection between prevention and treatment of disease, and therefore "sound public policy dictates that there should be a unity of administration for [public] health and medical care programs. The health department obviously is the one agency best fitted to do this job."[41]

Venereal disease was the perfect field for Parran's ambitions, since it muddied the distinctions between clinical medicine and public health. The Wasserman test, developed in 1906, was among the first blood tests used to screen for infectious disease. In 1909, Paul Ehrlich's "magic bullet" against syphilis, Salvarsan, became the first effective chemotherapy. Together, the Wasserman test and Salvarsan represented a historic advance in the fight against not only syphilis but also all infectious disease. But in an era when primary prevention of VD through condoms was socially and politically taboo, the next best way to control the spread of sexually transmitted diseases was to aggressively diagnose and treat them on a large scale. The promising new weapons against syphilis, therefore, collapsed the boundary between prevention—the bailiwick of public health—and the physician's claim on diagnosis and cure.[42]

Just as thymol had done for hookworm and DDT and chloroquine did for malaria, the powerful tools developed to fight syphilis also enhanced the prestige of public health. According to medical historian Allan Brandt, "scientific advances opened the way for state and local public health officials to take a more aggressive stand in the fight against venereal diseases and to encourage the growth of the public health field." Baltimore would be ground zero in that fight, especially after Parran won the passage of the 1938 National Venereal Disease Control Act. His campaign was the ideal vehicle for promoting both the horizontal integration of public health, medical care, and welfare services and the vertical integration of local, state, and federal health programs.[43]

In 1936, Parran helped J. Earle Moore, associate professor of medicine at the Johns Hopkins School of Medicine and head of the Johns Hopkins Hospital syphilis clinic, to secure an annual $10,000 training grant from the Social Security Act to establish the nation's first graduate training program in syphilis control. The program's graduates would lead the VD campaign and take it out into the countryside. Moore, arguably the most prominent syphilis expert of his generation, had worked closely with Parran when he headed the PHS Division of Venereal Disease. Both physicians were members of the Cooperative Clinical Group, whose study of syphilis treatment between 1928 and 1936 was an early example of organized therapeutic research. After the group published its initial studies in the relatively obscure PHS journal *Venereal Disease Information*, doctors paid them little attention and continued their own haphazard, unscientific treatment methods. Parran vowed to educate them on the value of public health research by "a concerted effort . . . for persistent propagandizing of the medical profession with the facts elicited by the studies." He soon was persistently propagandizing not just doctors but all of the American public, taking to the radio airwaves and the pages of popular newspapers and magazines to warn against the scourge of syphilis.[44]

The VD control training grant was the first of many federal training grants awarded to Johns Hopkins. Such grants would become a mainstay of medical and public health education programs at universities after the war. Moore and Parran then approached the Rockefeller IHD to request additional funding, but IHD officials rejected their original plan to base the program in the medical school, insisting instead that they revise the proposal "so that it has definitely a public health bearing." To receive Rockefeller funding, Moore would have to cooperate more closely with the School of Hygiene and the EHD to incorporate casefinding and epidemiological fieldwork.[45]

To direct the VD control program, Moore and Parran requested the IHD to assign Thomas B. Turner to Hopkins. Turner knew both men well. As a resident under Moore, Turner had taught the first VD control course at Johns Hopkins Hospital in 1930. Turner and Moore played instrumental roles in Parran's national campaign against syphilis, particularly in building the federal research juggernaut that evolved from the 1938 Venereal Disease Control Act and was later formalized as the PHS Syphilis Study Section. Parran also praised academic research on syphilis at Harvard, Vanderbilt, University of Pennsylvania, and University of Michigan.[46]

As a condition of continuing to pay Turner's salary at Hopkins, the IHD stipulated that he also direct a community syphilis control program that would expand on Frost's preliminary prevalence studies in East Baltimore. To address the lack of reliable data on nationwide trends in syphilis and their geographic and demographic variations, Rockefeller officials pushed Turner to conduct "an intensive piece of epidemiological work rather than an extensive undertaking involving much treatment but little of epidemiological value." In turn, Parran urged Rockefeller to support syphilis studies in diverse communities around the country to demonstrate "the practicability of applying various public health measures against syphilis" and to use methods that would "show beyond doubt the progress which may be expected by the application of the measures under consideration."[47]

In 1938, Moore, Freeman, and Huntington Williams convinced the city government to allocate $125,000 for a syphilis control program in Baltimore, including an EHD syphilis clinic (TB, by contrast, had received only $22,000 in additional city funding). The IHD approved support for this considerably strengthened plan for the Baltimore syphilis control program, which Parran hoped might become a model for other cities. Turner commented to his Rockefeller colleague, John Ferrell, "The set-up to which we have access here will be one of the most favorable places in the world to study syphilis."[48]

In 1938, the joint Medicine–Hygiene program to train physicians in VD control methods was formalized as the first specialized track in the MPH degree. The program involved three interrelated aspects: clinical experience, serology, and epidemiology. Students spent their mornings contributing to Turner's studies of prevalence and immunity in syphilis, either examining serological samples in the lab or doing fieldwork in the EHD with a social worker. Afternoons were devoted to patient care in the Johns Hopkins Hospital Syphilis Clinic. Turner's students learned the key methods and goals of a syphilis control program, particularly the need to treat both latent and active infections to prevent the spread of disease. The program's emphasis on clinical knowledge of disease for guiding public health control measures was consistent with the Rockefeller model but violated the medical profession's taboo against treating disease under public health auspices. But just as private physicians ceded responsibility for treating mental illness to state hospitals, they largely left to public health officers the job of casefinding among sexual contacts.[49]

The JHSPH program in VD control was originally conceived as a Johns Hopkins Hospital residency, and Moore and Parran had attempted to circumvent the hospital's discriminatory staff policy by requesting funding to establish a syphilis clinic at Provident Hospital, Baltimore's only general hospital for black patients. Their plan was for black physicians to receive their academic training at Hopkins but their clinical experience in an all-black patient setting. When no sponsors stepped forward, Parran arranged for the District of Columbia Health Department and Howard University (a historically black institution that was one of only three racially integrated medical schools in the country) to conduct a recurring three-month postgraduate course in syphilis control, with scholarships for black physicians funded by state VD control grants. Three days before the attack on Pearl Harbor, the PHS informed Dean Reed that JHSPH's two-month VD control course should admit black military medical officers, and Reed eagerly requested "application blanks for this group as quickly as possible." The course was, however, only offered a few times and admitted one black officer, a nurse in the Women's Army Corps.[50]

News of high rates of syphilis among recruits revived fears from World War I that VD would impede the fighting effectiveness of the armed forces. With manpower at a premium, the War Department assigned VD control officers to all major Army detachments, and Johns Hopkins stepped in to supply trained physicians. In response to reports that the spike in VD rates on training bases had been "traced directly to organized vice in adjacent municipalities," the Secretary of War asked the PHS to "cooperate with the Army in safeguarding the health of military personnel by suitable measures of extra-military area sanitation in connection with the present concentration of troops in the South." For the first time, VD control officers were given responsibility for both the civilian and military programs, including the inspection and surveillance of troop staging areas and ports of embarkation, which had never been within the scope of previous military VD control programs.[51]

In 1942, Turner was called to active duty as director of the US Army's VD control program. He rejected the traditional abstinence emphasis of Army policy as ineffective and approved the massive distribution of condoms among troops at the rate of up to 50 million per month throughout the war. Turner also authorized large-scale advertising campaigns aimed at convincing soldiers to protect themselves by using condoms or getting prophylactic treatment soon after having sex, but he had to fight widespread opposition from those who believed his programs encouraged promiscuity. Turner responded to his critics, "Some elements would have us discontinue the advocation of prophylaxis, which appears a little like removing the brakes from motor cars to prevent speeding." Condoms would, however, be used as a major tool of prevention in the military only for the duration of the war. The reluctance of military and public health leaders alike to embrace primary prevention in peacetime through the distribution of condoms or other prophylactic methods seems shocking by twenty-first-century standards, but this thinking remained dominant until the emergence of HIV in the 1980s removed any reluctance to discuss condoms and ushered in the modern age of "safe sex" campaigns.[52]

The national syphilis campaign and the civil rights movement both accelerated during World War II, prompting the School of Hygiene finally to admit its first African-American student, Reginald G. James (MPH 1946), who would also be the first black graduate of Johns Hopkins University. James, a PHS officer and Rockefeller Foundation fellow, had assisted the Alabama State Health Department in its VD survey and treatment program in rural Macon County, the home of Tuskegee Institute. He was certainly well qualified, but James succeeded where qualified black applicants had failed previously because the PHS, Moore, and Reed considered him a strategically valuable partner in the campaign against syphilis among blacks in the armed forces and the South.[53]

In 1946, Moore appointed Ralph J. Young as the first black house officer at the Johns Hopkins Hospital syphilis clinic. After finishing his residency, Young joined Maceo Williams on the BCHD staff and ran the EHD clinics for black patients under the supervision of C. Howe Eller (MPH 1933), the EHD health officer. Since the BCHD often combined its screening programs for TB and venereal disease, Young worked closely with Miriam Brailey (profiled in chapter 4) in the BCHD Bureau of Tuberculosis and E. Gurney Clark (MPH 1936) in the BCHD Bureau of Venereal Disease. With funding from JHSPH and the state and city health departments, Young established the East Baltimore Health Organization to encourage black residents to get screened for TB and syphilis, which supported both the BCHD's public health campaigns and the School of Hygiene's research and education needs. In 1952, he would break the color bar on the Maryland State Board of Health as well as the Hopkins medical faculty; in the early 1960s, Young joined the JHSPH faculty in the Department of Chronic Diseases.[54]

After James received his MPH in 1946, he returned to active duty in the PHS, and JHSPH began admitting African Americans to all of its degree programs. By contrast, black students were not admitted to the Johns Hopkins Hospital School of Nursing until 1952 or as candidates for the MD until 1963. Despite JHSPH's international diversity during this era, by 1961, the school had awarded degrees to only five black men and one black woman. Nationally, the only school that produced significant numbers of African-American public health graduates was North Carolina College, a black state school that, in partnership with the University of North Carolina School of Public Health, awarded more than 100 bachelor's degrees to health educators.[55]

The Parran–Farrand Report had urged more support for the new Division of Venereal Diseases at JHSPH, and the Rockefeller Foundation sponsored several additional faculty members during the war. In 1942, JHSPH appointed Moore as adjunct professor and head of the division, which cemented his influence and leadership within the school for the next 15 years until his death. Research and training on VD was further strengthened in 1947, when PHS officer John C. Hume (MPH 1947) was appointed assistant dean and director of the VD training program. As a young PHS officer, Hume had worked in the prewar VD campaign in Georgia, assisting Leroy Burney (ScM 1932) in establishing the first mobile VD clinic in the United States, which Burney nicknamed the Bad Blood Wagon. Burney and Hume represented the commitment of the PHS to extend effective control and treatment methods to the rural South, where disease rates were highest but treatment was nonexistent.[56]

The school's graduate VD control program advanced three fundamental goals: it promoted innovation in community public health; produced high-

TABLE 1.2
Prominent JHSPH Alumni in the Field of Sexually Transmitted Diseases

Harry Eagle	ScM 1929	Director, Johns Hopkins Venereal Disease Research Laboratory and Laboratory of Experimental Therapeutics 1927–1947; member, PHS Syphilis Study Section; scientific director, National Cancer Institute; chief, Experimental Therapeutics section of National Microbiological Institute; chief, Cell Biology Laboratory of NIAID
Leroy E. Burney	ScM 1932	PHS officer who established first US mobile VD clinic in Brunswick, Georgia, in 1937; led VD control in US Navy during World War II; US Surgeon General 1956–1961
Clarence A. Smith	MPH 1939	Director, PHS Venereal Disease Division
James K. Shafer	MPH 1943	Director, PHS Venereal Disease Division
Reginald G. James	MPH 1946	PHS officer in Venereal Disease Division; member, US Department of Health, Education, and Welfare's Ad Hoc Advisory Panel on the PHS Tuskegee Syphilis Study
John C. Hume	MPH 1947	Leader in the PHS and WHO VD and yaws campaigns; medical director, US Technical Cooperation Mission in India, 1955–1961; JHSPH Associate Dean 1961–1967; JHSPH Dean 1967–1977
Huan-Ying Li	MPH 1952	Led WHO campaigns against yaws in Indonesia and VD in Burma; applied TPI syphilis test in China; led in introducing multidrug therapy for leprosy in China

quality research that integrated epidemiological fieldwork, laboratory investigations, and clinical observation; and succeeded at attracting scores of physicians into public health careers. During its first four years, the Johns Hopkins VD control program trained 116 health officers from across the country. After JHSPH formalized the program in 1938 as the first specialty track within the CPH degree, VD control students represented one-third of CPH enrollment. Many JHSPH graduates rose to prominence in the domestic and global campaigns against VD (table 1.2).

Studies of the epidemiology of syphilis developed collaborations among JHSPH, BCHD, local physicians of all races, and even the Baltimore City school system, but community initiatives had their pitfalls. In late 1943, the EHD health officer, C. Howe Eller, proposed to conduct a VD survey in a high school, assisted by E. Gurney Clark, who had joined the JHSPH faculty in the Division of Venereal Diseases. The EHD Conference Committee, which reviewed all research proposals, recommended obtaining the cooperation of the School Board and area physicians. Patterson Park High School, an all-white school in East Baltimore, was selected to implement "the sex hygiene-venereal disease education side of the project." Williams, the Board of School

Superintendents, and the principal of the school approved the project, but it nearly self-destructed when Eller blundered by starting on Good Friday in a majority–Roman Catholic school, which deeply disturbed the headmistress. In 18 sessions over a period of five days, JHSPH student John D. Porterfield (MPH 1944) gave a 40-minute VD education talk to 750 students, who met in single-sex groups in the gym. Yet this blitzkrieg was akin to killing a fly with a sledgehammer: among the 80 percent of students whose parents permitted them to have blood tests, not a single student tested positive.[57]

Along with the epidemiology studies and laboratory research on syphilis control, the school played a central role in developing the methodology for randomized controlled trials to establish the safety, effectiveness, and optimal dosages for a host of new therapeutic substances. When Moore became head of the new PHA Division of Venereal Diseases, he was already a proponent of interdisciplinary collaboration in medical research. He and Turner seized the opportunity provided by the war to establish the first major Medicine–Hygiene research collaboration at Hopkins, involving the Department of Medicine and the Hygiene departments of Biostatistics, Bacteriology, and Venereal Diseases. Syphilis was uniquely suited to collaborative research because it presented a set of complex problems of great interest to clinicians, basic scientists, and epidemiologists. Like TB, diphtheria, and other common infectious diseases with severe, potentially fatal complications, syphilis was a social disease in the broadest sense in that it united medical and public health concerns. Between 1937 and 1949, Turner's lab received $140,000 from the IHD for research on immunity in syphilis. The school also received four major PHS grants during the 1940s for VD control research and training, totaling over half a million dollars (roughly $7 million in 2015).[58]

Until 1943, everything Turner and Moore had accomplished in the syphilis control program had been done without penicillin, but the largest VD grants to the school were for studies of penicillin therapy to treat early syphilis. Moore and other medical faculty worked closely with Lowell Reed and Margaret Merrell (ScD 1930) in Biostatistics, who provided crucial advice on experimental design and physiological reaction rates for most of the therapeutic drug studies at Hopkins. Their expertise in the application of statistical analysis for medical research made them JHSPH's most frequently sought collaborators. Merrell, the principal statistician for the penicillin trials and statistical consultant to the PHS and the US Army Surgeon General, emerged as one of the premier experts on statistical analysis for randomized controlled trials of therapeutic compounds. She and Reed helped to develop standard clinical protocols and follow-up procedures that would ensure comparability among the results of centralized, cooperative studies of large numbers of patients.[59]

Using the penicillin in syphilis studies as a guide, the PHS evaluated streptomycin to treat TB. Merrell's former Biostatistics colleague Carroll Palmer, director of the TB research programs for the PHS from 1942 to 1967, insisted that the evaluation adopt randomized controls. George W. Comstock (DrPH 1956), a brilliant TB epidemiologist like Palmer who joined the JHSPH faculty in 1962, observed that Palmer faced "considerable opposition" to conducting a controlled trial, but his success in carrying it out "went far toward insuring that the assessment of [streptomycin's] therapeutic value would be scientifically sound. In this way, a firm basis was established for subsequent trials of new chemotherapeutic regimens, each controlled by concurrent comparisons with the regimen found most effective by the preceding trial." Palmer became the leading expert on global TB epidemiology, directing TB research at the WHO from 1949 to 1955. His research refined the tuberculin screening methods used worldwide; he demonstrated that most weak tuberculin sensitivities were the result of infection with atypical mycobacteria, endemic in many regions. Palmer's studies of mycobacteria showed their capability to act as a natural vaccination against the disease.[60]

To prove penicillin's long-term efficacy in treating early syphilis, Merrell rounded up the clinical records of 15,000 patients who had been treated throughout the United States and then followed over a two-year period. In 1947, she announced her findings: 20 months after penicillin treatment, three-quarters of the patients had negative Wasserman blood tests and showed no clinical symptoms. Of the 25 to 30 percent of patients who still had positive blood tests, Merrell surmised that either the treatment had been ineffective or some patients may have been reinfected after treatment. To indicate the tremendous impact that penicillin treatment had on syphilis rates in the United States, mental hospital admissions for neurosyphilis showed a 60-fold decrease from 5.9 cases per 100,000 population in 1942 to 0.1 cases per 100,000 in 1965.[61]

In her many collaborations with clinical medical researchers, Merrell remained true to her public health training. In an era when clinical trials were still often conducted on very few patients without controls, she emphasized that "the final evaluation [of a drug] cannot be on patients but must be on the population. . . . A self-selected group of patients presenting themselves for observation, diagnosis, or treatment will not be representative of the general population. It may in fact give us almost no normal persons." Merrell, like Reed and Palmer, advised on statistical sampling for the EHD studies of disease over time in a general population. She was among the many JHSPH faculty who applied the discrete observations of a 1-square-mile section of East Baltimore to render a more scientific, data-driven view of the universe of health and disease.[62]

During the decade between the passage of the Social Security Act in 1935 and the end of World War II, the VD control program at Hopkins exemplified several important trends in public health education and knowledge. It used federal and philanthropic funding to dramatically expand training as well as research programs; it melded laboratory, clinical, and epidemiological research to achieve measurable reductions in the incidence and severity of disease; and it promoted intensive cooperation among Johns Hopkins medical and public health faculty, community doctors, and local health officials. Finally, the Hopkins syphilis control program in the EHD served as a catalyst for reorganizing and expanding the programs for the city of Baltimore and state of Maryland, for which Reed and Turner were appointed consultants.[63]

The Bioethics of Syphilis Research

Along with the achievements of the clinical trials of penicillin therapy for early syphilis and the military's VD prevention program, the antisyphilis campaign had another, deeply troubling legacy. Public health campaigns to fight disease by offering treatment, modifying environmental conditions, or conducting other types of interventions require significant resources and human effort, even as they pose potential risks to their intended beneficiaries. Wade Hampton Frost had written in 1923 that, to justify such campaigns, health officers (and, by extension, health policymakers) must have "more than a knowledge of [how] the specific organisms of disease [react] under the controlled conditions of the laboratory. It equally requires a knowledge of the community, of the psychology of the people, their social organization, the conditions and events of their everyday life. It requires that the knowledge of fundamental causes of disease be fitted together with the knowledge of people into a practical epidemiology, directly applicable to prevention." Frost—named for a Confederate general—had also mentored Ruth Rice Puffer and Miriam Brailey, who, like him, drew some of the earliest scholarly attention to racial disparities in health. He did not live long enough to teach Reginald James, the first African-American graduate of JHSPH.[64]

The School of Hygiene and Public Health, with its liberal reputation for welcoming international and political diversity, was the first Johns Hopkins University division to desegregate. Its faculty and alumni published pioneering studies of racial disparities in malaria, TB, syphilis, and other diseases. Yet, despite Moore and Parran's sincere efforts to open opportunities for black physicians at Johns Hopkins and in the PHS, they also advised the PHS on the Tuskegee Syphilis Study. The PHS, which funded and carried out the study in Macon County, Alabama, recruited 439 black men with late-stage syphilis as subjects and 185 as controls. Johns Hopkins University was not involved in funding, planning, or administering the syphilis research in Tuskegee at any point. Moore, while serving on the faculty of both the medical school and JHSPH, served as an independent consultant, and Parran, although he did not originate the study, allowed it to continue and expand during his tenure as surgeon general. Throughout the study, PHS physicians intentionally deceived the mostly illiterate men to continue to observe the natural history of the disease, telling them that they were receiving "special free treatment" for their "bad blood," in the form of diagnostic spinal taps, aspirin, and vitamins, but no effective therapy for syphilis.[65]

The initial purpose of the study was to compare the health of two otherwise similar groups of individuals, one with untreated syphilis and another without syphilis. This was a prospective cohort study of the natural history of a disease, which was a common tool for medical research in an era with few effective treatments. JHSPH researchers would continue to use and improve similar methods as the first step toward developing effective screening and treatment programs for newly discovered diseases such as AIDS. When the Tuskegee Study began in 1932, it had no clearly defined protocol and was not planned as a long-term study. Because the PHS did not then have an effective research review system, bureaucratic inertia allowed the study to continue until 1972, and it became the longest nontherapeutic medical study in history.[66]

During the Tuskegee Study's second decade (1942–1952), as noted above, the research protocols developed for the penicillin trials by Moore, Turner, Reed, and Merrell helped ensure the scientific validity and reproducibility of all subsequent JHSPH research and shaped the broader parameters of the randomized controlled trial. The PHS quickly applied the new methods to its trials of streptomycin for TB, but PHS researchers on the Tuskegee Study ignored such protocols. For example, 12 men in the control group who later tested positive for syphilis were switched into the syphilis group, which also compromised the original goal of only studying late-stage syphilis. For nearly 30 years after penicillin became widely available, the PHS failed to use it to cure the Tuskegee Study's participants.[67]

The syphilis research conducted by JHSPH in Baltimore bears many striking contrasts to the PHS study in Macon County, Alabama. In Baltimore, Moore and Turner focused on finding and treating patients with early syphilis, including those without apparent symptoms, and conducted follow-up case-finding and partner notification. They also developed effective educational interventions targeted to different population groups, and Turner's success in testing and applying these prevention methods in Baltimore led to his appointment as director of the US Army's VD control programs in military personnel as well as civilians. In the PHS Tuskegee Study, not only were the men denied treatment, but their wives, children, and sex partners also were not traced and few were treated. Researchers assumed the men were noncontagious since they

TABLE 1.3
Comparison of Syphilis Research at JHSPH and in the PHS Tuskegee Syphilis Study

	JHSPH Syphilis Research in Baltimore	PHS Tuskegee Study of Untreated Syphilis in the Negro Male
Basic parameters	Conducted in Baltimore in cooperation with the Baltimore City Health Department and the Johns Hopkins Hospital, 1936–1950; focused on finding and treating early and latent (subclinical) syphilis	Conducted in Macon County, Alabama in cooperation with the county health department, the PHS Bureau of Venereal Disease, and the Tuskegee Institute, 1932–1972; focused on observing effects of untreated, late-stage syphilis
Funding	Rockefeller Foundation, BCHD, PHS	Rosenwald Fund (pilot prevalence study), PHS
JHSPH involvement	Turner, Moore, and Eagle were principal investigators	Moore served as adviser, not investigator
Training	Venereal disease control MPH program trained numerous leaders for PHS, US military, and WHO	PHS and CDC trained numerous VD control officers on Tuskegee Study; many later rose to top leadership positions
Methods	Seroprevalence studies; prevention through education and prophylactic treatment; casefinding and partner notification; controlled trials of treatment with heavy metals (pre-1940) and penicillin (1942–1950)	Observed progress of disease over life span "to autopsy" in patients with late-stage syphilis compared with uninfected controls
Conclusions	Determined accurate prevalence and incidence rates in general population and highest risk groups to guide national STD control programs; established effective therapeutic protocols and dosages for penicillin treatment of early syphilis and gonorrhea; documented effectiveness of treatment for preventing disease transmission; established foundational methods for randomized controlled trials for evaluating all types of therapeutics	Untreated syphilis among African Americans caused its incidence to spiral and reduced black life expectancy by 17 percent
Race and gender aspects	All principal investigators were white physicians; African-American physicians from BCHD and private practice assisted in data collection; research subjects included both sexes and white and black races; data were analyzed by race and sex	All principal investigators were white physicians; African-American physicians from Tuskegee Institute and an African-American nurse assisted in data collection; research subjects were all African-American males

(*continued*)

TABLE 1.3 *(continued)*

	JHSPH Syphilis Research in Baltimore	PHS Tuskegee Study of Untreated Syphilis in the Negro Male
Informed consent and treatment	In keeping with common medical research practice in the 1940s, no formal consent was obtained from adult participants. Researchers obtained parental consent for blood tests on minors, under supervision of Baltimore City Public School officials. All patients with positive Wasserman tests were referred to BCHD clinics or Johns Hopkins Hospital for treatment.	No informed consent was obtained; researchers overtly deceived participants by claiming to offer free treatment for "bad blood"; administrators attempted to prevent participants from receiving penicillin through outside treatment programs.

were in the late stage of the disease, but their medical records contradict this. At least 16 deaths, and possibly many more, of Tuskegee Study participants were attributable to syphilis; 40 of the men's wives contracted the disease, and 19 of their children were born with congenital syphilis.[68]

Moore, the only JHSPH faculty member involved in any capacity with the Tuskegee Study, also chaired the 12-member PHS Syphilis Study Section. Moore and the other study section members from JHSPH, Reed, Turner, and Harry Eagle, served independently of their roles as Johns Hopkins University faculty and were not representing the university. In 1946, the PHS study section approved a grant proposal for an ill-fated project directed by John C. Cutler, then at PHS, who later enrolled at JHSPH (MPH 1950). Cutler's never-published research, conducted between 1946 and 1948, involved intentionally exposing 1,308 Guatemalan prison inmates, mental patients, sex workers, and soldiers to syphilis and gonorrhea. The participants were given blood tests afterward to determine whether they were infected, and Cutler's team administered penicillin to some, but not all, subjects with positive results to test the new drug's effectiveness as both a cure and a prophylactic against developing the disease after exposure. For this project and other serologic diagnostic studies of syphilis transmission and penicillin therapy, Cutler obtained the cooperation of the PHS, the Guatemalan government, and the Pan American Sanitary Bureau.[69]

During his subsequent career as a PHS officer, Cutler spent time working on the Tuskegee Study and dedicated himself to stamping out syphilis in the United States and abroad. Using findings from the Tuskegee Study, he emphasized to public health professionals that untreated syphilis among blacks caused its incidence to spiral and reduced black life expectancy by 17 percent, which justified continued federal funding for syphilis control efforts. Cutler would go on to serve as assistant US surgeon general, deputy director of PAHO, and chair of the Department of Public Health Administration at the University of Pittsburgh Graduate School of Public Health, where Parran was the founding dean. Another JHSPH alumnus, Leroy Burney, was among the many PHS venereal disease control officers whose training included a stint on the Tuskegee Study. As US surgeon general from 1956 to 1961, Burney, like his predecessors, allowed the study to continue.[70]

Ironically, the laudable desire to spare as many people as possible from disease in the *future* could become a justification for subjecting a small number of people in the *present* to pain and suffering, just as a general stoically decides to sacrifice the shock troops in a battle to win the wider war. But, as medical historian Susan L. Reverby reminds us, "It was allowable to use the 'other' as the foot soldiers." The tragedies of Tuskegee, Guatemala, and other breaches of bioethics hinged on power disparities at both the individual and community levels. These differentials do not always line up neatly as Good versus Evil but may more closely resemble Dr. Jekyll and Mr. Hyde—the same individual may be both resisting and accommodating ethically questionable science. For example, Reverby observed that "physicians in under-resourced communities often say yes to research because they have few other options and they triage the 'for right now' against the future. They remind us that the American doctors [of all races] involved [in the Tuskegee and Guatemala syphilis studies] believed they were doing good science for the common good. They thought it was their responsibility to protect the nation through this kind of research."[71]

The history of the Johns Hopkins School of Hygiene and Public Health is a compelling antidote to what Reverby calls "the monster doctors-are-infecting-the-vulnerable story[,] a powerful tale where our horror deepens as we expect to see the hapless victims and the evil scientist." Johns Hopkins was acknowledged as the foremost center of syphilis research, and the university and hospital contributed a disproportionate share of the knowledge necessary to treat the very common, often disabling, and potentially fatal disease. Yet, as this chapter has shown, Johns Hopkins was also a very powerful institution in a segregated city where both law and custom devalued black lives and rights.[72]

The Tuskegee Study is discussed further and compared with the school's later work in international health and family planning in chapter 13.

Conclusion

In the public health laboratories of Baltimore's Eastern Health District and the rural environs of the United States and Latin American South, JHSPH cooperated with the BCHD, PHS, and Rockefeller Foundation to develop novel programs to study and control communicable diseases. These programs built strengths in field observation, microbiology, zoonotic disease, medical ecology, and disease surveillance. By the late 1930s, the School of Hygiene and Public Health was a recognized national leader in biostatistics, parasitology, the biochemistry of nutrition, and the epidemiology of infectious diseases such as TB, syphilis, and diphtheria. Between 1920 and 1950, the southern public health campaigns brought down rates of malaria, hookworm, typhoid, and other epidemic diseases by broadly applying low-cost technology such as window screens, sanitary privies, chlorination of the water supply, ground and aerial spraying of insecticides, and building dams and earthworks to drain swamps. Likewise, the PHS campaign against syphilis, a disease that was most prevalent among the South's poor, medically underserved populations, drew upon the resources of the EHD and made JHSPH the leading center for syphilis research and training.

World War II brought new prosperity to the region and validated many of these southern-born solutions for global application. Defense industries such as the Westinghouse Electric Radio Division and Bethlehem Steel shipyards lifted Maryland's economy out of the Depression. Wartime federal contracts established ventures that launched Johns Hopkins University into national prominence, including the Applied Physics Laboratory and the cooperative clinical trials of penicillin in the treatment of early syphilis. Yet the war would also decisively unseat the South from its pivotal place in American politics and public health. With the return of peace, southern priorities—in both civil rights and disease control—increasingly yielded to national and international concerns.

CHAPTER TWO

School at War

During World War II, defense-related health initiatives and training programs benefited from unprecedented government largesse and strong bipartisan support. By the war's height in 1944, the federal budget had increased to 10 times its peacetime level in 1939. Wartime approaches to scientific research, vector control, and disease prevention became the prototypes for national and international postwar programs. The war also awakened the belief in US policymakers that controlling disease would stimulate economic and social development in foreign lands, which could be a powerful tool for maintaining peace and gaining allies. Although the Master of Public Health degree or its equivalent had existed at Johns Hopkins and other schools since the 1910s, it had still not really gained broad acceptance until the war provided the political will and funding to make the MPH the standard mark of professional competence for public health practitioners by 1950.[1]

This chapter tracks the school's wartime development in three related areas: specialized MPH programs that built on the success of the venereal disease control training program; the launch of the school's research on polio, which lay much of the groundwork for Jonas Salk's vaccine and gave JHSPH a decisive edge in vaccine development and evaluation; and the growth of collaboration between the schools of Hygiene and Medicine, formalized in the creation of the Medical Planning and Development Committee. By the time the Allies declared victory over the Axis in 1945, JHSPH had strengthened its place within the university and vis-à-vis the medical school and was poised to bring a public health perspective into the newly reorganized and expanded National Institutes of Health (NIH).

Expansion and Specialization of Public Health Education

In 1919, George E. Vincent, president of the Rockefeller Foundation, had dubbed the School of Hygiene and Public Health "A West Point for Health Officers." JHSPH lived up to the title more literally by training hundreds of graduates who either joined the military or directly aided the war effort in a variety of ways. The conflict was a catalyst for the school's leaders to improve and expand instruction, research, and the practical application of public health methods. Faculty members who were not on active duty were often advancing the war effort in Washington with officials from the War Resources Planning Board, War Manpower Commission, Works Progress Administration, Tennessee Valley Authority, National Research Council Division of Medical Sciences, and Naval Research Laboratory. Faculty also worked with the Rockefeller International Health Division to produce a yellow fever vaccine and study food supplies in occupied European countries. Hygiene faculty members advised the surgeons general of the Army, Navy, and PHS on communicable disease outbreaks at home and abroad, as well as helped shape public health training programs for military and civilian personnel.[2]

Among the most critical areas of wartime service was the Armed Forces Epidemiological Board (AFEB), which applied public health science to solve the tremendous day-to-day health challenges posed by armed conflict for both troops and civilians. The AFEB exemplified the optimal blending of basic science and applied research advocated by Surgeon General Thomas Parran and Lowell Reed. The AFEB sent numerous present or future Hygiene faculty members to tackle public health problems around the globe. From the Department of Epidemiology, Kenneth Maxcy was a senior AFEB consultant and member of the Typhus Commission, and John J. Phair (MPH 1933) directed the AFEB Commission on Meningococcal Meningitis. William W. Cort, chair of Parasitology, served on the AFEB Commission on Tropical Medicine and lectured on hookworm disease at the Army Medical School in Washington. Cort also chaired the Joint Committee on Military Medicine at Johns Hopkins and organized the Clinical Laboratory course for medical officers.[3]

The school's faculty and students worked extensively with refugees during and after the war, and some were themselves refugees. Ernest Lyman Stebbins (MPH 1932), who would succeed Reed as dean in 1946, had served during the war as New York City Health Commissioner under Mayor Fiorello

LaGuardia. LaGuardia was appointed in 1946 to head the United Nations Relief and Rehabilitation Administration, which opened doors for Stebbins to survey the war's devastating effects on Europe's health and recommend solutions. With the Health Advisory Committee of the International Red Cross Societies, Stebbins witnessed the impact of raging epidemics of tuberculosis and VD in Europe, where TB rates were four times as high as before the war and worst of all in Poland. He served on the executive committee and national board of governors of the American Red Cross and chaired its advisory board on health services. Stebbins toured 16 European countries in 1946 to survey medical aspects of the Red Cross civilian relief program and make recommendations for rebuilding local medical facilities. Under the US High Commissioner of Germany, Stebbins and Haven Emerson of Columbia University inspected public health facilities in refugee camps, factories, and water supply systems and then co-chaired a six-week series of public health planning institutes with German public health authorities to encourage adoption of American public health practices.[4]

JHSPH faculty joined Stebbins to address the needs of refugees, such as Cornelius Krusé in Sanitary Engineering, who was a member of the American Friends Service Committee delegation that met with President Truman to report on private humanitarian efforts to assist refugees. Paul Lemkau served on the psychiatry subcommittee of the American Red Cross Medical Advisory Committee and saw the organization's potential for shaping public opinion on mental illness: "The large membership and powerful educative force of the Red Cross makes its increasing interest in mental hygiene and psychiatric problems a magnificent resource for public education in these fields. . . . The study of the psychological effects of disaster will also be a probable outcome of the work of this committee." Lemkau was also a consultant to the psychiatric outpatient clinics of the VA Department of Medicine and Surgery. During Stebbins's deanship, JHSPH appointed several German Jewish faculty who had fled from the Nazis, including Manfred Mayer in Bacteriology, Abraham M. Schneidmuhl (MPH 1959) in Mental Hygiene, and Ernest Bueding in Pathobiology.[5]

European Jewish refugees also enrolled at JHSPH after the war, such as Alberta Szalita-Pemow (ScD 1950), a physician and neurologist from Warsaw, Poland, who received a scholarship from the National Council of Jewish Women for outstanding women who would return to Europe to rebuild war-torn Jewish communities. Her husband and children were killed in Hitler's purge of Polish Jews, and she had helped to care for Jewish patients in Russia and Poland before the war and in France during and after the war. While still a Hygiene student, Szalita-Pemow joined the staff of the Chestnut Lodge asylum near Rockville, Maryland, where she was electrified by the "extraordinary atmosphere" that was "bursting with the ideas and struggles of a group of sharp-minded, brilliant people totally devoted to the challenging and difficult task of the treatment of schizophrenia." With another Jewish refugee psychoanalyst, Frieda Fromm-Reichmann, Szalita-Pemow established a clinical research group that produced some of the first studies of the use of psychoanalysis in treating schizophrenia, including the therapeutic use of intuition.[6]

Consulting relationships with national scientific and defense agencies further strengthened the faculty's extensive network of contacts with agencies such as the Baltimore City Health Department, state health departments, and PHS. Maxcy observed, "The stimulation emanating from this [consulting] activity cannot be overrated. It keeps the [departments of epidemiology and biostatistics] in active touch with new studies which are going on in the field and it serves as a rich source of current material for teaching purposes." In addition to strengthening research and instruction, consulting activities opened new employment channels for the school's graduates. JHSPH received such a large volume of job announcements from health agencies, universities, and the military that Reed apologetically stated to one official, "The demand for medical men trained in public health is so great that at the moment I can't suggest the name of any of our graduates who would be available for the vacancies you have." Foreign health officials also petitioned the school to send its graduates. JHSPH received so many highly qualified applicants in response to the wartime campaigns to promote careers in public health that Reed declared it the school's duty "to cooperate with the public health movement in its rapidly growing training program," even if it meant running double sessions.[7]

The military's sudden demand for trained public health professionals to protect the health of troops and civilians accelerated the changes in graduate public health education triggered by the Social Security Act and the Parran–Farrand Report (detailed in the Prologue). The US Army's priorities guided JHSPH in expanding the preventive medicine program and establishing the first MPH specialty tracks in VD control, mental hygiene, sanitary engineering, and industrial hygiene. Hopkins was responding to the demand for new training programs in growing fields but also resisting the trend toward the balkanization of these programs in separate professional schools. Wartime mobilization not only disrupted academic programs in schools of public health but also thinned the ranks of public health workers just as the demand increased for sanitation and disease control in the boomtowns that sprung up around military bases and defense production plants. The armed forces were eager to employ MPH graduates trained in VD control to keep soldiers "fit to fight" and in mental hygiene to screen recruits and treat mentally ill servicemen and veterans.

In 1943, Reed wrote John Ferrell to urge the Rockefeller Foundation to extend its support for additional teaching personnel at JHSPH for as long as possible, noting that "the moment the war is over, it is obvious that there will be a great rush to graduate training in the field of public health." Reed also helped guide the wartime discussions of institutional accreditation that culminated with the APHA Committee on Professional Education accepting responsibility to oversee accreditation of master's and doctoral programs. Schools of public health were first accredited in 1946, which increased the legitimacy—and marketability—of the schools' longer, more comprehensive degrees versus the shorter, more numerous programs and certificates offered outside schools of public health. Another important function of the Association of Schools of Public Health (ASPH) was working with the PHS and other federal agencies to develop new research and training initiatives and to lobby Congress for aid to public health education. The ASPH became a broker among the sometimes conflicting interests of state and local health departments, federal health agencies, and schools of public health.[8]

Although defense priorities shaped the direction and volume of public health degree programs, educational reform was also spurred by changes in public health practice. The APHA Subcommittee on Local Health Units issued its recommendations in *Local Health Units for the Nation* (1945). The report's main proposal was to extend full-time modern public health services to include the remaining 40 million Americans (30 percent of the population) who still lacked them. The report's boldest suggestions involved changing not the core mission of public health departments but the composition of their workforce. For the first time, the supply of full-time health officers and sanitary engineers was deemed adequate, and the committee even advocated the dismissal of the existing 4,300 part-time health officers, many of whom were still untrained in public health. But for other types of workers, the report advocated doubling the number of public health nurses and clerical/statisticians; tripling the number of dentists, technicians, and unskilled laboratory workers; and increasing by more than 10 times the present force of dental hygienists and health educators. If these measures were implemented and state and local governments cooperated to boost the national average per-capita spending on public health from $0.61 to $0.97, the entire population could benefit from adequate public health services provided by full-time health departments.[9]

The committee's recommendations were realized with the tailwind of defense-related health spending and a postwar economic boom that boosted tax revenues, and the public health workforce steadily expanded during and after the war. During the first five postwar years, state health agencies increased their workforce by 16 percent, but these workers were concentrated in relatively few states, with 40 percent of full-time public health physicians employed by only five states. By 1950, the three fastest growing categories of workers in state health agencies were medical and psychiatric social workers, nutritionists, and health educators. Nearly 1,400 physicians and over 3,000 nurses were enrolled in public health training programs, about one-third of them in accredited programs lasting at least one year. The number of US and Canadian graduate public health programs grew from 10 in 1934 to 17 by 1948, quadrupling the production of degrees.[10]

Despite the Parran–Farrand Report's recommendations, public health practitioners and educators continued to disagree about how new degree programs should be structured, what types of students should be encouraged to enroll, and what courses, field experience, and other requirements should be standard for public health professionals. The profession's heterogeneity compounded the difficulty of establishing uniform standards, as indicated by the APHA's array of special sections (listed in the prologue, table 4). Potential applicants had to choose among 18 types of public health degrees offered by 45 different institutions, mostly at the bachelor's level in schools of nursing and engineering. In 1945, the *American Journal of Public Health* editorialized against "minutely specialized degrees" and warned that "if every school gives a specific degree in each possible specialty, the public will be completely confused and the value of all academic degrees will be threatened."[11]

In the postwar environment of widespread political support and federal funding for public health, state legislatures clamored to found schools of public health. The 1946 Hill–Burton Hospital Survey and Construction Act provided funds to enable states to conduct comprehensive planning surveys to determine needs for the health workforce, facilities, and services; state legislators used these data to bolster their case for creating and expanding health professional training programs at state universities. The PHS Bureau of State Services provided support to states that wanted to participate in the Hill–Burton program, including a template to assist legislators in drafting state health plan legislation as well as public relations materials to generate public support through billboards, newspaper ads, posters, and radio spots.[12]

Under such conditions, the balance of public health graduates shifted definitively from private to public universities. By 1956–1957, the first four state schools were also the largest and awarded over half of all graduate public health degrees. Physicians remained a majority of enrolled students at Hopkins, Harvard, and the University of Toronto, all private, Rockefeller-endowed schools allied closely with medical schools. But at many state schools, the medical school was not even located on the same campus, and student bodies were more multidisciplinary, welcoming nurses and social workers along with physicians, basic scientists, and engineers. Outside medicine's shadow, the state schools of public health were both freer to innovate in their curricula and more vulnerable to financial pressures.[13]

Not only did schools of public health multiply, but they also broadened and deepened their degree offerings and course content. The success of the Hopkins VD control training program prompted the PHS and JHSPH to create more specialized MPH tracks based on the same formula. During the school's early decades, the departments of Sanitary Engineering, Medical Zoology, and Helminthology had emphasized environmental approaches that were best suited for rural diseases of poverty. As America's accelerating industrial development created new environmental hazards and reshaped the urban landscape of large, aging cities such as Baltimore, the school had downplayed occupational health and thus the Department of Physiological Hygiene remained small and struggling. World War II elevated the public health importance of both sanitary engineering and two major types of noncommunicable disease: mental illness and industrial health and safety. The school established specialized training programs in all three of these areas, which built on the Progressive-era "positive environmentalists" who had advocated public investment in a wide range of moral and sanitary reforms, from sewer systems, garbage collection, drinking fountains, and bathhouses (to promote cleanliness and temperance) to child guidance centers, schools, and playgrounds (to provide wholesome environments for children and to help mold them into model citizens and workers).[14]

As an MPH specialty track, mental hygiene was an attractive choice to follow VD control, since it also forged ties between the School of Hygiene and a prominent medical school department that promoted the blending of epidemiological and clinical approaches. Hopkins was home to two of the national mental hygiene movement's founders: William Henry Welch, who had served as president of the National Committee for Mental Hygiene, and Adolf Meyer, the Swiss psychiatrist whom Welch recruited to direct the Phipps Psychiatric Clinic at Johns Hopkins Hospital. Welch had wanted to include mental hygiene among the school's original departments, but the field did not fit easily within the framework of laboratory-based science dedicated to fighting infectious disease.[15]

In May 1941, Lowell Reed, Allen Freeman (chair of Public Health Administration), and Hopkins psychiatrist Paul V. Lemkau met with Victor H. Vogel, assistant chief of the PHS Mental Hygiene Division, and representatives from the Mental Hygiene Society and the Maryland Commissioner of Mental Hygiene. The participants outlined a new graduate program in mental hygiene for psychiatrists, the first of its kind. Vogel pledged to send four PHS officers on Social Security fellowships and agreed to supervise clinical training with the assistance of Leo Kanner, who had founded the first child psychiatry clinic in the United States in 1930 at the Johns Hopkins Hospital's Harriet Lane Home for Invalid Children and published the specialty's first textbook, *Child Psychiatry*, in 1935. Kanner's 1943 paper, "Autistic Disturbances of Affective Contact," established the basis for diagnosing autism, among the developmental disabilities that would become a dominant focus of JHSPH research in the 1950s. In the fall of 1941, the first group of mental hygiene MPH students enrolled at JHSPH. At that time, approximately one of every 263 Americans lived in state mental institutions, and in New York State, over a quarter of the state's annual budget went toward caring for mental patients.[16]

Lemkau was appointed to the Public Health Administration faculty as the first director of the Division of Mental Hygiene. The young Lemkau had just completed a five-year residency under Meyer and retained a joint appointment in Psychiatry, but from the beginning, he channeled the mental hygiene program toward community epidemiology and spent little time at the medical school or hospital. He and other mental hygiene leaders were consciously trying to transcend the limits of mental hospitals and to identify and treat early mental illness through programs in schools and colleges, child guidance clinics, and other outpatient settings. Students in the VD control program divided their time between lab work, the Johns Hopkins Hospital syphilis clinic, and the EHD; by contrast, mental hygiene students worked exclusively in the EHD, reflecting the mental hygiene philosophy that mental illness was preventable and caused as much by social maladjustment and environmental factors as by somatic disorders.[17]

The MPH bacteriology requirement made more sense for syphilologists than psychiatrists, however. William W. Ford, chair of Bacteriology from 1923 to 1938, was fond of saying, "Give the student a stool and he will learn bacteriology." Such a statement might have prompted the MPH mental hygiene students to pull out their Sigmund Freud instead of a microscope. The bacteriology course taught topics including the morphological, cultural, and serological identification of infectious disease agents; principles of disinfection; methods of isolating and enumerating bacteria; and the physiology and chemistry of microorganisms.[18]

When the PHS asked the school to waive the required MPH bacteriology course to enable officers to concentrate on mental hygiene courses, the JHSPH Advisory Board refused. Board members countered that the course had already "been stripped of a great deal of bacteriological technic [sic] which it contained in previous years," and the mental hygiene students would still need to understand "the principles of bacteriological and virus disease as they relate to epidemiology and to public health in general." The board felt that a bare minimum of half the academic year should be devoted to common requirements "if the general public health course is to serve its purpose of developing general public health concepts in people with as varied interests as medical health officers, psychiatrists, sanitary engineers, public health nurses, etc." Although the Advisory Board prevailed for the time being, the addition of more specialized tracks brought increasing pressure to reduce the time allotted to common public health courses in the intensive MPH schedule.[19]

The first class of MPH graduates in mental hygiene included psychiatrist Robert H. Felix (MPH 1942), who recalled taking a biostatistics course from Lowell Reed. "Oh, God, how he would lay into us about the lousy statistics in medicine and he would use mental health as the most horrible example. He would take a journal article and give you the data and conclusions, and then he would go back and tear it to shreds. Then the guys [in class] would kid me, and I decided God, if I ever had the chance, one thing I would do was develop the finest mental health statistics department in the world."

Felix was appointed director of the PHS Division of Mental Hygiene in 1944 and helped to shape the National Mental Health Act of 1946, which channeled federal resources into psychiatric research and training programs. The act also created the National Institute of Mental Health (NIMH), whose training grants provided more generous stipends for psychiatry residencies to increase the number of physicians entering the specialty, including community mental health. When NIMH was formally organized in 1949, Felix was its first director, and he quickly hired Reed's star student, Morton D. Kramer (ScD 1939), as head of the Biometrics Branch. Mental hygiene was the major exception to public health's neglect of chronic disease during this period; NIMH was the exception to the NIH's general neglect of prevention and epidemiology.[20]

In addition to mental hygiene, JHSPH also created programs to meet increased military and civilian demand for sanitary engineers and industrial hygienists. Abel Wolman, chair of Sanitary Engineering in the schools of Hygiene and Engineering, oversaw the efforts of the US Army and PHS to recruit additional sanitary engineers to manage the exponential wartime growth of approximately 250 military or defense industry areas, where more than 500 PHS personnel had been assigned to emergency field duty within six months after Pearl Harbor. Kenneth Maxcy served with Wolman on the National Research Council sanitary engineering committee and warned of "the danger to our own people from infectious disease as a result of disturbances due to the war," particularly major population shifts. The armed forces mustered 16 million troops on training bases, and nearly 1 million civilians migrated to work in war-related industries such as the Baltimore shipyards, which wreaked havoc with existing water and sewer systems. Amendments to the Lanham Wartime Housing Act of 1940 provided significant federal funding for public works sanitation projects in war-affected areas, creating an urgent need for the expertise of sanitary engineers.[21]

With one-third of civilian doctors engaged in the war effort, the conflict precipitated a renewed appreciation for the contributions of sanitary engineers and other nonphysician fields of public health, while also elevating the importance of interdisciplinary teamwork. Before the war, nearly all members of the PHS Commissioned Corps had been physicians and surgeons, and the PHS employed sanitary engineers as civilians. The Public Health Service Acts of 1943 and 1944 incorporated Parran's recommendation to expand the professional categories eligible for PHS commissions, including sanitarians. Their duties encompassed malaria control in the southern United States and abroad and environmental health services for federal public housing projects, such as water and sewage systems, food sanitation, and insect and rodent control. Similar changes at Hopkins brought more sanitary engineering students into the School of Hygiene and Public Health. They had received degrees and taken most coursework through the School of Engineering on the Homewood arts and sciences campus until 1946, when JHSPH began offering the ScM and ScD degrees to sanitary engineers.[22]

To help Wolman expand the program, the school appointed Cornelius Krusé, known for his work with the PHS Malaria Control in War Areas program to combat malaria via aerial application of DDT. Krusé's wide-ranging professional experience with vector control efforts earned him spots on the Armed Forces Epidemiology Board Commission on Environmental Health and the WHO Expert Committee on Insecticides. His methods of controlling mosquitoes in reservoirs were adopted by the WHO Vector Biology and Control program. Krusé took over the lion's share of the teaching load in sanitary engineering, freeing Wolman to globetrot as a consultant. Krusé's student and colleague Kazuyoshi Kawata (DrPH 1966) praised Krusé's technical skills. "In the laboratory we would say, 'He has hands.' In lab courses, we would find him titrating, pipetting, operating the pH meter or the gang mixers right along with the students." Krusé also advised the Tennessee Valley Authority and state of Maryland on controlling air pollution from steam plants, coal mines, and institutional incinerators that burned radioactive wastes.[23]

Given the massive wartime expansion of overall manufacturing capacity and the proliferation of defense plants, industrial hygiene experienced dramatic growth during the 1940s. Carl M. Peterson, secretary of the American Medical Association (AMA) Council on Industrial Health, told Reed, "Requests are reaching us almost daily from practicing physicians who are interested in industrial health both as a contribution to the war effort and with a view towards a permanent career." JHSPH offered five courses in industrial hygiene with a combined 60 hours of lectures and an equal amount of time devoted to lab work, field trips, and clinical experiences in occupational diseases, all taught and supervised by Anna M. Baetjer (ScD 1924). She arranged for students to attend the public and private hearings of the Medical Board for Occupational Diseases of the Maryland State Compensation Commission, to participate in clinics on occupational dermatoses and arsenic poisoning at Johns Hopkins Hospital, and to visit the BCHD and area industrial plants.[24]

Baetjer should have been among the new generation of faculty leading JHSPH, but in the eyes of school administrators, her sex disqualified her as a potential department chair. After earning her doctor of science in Physiological Hygiene in 1924, Baetjer convinced her adviser William H. Howell to appoint her to the faculty, even though he only granted her the lowest salary allowable and warned her not to get married. After Howell's death in 1931, the Department of Physiological Hygiene remained without a permanent chair for nearly two decades, and throughout the 1940s, Baetjer was the department's sole faculty member. Physiological hygiene dealt with the environmental aspects of health and the effects of ambient conditions such as temperature, climate, humidity, noise, light, ventilation, radiation, and dust on human health and performance. The discipline, therefore, included evaluating and protecting the health of groups such as workers, schoolchildren, and others in institutional settings. With Wolman and Reed's moral support but little else, Baetjer built her program single-handedly during the war and served as a highly sought-after consultant to government, industry, and the military. She wrote to thank Reed in May 1941 for increasing her salary, which demonstrated Reed's "understanding of the work I am trying to do to keep this department as an active and valuable unit in the School. Sometimes I have felt discouraged but your constant interest in physiological hygiene and your advice have helped immensely." The scores of medical officers who enrolled at JHSPH gravitated toward her, dubbing themselves "Anna's boys."[25]

Baetjer emerged during the 1940s as a national leader in industrial hygiene and military medicine, later winning acclaim for her discovery that chromate dust caused lung cancer. She also was an important contributor to the Baltimore City Health Department's campaign against childhood lead poisoning, which achieved national fame for Huntington Williams. The health commissioner worked closely with medical and public health faculty at Johns Hopkins and the University of Maryland to document the sources of exposure, develop and test effective treatment, and implement the nation's first mass screening and abatement programs. The city's extensive casefinding program during the 1940s and 1950s uncovered several hundred children who had eaten or breathed lead paint particles that had flaked off from toys, furniture, or the walls of their homes, with much higher rates among poor black children, who were more likely to live in older, poorly maintained housing. At least 50

Baltimore children died of lead paint exposure between 1936 and 1951. Baetjer's detailed epidemiological studies of pediatric lead poisoning based on medical records and investigations of patients' home environments resulted in the first municipal ordinance banning lead paint inside homes, passed in 1951. Williams pushed the paint industry to stop manufacturing and advertising lead-containing paint for interior use, and in 1958 and 1959, Baltimore passed strict labeling laws, backed by investigations and threatened prosecution of local manufacturers and retailers who were caught in noncompliance. Yet, despite her accomplishments, Baetjer did not advance to the rank of associate professor until 1952 or to full professor with tenure until 1962. Only in 1983 would JHSPH appoint the first female department chair, Karen Davis, to lead Health Policy and Management.[26]

Polio

The wartime expansion of the syphilis, mental hygiene, sanitary engineering, and industrial hygiene MPH tracks had been part of a second-wave attack on the growing health problems of urban environments. The first wave had begun in the early 1900s, when less than 10 percent of Baltimore's families had private bathrooms, and the Baltimore Bath Commission had promoted public baths as "a public necessity and obligation." The commission made Baltimore a paragon of the national public bath movement by inducing the wealthy Louisville and Nashville Railroad magnate Henry Walters to donate funds to construct six bathhouses in poor neighborhoods around the city. One bathhouse was reserved for African Americans, which was an exception to Baltimore's general pattern of racial exclusion in that era. But after the city passed a law requiring all new homes to include bathrooms, growing prosperity and improving housing standards made private baths the norm rather than the exception. The public Turkish baths, where William Henry Welch had once steamed away his aches and pains, closed in 1955, and rising maintenance costs and dwindling usage led to the closure of the public bath system in 1960.[27]

The positive environmentalists at the turn of the twentieth century had been paternalistic toward the poor but had employed broad-based strategies to improve living and working conditions, including invoking government regulation to reign in the unhealthy practices of factory owners and slumlords. But as real estate and business interests stimulated the growth of both government and corporate funding for constructing new cities, towns, and neighborhoods, the goal of reducing disease rates became part of 1920s civic boosterism. Sanitation was no longer seen as a moral imperative to clean up filth and "the great unwashed" and became instead a practical problem of building the infrastructure systems necessary to supply population-dense cities with clean water and adequate waste disposal. Midcentury public health advocates were more focused on fighting infectious diseases among individuals and also more in-clined to seek voluntary cooperation from business, especially in the context of joint government-industry efforts to ramp up defense production.

The polio epidemics that began to hit America with regularity in the 1930s were a product of these developments. Like cholera and typhoid, polio was a disease of filth. Yet, ironically, the environmental sanitation reforms that vir-tually wiped out waterborne diseases merely reduced polio's endemicity in the population. Polio victims shed the virus in their feces, and without early expo-sure to the virus during infancy, American children who grew up in homes with indoor toilets and laundry facilities were vulnerable to polio epidemics that struck each summer with increasing frequency.

Beginning in the late 1930s, the search for a polio vaccine would dominate the headlines for two decades, and the successful trials of Jonas Salk's vaccine in 1954 would revolutionize American public health. On the surface, the cam-paign against polio was not crucial to national defense in the same way as efforts to prevent syphilis and mental illness among soldiers or to prevent industrial hazards among defense workers. But the war had an indirect yet significant influence on how the polio campaign played out through the 1940s and be-yond. Polio was also an infectious disease, like syphilis and TB, that had the potential to cause lifelong disability, characteristics it shared with noncommu-nicable chronic diseases.[28]

Like syphilis, polio was spread by healthy carriers who were infected but asymptomatic, but no simple, accurate blood test for polio existed that could be applied in mass screening campaigns the way the Wasserman test was for syphilis. Under William Henry Welch's emphasis on basic science research to drive public health advances, the School of Hygiene and Public Health had birthed the nation's first academic departments of both immunology (a found-ing department in 1917) and virology (established in 1925 as the Department of Filterable Viruses). But viruses were much more difficult to study than spiro-chetes, due to their small size (1/100th the size of a human cell) and the technical challenges of culturing live virus samples for observation and testing (unlike bacteria, which could be grown easily in a simple medium such as an agar plate, viruses required a growth medium with live cells). Victory over polio would require a completely new range of laboratory techniques and equipment.

Especially important was the newly introduced electron microscope, first used at JHSPH by a group of faculty recruited from the Rockefeller Institute for Medical Research, which had helped perfect the electron microscope's use in medicine and physiology. The group included Isabel M. Morgan, a highly innovative researcher in polio immunology, and Frederik B. Bang, who used electron microscopy to examine both parasitic organisms and cancer-ous viruses.[29]

In addition to strengthening the MPH curriculum and developing new specialty tracks in defense-related fields, JHSPH rose in prominence by excelling in the basic science of public health. At JHSPH, lab research on syphilis and polio radically deepened the faculty's knowledge of the immunology and pathology of bacterial and viral diseases, building the foundation for one of the world's most diverse and productive vaccine development programs. Syphilis and polio represented two distinct approaches to solving public health problems. The VD campaign employed mass screening and treatment programs that were almost entirely government funded and conducted by public health departments. The drive to control polio centered on privately funded researchers, based primarily at elite private universities, who focused on finding a vaccine. The dominant player in polio research was the National Foundation for Infantile Paralysis (NFIP), one of the disease-specific foundations that began to make large grants to academic researchers during the 1940s. Like the trials of penicillin to treat early syphilis as well as the experiments to identify antimalarial drugs, polio research would set an important precedent for the postwar multiplication of NIH institutes that focused on specific diseases or body systems, also known as categorical programs.

Among the early polio researchers was Kenneth Maxcy, who demonstrated the person-to-person transmission of polio and disproved the hypothesis that polio was a waterborne disease. Yet scientists still knew little about the immunology or etiology of polio. Some surmised that it was spread by a route similar to that of typhoid fever, whose victims ingested food contaminated by infected human carriers and flies. In some areas where DDT was used to control flies, cases of polio had also declined, which researchers from the Communicable Disease Center (CDC) erroneously attributed to DDT. The CDC even developed a cooperative program with state health departments in the late 1940s to use DDT to control polio, based on trial programs in New Mexico and Texas. After the bacillus Calmette–Guérin (BCG) vaccine was proven effective in preventing tuberculosis, the CDC also experimented with BCG to cure intestinal diseases. Because so few effective measures were available to prevent or cure most diseases, DDT and the BCG vaccine both exemplified the risk that new technology that proved effective against one disease might be abruptly shifted to attack another, even without evidence to support the technology's use in a substantially different context.[30]

By 1940, Thomas Parran and the PHS had made syphilis a cause célèbre, with federal legislation dedicated to stamping it out; funding for polio research was scarce. The NFIP, newly established by President Franklin Roosevelt and his law partner Basil O'Connor, so far had funded only one small project at Hopkins in the medical school's Division of Orthopedic Surgery. George Radcliffe, US senator from Maryland, served on the Senate Finance Committee and was also the NFIP state fundraising chairman. Radcliffe asked why Hopkins had not yet received research grants from the NFIP, and Alan Chesney, dean of Medicine, replied that "the University was rather hesitant to seem to seek a part." At the time, anti-Roosevelt feeling was extremely strong in Maryland, where the New Deal was viewed with suspicion as intrusive federalism that threatened both business interests and segregation. Some Marylanders viewed the NFIP as a political tool of FDR. Senator Radcliffe took credit for reinvigorating the state NFIP campaign and told JHU's president, Isaiah Bowman, "I thought it was rather bad psychology for Maryland to drop out of the picture for raising funds at a time when plans for Johns Hopkins to do research work [on polio] were in the making."[31]

In the medical school's Department of Anatomy, Howard A. Howe and his postdoctoral fellow David Bodian studied the ways poliovirus acted on the central nervous system and other aspects of the host–agent relationship in polio. At the University of Chicago, Bodian had earned a BS in zoology, an MD, and a PhD in anatomy, an education that gave him a unique, in-depth knowledge of virology and comparative anatomy that would aid in major breakthroughs in animal models, with important implications for fighting polio in humans. Bodian showed that the virus caused irreversible damage to motor neurons before clinical symptoms appeared. He also investigated the internal pathways of infection in humans and animals, the immunological response to infection, and the spread of the virus in populations. In 1941, Bodian and Howe confirmed that poliovirus entered through the mouth into the digestive tract, not the nasal passages, as conventional wisdom held. Despite these achievements, the Commonwealth Fund had terminated its support for Howe's lab, jeopardizing further progress on polio.[32]

Meanwhile, Thomas Turner's success in combining epidemiological and laboratory approaches to screen EHD residents for syphilis had influenced the national VD campaign and earned him an appointment as chair of Bacteriology in 1939. That year, Turner had published an important discovery of a new syphilis antibody (described further in chapter 3), and he now applied the same techniques to study the immunology of poliovirus. In 1941, he also outlined his plans for "a more comprehensive epidemiological study" of polio with the Department of Anatomy and Maxcy's Department of Epidemiology. Turner theorized that the presence of antibodies in a patient's blood would indicate past or present infection with the poliovirus, enabling physicians to diagnose polio at a much earlier stage of illness. With the assistance of Lawrence E. Young and Margaret Merrell, Turner developed a project to screen EHD residents for Lansing strain antibodies and then correlate these results with the occurrence of clinical poliomyelitis among the same population, using the comprehensive data collected by JHSPH and the BCHD. Reed sent a copy of Turner's NFIP grant proposal to Bowman with a cover letter stating, "We are in hopes that this grant will be the beginning of a really cooperative research program in this field."[33]

David Bodian later recalled that polio research featured "greater interplay and mutual stimulation during that period than you find in most fields," yet it was also one of the most competitive. At first, School of Medicine officials seemed to consider the modest polio research taking root in Hygiene as a potential asset to build a larger program based at the medical school. The medical school's director, Lewis Weed, was also chair of Anatomy and headed the National Research Council (NRC) Division of Medical Sciences. In late 1941, Weed wrote Basil O'Connor, chairman of the NFIP, that Maxcy's research program would "promise much in the way of advanc[ing] knowledge in this difficult field and the plan of starting in a relatively small way with a few competent investigations appears sound and logical. While the School of Medicine is only indirectly concerned in the undertaking (though one of the principal investigators will be drawn from its faculty), I can assure you of the extreme interest of the Medical Faculty in the program and of its desire to cooperate in every way to make the undertaking an outstanding success." Weed artfully suggested that "the National Foundation may see its way clear to finance this program of long-term research in its entirety so that the work of the small staff at the outset may be gradually expanded into a comprehensive study of the many facets of the problem, with a larger staff added when good men become available and when opportunities develop for an intensive attack upon some phase of the total investigation." He then made it clear that he expected the medical school to be included in an expanded polio research program at Hopkins: "All of us *in the medical group* at the Johns Hopkins would do our utmost to cooperate, were it possible to carry out this long-range program of work on poliomyelitis and related diseases."[34]

Reed, Turner, and Maxcy's hopes of "a really cooperative" polio research program were realized in spades, but the cooperation was among Hygiene departments, not with Medicine. Maxcy was a formidable contestant for grant funding, since he was a member of the NFIP Committee on Epidemics and Public Health, chaired the APHA Committee on Research and Standards, and served with Reed on the PHS National Health Advisory Council. In January 1942, O'Connor gave the JHSPH researchers unofficial word that they would soon receive a then-colossal $300,000 five-year grant from the NFIP. The grant saved Howe's polio research lab, and he transferred his lab and faculty appointment to the Department of Epidemiology. He immediately recruited Bodian, who had meanwhile left Hopkins. Bodian would also work with Robert C. Mellors to make key discoveries regarding nerve regeneration in polio victims.[35]

When the NFIP formally announced the grant to JHSPH in July, it was the largest award since the foundation's creation in 1938. The Center for the Study of Infantile Paralysis and Related Viruses was the first major university polio research center and also the first research center to be established at JHSPH. For many years, it was the only one; not until the early 1960s did the school establish the Training Center for Public Health Research in Hagerstown, Maryland, and three international health research centers in South Asia. In his public announcement of the grant, O'Connor employed language that would be echoed in every subsequent JHSPH research center proposal: "This center at Johns Hopkins is the product of the ideas of many investigators . . . with widely diverse backgrounds [who can pool their talents] in a concentrated attack upon the problems of the disease." With its force of epidemiologists, virologists, serologists, neurologists, and biochemists mounting a coordinated attack, Johns Hopkins University was "an ideal place" for a center that would facilitate polio research "on a comprehensive scale and on a long time basis."[36]

O'Connor emphasized that wartime conditions made it "highly desirable, if it can be accomplished without sacrificing defense interests, to keep a nucleus of scientists at work on the problems of infantile paralysis which are so important to human welfare, with the hope that, when peace is accomplished, contemplated expansion on this field may be rapidly consummated." The NFIP was explicitly preserving scientific expertise during a time of national emergency, when available resources would normally be diverted to the war effort. This rationale rejected the conservative strategy of freezing "nonessential" civilian research activity, instead framing polio research as a universal endeavor that might be used for postwar aims.[37]

The year 1942 was a landmark year for polio research, and JHSPH was at the forefront. Howe and Bodian published a breakthrough article in the *Journal of Pediatrics* on the penetration of the poliovirus from the gastrointestinal tract in the chimpanzee, thereby challenging the common notion that polio was contracted through the respiratory system. This discovery was recognized with the 1942 Mead–Johnson Award for Research in Pediatrics. The duo capped the phenomenal year with the publication of *Neural Mechanisms in Poliomyelitis*, which summarized their own work at Hopkins and introduced researchers to the new knowledge of neurology and immunology in polio. Bodian, Howe, and Mellors also took on significant teaching loads and anchored a dynamic new virus research training program that increased Epidemiology's output of Doctor of Science in Hygiene graduates.[38]

The principal polio investigators at Hopkins were in the School of Hygiene and Public Health, not the School of Medicine, a distinction that was rarely made in the media or among most scientists. At the medical school, Lewis

Weed clearly still had designs on a more elaborate facility. He described Hygiene's new polio lab as merely "adequate" and told Bowman in August 1944, "I do not think we [the medical school] need have any worry about appropriations from the National Foundation. . . . I am keeping in close touch with Basil O'Connor. In fact, the [National] Research Council is now doing a job for him." Weed, joined by Edwards Park, the current chair of Pediatrics, and Francis Schwentker, who would become chair in 1946, lobbied Bowman to hurry up with reorganizing the medical school so that they could capitalize on the NFIP's plans to establish a university-based polio research center with a full-time staff.[39]

Instead, Bowman threw the medical school a curve. The week before he was scheduled to meet with O'Connor, Bowman told Park that the reorganization would have to wait until after the war. The medical school would not "play a significant part in the decision concerning the location of the [polio] laboratory here because Dean Reed and I, as well as officers of the School of Medicine, have discussed forms of cooperation so thoroughgoing that for the purposes of a major enterprise organization presents no difficulty whatever." At the meeting with O'Connor, Bowman expressed his excitement over Bodian and Howe's studies of modes of transmission, immunity, and the interaction of the virus with nerve cells as well as Maxcy's plans to develop a vaccine project the next year. Contrary to the School of Medicine's hopes, it did not receive one of the NFIP's large early grants to establish polio virology laboratories at major research universities. The NFIP shifted its emphasis to support investigations of the epidemiology of polio at Yale and Michigan, and the JHSPH Department of Epidemiology received a second major grant in 1946 to establish the Division of Neurobiology and Neurotropic Virus Diseases.[40]

The Medical Planning and Development Committee

The "thoroughgoing form of cooperation" to which Bowman had referred was the genesis for the Medical Planning and Development Committee. At the close of 1945, Turner observed that even though the schools of Hygiene and Medicine each had "a well-defined area of activity within the University, . . . in recent years shadow zones have developed." He twice warned of the dangers of "unhealthy competition" even as he predicted that the "force of events as well as our own best interests will draw these three institutions [JHSPH, the medical school, and Johns Hopkins Hospital] more closely together." Throughout 1944 and 1945, Turner, Reed, Wolman, Maxcy, and J. Earle Moore (who held appointments in both schools) lobbied Bowman to pursue joint planning and development for the medical institutions via a permanent administrative body to review common goals, problems, and interrelationships. Such proposals would have been unthinkable before the war; now, JHSPH was leveraging the national recognition it had accrued with the syphilis, malaria, and polio research programs.[41]

To begin addressing the postwar needs of the medical institutions, Bowman convened a series of joint committees that began meeting in May 1944. In his initial charge to the Special Committee on Organization and Policy, Bowman sized up the challenges ahead for research and education that would require "an all-out effort to secure substantial additions to our present assets."[42] One of the committee's first tasks was to outline a proposal for developing the medical institutions, particularly construction to replace obsolete facilities and provide adequate, modernly equipped space for teaching, research, and patient care. In late 1945, Lewis Weed, director of the medical school, requested reports on the present status and future needs of medical school departments from all chairs and other selected medical and public health faculty. Weed had specifically asked for comments on the School of Hygiene's relationship to the medical school, but none of the department chairs even mentioned JHSPH, and their reports instead focused inward on the severe overcrowding of the hospital and medical school. In contrast, the broad-minded responses of Hygiene faculty envisioned JHSPH as a fully integrated partner with the hospital and medical school in a unified academic medical center, led by a single director responsible to the president.[43]

Such visions of cooperation were by no means unprecedented. As a member of the Rockefeller Foundation's site selection committee for the first school of public health, William Henry Welch had proclaimed in 1915, "It is of the utmost importance that hospitals should be more linked together with all the agencies which are concerned with public health work." The combined clout of Johns Hopkins Hospital and the medical school under Welch had helped Baltimore to win the competition. Yet public health departments, including Baltimore's, continued to approach disease from either a microscopic or population perspective, largely apart from the care of individual patients.[44]

Turner was hopeful that Johns Hopkins could finally realize Welch's vision for making the hospital a valuable resource for public health: "No one doubts the functional essentiality of the Hospital to the School of Medicine. Yet few fully appreciate to what extent the Hospital holds rich teaching material for the School of Hygiene, or perhaps the extent to which this material is even now being utilized." Turner even proposed that the chair of Public Health Administration should receive a hospital appointment like the heads of the medical and surgical departments, which would foster "the advancement of learning as applied to the broad fields of medical care and public health." He concluded, "The great potentialities of the Hospital are only beginning to be realized . . . for exerting even greater influence locally, nationally, and internationally."[45]

The context of wartime cooperation to achieve national goals distinctly influenced both polio research and the discussions of future plans for the Johns Hopkins medical campus. The themes of systematic planning and collaboration for the common welfare also shaped congressional debates on the Hill–Burton Hospital Survey and Construction Act, conceived in part as an alternative to national health insurance that was acceptable to organized medicine. Under Parran, the PHS used federal grants as an incentive for comprehensive statewide surveys of medical and public health needs, with the stipulation that state health departments be charged with the authority to carry them out. Federal policy thus promoted a new role for public health agencies as coordinators of efforts to evaluate and plan medical and hospital care on a population level. In states with schools of public health, the schools played key advisory roles in state health planning.[46]

One controversial aspect of this burst of planning activity was the organization and implementation of government-funded health services. Haven Emerson, professor of public health administration at Columbia, stridently opposed entering the realm of medical care, whether in public policy or by creating a new section in APHA. Emerson defended the primacy of the long-established "basic six" local health services (vital statistics, control of communicable diseases, environmental sanitation, public health laboratory services, maternal and child hygiene, and health education), which carefully preserved the accepted division of labor between preventive public health and curative clinical medicine. Health departments used newly developed laboratory tests to diagnose infected individuals but referred them to physicians for treatment. Quarantine and vaccination were the main methods used to control most common communicable diseases, such as smallpox, TB, and diphtheria.[47]

Yet the passage of the Hill–Burton Act in 1946 proved to be a major catalyst for moving public health into the clinical realm, as a variety of political and economic forces both pushed and pulled public health outside its traditionally circumscribed role of preventing and controlling infectious disease. In some states, Hill–Burton brought hospital care under the aegis of the state health department; in all states, it substantially increased the number of government-owned hospitals as well as the overall proportion of beds in public hospitals, particularly teaching institutions affiliated with medical schools. Construction programs were a prime example of how postwar federal spending broadened the scope of public health beyond the traditional limits of the local health department. Hill–Burton also created the Hospital and Medical Facilities Study Section, which offered the first formal federal support for health services research to plan and evaluate medical care systems on a population basis. As chapter 4 will show, JHSPH responded to these changes during the 1950s by developing new initiatives that used outpatient clinics and government health programs to advance research and train students in interdisciplinary settings.[48]

In the Hill–Burton hearings, PHS officers and allied reformers had proposed medical centers that housed medical schools alongside hospitals, group practices, and outpatient and public health services. Parran's successor, Surgeon General Leonard Scheele, described "the medical center of the future," which would be "the hub of continuous research and education, as well as of medical and public health services to outlying areas." A central mission of the new medical centers was to expand outpatient clinics that would complement and coordinate existing preventive and curative health services.[49]

Wolman envisioned the Johns Hopkins medical center as not just a health services hub for Baltimore but also an opportunity for the university to broaden its vision for the medical campus to encompass the surrounding East Baltimore neighborhood. As chair of the Maryland State Planning Commission, Wolman had managed Maryland's conversion to wartime production and had guided subsequent postwar planning. He urged university leaders to engage in comprehensive planning to rehabilitate the medical campus and its environs, in cooperation with the City Planning Commission and municipal agencies for health, housing, urban redevelopment, welfare, and public works. The new federal public housing and hospital construction legislation would, Wolman predicted, result in the construction of facilities on "a scope perhaps far beyond our present planning."[50]

As founder of the VD control program at Johns Hopkins, J. Earle Moore had worked closely with Parran and JHSPH for a decade. Moore voiced the heresy that "the existence of the Johns Hopkins University and Hospital as two separate corporations should terminate, if this is legally possible, in order to consolidate planning for the future and to eliminate unnecessary expense of operation; and the two institutions should become a single Corporation, with a single Board of Trustees." By proposing to merge the hospital and university, Moore may have intended to clear a place for JHSPH at the table of clinical care, since under the existing arrangement, the medical school had exclusive rights to research and teaching activities within the hospital. Maxcy wanted to go one step further than Moore, to also include the BCHD in the formal organization of the medical center, since he envisioned a full range of community health services modeled on and dramatically expanding the scope of the EHD. Maxcy urged the medical institutions to formulate a "precise and objective definition of the medical <u>service</u> function which this center can be expected to perform for (a) the city of Baltimore, (b) the state of Maryland, and (c) the United States and foreign countries."[51]

After its faculty had all returned from active duty, the school kicked into high gear to fill the renewed demand for public health personnel and recoup wartime losses of staff and enrollment. The East Baltimore campus was bustling with activity and extremely crowded with students, faculty, and patients. Buildings seemed to be literally bursting at the seams and awaited long-delayed renovation and expansion. Reed's deanship ended in 1946, when the Johns Hopkins Board of Trustees created the new position of vice-president of the university and Johns Hopkins Hospital. The university's leaders appointed Reed, in recognition of his role in raising Hygiene's national profile and fostering cooperation with the medical school and other divisions. Moore, Maxcy, and Wolman's expansive vision of a Hopkins medical center that integrated the resources of the university, city, and private health system had gone too far toward government-controlled health care to suit their medical school colleagues. But, based on the collaborative ideas put forth by JHSPH faculty, university administrators did establish a permanent Medical Planning and Development Committee (MPDC) in January 1947. With Vice-President Reed as chair, the MPDC also included the deans of Medicine and Hygiene and the director of the hospital.[52]

Reed's new position gave him an excellent base for fostering new joint collaborations and pursuing additional philanthropic funding. The School of Hygiene's organization had been disrupted by the war and further shaken by the deaths or retirements of five of the 10 department chairs between 1940 and 1946. Several departments were either merged or eliminated, and by 1948, only eight departments remained. That year, Reed estimated that at least $150,000 in new annual income was needed, to which the Rockefeller Foundation agreed to contribute $75,000 per year for 10 years with an equal match required from the university. The foundation stipulated, however, that it would end its support for individual research projects at JHSPH and would not renew the development grant when it expired.[53]

From the school's founding in 1916 through 1922, the Rockefeller Foundation had granted JHSPH just over $7 million, including a $5 million endowment. It granted another $1.2 million through 1949 for research projects on malaria and hookworm and to support the EHD (including studies of syphilis, diphtheria, mental hygiene, and rodent control), as well as developmental aid to hire more teaching faculty. Beginning in the late 1930s, the school had diversified its income sources with grants from smaller private foundations, including the Commonwealth Fund, Milbank Memorial Fund, and NFIP, as well as federal grants from the PHS and the US military.[54]

In the radically altered postwar environment for philanthropy and international development, Rockefeller officials moved to pull the foundation out of longstanding research and training programs in domestic medicine and public health. In 1950, the Rockefeller International Health Division announced its decision to end any further operational support for the schools of public health at Harvard and Hopkins. The IHD appointed a commission to review its organization and goals and make recommendations for the future. Parran, who now served as a Rockefeller trustee, was among the 10 representatives from within the foundation. Among the 12 external members from various fields, three represented public health: Reed and Maxcy from Hopkins and Hugo Muench of Harvard. Between 1916 and 1959, when the final development grant expired, the Rockefeller Foundation had awarded a total of $9 million to JHSPH. At schools of medicine and public health worldwide from 1913 to 1951, the Rockefeller Foundation had disbursed just over $100 million through its International Health Division and nearly $124 million through the Division of Medical Sciences. After a year of deliberation, the commission determined that these two oldest divisions should be merged to form a Division of Medicine and Public Health.[55]

The new division would now make modest grants rather than major institutional endowments and would concentrate on four areas: the advancement of professional education in medicine and public health in developing countries; the improvement of the quality, organization, and financing of medical care in the United States; the investigation and control of insect-borne viral diseases; and the development of the health sciences. So ended nearly 40 years and a quarter-billion dollars of Rockefeller Foundation support for William Henry Welch and Simon Flexner's model of medical and public health research. At Rockefeller and elsewhere, American philanthropy broadened its concern beyond national borders to include international issues, particularly population growth and scientific methods for expanding agricultural production. These new programs aimed to address the related threats of global famine and political turmoil, which many observers feared might reignite another world war.[56]

Reed contended in his final Rockefeller Foundation grant proposal that "there is ample evidence that public health is becoming more and more a social science. The social implication of disease and disability is better recognized than it was when the infectious diseases played a predominant role in all public health thinking in the United States." Reed's evaluation of public health at midcentury represented a major departure from Welch's emphasis on the basic sciences as the engine of medical and public health progress. The Rockefeller Foundation's 1951 annual report seconded Reed's ideas: "The old idea that biophysics and biochemistry would eventually unravel all the problems of health and disease is less tenable today than was the case 40 or 50 years ago." Rockefeller officials responded enthusiastically to both the MPDC and Reed's proposal for a new medical care division at JHSPH, which they predicted would "place Johns Hopkins in the lead of other medical environments in this country in the evolution of new service facilities for its community, especially as the

School of Hygiene is more and more taking the leading role in the formulation of plans."[57]

Conclusion

The JHSPH leadership team of Lowell Reed, Thomas Turner, J. Earle Moore, Kenneth Maxcy, and Allen Freeman had launched the school's highly successful research and training programs in syphilis, polio, and mental hygiene. Reed and Thomas Parran had served together during years of national crisis on the Rockefeller IHD Board of Scientific Directors and a variety of national committees. Their vision for public health had been tested and validated in the crucible of World War II, which had vastly increased the scope and resources of the PHS, strengthened and expanded the nation's schools of public health, and cemented Johns Hopkins' national leadership role in public health training and research. Parran stepped down as surgeon general in 1948 to become the founding dean of the University of Pittsburgh Graduate School of Public Health. Reed retired as vice-president of Hopkins and chair of the MPDC in 1951, only to be called back into university service as president a few months later.[58]

The war had ushered in dramatic improvements in both American standards of living and in malaria control and treatment methods. In 1949, the CDC declared that malaria had been eradicated in the United States, and in 1952, the National Malaria Society voted itself out of existence. American schools of medicine and public health responded by deemphasizing tropical diseases in their research and curricula. The School of Hygiene's geographic advantage was no longer its access to southern diseases of poverty but instead its proximity to the national health agencies and decisionmakers in Washington, DC. During the war, Reed, Parran, and their allies had confirmed that national defense was a compelling justification for publicly supported programs in health services, research, and education, which initiated a long, upward trend in federal funding. By 1950, the federal government would become the school's largest source of income. The era of the lone health officer hunting down deadly microbes and parasites was over, and public health redefined its mission for the atomic age.[59]

CHAPTER THREE

Postwar Public Health Science

In August 1945, President Harry S. Truman gave the order to detonate two atomic bombs over Hiroshima and Nagasaki, Japan, hastening the Japanese surrender that ended World War II. The Manhattan Project, which had invested 1.9 billion (approximately 25 billion in 2015) in taxpayer dollars to build four bombs, had harnessed the collective brainpower of nuclear physicists to develop American atomic capability at an unprecedented speed. The Manhattan Project instantaneously brought science to the center of national policy. Like the manned *Apollo* space flight to the moon a quarter century later, the Manhattan Project became a shining icon of the limitless potential of scientific research, generously backed by federal dollars, to solve the biggest problems facing humankind.[1]

The most oft-cited exemplar of this mind-set was Vannevar Bush, director of the federal Office of Scientific Research and Development, the agency that had overseen the collaborative public–private effort to apply existing scientific knowledge to solve technical problems involved in prosecuting the war. In *Science: The Endless Frontier* (1945), Bush opened with the miracle of wartime penicillin production and made "The War against Disease" the centerpiece of his call to increase public support for scientific inquiry. He wrote, "The death rate for all diseases in the Army, including the overseas forces, has been reduced from 14.1 per thousand in the last war to 0.6 per thousand in this war. Such ravaging diseases as yellow fever, dysentery, typhus, tetanus, pneumonia, and meningitis have been all but conquered by penicillin and the sulfa drugs, the insecticide DDT, better vaccines, and improved hygienic measures. Malaria has been controlled." He attributed these "striking advances" to the availability of "scientific data accumulated through basic research." William Henry Welch could not have said it better.[2]

The scientific contributions to winning the war had represented an exceptional surge of activity and achievement, and President Franklin D. Roosevelt had urged Bush to ensure that they continued and expanded in peacetime. Bush advocated the establishment of a system of federal grants to medical schools and universities because "traditional sources of support for medical research, largely endowment income, foundation grants, and private donations, are diminishing, and there is no immediate prospect of a change in this trend." Yet public sponsorship should not interfere with, in Bush's words, "the supreme importance of affording the prepared mind complete freedom for the exercise of initiative." He called scientific progress an "essential key to our security as a nation, to our better health, to more jobs, to a higher standard of living, and to our cultural progress." Health reform advocates would eagerly adopt Bush's language, and one of the defining characteristics of postwar public health policy would be the common use of national defense as a justification for government investment in public health.[3]

Fred Soper (profiled in chapter 1) provides an excellent case in point. He became such an enthusiastic apostle of the new insecticide DDT that, in 1948, Soper proclaimed to 2,000 scientists and physicians gathered from 21 countries at the Fourth International Congress of Tropical Diseases and Malaria, "It is a safe statement that at least 90 percent of the malaria of the world can be wiped out in the next ten years, and that's conservative." He estimated that this malaria-fighting equivalent of the Manhattan Project would cost about $280 million above regular health spending by governments in tropical countries. US Secretary of State George C. Marshall justified the expense in dynamic terms: "Little imagination is required to visualize the great increase in the production of food and raw materials, the stimulus to world trade, and above all the improvement in living conditions, with consequent social and cultural advances, that would result from the conquest of tropical diseases." Controlling malaria would, according to proponents, pave the way for economic development on a national and global scale.[4]

Both America's postwar faith in science and the rapid-fire successes of "wonder drugs" such as penicillin and cortisone (introduced in 1949) primed the federal funding engine for scientific and medical research. Federal expenditures for research and development grew more than 22 percent annually during the 1950s, nearly three times the growth rate of overall federal spending, but the budget for the NIH outpaced all other types of federally supported research. In the 1950s, the NIH replaced the Rockefeller Foundation as the world's largest single funder of biomedical research and has remained so until today, although overall spending on health research and development by industry would overtake that by government after the late 1980s.[5]

Thomas Parran's successor as surgeon general, Leonard Scheele, had previously directed the National Cancer Institute, and he accelerated the importance of medical research as the top priority of the PHS. When Scheele was appointed in 1948, the budget of the National Institute of Health was only $37 million, but within a year, the agency had been renamed the National Institutes (plural) of Health. The reorganized NIH oversaw the National Cancer Institute, added new heart and dental institutes, and received $40 million from Congress to build a research hospital on the Bethesda, Maryland, campus. When Scheele stepped down in 1956, NIH expenditures had grown to nearly $100 million. By 1965, they would reach $1 billion, nearly half the total PHS budget. Scheele's apolitical style contrasted dramatically with Parran's activism, and Scheele withheld his support from the final attempt to pass the Wagner–Murray–Dingell national health insurance bill in 1948. He preferred to remain professionally nonpartisan and warned PHS officers that they should follow suit.[6]

Ernest Stebbins would not enjoy the same close partnership with Scheele that Reed and Moore had forged with Parran. When Stebbins arrived in Baltimore in 1946, he was only 44, the youngest dean ever to head the Johns Hopkins School of Hygiene and Public Health. He was also the first dean born in the twentieth century and the first to hold an MPH. Every dean since Stebbins has been, like him, a white male physician and JHSPH alumnus who was recruited through a national search. Stebbins, an Iowan known as "Stebbie," led JHSPH for 21 years, from 1946 to 1967, and remains its longest-serving dean.

Chapters 3 through 6 cover the first 15 years of his tenure, which was dominated by the school's national leadership in syphilis and polio research and Stebbins's efforts to strengthen collaboration among JHSPH, the medical school, and Johns Hopkins Hospital. Stebbins addresses his two main challenges as dean: expanding the school's teaching and research programs beyond the traditional emphasis on infectious and nutritional diseases, and pursuing federal funding in the wake of the Rockefeller Foundation's withdrawal from the field of academic public health. Chapter 3 explores the pros and cons of the new research models put forth by the National Foundation for Infantile Paralysis and the NIH, using as examples the JHSPH programs in polio, syphilis, chronic disease, and pathobiology. Chapter 4 focuses on the ups and downs of the relationship between JHSPH and the Baltimore City Health Department, highlighting Stebbins's role as chair of Public Health Administration (PHA), a fast-growing, multidisciplinary department whose faculty was perfecting the randomized controlled clinical trial, tracing the origins and prevalence of developmental disabilities, and training public health professionals to lead national and international health agencies. In chapter 5, the chair of Pathobiology, Frederik B. Bang, translates his ideas on the biology of populations into a new course that displaced microbiology as the MPH science requirement and incited rebellion among the basic science faculty. In chapter 6, the JHSPH faculty hammers out a new paradigm for public health research at the height of the Cold War, as public health leaders sought a new professional identity and funding sources by "waging health" on behalf of American defense and foreign policy objectives.

The Polio Decade

Along with the Rockefeller endowments he secured, William Henry Welch's legacy to Johns Hopkins was his conviction that the modern advancement of medicine and public health against disease must be grounded in basic science research. As the previous chapters have shown in the cases of both syphilis and polio, this emphasis at times threatened to overshadow both clinical and epidemiological perspectives in favor of the wet laboratory methods of chemical and microscopic analysis. During the 1950s, the federal government increased its expectations for research grant recipients to pursue highly applied work that could be politically justified as serving national interests, and in the 1960s, this rationale would be even more emphasized for grantees of the new US Agency for International Development. This presented a structural conflict with universities' sacrosanct principle of academic freedom and with scientists' deep commitment to following their curiosity wherever it may lead, or "science for science's sake."[7]

Through the 1940s, the fields of medicine and public health had stood on relatively equal footing during a period when cooperation in national health policy, biomedical research, and clinical studies reached new heights. At Johns Hopkins, basic science research on major communicable diseases benefited from the permeability of disciplinary barriers among JHSPH departments as well as between Hygiene and Medicine. Studies of syphilis and polio provided a platform for two of the school's most influential leaders, Kenneth Maxcy, chair of Epidemiology, and Thomas Turner, chair of Bacteriology.

Like Maxcy, Turner was a physician–scientist equally accomplished in the fields of bacteriology and epidemiology. Before coming to JHSPH, both men had honed their clinical and epidemiological skills in major disease control campaigns, Maxcy with the PHS malaria and typhus programs in the southern United States and Turner as a Rockefeller IHD officer combating syphilis and yaws in the Caribbean and Latin America. Just as Turner had mastered the clinical and epidemiological aspects of syphilis under Moore, he would branch out with Maxcy to learn the fundamentals of polio, going on to make major contributions to understanding the immunology of both diseases. During the war, Turner began serving on the PHS Syphilis Study Section with Moore and Dean Reed, and in the late 1940s, he joined the scientific board of the NFIP with Maxcy and Dean Stebbins.[8]

Turner, Moore, and Maxcy all pursued medical collaborations on diseases of mutual interest such as syphilis and polio, but their research was fully compatible with broader public health priorities, such as Parran's crusade to bring syphilis, the "shadow on the land," into the spotlight of scientific research and treatment. Faculty who could not relate their basic research to public health practice did not long remain at the school. For example, Reginald MacGregor Archibald succeeded E. V. McCollum as chair of Biochemistry from 1946 to 1948 but returned to a senior position at the Rockefeller Institute for Medical Research because "he found it difficult to develop a meaningful bridge between his basic research interests [in calcium metabolism] and the more pragmatic interests in nutrition of the public health students." In many ways, JHSPH had a freer and more conducive atmosphere for research than did the medical school, a difference that attracted a considerable number of medical researchers to Hygiene over the years.[9]

Public health researchers in the basic science disciplines arguably enjoyed the best of all worlds: like their laboratory science colleagues at the Rockefeller Institute or the PHS Hygienic Laboratory, they were free to pursue abstract knowledge without the pressures of patient care responsibilities, yet they could claim to be advancing the welfare of humanity on a large scale in ways that other basic scientists, isolated in their labs, and clinical researchers, limited to their relatively small groups of patients, could not. The training of physicians strongly emphasized the value of the practitioner's accumulated experience. The individualistic culture of medicine was counterbalanced by the population basis of public health, which relied on the analytic methods of biostatistics and epidemiology. Because public health researchers could conduct investigations in both the laboratory and in populations, their conclusions were inherently more generalizable, and therefore scientifically valid, than studies of a few hospital patients.

Schools of public health, along with private research institutes, government laboratories, and specialty clinics, were among the variety of institutions that pursued biomedical research alongside university medical schools. Medical historian Harry M. Marks notes that "this organizational diversity permitted researchers to 'experiment' with various strategies for linking the scientific work of the laboratory with the problems seen in the clinic," and also with the health problems of populations. The postwar rise of American wages and health insurance coverage enabled medicine to develop into a politically powerful profession. In addition, Cold War competition for scientific supremacy over the Soviet Union helped to sustain an explosion of federal funding for biomedicine that drove a steady expansion of American medical schools and their domination of therapeutic research. Schools of public health like Johns Hopkins, with strong ties to medical schools, therefore felt increasing pressure to follow the example of research-intensive medical schools.[10]

In the race for the polio vaccine, the School of Hygiene would surpass the School of Medicine in a major field of biomedical research, and Isabel Morgan was one of Hygiene's most prized assets. Until her arrival in 1944, all the principal actors in the syphilis and polio research programs at Johns Hopkins had been male. Since the founding of JHSPH, the faculty had included many women, concentrated in Biostatistics, Epidemiology, and the basic science departments. But most held entry-level positions, and by 1960, only six women (most of them single) in the school's history had been appointed associate professor. In 1957, JHSPH finally appointed its first female full professor, biostatistician Margaret Merrell, just before she retired. The School of Hygiene, in this instance, lagged far behind the medical school, where Florence R. Sabin had become the first female full professor in 1917.[11]

Morgan, during a brief but highly productive career in Epidemiology from 1944 to 1949, conducted critically important research on a polio vaccine, using first live virus (which produced stronger immunity but posed the risk of vaccine-associated polio) and then killed virus (which was safer but might not be strong enough to produce immunity). Polio historian David Oshinsky argues that the Bodian–Howe–Morgan team "did more to unravel the mysteries of polio than any other group" and was also in the best position to make rapid progress on a vaccine. By mid-1947, the JHSPH polio research center had received nearly a quarter-million dollars and would soon receive another $425,000, making it the most heavily backed NFIP-funded university center. In June 1947, *Time* magazine reported the trio's announcement that trials in monkeys showed their new live-virus vaccine had produced "solid immunity," performing better than any other vaccine to date. After four injections into the muscle, 100 percent of the monkeys had demonstrated immunity to "thousands of times the lethal dose of polio" and remained immune even when the virus was injected directly into their brains.[12]

The live-virus vaccine, however, was dangerous to test in humans. *Time* noted, "A promise of cures or preventives for infantile paralysis has backfired so often that researchers are gun-shy." Morgan subsequently demonstrated the effectiveness of immunization with a killed-virus vaccine, which most virologists until that time had thought impossible, since the immune response is typically triggered only by the presence of live virus. Between 1949 and 1951, Howe and Morgan showed that the safer killed vaccines, containing virus that had been inactivated in formaldehyde, were similar to live vaccines in producing antibodies and immunity in monkeys and chimpanzees. Bodian further concluded that injections of an antibody-containing blood product, gamma globulin, produced low levels of antibodies that were still effective in preventing paralysis in monkeys.[13]

Bodian developed the chimpanzee model that was instrumental in solving the puzzle of polio transmission and developing an effective vaccine. He, Howe, and Morgan grew very attached to the chimps (see photo gallery) and broke standard protocol by referring to them by names like "Zombie" and "Bozo" or by the pronouns "he" or "she" instead of "it." One expert called the chimpanzee model "a conspicuous step forward," since chimps' reaction to the virus was closer to humans' than that of any other animal. By 1955, the NFIP had purchased 30,000 primates from India and the Philippines. The polio research lab animals in Epidemiology cost $59,300 annually, the largest research budget item in the school. Bodian knew more about poliovirus infection in humans and primates than anyone else in the country, and his procedures for tracing its passage through the primate nervous system made his laboratory central to the adjudication of claims about the presence of active virus, either in communities or in contaminated vaccines.[14]

Maxcy, Turner, Bodian, and Stebbins served on a variety of key NFIP committees and provided expert guidance to scientists at other institutions, particularly Jonas Salk at the University of Pittsburgh, and to the many agencies involved in the national campaign. In addition to his scientific acumen, Bodian's personal skills as an arbitrator and leader made him a vital committee member. The most important advisory body within the NFIP was the Virus Research and Epidemiology Committee that oversaw research dealing with poliovirus and with vaccine development. In a January 1948 meeting, Turner suggested that the established procedure for typing viruses (i.e., identifying how many different strains, or types, of poliovirus existed) could be reversed to save time and monkeys. The existing method involved infecting monkeys with viruses of a known type, waiting for them to recover and develop immunity to that type, and reinfecting them with an unknown virus to see if it belonged to the known group or not. Instead, Turner advocated infecting the monkey with an unknown virus and then checking its blood against samples of known viruses, a suggestion that proved critical in confirming which types of virus were needed for an effective vaccine. Bodian had been the first to hypothesize that there were at least three types of virus, and he, Howe, Morgan, and Turner threw themselves into the NFIP's cooperative laboratory effort to type wild poliovirus strains. In 1949, Bodian and Morgan published their finding that there were only three immunological types of poliovirus, which explained why previous vaccines that only protected against a single strain had failed.[15]

After Morgan married in 1949, she left Johns Hopkins and moved with her husband to New York City. The School of Hygiene lab's progress on a vaccine halted, since Howe and Bodian were more interested in the pathology of polio. Oshinsky asserts that if Morgan had stayed at Hopkins, she might even have beat Jonas Salk to developing an effective polio vaccine, since she had a significant head start and the resources of Hopkins' first-rate lab. Oshinsky paints Morgan's decision as a hard choice between family and professional achievement: "But in 1949, in the prime of her career, the 38-year-old Morgan left Johns Hopkins to marry and become a homemaker. . . . She died in 1996, without ever returning to polio research." Most people, including those at Johns Hopkins, also believe that Morgan never worked in science again after her decision to resign from the Department of Epidemiology.[16]

In fact, she continued her work on polio, publishing four more articles in major peer-reviewed journals on the topic in the 1950s under her married name, Isabel Morgan Mountain. Mountain's parents were both gifted scientists at Columbia University, where her mother, Lillian Vaughan Morgan, had developed the first primate polio vaccine and her father, Thomas Hunt Morgan, had pioneered the fruit fly *Drosophila* model to study chromosomal structure. Thomas Morgan received the first Nobel Prize to be awarded for genetic research (in 1933), but he was also a patrician who had marginalized his wife's career in deference to his own. Isabel would not repeat her parents' mistakes. She continued her research in microbiology at Columbia, where she earned a master's degree in biostatistics in 1961. Mountain published 25 peer-reviewed articles during her post-Hopkins career, including work on the links between air pollution and illness in urban environments, as well as on tumorigenesis and cancer chemotherapy. In the mid-1960s, she joined the Sloan–Kettering Institute for Cancer Research, and in 1967, Mountain even published one of the first scientific articles on sex-linked inhibition of tumors (completely unheard of at that time, sex-based biology became a research strength at JHSPH decades later).[17]

By the time Isabel Morgan left Hopkins in 1949, Bodian had already made more fundamental contributions to polio research than anyone else, yet one polio historian described him as "a man for whom gratification lay in work and thought rather than prerogative or empire." In 1952, Bodian and Dorothy Horstmann of the Yale School of Medicine demonstrated the existence of a brief viremic phase during which the poliovirus traveled through the bloodstream before it produced its drastic effects on the nervous system, giving vaccines an opportunity to act. These findings paved the way for Salk to proceed with human field trials of killed vaccine.[18]

Bodian and Turner had played critical roles in assisting Salk, and they risked their reputations to defend Salk's 1953 proposal to conduct a field trial with a killed vaccine. The NFIP originally had planned to conduct the trial between November 1953 and May 1954, but many scientists objected, insisting that the vaccine was not yet safe enough for a large-scale field trial in humans. On April 24, 1954, when the Advisory Committee met to determine the final fate of the vaccine trial, Bodian interpreted findings of paralysis in mice after injection with the vaccine and concluded that the paralysis was unrelated to human polio, thus convincing the NIH to allow human testing. With newspaper reporters and photographers waiting expectantly outside, Turner, Bodian, Stebbins, and the rest of the Advisory Committee voted to approve the trial on April 25, 1954, and Howe directed one of the nine teams in the historic Salk vaccine trial.[19]

The NFIP continued in the tradition of health-oriented philanthropies such as Rockefeller, Rosenwald, Commonwealth, and Milbank by fostering an elite collaborative nexus among the PHS, academia, and nonprofit foundations, which created a reserve of problem-solving expertise when crises arose. In 1955, dozens of children contracted polio after being vaccinated with the newly approved Salk vaccine. In the Epidemic Intelligence Service at the Communicable Disease Center (EIS), a team of investigators led by Alexander Langmuir (MPH 1940) analyzed data from the new nationwide disease surveillance system to discover a pattern: the polio cases were all in children vaccinated with a batch of vaccine manufactured by Cutter Laboratories. Bodian and several other NFIP-funded researchers joined the PHS committee that tested the vaccine and determined it had been contaminated with live virus due to inadequate quality control procedures. The committee also devised new safety protocols to ensure that from then on, all virus particles were inactivated during vaccine preparation.

The crisis, known as the Cutter Incident after the company that produced the contaminated vaccine, was a critical moment in the history of immunization. Without the disease surveillance and epidemiological fieldwork of the EIS, many more children could have been afflicted with polio and its disabling aftereffects, forever ending the promise of wiping out polio and other vaccine-preventable diseases. And without the remarkably deep knowledge of poliovirus and virology gained from NFIP-funded research at JHSPH over the past 17 years, Bodian and the PHS committee could not have regained the public's trust in the safety of the Salk vaccine.[20]

During the 1940s and 1950s, the Department of Epidemiology was almost wholly subsidized by the NFIP. The organization also contributed substantially to research in the departments of Bacteriology and Biochemistry, making polio the school's single largest research program during that era. The NFIP was also among the first granting organizations to embrace the concept of indirect costs, which proved to be an increasingly important source of revenue for higher education, particularly in the health sciences. Indirect costs were those not directly associated with the granting activity, such as administrative and facilities expenses, often explained as "keeping the lights on." The school first recovered indirect costs in 1949–1950, and by 1955, they represented more than 10 percent of its total income.[21]

Turner expressed his ideas on the NFIP's future in a 1955 letter to its president, Basil O'Connor, with whom Turner enjoyed a close personal as well as professional relationship. Turner connected polio research to his own broad-gauged scientific philosophy: "The problem of poliomyelitis constituted a medical microcosm with many medical fields to cultivate—a transmissible disease and an acute infection calling forth the disciplines of virology, immunology, and epidemiology; a chronic disease, involving the fields of neuro-muscular and respiratory physiology; a handicapped individual with somatic, psychic, and sociological problems to be solved; a crippled person, mostly not isolated in an institution but a member of society invoking pity on the one hand and fear on the other. By the fruits of experience the National Foundation has some understanding of the potentialities in these varied approaches to medical problems." Turner may have recognized polio's multifaceted nature, but he and the polio scientists at JHSPH largely confined themselves to the lab. Maxcy first requested approval from the JHSPH Advisory Board to conduct polio research on human subjects in 1952, a full 10 years after the laboratory research program began.[22]

The syphilis and polio programs had brought the laboratories and leadership of Turner, Howe, and Bodian from Medicine to Hygiene and had also made J. Earle Moore a key Hygiene advocate. As had been true with the JHSPH syphilis and malaria programs, the NFIP took many of its operating principles and personnel from the Rockefeller Foundation. Thomas M. Rivers, Maxcy's medical school roommate at Hopkins, was both director of the Rockefeller Institute and vice-president of medical affairs for the NFIP. But Turner complained that established foundations such as Rockefeller and the Commonwealth Fund unduly hampered academic medical research by making grants that were "usually intended for purposes that appealed more to the donor than to the recipient." Rivers, Maxcy, Turner, and Bodian ensured that the NFIP gave comparatively free rein to individual researchers to do basic science research that charted new territory and might not have immediate application, which influenced the extramural research grant program then being launched at the NIH. Yet epidemiology was given lower priority at the NIH than at the NFIP, which carried on the traditions of epidemiological fieldwork at the Rockefeller IHD and the PHS Hygienic Laboratory.[23]

The NIH Model of Public Health Research

The Center for the Study of Infantile Paralysis and Related Viruses was the prime but certainly not the only example of the explosion of basic science lab research at JHSPH. Maxcy and Turner both had an excellent grasp of the postwar direction of medical and public health research, especially its funding mechanisms, at a critical time when the Rockefeller Foundation stepped aside as the school's main sponsor. Disease-specific foundations such as the NFIP, American Cancer Society, and American Heart Association fervently promoted a new research model that prioritized investigator-driven projects to discover new cures. Known as the categorical disease model of medical research, it received the lion's share of funding and media attention and displaced the interdisciplinary studies where laboratory science, clinical observation, and field-based epidemiology had been more nearly equal partners. The same was true at the NIH, where the categorical disease model privileged research that used laboratory-based technology for basic science investigations of both communicable and chronic diseases.

The NFIP began the school's upward trend in externally sponsored research, but the NIH decisively tipped the balance toward one of the most important turning points in JHSPH history. In 1950, for the first time, a majority of the school's external funding came from federal grants and contracts from the PHS (which then included the NIH and CDC), National Science Foundation (NSF), and the US Departments of State and Defense. Government agencies had provided 46 percent of funding for sponsored projects at JHSPH in 1948–1949. The following year, the government share jumped to 54 percent, due to slight declines in Rockefeller Foundation funding and increased PHS support for the Venereal Disease Consultation and Research Service and new training grants in mental hygiene and deafness prevention. By 1955–1956, total sponsored research at JHSPH topped $1 million, with the two largest grants coming from the NFIP in Epidemiology and the NSF for immunologist Manfred Mayer's research on cytotoxic reactions mediated by antibody and complement. Johns Hopkins had, by far, the most well-funded research program of any of the 13 schools of public health in North America.[24]

As chair of the JHSPH Department of Bacteriology from 1939 to 1957, Thomas Turner embodied the evolution of basic science in public health generally, as well as in the relationship between the schools of Medicine and Hygiene. Turner succeeded in making Bacteriology a research powerhouse with strong connections to many departments in both schools. He saw himself as a standard-bearer for Welch's dedication to the laboratory ideal in public health. In 1939–1940, the JHSPH budget had been distributed relatively equally among the 10 departments, but Turner accelerated the shift to federal funding that upset the existing fiscal equity among the school's departments.

During the heyday of the syphilis and polio programs, the Department of Bacteriology fostered multipronged research in the field, lab, and clinic. As Turner's influence and the PHS's research budget both rose rapidly, he arranged in 1946 for the transfer of the Venereal Disease Research Laboratory from Johns Hopkins Hospital to his department. The lab, which had overseen the landmark clinical trials of penicillin in early syphilis, was renamed the PHS–Hopkins Laboratory of Experimental Therapeutics, and its longtime director, Harry Eagle (ScM 1929), joined the Department of Bacteriology to teach the immunology course and electives on chemotherapy. Eagle proposed a new doctor of science program in chemotherapy research that would have been the first of its kind, but Turner denied Eagle's request for additional compensation for himself and his teaching staff. At the end of 1947, Eagle resigned to become scientific director of the National Cancer Institute, and the PHS transferred its remaining personnel and equipment to the University of North Carolina. There, John J. Wright (MPH 1939) and Cecil G. Sheps were beginning important epidemiological studies of venereal disease casefinding and congenital syphilis.[25]

Considering that drug research, particularly penicillin therapy for syphilis, had garnered such acclaim and funding for Hopkins and that Turner and J. Earle Moore had been its central figures, why did Turner essentially run Eagle off and deny him the chance to pursue this promising avenue? After Eagle left, Turner reorganized the department into four divisions. Turner headed Spirochetal Diseases and Thomas G. Ward (ScD 1941, ScM 1940) oversaw Virus Diseases. To launch two new divisions, Turner recruited faculty who shared his priority on basic science research: Carl Lamanna from Cornell headed the Division of Bacterial Diseases, and Manfred Mayer from Columbia University headed the Division of Immunochemistry.[26]

Instead of the research and teaching program in the science of chemotherapy that Eagle proposed, which probably would have turned toward cancer, Mayer's Division of Immunochemistry built significantly on the prewar research on the hemolytic action of complement in the JHSPH Department of Immunology, which had been absorbed into Bacteriology when its chair, Roscoe Hyde, died in 1942. The complement system comprises a group of proteins in the blood (or serum) that helps the immune system fight infections and destroy foreign substances. Complement tests are blood tests that measure the activity of the nine major proteins in the system, and hemolytic refers to hemolysis, or destruction of red blood cells, by the complement proteins. The prewar work of Hyde's department—the first academic department of immunology in the world—and the postwar contributions of Mayer's team were groundbreaking for medicine and public health, because they made possible many of the critical diagnostic tests for infectious and certain types of chronic disease, including kidney disease and autoimmune diseases.[27]

A key difference between Eagle and Mayer was that Eagle's chemotherapy work required experimentation in both the lab and with human subjects, while Mayer's relied solely on animals or the new test-tube tissue culture techniques then being developed at Hopkins by George Gey, among others. Mayer's team did use animal red blood cells to study immunity in cancer but primarily worked to identify the individual components of the complement system. Mayer had studied with the most prominent immunologist of the day, Michael Heidelberger, with whom he published a series of articles on new blood tests and vaccines for *Plasmodium vivax* malaria. Applying his knowledge of malaria vaccines to polio, Mayer worked on an improved blood test for polio using highly purified antigens, or foreign pathogens that induce an immune response that produces disease-fighting antibodies. In a series of four articles in the *Journal of Immunology*, Mayer's lab showed that the purer antigens were superior to the previous types of crudely derived tissue culture fluids, which contained unreliable levels of infective virus particles and so could be insufficient for producing an effective vaccine. The tissue culture fluids also contained nonviral contaminants that could invalidate test results.[28]

By integrating virological, chemical, and immunological analyses, Mayer's group measured the efficacy of various methods of virus purification and identified methods that produced high-purity, high-yield polio antigen that retained its infectivity. Mayer also showed that using highly purified antigens in complement fixation blood tests yielded more reliable, easier-to-read results than previous tests. From 1952 to 1958, Mayer's lab received nearly $300,000 in NFIP funding, more than any other Hopkins investigator except the Bodian–Howe–Morgan group. One of Mayer's most brilliant students was Bernard Roizman (ScD 1956), who held a faculty appointment in Microbiology from 1956 to 1965. He identified several viral genes and proteins and worked with Mayer and Roger M. Herriott, chair of Biochemistry, to determine the structure of viral DNA. He defined the basic principles of herpes simplex virus gene regulation, as well as the molecular mechanisms by which the virus regulates expression of its genes. Roizman joined the faculty in the Department of Molecular Genetics and Cell Biology at the University of Chicago, which he chaired from 1985 to 1988. He is considered the world's foremost expert on herpes simplex virus, and many of his genetic engineering techniques are still applied in labs today.[29]

Despite Turner's affinity for the medical school, he gradually lost his zeal for incorporating patient care into public health research and devoted himself fully to the laboratory. Turner had been selected to lead the Hopkins syphilis control program in 1936 because he was "thoroughly acquainted with both the clinical and field aspects of syphilis control." He had promised the Rockefeller Foundation that he was interested in syphilis "as a public health problem" and that laboratory research "would be incidental." But soon after coming to Hopkins, Turner had asked to move his lab from the medical school to larger quarters in the JHSPH Department of Bacteriology. With IHD grants, he renovated his new lab and broadened the scope of his research on humoral immunity in syphilis (in contrast to cellular immunity, humoral immunity was mediated by antibodies found in extracellular fluids). In late 1938, Turner asked to be relieved of his clinical and teaching duties in the VD control program to turn his attention to research on immunity in syphilis. After being appointed chair of Bacteriology in 1939, Turner divested himself of clinical duties and wrapped up his community study of syphilis in the EHD. By 1950, he had completed his last epidemiological studies, on the Lansing strain poliovirus (one of the most common virus types) in EHD residents. From then on, he was strictly a laboratory man who equated quality research with bench work.[30]

In 1952, Turner discarded his department's original title of Bacteriology, which evoked "the activities of an earlier day in which immunology and virology were scarcely included," and renamed it Microbiology to "better categorize [the department's students] in the stream of modern scientific endeavor." To house the additional research activity and teach bacteriology and immunology courses to medical students, the department occupied classroom space on the sixth and seventh floors of the medical school's Pathology Building. Turner noted in 1952 that "it would be to our advantage to have [extra space on the sixth floor] occupied . . . by investigators who are working on subjects more or less related to bacteriology." Microbiology's drift into the medical school's orbit was further abetted by the arrival in 1955 of microbiologist W. Barry Wood to succeed Lowell Reed as vice-president of the Hopkins medical institutions. Wood was also a full professor in Turner's department.[31]

Historians of public health in the 1950s have, somewhat unfairly, accused faculty and professionals of foot-dragging and being overly fearful of change. An alternate interpretation is that they had a clear-eyed appreciation of what they stood to lose by chasing after the moving targets of federal grant requirements, whether for research or state and local health programs. The rise of externally funded research at JHSPH had drawbacks that troubled even Tommy Turner. He wrote to Stebbins in 1950 that, since funding agencies specified the purpose of every dollar granted and expected schools to furnish salaries for principal investigators, it was difficult to offer competitive salaries or to find support for junior faculty just starting their research. Turner identified the department's strength "in the alert group of young associate professors who already have attained national standing in their particular fields. So long as the School must depend largely upon outside funds for research this constitutes the best insurance that we shall continue to attract a fair share of support." Yet he complained that members of his department earned "considerably less than many county health officers or laboratory division chiefs in this country," a lament upheld by the statistic that 10 percent of advertised science faculty positions in schools of public health remained vacant. Turner also warned that, without unrestricted department funds for new research to lay the groundwork for later outside support, "the enforced limitation of student research to that supported by categorical grants may, I fear, turn out to be a self-sterilizing process."[32]

While Turner wanted more unrestricted freedom for himself and his students to pursue their own research paths, Lloyd E. Rozeboom (ScD 1934), professor of parasitology, alleged that "the grant in aid program is in part responsible for some of our teaching difficulties," since time with students infringed on research and forced faculty to choose between classroom responsibilities and obligations to funding agencies. Rozeboom glumly observed in 1957, "If our future is to depend largely upon the grantmaking agencies, one wonders whether it would be better to make this school an institute for public health and medical research, and discontinue all formal course work." Rozeboom's forecast was reminiscent of the Rockefeller Institute for Medical Research, one of Welch's inspirations for the School of Hygiene. Frederick T. Gates of the Rockefeller Foundation had envisioned the Institute as "magnificently endowed, devoted primarily to investigation, making [medical] practice itself an incident of investigation." Hopkins and other schools of public health also seemed to be headed toward making both teaching and public health practice "an incident of investigation." During the postwar decade, instructional budgets at most schools of public health stagnated while research budgets rose. These trends made it increasingly difficult to attract and retain talented faculty.[33]

The promise and tensions inherent in basic science collaborations between Medicine and Hygiene were borne out in Turner and Moore's initiation in 1950 of a major new lab research initiative to improve syphilis screening. Physicians knew that at least some patients who were not infected with syphilis had false-positive Wasserman test results—as many as 25 percent of all positive Wasserman results were false. This was a serious problem, not only in terms of wasted resources for testing, but because individuals with false positives unnecessarily underwent the toxic treatment, which in the pre-penicillin era involved a year of injections with compounds containing arsenic and mercury. Robert A. Nelson Jr. in Turner's lab, with Manfred Mayer, developed a syphilis test in 1949 with much greater specificity, which became the most important postwar breakthrough in VD research at Hopkins.

The *Treponema pallidum* immobilization (TPI) test was an outgrowth of Turner's 1939 discovery of an immobilizing antibody in the serum of syphilitic rabbits, which he later discovered was uniformly present in human patients with untreated syphilitic infection, especially in the secondary and tertiary stages. When exposed to an infected blood sample, the antibody immobilized *T. pallidum*, the organism that causes syphilis, thereby demonstrating that the presence of the disease had triggered an immune response. Unlike the antibody detected by the ubiquitous Wasserman test, Turner's immobilization antibody was absent from the sera of patients with other chronic conditions, such as leprosy and lupus, that triggered biologic positive Wasserman results.[34]

Moore expressed his excitement about the new TPI test to the head of the Cuban Ministry of Health and Social Welfare. He requested the cooperation of the national leprosarium in obtaining serologic samples for testing at Hopkins, and wrote, "It is of the utmost importance to the further study of the immunology of syphilis and of leprosy to apply the new test to a carefully selected series of lepers, including a substantial number of those in whom syphilis can be excluded, as nearly as possible, as well as a few known simultaneously to be infected with syphilis." Turner received funding from the WHO to establish the International Treponematosis Laboratory Center in the Department of Microbiology.[35]

Soon, the department was receiving requests for the test from organizations around the world, such as the Medical Research Institute of South Africa, which wanted to determine the proportion of false positives among the Bantu population. By 1953, the TPI Lab used 100 rabbits annually for clinical runs to test over 1,000 blood samples. Only half of the runs performed were successful, so each blood sample was tested an average of three times to achieve valid results. As demand for the test increased, so did the tension between Turner, who wanted to emphasize "pure" basic science research, and Moore, who believed that the TPI Lab should support the clinical treatment of VD patients at Johns Hopkins Hospital. Moore argued that the lab's data were meaningless without clinical application, while Turner protested that Moore (who had secured the majority of funding for the lab from the NIH, WHO, and private corporations) was using the Microbiology faculty as "lab technicians" and that their primary research was suffering because of the high volume of requests for the complicated, expensive, and time-consuming TPI tests for hospital patients. In 1955, Turner mused, "[Basic science] medical research has caught the public's fancy and may be as appealing as patient care. Moreover, large programs of medical research can be supported with substantially smaller amounts of money than large programs involving patient care."[36]

Rumblings of discontent began among JHSPH scientists in the summer of 1955, when Bodian dissolved his joint lab with Howe, his one-time mentor and colleague of more than 15 years. To Howe's great dismay, Bodian moved his lab and equipment back to Anatomy to study the pathology of polio. Bodian's essential role in laying the scientific foundation for the Salk vaccine had garnered unprecedented funding and acclaim for JHSPH, and he would be elected to the National Academy of Sciences in 1958. Yet he remained untenured until 1955, due to the JHSPH policy of only granting tenure and full professorships to department chairs. In 1956, Turner engineered Bodian's transfer from Epidemiology to Microbiology to head the Division of Viruses Diseases. Bodian, Turner, and Manfred Mayer were the School of Hygiene's biggest grantees, with a total of $2.1 million in NFIP research grants, three-quarters of which went to the Department of Epidemiology. Polio was the medical success story of the 1950s, but the school could not meet the Polio Research Lab's need for better equipment and larger facilities, particularly the quarters required for its large colony of animals.[37]

Environmental Medicine faculty members were also distraught at the loss of their well-regarded chair, Joseph Lilienthal (profiled in chapter 6). Without him, the faculty who originally had come from the physiology division of the Department of Medicine began to cut their ties to Hygiene. In 1957, the medical school advisory board voted to withdraw from the joint Department of Environmental Medicine. After prolonged wrangling between Moore and Turner, the TPI Laboratory in the Department of Microbiology was closed on June 30, 1957, and the TPI test was replaced by the *T. pallidum* complement fixation test, performed in the Serologic Laboratory of the Johns Hopkins Hospital. The new test was equally accurate but much simpler to perform, did not require sterile blood specimens, and was not affected by antibiotic treatment. It also effectively ended two decades of cooperation on VD research between Medicine, Hygiene, and the Johns Hopkins Hospital.[38]

During JHSPH's first 40 years, research and teaching had been centered on the great plagues of public health: hookworm, syphilis, polio, TB, and malaria. But as the 1950s wore on, these diseases faded in the memories of most Americans. Yesterday's epidemics seemed destined for extinction, and faculty advised entering students to seek other fields to conquer. Andrew Spielman (ScD 1956) remembered a conversation over a beer in a Baltimore bar with his graduate adviser, Lloyd Rozeboom. The great medical entomologist admitted feeling guilty about encouraging the young scientist to enter the field of public health entomology, which he predicted would be eliminated in a matter of years by

DDT. Spielman ignored Rozeboom's advice but emulated his career by joining the faculty of the Harvard School of Public Health as an expert on vector-borne infectious diseases.[39]

JHSPH epidemiologist Miriam Brailey (profiled in chapter 4) wrote poignantly in 1958, "My specialty is a narrow one and I can stay on here only as I succeed in getting the annual grant for my work in tuberculosis. Tuberculosis is not exactly disappearing in Baltimore, but it no longer calls for home treatment and the kind of pioneering approach to the problem which was so important when chemotherapy was just beginning to be used. In a relatively short time, probably before I will be sixty-five, the possibility of not being able to get the grant because of diminishing numbers of tuberculosis patients seems to me very real." Brailey left the JHSPH faculty in 1959 to join a religious community founded by the Society of Brothers, or Bruderhof. In fact, TB continued to be both a serious public health problem and a source of grant funding, as demonstrated by the JHSPH faculty's research, including Richard L. Riley's work on irradiating air ducts to prevent TB and George W. Comstock's studies of isoniazid therapy for TB among Alaskan Eskimos.[40]

The school was gradually drifting away from its original moorings in infectious and parasitic diseases. Without Rockefeller Foundation funding, syphilis, polio, malaria, or even hookworm, what was a school of public health to do?

Early Chronic Disease Research and Teaching

In 1927, Frost was the first to apply the term *epidemiology* to nonepidemic disease such as tuberculosis and noninfectious conditions such as nutritional deficiency. A decade later, he declared to the APHA Epidemiology Section that the methods of epidemiology applied to all diseases and health hazards. The school's work in the EHD on tuberculosis and syphilis became the foundation for its approach to noncommunicable diseases such as cancer and heart disease. But after World War II, at Hopkins and elsewhere, medicine and public health were increasingly diverging in the realms of both academic research and professional practice.[41]

In the postwar decades, cancer received the lion's share of chronic disease funding and scientific scrutiny. By 1952, all US medical schools were receiving research grants from the National Cancer Institute (NCI), but schools of public health were slow to apply, even after the NCI's R. F. Kaiser told deans in the Association of Schools of Public Health that his agency wanted to make cancer control training grants to all schools of public health. Of the 10 schools, only those at Harvard, Yale, and University of Michigan were current grantees, along with the public health nursing programs at Teachers College at Columbia University and University of Minnesota. Given the relative disinterest from the public health sector in cancer research and teaching, by 1960, NCI's budget of $91.6 million went primarily to medical research. The PHS allocated only $3.6 million for grants to support cancer prevention programs in state health departments. Likewise, heart disease control received only $1.5 million. Chronic disease in general did not become a major focus of national public health efforts until after 1960. That year, cancer and heart disease control combined still received only $5.1 million (6 percent) of the $83.6 million available for PHS grant-in-aid programs to state and local health departments.[42]

These trends were also in evidence at Johns Hopkins. By 1950, the majority of medical faculty publications eschewed infectious disease and public health issues, dealing instead with chronic disease, especially heart disease and the effects of cortisone, as well as asthma, diabetes, and pulmonary conditions. Pediatrics, which had traditionally investigated childhood infectious and nutritional diseases with major public health implications such as TB, diphtheria, and rickets, was now entirely focused on noninfectious conditions, particularly congenital heart defects. Even the Department of Preventive Medicine, whose chair, Perrin H. Long, had pioneered in the development of antibiotics, became preoccupied with the new wonder drug cortisone and experimental chemotherapy for cancer. In 1946, when the American Cancer Society announced the first 130 recipients of its inaugural individual research grants, Long received the largest award by far. By 1948, Long's department had grown to a full-time staff of 13 and six lecturers, and his work on cancer increased Preventive Medicine's grant funding to rank third among School of Medicine departments.[43]

Such changes in the medical school resulted from (1) the epidemiological transition from infectious to chronic disease as the leading cause of death and disability in America and (2) the NIH's overall tendency to deemphasize interdisciplinary research on prevention and community health in favor of narrower lab and clinical research on therapies for noncommunicable disease (infectious diseases were the specific purview of only one NIH institute, the National Institute of Allergy and Infectious Diseases). In light of these trends, the overall reluctance of public health practitioners and academic faculty to branch out beyond infectious disease weakened the basis for collaboration with medical colleagues.

Yet the postwar decades also need to be reframed against a different model than the "epidemiological transition" from infectious to chronic disease that has so dominated the history of public health. While there was undoubtedly a shift in the leading causes of mortality from infectious to chronic diseases, it had already occurred in the United States by 1910, when heart disease surpassed TB and pneumonia as the most common killer. During the decades before World War II, overall mortality rates declined sharply as living standards rose and public health and medical professionals instituted more effective methods of preventing, controlling, and treating communicable disease. But the epidemiological transition was more clear-cut in mortality than in morbidity, which evidenced greater variations by race, class, region, and rural-urban residence. Moreover, the category of "chronic disease" was ill-defined, since the etiology and treatment of the most common chronic conditions, including heart disease, cancer, stroke, and arthritis, were still largely unknown.

Although schools of public health were slower to embrace the campaigns against chronic disease, they did pursue answers to other noninfectious health problems. As subsequent chapters will explain, JHSPH launched specialized degrees and studies during the 1950s in areas such as aviation medicine, radiological health, the health implications of housing, community mental health, operations research as applied to public health and medical services, and organization of primary health care programs under the auspices of government, public schools, and industry. None of these new initiatives at Johns Hopkins and other schools of public health fit neatly into categories of either infectious or chronic disease; in fact, several did not deal primarily with disease of any type.[44]

The first step toward mounting an effective public health response to chronic disease was to measure accurately its occurrence in the general population. The first studies to estimate the overall incidence (or rate of first attack) and prevalence (number of cases of active disease at a particular time) of chronic disease and disability in the United States were the PHS National Health Survey, which included a Baltimore component, and the five-year East Baltimore Longitudinal Study, conducted from 1938 to 1943 by JHSPH, the PHS, and the Milbank Memorial Fund. The East Baltimore Study used methods developed by Reed and Frost for in-depth, long-term cohort studies of TB in the EHD. One of the most influential publications from this research was Frost's 1940 article, "The Age Selection of Mortality from Tuberculosis in Successive Decades," which defined modern epidemiology as an analytical science closely integrated with biology and medicine. Kenneth Maxcy used these longitudinal cohort study methods to help his student, Gilcin Meadors (MPH 1946), frame the initial parameters of the PHS Framingham Heart Study, which sought to determine the predisposing factors in heart disease by studying a healthy population, using long-term follow-up with clinical and laboratory data. Meadors served as the Framingham Study's first principal investigator while he was still at JHSPH.[45]

During the height of JHSPH research on polio in the 1950s, faculty in Public Health Administration and Epidemiology gave little attention to cancer or heart disease but instead initially modeled their approach to chronic disease on tuberculosis and syphilis, which both blurred the boundary between acute and chronic conditions. J. Earle Moore, head of the PHA Division of Venereal

Diseases, had done foundational work in the chronic aspects of syphilis and authored the classic textbook *The Modern Treatment of Syphilis* (1933). At the same time that Reed and Frost were developing the historical (or retrospective) cohort study to measure and predict TB mortality throughout the life span, Moore was using longitudinal (or prospective) patient studies to evaluate the effectiveness of various forms of chemotherapy for syphilis. Both these approaches, developed at Johns Hopkins and other research centers, became fundamental tools for chronic disease research. In 1953, Moore revamped the *American Journal of Syphilis* to become the *American Journal of Chronic Diseases*. He similarly renamed the Division of Venereal Diseases and the Department of Medicine's VD clinic in 1956.[46]

Likewise, the school's research and teaching in Epidemiology reflected the longstanding primacy of TB under chairs Wade Hampton Frost, Kenneth Maxcy, and Philip E. Sartwell (Sartwell was also president of the Maryland Tuberculosis Association). While the introductory Principles of Epidemiology course focused on acute infectious diseases, the Statistical Methods in Epidemiology course (taught jointly by Biostatistics and Epidemiology) used tuberculosis as "the principal illustrative chronic disease." After he succeeded Maxcy as chair of Epidemiology in 1954, Sartwell noted, "The day when a John Snow could virtually unaided prove the contagiousness and solve the problem of transmission of a disease has passed." Research in epidemiology had become a lengthy, costly group effort that "involve[d] much interdisciplinary planning and cooperation." The challenges of both polio and chronic disease had greatly and permanently increased the complexity of departmental activities.[47]

Before joining the Epidemiology faculty in 1947, Sartwell, a native of Massachusetts, had earned an MD from Boston University and an MPH from Harvard. From 1938 to 1943, he was assistant director of the Massachusetts Department of Health Division of Tuberculosis, and he served the next four years as an epidemiologist for the US Army Office of the Surgeon General. Immediately after the war he went to Germany to assess the TB outbreaks in the American Occupation Zone. Sartwell, who chaired Epidemiology from 1954 to 1970, helped to found the Maryland Public Health Association in 1955 and served as its first president. He also chaired the APHA Epidemiology Section, served as editor-in-chief of the *American Journal of Epidemiology* from 1957 to 1958, and cofounded *Epidemiologic Reviews* in 1979 with Neal Nathanson.[48]

As the polio research lab was winding down, Sartwell appointed Winston H. Price to replace David Bodian, and the Division of Neurobiology and Neurotropic Virus Diseases was renamed the Division of Medical Ecology. Price remained focused on virology but switched from polio to influenza and broadened the division's scope to include more clinical and field work, notably clinical trials led by Raymond Seltser (MPH 1957) that showed that the CDC's vaccine against the 1957 Asian flu was 60 percent effective. Faculty in the departments of Microbiology and Biochemistry also worked on the basic science of influenza, and Biochemistry chair Roger Herriott studied the genetics of *Haemophilus influenzae* bacteria and emerged as an early national expert in molecular genetics and DNA. Herriott had originally recruited Price in 1951 from the Rockefeller Institute of Medical Research, and they collaborated to explore the origin and properties of bacterial viruses, which led to their introducing the university's first courses on DNA. As the school transitioned from studying polio to studying influenza, its strength in virology remained squarely within infectious diseases. Yet by reconfiguring research programs in Epidemiology to emphasize clinical epidemiology and medical ecology, Sartwell forged stronger ties between the department and the medical school than had been the case under Maxcy. Herriott's work also allowed the departments of Microbiology and Biochemistry to branch out into genetics, using the powerful new tools of molecular biology.[49]

Like Reed, Frost, and Moore, Sartwell distinguished himself as one of the early epidemiologists of chronic disease. With Biostatistics colleague Margaret Merrell, he wrote an insightful 1952 *American Journal of Public Health* article on the variable nature of chronic disease and how it complicated conventional prevalence and incidence figures, since they had been designed to describe acute illnesses. Understanding rates of progression through multiple stages of chronic diseases such as cancer, heart disease, or diabetes was as important as knowing how many people suffered from each disease in all its forms. Sartwell and Merrell also proposed to study the relationships between incidence rates and the progression of disease in populations: for example, did diabetes progress more rapidly in patients within a high-incidence population? The authors identified disability resulting from chronic disease as "a more meaningful index in many conditions than any clinical or laboratory test yet devised," since many chronic diseases remained poorly defined and classified. They also warned against misinterpreting apparent disparities or increases in morbidity rates for diseases such as TB and syphilis, since mass survey techniques had enabled the discovery of more cases of disease at much earlier stages than previously.[50]

While Epidemiology remained focused on the infectious diseases of polio, TB, and influenza, Hopkins biostatisticians made crucial contributions to constructing the case against cigarette smoking as a cause of lung cancer, particularly in developing new methods of causal inference to identify and quantify risk. The first to do so was Raymond Pearl, who prematurely declared in 1928 that he had found the cure for cancer. In his examination of autopsy records, Pearl had observed a negative association between cancer and TB mortality and concluded that perhaps TB protected against cancer. He even conducted trials for a year to test the efficacy of treating terminal cancer patients with tuberculin. Pearl redeemed himself with a 1938 article in *Science* that used the family history records of nearly 7,000 white males to prove that "the smoking of tobacco was statistically associated with the impairment of life duration, and the amount of this impairment increased as the habitual amount of smoking increased."[51]

These two contrasting episodes illustrate important differences between the tradition of clinical and laboratory investigation upon which Johns Hopkins was founded and the new epidemiology of chronic disease that took hold after 1945. In the first instance, Pearl had been blinded by the reductionist promise of lab and clinical methods to match precisely a specific disease with its unique cause or cure. In the second, he relied on statistical inference to determine what could not be proved either in the laboratory or in direct experimentation on humans. Although Pearl died in 1940, his interest in the relationship between heredity and environment as factors in disease and life expectancy, the forerunner of today's field of epigenetics, flourished in the Department of Biostatistics and later became an important line of inquiry in Environmental Health Sciences.

Pearl's student Morton L. Levin (MPH 1933) was a gifted biostatistician who conducted the first case-control study of smoking and lung cancer in the United States. Frost, who believed that cancer was a viral disease, had dispatched Levin to become the only cancer investigator for the New York State Department of Health during the 1940s. Levin collected detailed information on patients' smoking histories, including years of smoking and number of cigarettes smoked daily, and compared them to their medical records over a 10-year period. He concluded that heavy smokers were 10 times as likely to develop lung cancer as were nonsmokers, and the length of smoking history was positively related to the age-adjusted risk of lung cancer. His rigorously systematic, controlled study of lung, lip, pharynx, esophagus, colon, and rectal cancers in relation to types of smoking was the first to test associations between cancer site and method of tobacco use. Levin noted that statistical significance was achieved for cigarette smoking and lung cancer and for pipe smoking and lip cancer. He quit smoking and published his findings in 1950 articles in the *Journal of the American Medical Association* and *Cancer*, which attracted the attention of American researchers alongside the publications of British epidemiologists Richard Doll and Bradford Hill. These studies confirmed the dose–response effect of cigarette smoking first noted by Pearl.[52]

Just as Pearl, Reed, and Frost had shaped Levin's approach to chronic disease epidemiology, he in turn trained Abraham M. Lilienfeld (MPH 1949), who worked as an epidemiologist under Levin, now serving as assistant commissioner at the New York State Department of Health. As a faculty member in PHA from 1950 to 1954, Lilienfeld contributed to the school's path-breaking studies of premature birth and developmental disability (discussed in chapter 4). During this period, he also formed several relationships that would influence his career in chronic disease epidemiology. William Cochran and Irvin D. J. Bross in Biostatistics helped Lilienfeld to develop his statistical reasoning ability. As an instructor in the first officer training course for the CDC's Epidemic Intelligence Service (see chapter 6), he met EIS director Alexander Langmuir. In 1952, Langmuir initiated national trials of gamma globulin, a blood product containing antibodies, to determine whether it reduced the severity of paralysis in polio. Langmuir named Lilienfeld to direct the new National Gamma Globulin Evaluation Center. Although the trials were inconclusive, gamma globulin would subsequently be adapted for the clinical management of other diseases, including measles, viral hepatitis, rubella, and varicella, and, more recently, immunodeficiency.[53]

In the mid-1950s, Lilienfeld and Levin collaborated on a landmark survey of chronic illness morbidity. One of the most fundamental obstacles to controlling chronic disease was a woeful lack of data, particularly on morbidity. Most noninfectious chronic diseases were not reportable, and as late as 1980, only three states—New York, California, and Connecticut—had established cancer registries that allowed analysis of long-term trends in incidence. Before 1950, the only scientific large-scale morbidity surveys of the general population had been conducted by the PHS, two on a nationwide basis and four in cities or counties. The smaller scale of the local surveys permitted more detailed household interviews that were repeated at regular intervals over a year or more, including the intensive monthly surveys of illness in the EHD mentioned above.[54]

But the gold standard of morbidity surveys were those conducted by the Commission on Chronic Illness, established in 1947 by the AMA, American Hospital Association, American Public Health Association, and American Public Welfare Association. In a joint statement, spokesmen for the groups declared that "the basic approach to chronic disease must be preventive. Otherwise the problems created by chronic diseases will grow larger with time, and the hope of any substantial decline in their incidence and severity will be postponed for many years." Stebbins served on the commission, whose first two directors were JHSPH alumni who went on to become senior state health department administrators. Levin was appointed the commission's first director in 1950. Maryland State Department of Health Deputy Director Dean W. Roberts (MPH 1948) took over from Levin in 1952.[55]

In 1953, the new JHSPH Division of Chronic Diseases was boosted by a PHS training grant in cardiovascular disease control and by the Commission on Chronic Illness's decision to relocate its offices to Baltimore. From 1953 to 1956, the commission's headquarters moved from the AMA offices in Chicago to the seventh floor of the Hygiene building, and Roberts was appointed as a lecturer in PHA. JHSPH faculty worked closely with the commission's staff to conduct an intensive study of chronic illness in 4,000 families in Baltimore, chosen as a representative urban area. The Baltimore study included an evaluation of multiphasic screening techniques as well as surveys of prevalence figures and nursing home utilization.[56]

The Commission on Chronic Illness also conducted a study in the rural community of Hunterdon, New Jersey. Like the five-year EHD surveys from 1938 to 1943, the Baltimore and Hunterdon surveys were correlated with detailed clinical evaluations of a representative sample of those interviewed. Four published volumes provided detailed analysis of the development and application of chronic disease screening methods, as well as the pros, cons, and optimal format for household interviews. The commission documented the presence of chronic diseases in a "tremendously high proportion of the population," of whom very few patients "had a condition preventable with current knowledge." Its methods and findings were a model for all subsequent research in chronic disease epidemiology, including the surgeon general's reports on smoking and health and the cancer prevalence studies conducted by the JHSPH Division of Chronic Diseases (explored in chapter 11).[57]

Biostatistics provided the foundation for studying not only cancer but all types of chronic disease, and the Biostatistics faculty included some of the school's most gifted teachers. Margaret Merrell's Statistical Methods in Epidemiology course introduced students to statistical methods for systematic field investigations of chronic diseases, and they consistently rated it as one of the school's best courses. She creatively used real-life raw data to construct problems that engaged students in interpreting current public health trends. They measured survivorship and cumulative mortality, by cause, using data from a longitudinal study begun in 1935 of the effectiveness of the BCG vaccine in American Indian children. Another problem analyzed age distributions and compared mortality between the vaccinated and control groups to judge the long-term effectiveness of vaccination. Merrell's students tracked time and age changes in male death rates from lung cancer, which had increased fivefold from 1931 to 1951, and used birth cohort analysis to plot the age-specific death rates on a curve and predict future trends.[58]

William Gemmell Cochran, who succeeded Reed as chair of Biostatistics in 1948, requested a salary increase for Merrell, whose value to the department he found "difficult to overestimate. . . . She is the outstanding teacher in the department and carries the great bulk of the teaching load in addition to handling much of our most important consulting work and playing a prominent part in the direction of research by students." Merrell's student Helen Abbey (ScD 1951) joined her on the Biostatistics faculty in 1949. Like Reed and Merrell, Abbey was known for her research on the design and statistical analysis of epidemiologic studies, but she also was among the school's earliest genetics researchers. In 1959, she coauthored one of the first studies of heredity in breast cancer among 200 probands (the first-affected family members to seek medical attention). Always accompanied by her Pomeranian, Peppy, Abbey taught biostatistics to over 4,000 students and read over 700 doctoral theses. The conventional wisdom at the school was that if you parachuted anywhere on earth, you would land within 50 miles of a former student of Helen Abbey. Many of them went on to become major figures in medicine and public health, including Victor McKusick, Bernice Cohen, Alfred Sommer, Marie Diener-West, and Michael J. Klag, all of whom held joint appointments in the schools of Hygiene and Medicine.[59]

Cochran was an authority on sampling and the analysis of variance, just as multivariate analysis was emerging as a critical tool of risk factor epidemiology. Under Pearl and Reed, the Department of Biostatistics had focused on vital statistics and demography, but Cochran's work on sampling theory, especially sampling in human populations, brought the department into the modern era of biostatistics and epidemiology. He introduced biostatistics courses on advanced sampling techniques and experimental design, and his textbooks on these subjects went into multiple editions over the next three decades. The importance of sampling to biostatistics and all biomedical research cannot be overstated, since sample size and selection are two of the most important factors in detecting a valid association and, therefore, determining how much time and funding will be needed for a research project. Cochran's work on strengthening the common chi-square test to determine the independence of two nominal variables became a key element of the statistical basis for linking smoking with lung cancer.[60]

The Reed–Frost model and other epidemiological models had been deterministic, but in the 1950s, Cochran was among the biostatisticians who developed theories of stochastic processes, which introduced elements of uncertainty to explain more realistically the ways disease spreads in a population. One such model drew from the catalytic process in chemistry, where a fraction of reacting molecules is converted during each time interval over the course of a chemical reaction, to explain how the relative prevalence of disease shifted as more individuals in the population were exposed to a communicable disease. The catalytic epidemic model was modified with differential equations to account for situations where some percentage of the population did not react after exposure, such as to measles or whooping cough. Catalytic processes were capable of operating in two opposite directions simultaneously, whereby reactions could be reversible. Further complexity was added by introducing multiple stages of change with varying rates of transition, which was used to explain phenomena such as survival data among patients with hypertension.[61]

From the late 1930s until the late 1950s, JHSPH faculty in Public Health Administration, Epidemiology, and Biostatistics based their approaches to chronic disease almost entirely on existing methods for studying infectious diseases, particularly syphilis and TB. The main exception was the work of Biostatistics faculty and alumni on smoking and lung cancer, which provided one of the earliest and strongest examples of the dose–response relationship, one of the fundamental principles for determining causality in observational studies, as opposed to clinical trials. During the 1950s, the school's teaching and research also began to incorporate insights from genetics, both human and viral, and to pay greater attention to morbidity and the social and organizational challenges associated with long-term illness and disability. But it was not until the late 1950s that JHSPH wholeheartedly followed its medical brethren into the realm of chronic disease research that went beyond quantifying the scope of the problem and began seeking workable methods of prevention and treatment. As we shall see in chapter 11, this move was warmly welcomed by NIH grant reviewers.

The Department of Pathobiology had one foot in the school's glorious past in parasitology and one foot striding forward into the future of cancer research that combined innovative, interdisciplinary thinking with high-quality (and highly fundable) bench science. The Department of Parasitology's wartime transition from domestic to international health became permanent. After 1945, most US schools of medicine and public health suspended their teaching and research programs in tropical diseases, since they were no longer considered serious domestic threats. As noted above, federal research funding shifted decisively toward chronic diseases, although defense agencies such as the Office of Naval Research continued to support research on tropical diseases due to their military importance.

Frederik B. Bang, like NIH director James Shannon, came to cancer research from the campaign against malaria. Bang had joined the Department of Medicine at Johns Hopkins in 1946, where he supervised parasitology courses for medical students and conducted electron microscope studies of viruses. His research emphases included anopheline mosquitoes, malaria treatment, and the epidemiology, treatment, and control of schistosomiasis, second only to malaria as the most devastating parasitic disease. Bang had investigated schistosomiasis, transmitted by worm-carrying snails, on Leyte Island in the Philippines, and he enthusiastically supported the new faculty exchange program between JHSPH and the University of the Philippines, funded by the Rockefeller Foundation and the WHO.[62]

After W. W. Cort's retirement in spring 1953, the School of Hygiene announced Bang's appointment as the new professor and chair of Parasitology. Despite Bang's solid medical research credentials and background as an Army Medical Corps officer in the Pacific campaign against parasitic diseases, news of his appointment caused an unprecedented firestorm among Parasitology faculty and alumni, who protested that Bang was not a national leader in parasitology or even active in the field's professional organizations. Within the department, many had considered Gilbert F. Otto (ScD 1929) or Lloyd Rozeboom as the most promising successors to Cort, and Otto promptly left Hopkins for a productive career in industry. An outraged Marion M. Brooke (ScD 1942), director of the CDC's Parasitology and Mycology Laboratory, demanded a personal appointment with Dean Stebbins and President Detlev Bronk. Don E. Eyles (ScD 1950), director of the NIH Tropical Diseases Laboratory, and William D. Lindquist (ScD 1949) at Michigan State University both wrote to urge Dean Stebbins to reconsider the decision in light of the strong and unanimous disapproval among alumni as well many leading parasitologists. Lindquist asked how the alumni could be expected to continue giving to the School of Hygiene "when we have our faith shattered by such an ill-advised selection to head that illustrious department?"[63]

Stebbins stood by the search committee's decision despite the initial outcry. Bang stayed and took the Department of Parasitology in uncharted directions that deeply chagrined Turner and other science faculty. Bang's new catalog statement called parasitology "A Biology of Disease" that studied "the phenomenon of parasitism" involving both extracellular and intracellular parasites from biological as well as medical perspectives. Bang also advertised the "variety of specialized techniques" not typically found in parasitology labs, including facilities for biochemistry, tissue culture, and electron microscopy (a special interest of Bang's since his days at the Rockefeller Institute for Medical Research, which pioneered in its development). His vision for the department represented such a significant departure that he renamed it Pathobiology in 1955.[64]

Bang's career, like Turner's, epitomized the counterpressures on postwar basic science research in public health to emulate the medical model while also remaining true to preventive and population-based methods of fighting disease. When Bang left the Department of Medicine for JHSPH, he had come under fire for his background as a clinical medical researcher without sufficient formal training in the quintessential public health discipline of parasitology. As time went on, he would alienate his more medically oriented basic science colleagues in Microbiology, who were appalled by Bang's interdisciplinary, unorthodox, pan-species approach to understanding the behavior of disease in populations. Under Bang, the Department of Pathobiology developed a uniquely public health–oriented research program of studying the effects of disease in populations of creatures ranging from mosquitoes, rats, and turtles to foxes, penguins, and polar bears. By drawing from the disciplines of field biology, ecology, and zoology, pathobiology adapted concepts of interactions within and among animal populations and applied them to an analysis of disease in human populations.

Bang was not only a broad-gauged thinker but also a gifted laboratory investigator whose research on cancer helped win back skeptics on both sides of Wolfe Street. Early cancer research in Hygiene was indistinguishable from that conducted in the medical school and focused on understanding "the structure, the properties and the growth of normal and malignant cells, and the reactions of cells and tissues to different internal and external conditions," including hormones, viruses, radiation, and airborne particles. Bang's department would introduce critical new perspectives on cancer by studying both the molecular mechanisms and environmental epidemiology of oncogenesis.[65]

Bang collaborated with cell biologist George O. Gey, director of the Finney–Howell Cancer Research Laboratory at the Johns Hopkins Hospital, who developed the HeLa cell line adopted worldwide for tissue culture research. "Examination of the cells is the first thing to do," Bang wrote in 1958, "and yet there has been relatively little of this; and of this, in turn, a large part has been forgotten or ignored." Gey was a lecturer in Pathobiology who assisted in teaching the Host–Cell Parasitic Relationships course, which dealt with parasitic relationships between an intracellular agent and its host cell. Students first studied the structure of normal cells in tissue culture and under the electron microscope, which at the time were revolutionary new tools. Students then learned how the cells responded to large parasites such as trichina, leishmania, toxoplasma, and smaller agents such as psittacoid and tumor viruses.[66]

As the only infectious agent among a raft of potential carcinogens, viruses were an atypical branch of oncology research, but one particularly well suited for the School of Hygiene's expertise in developing and applying effective animal models. Polio research had provided the foundation for JHSPH to build an unsurpassed knowledge base in virology and vaccine development and evaluation. The Department of Pathobiology built on this foundation by fostering both basic and ecological field research on the role of viruses as cancer agents, particularly the Rous tumor virus in birds, one of six viruses known to cause in vitro carcinogenesis.[67]

Keerti V. Shah (MPH 1957, DrPH 1963) examined the classical pathogen–host–environment triangle by studying simian virus 40 (SV 40), an oncogenic polyomavirus that had accidentally contaminated lots of both the Salk (inactivated) and Sabin (live) polio vaccine administered in the United States in the late 1950s. In North India, Shah observed the ecological interaction of humans with rhesus monkeys, who often had antibodies to some human respiratory viruses as well as to measles and parainfluenza, indicating a possible human-to-monkey transfer of virus infection. Hypothesizing that humans could be infected with SV 40 in areas where they lived in close association with rhesus monkeys, Shah tested for antibodies to SV 40 and other simian agents, as well as to the SV 40 tumor antigen, in blood samples from hospitalized cancer patients and residents of North Indian villages. But after four decades of research on the connections between SV 40 virus and various types of cancer in humans, Shah concluded that SV 40 was not a human carcinogen. His in-depth exploration of polyomavirus did, however, lead to a far more revelatory finding about a related type of small DNA virus, papillomavirus. In 1999, Shah's lab would publish the results of research demonstrating that infection with any one of a subset of mucosal human papillomaviruses (HPVs) that inhabit the human genital tract is the primary catalyst for the eventual development of invasive cervical cancer.[68]

Like Bodian, Howe, and Morgan in polio research, Bang and Shah's wide-ranging, creative approaches drew upon animal models and united the best of clinical, field, and lab methods. Bang considered cancer-causing viruses a form of parasite, and his research balanced infectious and chronic disease, especially cancer. In the early 1950s, when he was still in the Department of Medicine, Bang had studied the destructive effects of viruses on normal and malignant living cells in tissue cultures and discovered that horse encephalitis virus destroyed certain strains of cancer cells without harming normal cells. The medical school appointed him to the Joint Committee on Cancer Teaching and Research, and he continued to serve on the committee after moving to JHSPH. Bang's research with Heinz E. Carrer on the biology of the mammary tumor virus in mice received long-term funding from the NCI, and Pathobiology also received NIH training grants from both the NCI and the National Institute of Allergy and Infectious Diseases. Bang served on the National Science Foundation Developmental Biology Study Section and the American Cancer Society's Committee on Therapy, and by 1960, his success in attracting NIH and PHS funding had made Pathobiology the school's top grant recipient, with 40 percent of all external funding.[69]

Conclusion

During the 1950s, the School of Hygiene and Public Health underwent a major shift in both its funding streams and its research emphases, from private foundation funding for investigations of infectious disease to federal grants and contracts for projects on noncommunicable disease as well as health problems outside the realm of somatic disease. This was not a clear-cut process, and the school continued to receive private grants from foundations such as the Ford Foundation, which would be a major supporter of JHSPH population planning

TABLE 3.1
New Categories of PHS and NIH Funding at JHSPH, 1950–1960

Department	Investigators	Communicable Disease	Noncommunicable Disease	Nondisease
Bacteriology/ Microbiology	Thomas Turner, Robert Nelson	Syphilis		
	Manfred Mayer	Immunology of complement system		
Biochemistry	Roger Herriott, Winston Price Bacon Chow	Genetics of *Haemophilus influenzae*		Enzyme and protein biochemistry
Biostatistics	William Cochran Rowland Rider		Maternal complications and developmental disability	Biostatistics training
Environmental Medicine	Joseph Lilienthal, Richard Riley			Lung physiology, aviation medicine
	Anna Baetjer		Occupational lung cancer	
	Samuel Crowe			Audiology and speech; nasopharyngeal irradiation to prevent deafness
	Russell Morgan, Clifford Beers			Radiation hazards
Epidemiology	Winston Price	Influenza and common cold		
	Philip Sartwell, Winston Price, Raymond Seltser	Evaluation of 1957 Asian influenza vaccine		

Parasitology/ Pathobiology		Schistosomiasis Malaria	Cancer virology	Rodent ecology; Polar and North American waterfowl
	David E. Davis, Frederik Bang, Keerti Shah, Ernest Bueding, Lloyd Rozeboom, Everett Schiller, William Sladen			
Public Health Administration	Ernest Stebbins			PHA training
PHA Public Health Nursing	Ruth Freeman			Public health nursing training
PHA Venereal/ Chronic Disease	J. Earle Moore, Abraham Lilienfeld		Cancer, heart disease, Premature birth and neonatal care	
PHA Maternal and Child Health	Paul Harper		Premature birth and neonatal care	School health
PHA Mental Hygiene	Paul Lemkau, Benjamin Pasamanick, Hilda Knobloch		Premature birth and neonatal care	Mental health training

programs in the 1960s. Still, a permanent trend had emerged that continued into the twenty-first century: since 1960, more than three-quarters of the total JHSPH budget has always come from federal sources.

This trend was not confined to the science departments, but as this chapter has shown, basic science research had long enjoyed a privileged status at Johns Hopkins, and that status was challenged by the perception (although not the reality) that infectious diseases such as malaria, syphilis, polio, and TB had been all but conquered. The school had been a "magic bullet factory," producing and/or evaluating many of the century's most powerful tools and tests for preventing disease in populations, such as vitamin D, penicillin, DDT, antimalarial drugs, the TPI test, and the diphtheria–pertussis–tetanus (DPT) and Salk polio vaccines. The shift away from a singular emphasis on infectious and parasitic disease—"bugs and drugs"—and toward a less binary, more multicausal understanding of health and illness as a continuous spectrum was akin to the postwar conversion of defense production to a diversified peacetime economy.

The accompanying turn toward NIH grants, although it had begun in the 1940s with syphilis research in the departments of Microbiology and Biostatistics, accelerated in the late 1950s with support for projects on chronic disease in the departments of Biostatistics, Chronic Disease, Environmental Medicine, and Pathobiology (table 3.1). Cancer was the foremost topic among these projects, which continued the tradition of in-depth lab and field work while also expanding the school's capacity for clinical epidemiology, particularly under Lilienfeld in Chronic Disease. Yet, as the following chapters will explore, the rise of federal support at JHSPH lifted many boats in addition to chronic disease, including mental health (which also had chronic aspects), prenatal and primary care, aviation medicine, and radiation hazards. The 1950s marked the school's transformation into a research grant electromagnet, capable of attracting all of the most precious categories of funding metals: defense, foreign aid, biomedicine, child health, population control, environmental hazards, and health services planning and evaluation.

CHAPTER FOUR

The School and the City

In an era of grand crusades—against syphilis, polio, and totalitarianism—Ernest L. Stebbins was the public health equivalent of a Hollywood movie star. As a student at Rush Medical College in Chicago, Stebbins originally had intended to pursue surgery but was persuaded to go into public health by his roommate, L. T. Coggeshall, a globetrotting malaria expert and Rockefeller Foundation fellow. After earning an MPH at Johns Hopkins, Stebbins worked as a district health officer and epidemiologist for the New York State Health Department, then headed by Thomas Parran. In 1942, Parran backed Stebbins's appointment as New York City Health Commissioner and Professor of Epidemiology at Columbia's DeLamar Institute of Health. From 1942 to 1946, Stebbins ran the nation's largest public health unit, which served 7.5 million people. Albert Deutsch praised him in *PM* as one of the best health commissioners in the city's history, and the *New York Times* called Stebbins the latest in "a remarkable succession of Commissioners of Health" whose department was making strides to advance public health research. Abel Wolman, one of Stebbins's JHSPH professors, called him "a missionary of public health. Not flamboyant, a noiseless worker, a gentleman, an advocate." Wolman advised Stebbins on the formidable problem of maintaining sanitary conditions in New York City's restaurants, where Stebbins complained he could not find a clean glass of water.[1]

Stebbins would bring to fruition Reed's plans for greater cooperation among the Hopkins medical institutions and government health agencies. He and Reed served on the National Health Council of the Public Health Service, of which Stebbins was president in 1951. Stebbins was elected president of the APHA in 1966, after serving as a member of the Governing Council and secretary of the Epidemiology Section. He also advised the Maryland Health Department and those of numerous other states. In Delaware, for example, he helped establish the nation's first statewide public health training program for physicians.[2]

At Johns Hopkins, Stebbins built on Reed's efforts to foster the growth of the MPH program and continued the quest for stable operational funding to support more students, but the main educational challenges remained those identified in the 1939 Parran–Farrand Report: facilitating the interdisciplinary training of public health professionals, improving and expanding students' opportunities for practical experience in public health agencies, and recruiting top medical students into public health through undergraduate teaching of preventive medicine. Stebbins would meet these goals at Hopkins via new programs that brought Hygiene students and faculty into a broader spectrum of public health practice environments and broached the uncharted territory of the Johns Hopkins Hospital.

The Rise of the Eastern Health District and the Baltimore Medical Care Plan

William Henry Welch had groomed two of Maryland's most influential twentieth-century public health leaders, Huntington Williams (DrPH 1921) and Robert H. Riley (DrPH 1922), who had both studied under Welch as medical students at Johns Hopkins and had then earned doctorates at the School of Hygiene. Both played crucial roles in the early development of JHSPH, Williams primarily through the EHD and Riley through various consulting projects, such as enlisting JSHPH faculty to conduct a comprehensive review of the Maryland Department of Health in the late 1930s. Under Riley's leadership from 1928 to 1955, Maryland became the first state to establish full-time local public health units in every county. Maryland also boasted one of the first extensive chronic illness programs and the only state network of six branch bacteriological laboratories. Johns Hopkins was a critical state resource that helped Maryland and Baltimore to rise to the top of national rankings in both public health and medical services. Health personnel in Maryland, California, New York, and the District of Columbia remained at the forefront of public health innovation and, not coincidentally, at the top of the salary scale as well.[3]

When Huntington Williams was appointed health commissioner in 1931, he had been Welch's favorite son, charged with healing the rift between the school and the Baltimore City Health Department that had delayed the founding of the EHD for several years. Elizabeth Fee described the young Williams, who "brought new energy to the job. Whereas some commissioners of health owed their loyalty to a political leader, a party machine, or to the economically powerful, Williams owed his first loyalty to Welch who had groomed him, to his Hopkins professors who had taught and inspired him, and to the example of Hermann Biggs [New York State Commissioner of Health] who had demonstrated what an effective public health organization should be. Williams was determined to show them all what he could do if given the chance." He confirmed his mentors' faith in him by making Baltimore a national model in key areas such as syphilis control (discussed in chapter 1), tuberculosis control, mental hygiene, and childhood lead paint poisoning, all in close collaboration with Johns Hopkins medical and public health faculty.[4]

After Welch's death in 1934, Williams worked to develop and expand the EHD with JHSPH deans Wade Hampton Frost, Allen Freeman, and Lowell Reed, who were all widely respected in Baltimore political circles. In 1935, Williams made Baltimore the first city in the nation to provide free diagnostic tests to measure blood lead levels in cases of suspected lead poisoning. Williams enlisted JHSPH's Anna Baetjer to visit the homes of children with high blood lead levels to confirm the source of exposure. Under Williams's leadership, Baltimore became the only US city to establish a central diagnostic and reporting mechanism for lead poisoning, and he also instituted extensive public education campaigns and passed lead paint labeling laws that made the BCHD a leader in efforts to identify and address the problem of childhood lead paint poisoning.[5]

TB, like lead paint poisoning, was associated with substandard housing conditions and poverty, which put Baltimore's black children at disproportionate risk. Before the war, Freeman had surveyed Baltimore's facilities for preventing TB, which were sorely lacking, given the city's high rates. TB was the second-ranked killer among Baltimore's black population and seventh among whites, reflecting racial differentials in income and housing conditions. Freeman had recommended that the city expand the Bureau of Tuberculosis budget, including funding for a full-time director (up to this point, the position had been federally funded on a part-time basis). The Baltimore City Council voted in 1941 to approve $22,000 in additional funds, of which $7,000 was designated for a new diagnostic clinic at the Druid Hill Health Center for black West Baltimore residents, the third TB clinic established by the BCHD. Pediatrician Miriam E. Brailey (DrPH 1931) was the first woman on the Epidemiology faculty and, in 1941, Commissioner Williams appointed her to head the BCHD Bureau of Tuberculosis.[6]

Brailey was another Frost and Reed protégée who, like Ruth Rice Puffer, addressed the black–white health divide. In November 1942, she initiated a TB screening program in the EHD. The initial chest X-rays from pediatric patients provided data for Brailey's research on the prognosis for children who tested positive. She also helped design Maryland's new TB control program, which extended the screening program statewide. Although black physicians and laypeople had been crusading for years to raise awareness of racial disparities in TB mortality rates and hospital beds, Brailey took up this message and gave it strong official backing. At public forums in Baltimore, at the first conference of Negro Tuberculosis Workers at the Howard University School of Medicine, and in journals such as the *American Journal of Public Health*, she emphasized the need for improved funding for services and outreach to Maryland blacks, who suffered four times higher mortality from TB than whites but were allotted only one-third as many sanatoria beds per capita.[7]

Brailey went on to publish one of the first major studies of pediatric TB as well as racial disparities in infectious disease, *Tuberculosis in White and Negro Children: The Epidemiologic Aspects of the Harriet Lane Study*. Based on her research with School of Medicine colleague Janet Hardy, the book analyzed statistics on racial disparities in initial morbidity, development of extrapulmonary tuberculosis, and mortality from tuberculosis over a 15-year follow-up period. Frost, Freeman, and Brailey's foundational work on TB was just one example of how the EHD studies influenced the questions and methodology of epidemiological research and contributed to American epidemiology's postwar shift toward emphasizing chronic disease.[8]

At the same time that Williams's star was on the rise in Baltimore and nationally, public health leaders at JHSPH and in the federal government were beginning to transgress the traditional boundaries between clinical medicine and public health. In 1938, Josephine Roche, assistant secretary of the Treasury for Public Health (the PHS was at this time under the Treasury Department), had advanced the iconoclastic argument that "the treatment of the sick was no less a responsibility of health officers than the prevention of disease." Roche chaired President Roosevelt's Interdepartmental Committee to Coordinate Health and Welfare among five federal agencies, and she asked the leadership of the APHA to establish a committee to cooperate with the federal government and the medical profession to plan for a federally sponsored indigent care program. New Deal reformers like Roche and Parran promoted both the horizontal integration of public health, medical care, and welfare services and the vertical integration of local, state, and federal health programs. Riley was also a formidable New Dealer who served on the US Department of Labor's Advisory Committee on Child Welfare under the Social Security Act (SS), as president of the Conference of State and Provincial Health Authorities of North America, and as chair of the Surgeon General's Committee on Venereal Disease.[9]

As discussed in chapter 2, JHSPH leaders were advancing the same ideas that had percolated during the Hill–Burton hearings for cooperative health programs among government, private, and academic institutions. Reed, Wolman, J. Earle Moore, Thomas Turner, and Kenneth Maxcy challenged the Johns Hopkins Medical Institutions to consider plans for a medical center in East Baltimore that would formally integrate the hospital and university with city health department services and local private medical and hospital care. Wolman chaired the nine-member APHA committee, which also included Harry S. Mustard, the EHD's first director who now headed Columbia University's DeLamar Institute of Public Health. Wolman's committee met with Roche to discuss the proposals advanced by the 1938 National Health Conference to expand federal–state cooperation under SS and to formulate a national health program. The APHA committee maintained that the state health department was best qualified to administer and orchestrate such a program, which should build on existing preventive health services.[10]

Parran called on medical and public health leaders to contribute "the best professional thinking" to create a new health system that coordinated the government, business, and nonprofit sectors. He claimed that physicians and the public had already accepted the essential connection between prevention and treatment of disease, and therefore "sound public policy dictates that there should be a unity of administration for [public] health and medical care programs. The health department obviously is the one agency best fitted to do this job." Under Parran, the PHS used federal grants as an incentive for comprehensive statewide surveys of medical and public health needs, with the stipulation that state health departments be charged with the authority to carry them out. Federal policy thus promoted a new role for public health agencies as coordinators of efforts to evaluate and plan medical and hospital care on a population level. In states with schools of public health, the schools played key advisory roles in state health planning.[11]

In defense of these goals, Parran testified before Congress on behalf of the 1939 Wagner National Health Plan Bill and its successor, the Wagner–Murray–Dingell Bill, which included comprehensive national health insurance. He also encouraged PHS staff to develop federally sponsored experiments in single-payer group medical care through the Farm Security Administration and the wartime Emergency Maternity and Infant Care program. The Wagner Bill won support from Reed, Wolman (APHA president in 1939), and the eminent Johns Hopkins medical historian Henry Sigerist, as well as from APHA executive secretary Reginald Atwater (DrPH 1921), Joseph Mountin, and Michael M. Davis, all of whom would be instrumental in forming the APHA's Medical Care Section in 1948.[12]

Such proposals sparked controversy in both medical and public health circles. Haven Emerson, professor of public health administration at Columbia, stridently opposed entering the realm of medical care, whether in public policy or by creating a new section in APHA. Emerson defended the primacy of the long-established "basic six" local health services (vital statistics, control of communicable diseases, environmental sanitation, public health laboratory services, maternal and child hygiene, and health education), which carefully preserved the accepted division of labor between preventive public health and curative clinical medicine. On this point, Williams was much closer to Emerson than to Parran. Williams told the *Baltimore Sun* that he opposed shifting the BCHD's emphasis from prevention to treatment and was "convinced that in the next 150 years, the department can make just as great strides in primary preventive medicine as have been achieved in the last 150 years. I am also convinced that if great care is not taken to avoid placing administration of large curative medical services, hospitals and otherwise, in the hands of the department, it will not be free to do what it should in the many untilled fields of preventive medicine."[13]

One important factor underlying Williams's hesitancy to embrace the expansion of individual health services under public health departments was the extremely conservative stance of Baltimore's physicians, with whom Williams had to maintain positive relations. The American Medical Association, with *Journal of the American Medical Association* editor Morris Fishbein as its most visible spokesman, vehemently opposed New Deal and wartime health programs that increased government involvement in clinical medicine and fostered its cooperation with public health. Fishbein tirelessly warned that "socialized medicine" would undermine the twin pillars of the American private health system, the doctor–patient relationship and fee-for-service practice. While *socialized medicine* commonly referred to national health insurance, the term had many overlapping meanings, ranging from group insurance plans, whether public or private, to all forms of government-sponsored health services. As rural health expert C. Horace Hamilton pointed out, use of the term *socialized medicine* was "designed to decide the issue on the basis of popular prejudice against socialism in general rather than on the basis of facts and logic. If public health care is socialism, then we . . . could just as well speak of socialized highways, socialized education, socialized postal service, or socialized fire protection."[14]

Maryland exemplified the role of state and local politics as catalysts in the development of public health research and training programs. JHSPH faculty and alumni worked with Riley to revise and dramatically expand the state's medical care program for welfare recipients. To convince Maryland physicians that the Department of Health should do more to extend health care to the poorest citizens, Riley argued that a physician-led, state-level program would act as a foil against the threat of national health insurance legislation. He also relied on the strong reputation and persuasive skills of Abel Wolman, whose experience in planning the water and sanitation systems for Baltimore City and the state was excellent preparation to chair the Maryland State Planning Commission. Wolman served on its Committee on Medical Care, which carried out the medical society's request to conduct a comprehensive survey of medical care and facilities and then determine the need for and costs of indigent care. After the committee sent its recommendations to the Maryland General Assembly, Allen Freeman helped to author the enabling legislation and secure its passage in 1945. After he retired from the faculty, Freeman led further legislative reform to enact a major reorganization of the state health department in 1951.[15]

In Maryland and other states, planning for indigent care reflected the priorities of state medical societies and legislatures by minimizing state control and according local health officers and physicians maximum latitude. A history of Maryland's medical care plan later proclaimed, "On the initiative of its doctors, Maryland set out to prove that a state can solve its own health problem without Federal aid or Federal intervention." When representatives of the Committee on Medical Care explained the new plan in 1944 at the annual conference of the Maryland State Department of Health, they stressed the authority of county health officers to develop and administer the program. This feature simultaneously assured physicians and legislators that the plan would not usurp local autonomy even as it incorporated Riley, Wolman, and Freeman's belief that public health should move into the field of medical care. After the war, JHSPH faculty and alumni worked to enact further state health reform, particularly in the areas of mental health and maternal and child health, which reinforced the school's government consulting role and fostered new field training assignments for the growing number of students.[16]

Baltimore City administered its own health department independently of the county-based programs under the aegis of the Maryland Health Department, and the state Medical Care Program excluded Baltimore. In 1944, the Maryland State Committee on Medical Care appointed Lowell Reed to chair the Committee to Study the Medical Care Needs in Baltimore, which recommended that the city's hospitals should establish medical centers to provide home and ambulatory medical care through the integration of hospital outpatient departments, local physician services, and health department clinics. This organization would achieve "a most desirable coordination of medical resources" that "would have a distinct educational value and tend thus to raise the level of medical care for the whole community." Reed's committee also proposed a comprehensive plan for Baltimore City's welfare recipients, including preventive, diagnostic, and therapeutic services, as well as dentistry, nursing, and rehabilitation. The plan was guided by data from JHSPH's monthly home survey of illness in the EHD, conducted among 1,500 families between 1938 and 1943. The Maryland General Assembly appropriated funds to start the program on June 1, 1947, and the BCHD established a Medical Care Section to carry it out.[17]

Yet the EHD itself was changing. In the 1940s, both the Baltimore city and Maryland state health departments enjoyed relatively ample budgets and were in the national vanguard among public health agencies. Under Williams and Riley, both health agencies had contributed personnel and funds toward the support of JHSPH programs such as syphilis and TB control, maternal and child health, and mental hygiene. From 1940 to 1945, JHSPH faculty had published 32 articles based on research in the EHD. At its peak in 1951, the EHD employed a full-time health officer, three part-time health officers, eight support staff, 31 nurses, and a full range of consulting specialists in pediatrics, obstetrics, mental hygiene, and radiology.[18] But the wartime draft and defense industry jobs caused substantial outmigration from the district, which largely invalidated the baseline population data that had been laboriously and expensively collected during the decade before the war. Turner observed in his history of the Johns Hopkins Medical Institutions that the EHD "reflected the growing social instability of large urban centers, and the high hopes entertained that this district would become a teaching area for the School of Hygiene, somewhat analogous to The Johns Hopkins Hospital for the School of Medicine, foundered on the shifting sands of its mobile population."[19]

Under Parran, federal policy had emerged as a powerful instrument for improving both rural and urban health. Yet government interventions outside the realm of health had already begun to distort the racial and economic balance of inner-city communities. Beginning in 1937, the federal Home Owners' Loan Corporation had assigned grades to neighborhoods to determine their suitability for mortgage lending. On the maps of each city in the nation used by banks to process mortgage applications, black and Jewish neighborhoods were color-coded red (known as "redlining") to denote "detrimental influences in a pronounced degree, undesirable population or an infiltration of it." After the war, federal policy underwrote construction costs and mortgage insurance for millions of new homes, as well as for the highways, water and sewer systems, and other infrastructure that promoted suburbanization. Although Reed and other administrators of the medical institutions attempted to foster East Baltimore's redevelopment, their top priority was to relieve cramped conditions and outdated facilities on the campus itself. The redlined environs of the medical campus deteriorated as East Baltimore transitioned from a stable, ethnically diverse, working-class enclave to an impoverished, majority-black district. As the skyline of the medical institutions rose higher with each passing year, the surrounding neighborhood lost more of its social capital as businesses and families left for greener suburban pastures.[20]

Stebbins and Williams Square Off

As the EHD and the school both expanded, competition erupted between Williams and Stebbins over jurisdiction and funding. On the basis of his extensive epidemiological research on syphilis in the EHD, Turner had called the unique collaboration among JHSPH, the Johns Hopkins Hospital syphilis clinic, and the BCHD "one of the most favorable places in the world to study syphilis." But during the war, the PHS had to circumvent Williams to disburse federal funds for VD control training at Hopkins and the University of Maryland. Williams was suspicious of federal control and so protective of the BCHD-run clinics that he had, according to the head of the PHS Venereal Disease Division, "absolutely refused up to the present time to aid any of the excellent unofficial clinics which exist in Baltimore and [the PHS had] been unable to influence him."[21]

Williams and Stebbins held conflicting views on the government's proper role and scope in public health, particularly at the federal level. Stebbins was a protégé of Parran, and while Stebbins was New York City health commissioner, he had also enjoyed the support of Mayor Fiorello LaGuardia, a prolabor advocate of an expanded governmental role in health care and a member of the National Association for the Advancement of Colored People Board of Directors. Stebbins was among the more liberal APHA leaders who advocated a greater role for public health agencies in administering medical care and coordinating private and public health services with those of welfare agencies. TB was the city's top public health problem, causing 3,000 annual deaths. Stebbins supported established control methods such as isolating infectious cases and increasing early diagnosis efforts. He also sought to reduce the city's high TB morbidity and mortality by providing adequate medical care for all TB patients and expanding programs to supply adequate food, housing, and supplemental care. In addition, the New York City Health Department was at the forefront of expanding individual health services through the wartime federal Emergency Maternity and Infant Care Program as well as rapid treatment centers to implement newly available methods of penicillin treatment for syphilis and gonorrhea, supported by an intensive casefinding and follow-up program.[22]

Stebbins had engaged in New York's rough-and-tumble politics and fired people when he thought they deserved it. Under him, New York was the first major city to introduce public education programs on sex and birth control. But in Baltimore, Stebbins was a liberal outsider in a conservative, segregated city that was still not ready for sex education in the public schools. He was the first JHSPH dean who had no personal connection with William Henry Welch, and he lacked experience with the powerful antifederal sentiment and political machines that ruled Baltimore. City health officials and residents punctured the new dean's hopes for a population health laboratory that would serve local health needs while training students and generating cutting-edge scholarship.

In July 1947, the School of Hygiene and the BCHD conducted the fourth and what proved to be the last comprehensive census of the EHD. This would be the most extensive survey ever, since the EHD had been enlarged to encompass a population of 110,000, nearly twice the 60,000 residents of its original square mile. The survey was conducted in the heat of summer by seven full-time private nurses and 80 BCHD nurses working on a part-time basis as their duties permitted, with the assistance of local college students and JHSPH graduate students. Williams informed readers of the *Baltimore Sun* that information collected from the survey "will be of great assistance to the Baltimore City Health Department in setting up the new medical care program which will be inaugurated on September 1, when the newly erected medical care section of the department begins to operate."[23]

The survey provoked unprecedented negative reactions from both BCHD nurses and EHD residents. Two dozen BCHD nurses gathered at a public meeting to complain that participating in the survey was "not a nursing job" and was deterring them from their essential duties in the district. Lilly Jackson, an active NAACP member, came to represent "the colored nurses." In his hand-written notes from the meeting, Williams jotted that the survey was "destroying relations of H[ealth] D[epartment] with people of EHD—they grumble," and he worried that it would also hamper future relations between the city and the health department. One nurse apparently lost her composure during the meeting, and Williams rendered an underlined judgment: "Tears. Relieve her." Under the headline "Nurses Claim Dr. Williams 'Browbeater,'" the *Baltimore Afro-American* reported that "about two dozen irate nurses appeared before the City Council Ways and Means Committee today and charged that Dr. Williams ruled his department with an iron hand and kept the nurses from complaining to the City Service Commission."[24]

Williams had boasted that "nowhere else in the world has a given population been kept under observation for such a long period of time and the impact of diseases, especially those of a chronic nature, on the family studied so carefully." The JHSPH Department of Biostatistics provided each census taker with "Instructions for Enumerators," which specified,

> It will be necessary to go in and out of each alley, passageway or court in the block and to be certain not to miss any person who lives within the block. Particular attention must be paid to the possibility of missing families or single persons who may be living in such places as garages, shacks, basements, and upper floors of public or semi-public buildings. . . . Do not conclude that a place is vacant because no one is at home. A neighbor or landlord should be questioned about it. It must be understood clearly that a schedule must be made for every house, or apartment, whether or not it is being occupied at the time the visit is made.[25]

By 1947, East Baltimore residents were growing weary of the attention. An anonymous postcard informed Williams curtly, "Sir: I want no nurses coming in to ask my family unnecessary questions. Take care of city health and stop wasting time." Another resident called the survey questions a "lot damfool stuff how many wifes how many child how many bath how many toilet, nuts." In an early and forceful example of "maximum feasible participation of the poor," the writer told Williams, "We got some things to ask to. How many branes you got, why you waist our time? All us in my blok, we go gather, ask Mayor Tommy [D'Alesandro] if you crazy, what you get pay for why use tax pairs money, why he don't kick you out." Another resident made a similar threat to "take it up with the Mayor and our councilman to see if he can get us a new health commissioner" and told Williams, "You go count the toilets out in whatever part of town you live in and we will take care of ours," a reference to the detailed survey questions intended to determine the population's living standards by asking about each household's sanitary facilities and plumbing, such as the number of bathtubs and toilets. The writer concluded, "Just because we are poor people we don't have to tell you and your nurses our private business." An East Baltimore woman wrote to object that a BCHD nurse had asked if she had divorced her husband, which offended the woman's Catholic beliefs. She concluded her letter, "You keep nurse way <u>for good</u>. I wont open door."[26]

In the aftermath of the survey, three Epidemiology faculty members who had played key roles in the EHD resigned. Martin Frobisher (ScD 1925), who had directed the EHD Laboratory since it was established in 1932, became founding director of the National Microbiological Institute, and EHD director Harry Chant was named the first head of the Medical Care Clinic at Johns Hopkins Hospital. Alexander Langmuir left in 1949 to direct the Epidemiology Section of the CDC. This left the Department of Epidemiology short-staffed just as Maxcy's health began to fail and qualified faculty were extremely scarce.

For much of the 1950s, the department would narrow its focus almost entirely to polio.[27]

The EHD survey was also a major political blow to Williams, who began to view both JHSPH and the Baltimore City Medical Care Program as sources of major administrative headaches. He now opposed using BCHD clinics for teaching purposes and only allowed Hygiene students to observe rather than treat patients. In a 1949 letter to Mayor D'Alesandro, Williams acknowledged that "sharp differences of opinion between the City Health Department and the School" had arisen regarding "how many students should be permitted to observe and participate in Health Department service clinics," since too many students could "well disturb the service nature of the clinic and turn it into a teaching clinic where the necessary work load is, to some extent, jeopardized." Stebbins and Paul A. Harper (MPH 1947), head of the school's Division of Maternal and Child Health, scrambled to negotiate new field training agreements with the Maryland State Health Department, rural clinics in Anne Arundel and Baltimore counties, and the city and county schools of Baltimore.[28]

Stebbins attempted to win back Williams's support by appointing him as an adjunct professor of public health administration and director of field training, but the move did not improve relations between Hopkins and the EHD. Plans for the new EHD headquarters building were scaled back until Stebbins told Williams in 1949 that it was "more and more apparent that the projected building would provide inadequate space for the full development of the cooperative service and teaching program in which I am sure we are both greatly interested." Stebbins had hoped to duplicate the arrangement he had enjoyed as health commissioner of New York City, where the City Health Department shared a building with the DeLamar Institute of Public Health at Columbia. He pushed for a larger EHD headquarters building located in the same block as the School of Hygiene, with land and additional funds provided by the university, which "would make possible a far closer relationship between the Baltimore City Health Department and the School of Hygiene, and the Eastern Health District could then become a really outstanding example of City and University cooperation for the benefit of the citizens of Baltimore." Stebbins emphasized the benefits for in-service training of BCHD employees and for research in administration that "would result in significant advances in general public health practice that would be of great value to the City of Baltimore and to the country as a whole."[29]

But Williams resisted what he considered the School of Hygiene's smothering influence. In a meeting with Stebbins, Williams opened a map of East Baltimore and traced his finger along a boundary four blocks from all sides of the Johns Hopkins medical campus. He told Stebbins that he would never approve a building inside the line. Under the new $8 million hospital and health center loan approved by Baltimore voters in November 1948, the BCHD favored building on the city-owned block bounded by Bond, Orleans, Bethel, and Jefferson streets. Williams confided to Mayor D'Alesandro, "The experiences of the past fifteen years have shown the City Health Department that it cannot administer the Eastern Health District as part of its normal official city-wide administrative responsibility in a satisfactory manner if the district building is too directly connected by location with the University buildings. The staff psychology, the public psychology and the feeling of the people living in the district, and this applies particularly to the general medical practitioners, white and Negro, living in Wards 4, 5, 6, 7, and 10, which constitute the greater part of the Eastern Health District, is affected by the location of the Health District building." Williams was "convinced, after years of careful study and analysis," that the interests of the BCHD and JHSPH were best served by a healthy degree of physical separation. After George A. Silver (MPH 1948) resigned as EHD director in 1951, the position was vacant for years at a time. Silver would later serve from 1966 to 1968 as Deputy Assistant Secretary for Health and Scientific Affairs.[30]

In spring 1949, another political fiasco added insult to the already injured relationship between the school and the Health Commissioner. The Maryland General Assembly passed the Maryland Subversive Activities Act, known as the Ober Act, which made it a felony to advocate overthrowing the state or federal government "by revolution, force, or violence" and also required city and state employees to affirm that they were not members of any subversive organization, domestic or foreign. One of the Ober Act's first casualties was Miriam Brailey, director of the BCHD Bureau of Tuberculosis. Brailey, a Quaker who advocated interracial cooperation and world peace, called the Ober Act "contrary to the fundamental principles of Christianity" and "a law which persecutes minorities," since the American Communist Party's egalitarian philosophy and rejection of racism attracted many black members. Commissioner Williams had not even read the law yet when Brailey first told him that she would not sign the oath. She wrote to her former student and BCHD colleague Charlotte Silverman (MPH 1942, DrPH 1948), "I laugh that he had the effrontery to insist on giving me a copy of the [Ober Commission] Report. But he is on the spot. He and his lawyer brother are friends of Ober's and believe in suppression of unpopular minority views." Although Brailey believed that Williams "really liked the publicity," she did not think he would actually fire her. Pediatrics chair Edwards Park, Brailey's former boss at the Harriet Lane Home and a frequent Hygiene collaborator, was a sponsor of the Maryland Civil Liberties Committee's campaign against the Ober law, and Brailey noted thankfully, "Good old JHH very friendly."[31]

The *Baltimore Sun* and many prominent citizens rallied in support of Brailey, who told Silverman, "No one is more surprised than I at the remarkable reporting by the *Sun* and the general wide-spread approval." The reformist judge Joseph Sherbow, who presided over the Supreme Bench of Baltimore, gained national attention when he declared the law unconstitutional, but the Maryland Court of Appeals reinstated the law in February 1950. Brailey's colleague Ralph W. Ballin protested to the *Baltimore Sun*, "No Marylander—and that includes Dr. Huntington Williams—has ever had any reason to believe that Dr. Miriam Brailey, the head of the Bureau of Tuberculosis, is a Communist or has any Communist leanings." Calling Brailey "a nationally known authority" whose "services to the city have been invaluable," Ballin criticized the Ober Act for threatening "to rob the citizens of Baltimore of one of their most valuable servants." On March 26, 1950, Williams fired Brailey, who filed a lawsuit against the city of Baltimore to contest the law. Brailey lost the case after the Maryland Supreme Court upheld the Ober Act, which prompted Stebbins and Kenneth Maxcy to invite her to rejoin the Epidemiology full-time faculty in early 1951 as an assistant professor with joint appointments in Pediatrics and Medicine. Yet not until 1969 did decisions by the US Supreme Court and Maryland District Court void the Ober Act as unconstitutional.[32]

The politics of McCarthyism was but one of the points of contention between Williams and Stebbins. Another was the proper role of public health departments in providing personal health services and whether to accept federal and state aid to support expanding those services. In 1953, the APHA Committee on Professional Education acknowledged the changing nature of public health practice by changing the title of the Subcommittee on Field Training to the Subcommittee on Clinical Training. In addition, the APHA committees on State Health Administration, chaired by Maryland State Health Commissioner Robert Riley, and Administrative Practice, which included Paul Harper and Paul Lemkau from JHSPH, formally revised the responsibilities of state health departments to include civil defense and disaster response, rehabilitation of disabled persons, and the early diagnosis of chronic as well as communicable diseases. Preventive measures were broadened to include arresting the progress of disease as well as its onset, thereby incorporating curative treatment. In the Committee on Administrative Practice's organizational plan prototype, state health departments could consider adding divisions of mental health, dental health, social work, alcoholism, chronic disease, and medical care, according to the specific needs of their populations. A primary duty of the state health department was to plan and evaluate the programs of state and local agencies as well as to coordinate the efforts of all voluntary and professional organizations involved in public health.[33]

As their responsibilities expanded, state health departments did receive increased appropriations in nearly all states, but the largest and wealthiest states increasingly outpaced the rest in regard to salaries, quality and range of services, and adaptability to change. For example, from 1942 to 1957, the state health department budget for New York rose from $5 million to $55 million, and in Maryland, it rose from $1 million to $22 million. The main source of financial strain on state and county health departments was increased responsibilities and population growth alongside modest increases in funding. But the perception of hard times in public health agencies was also relative to the unprecedented postwar expansion of real wages, particularly in the fields of medicine and industry in direct competition with public health. Overall federal public health spending increased, both within the PHS and in agencies such as the Office of Vocational Rehabilitation, Food and Drug Administration, and Children's Bureau.[34]

In many ways, local health departments struggled most, particularly in declining urban areas, as they stretched their budgets and attempted to recruit qualified personnel with unattractively low salaries. A 1956 National Health Council survey of community health officials identified adequate financial support as by far the most important need. Between 1950 and 1970, suburbanization depopulated the nation's largest cities and eroded their tax bases, which was particularly pronounced in Baltimore. A PHS regional medical director identified the changing mission of local health departments "from their traditional role of providing direct services to a relatively small segment of the population to one of acting as a catalyst for all community services that have a health role: i.e., hospitals, physicians, voluntary health agencies," yet this more expansive responsibility coincided with shrinking resources for many municipalities. The EHD budget was slashed from its 1951 peak of $132,165 (including $15,150 from JHSPH) to $58,100 by 1961. The reduction was even more severe, considering that the district had been enlarged from 110,000 residents in 1950 to include over 333,000 residents in a 24.2 square mile area by 1957.[35]

In 1954, the city finally completed a modest two-story building for the EHD on Caroline Street, four blocks from JHSPH (and outside Williams's proclaimed boundary). The Somerset Health Center, opened with such fanfare a decade before to serve the needs of black East Baltimore residents, was closed and the city consolidated and desegregated the EHD clinics in the new building. The JHSPH Division of Mental Hygiene moved into the new structure, but Williams's desire for separation had, in general, prevailed over Stebbins's hopes for cooperation. John Black Grant (DrPH 1921) of the Rockefeller Foundation noted in 1958, "Apparently, the usefulness of the Eastern Health District [to the School of Hygiene] has markedly deteriorated, partly because of relations with Dr. Huntington Williams, and also because of the mediocre quality of the present director."[36]

In 1956, Williams described the Baltimore City Health Department as "crumbling." He also found that his political power was waning when he opposed the city council's attempts to pass legislation on issues such as compulsory polio vaccination and lead paint labeling. Councilman Richard D. Byrd charged that Williams rejected any proposal that did not originate in his office, and the *Baltimore Sun* proclaimed that the council was "in a general revolt against the city health commissioner." The city Board of Estimates demanded to know why the Health Department was "flat on its back," which Williams blamed on vacancies in key positions that could not be filled due to low salaries, especially for physicians to direct bureaus and to staff clinics. He asked the city for substantial raises for health department staff, but Charles L. Benton, the city's budget director, and other members of an investigative subcommittee confronted Williams about why he had not taken steps to qualify for an estimated $1 million in available federal and state aid for local health services. In the 1930s, the state had originally subsidized newly established county health departments with Social Security Act funding to raise them to the level of services in Baltimore City, but after the city's fortunes began to falter, Williams had delayed seeking outside assistance that might threaten the BCHD's autonomy.[37]

In response to growing concern over Williams's administration, Stebbins chaired special committees appointed by Mayor D'Alesandro in 1956 to study the administrative structure of the Baltimore City Health Department and by Maryland Governor Theodore McKeldin in 1957 to investigate the financing of local health services in Maryland, particularly in regard to problems surrounding state aid to Baltimore City. The recommendations of Stebbins's committees resulted in a major reorganization of the BCHD and its administration of the state Medical Care Plan. The reorganization reduced the authority of the health commissioner by creating four major divisions headed by assistant commissioners. Mayor D'Alesandro had delayed reappointing Williams until he saw Stebbins's report, and in 1958, Williams capitulated to accepting state aid for local health services in Baltimore City. Williams retired in 1961 after 30 years as health commissioner of Baltimore. From 1931 to 1947, everything had seemed to go his way, but during the second half of his tenure, he had watched both his power and the health department budget decline.[38]

Public Health Administration

Maternal and child health, TB, VD, and mental health had been the focal points of Stebbins's wartime leadership of the New York City Health Department. At JHSPH, he applied this experience to his leadership of PHA from 1946 to 1961. Before the war, collaboration between schools of medicine and public health had centered on basic science research with broad applications for infectious disease; after the war, collaboration shifted to the clinic, which also opened new research and field training opportunities for JHSPH. New

TABLE 4.1
MPH Specialty Programs Established at JHSPH, 1938–1954

MPH Specialty	Year Established	Sponsor
Venereal Disease Control	1938	Rockefeller Foundation/US Public Health Service
Mental Hygiene	1941	US Public Health Service (later NIMH)
Hospital Administration	1947	Kellogg Foundation
Vertebrate Ecology	1947	US Public Health Service
Maternal and Child Health	1948	US Children's Bureau
School Health	1949	US Children's Bureau
Audiology and Speech	1949	US Children's Bureau
Tuberculosis Control	1949	National Tuberculosis Association
Environmental Medicine	1950	US Public Health Service/US Air Force
Public Health Nursing	1950	US Public Health Service
Chronic Diseases	1954	US Public Health Service
Effects of Housing on Health	1954	US Public Health Service

state and federal categorical health programs underwrote the establishment or expansion of a wave of specialized MPH tracks and divisions (table 4.1), most of which were based in PHA. Stebbins, the last dean to also chair a department, made PHA an engine of growth and innovation that showcased the best new methods in public health teaching and practice.

The composition of the JHSPH faculty and curriculum changed accordingly, and the number of hours MPH students spent in the laboratory slowly declined to accommodate material from outside the basic sciences. The percentage of elective hours allotted to public health administration courses at Hopkins increased from 15 percent in 1936 to nearly 40 percent by 1954. Among schools of public health nationally, this subject captured the largest number of hours in course schedules. Biostatistics was second, followed by environmental sanitation, microbiology, hospital administration, public health education, epidemiology, and parasitology–tropical public health.[39]

Despite the strong growth of basic science research funding in the departments of Biochemistry, Environmental Medicine, Epidemiology, and Microbiology, they were dwarfed by the least basic science–oriented department, PHA, in terms of research as well as faculty size and enrollment (table 4.2). Under Stebbins, PHA mushroomed from only two faculty in 1936 to three senior and 17 junior faculty by 1954, all of whom taught in the MPH program. At most schools of public health, the MPH was awarded on a departmental basis; at Hopkins, it remained a schoolwide degree. Students in the introductory PHA course devoted nine hours each week to solving real-world problems, such as setting up a record system and plan of fiscal and office management for a local unit servicing a population of 50,000, evaluating Washington

County's health needs and programs and presenting recommendations for their future development, outlining a health department program for accident prevention, or developing a plan for hospital–health department relationships in a governmental unit.[40]

During the postwar surge of cooperation among the Johns Hopkins Medical Institutions, one of Stebbins's first moves as dean had been collaborating with Edwin L. Crosby, director of the Johns Hopkins Hospital, to found the graduate hospital administration program in 1947 with a grant from the Kellogg Foundation. During the first third of the twentieth century, the profession of hospital administration had shifted from female graduate nurses to male nonphysicians. Beginning with the first graduate program in hospital administration established by Michael M. Davis at the University of Chicago in 1934, most schools drew upon existing accounting, business management, and public administration techniques and focused on the needs of the community voluntary hospital.[41]

The Hopkins hospital administration program was unique in several respects. It maintained the characteristic Hopkins emphasis on training physicians for "the role of the future, the public health officer-hospital administrator," a hybrid for which Stebbins and Crosby anticipated increasing demand as communities across the country integrated their public health and medical care programs. The hospital administration MPH track, therefore, required an MD or

TABLE 4.2
Evolution of JHSPH Departments, 1936–1954

1936	No. Faculty	1954	No. Faculty
Bacteriology	5	Renamed Microbiology in 1951	9
Biochemistry	5	Biochemistry	5
Biology	4	Dissolved in 1940	0
Biostatistics	2	Biostatistics	5
Epidemiology	5	Epidemiology	3
Immunology	4	Dissolved in 1946	0
Helminthology	2	Merged to form Parasitology in 1942	4
Protozoology and Medical Entomology	2		
Physiological Hygiene	1	Reorganized as Environmental Medicine in 1950	6
Public Health Administration	2	Public Health Administration	20
Sanitary Engineering	2	Sanitary Engineering	2
Total	34		54

a background in biology, chemistry, and physics, as well as previous public health experience. After Crosby left in 1952 to direct the newly founded Joint Commission on Accreditation of Hospitals, the hospital administration program was a relatively low priority for his successor, Russell A. Nelson, who considered Hygiene a minor player within the Hopkins medical institutions.[42]

Stebbins established the Division of Hospital Administration in 1952 under the full-time direction of Paul A. Lembcke, who published some of the earliest research analyzing medical outcomes among hospital patients. In January 1955, the Commission on University Education in Hospital Administration, which was sponsored by the Kellogg Foundation and the Association of University Programs in Hospital Administration, conducted a site visit at Johns Hopkins. The evaluation team opened their report by rejecting the program's core assumptions that hospitals were "a major public health resource" or that a significant number would ever be run by health officers. The report's authors insisted that hospital administration should be taught in schools of business administration since hospitals were "a form of business enterprise organized to achieve certain social goals." The evaluators also alleged that schools of public health with "a desire to capitalize the opportunities to get promising students" had created experimental hospital administration programs that produced graduates for whom there was "no tangible market demand." Three-quarters of the JHSPH hospital administration students were over age 35, which the accreditation report described as "elderly."[43]

According to the Commission on University Education in Hospital Administration, the negative influence of a public health philosophy was "without question most noticeable in the Johns Hopkins program," whose curriculum penalized students by training them in the core public health disciplines rather than in practical management. One graduate of the program agreed, rating it "weak and unsatisfactory," and urged the school to "either develop or abandon the program." After the damning evaluation of the hospital administration program, the department continued to offer two courses, but Stebbins quietly eliminated the division and Lembcke spent a year in the Philippines at the Institute of Hygiene.[44]

A few months after the hospital administration site visit, JHSPH biostatistician Margaret Merrell chaired a subcommittee of the Applications and Curriculum Committee that surveyed alumni opinion on how to improve the MPH program. The subcommittee concluded "that our program was not leading or even keeping up with the public health field, that our science courses needed sharper focus, that sociology, philosophy of public health, and modern principles of administration should be presented." Its most serious criticism was "that the actual teaching receives such casual consideration within the multiplicity of staff activities, that it is not of the quality worthy of a graduate school." Students and alumni also requested the Department of PHA to incorporate modern management principles into its courses and suggested introducing instruction in public relations, personnel issues, and methods of organizing and implementing programs in research and community outreach.[45]

The two 1955 reports identified problem areas that were echoed by students, faculty, and outside observers' evaluations of the MPH program in general, including admissions requirements, age and composition of students, and the curriculum's lack of relevance to current practice. Perhaps the first skirmish in the coming war to reform the MPH curriculum was over the ideal quantity and quality of basic science courses for physicians who would not be primarily engaged in laboratory research. Beginning with the PHS's 1941 request to exempt its officers in the MPH mental hygiene specialty track from bacteriology, there was increasing pressure to reduce the amount of time devoted to the basic sciences, particularly lab work, to make room for public health administration and other emerging fields.

The hospital administration program had attempted to forge new cooperative relationships between JHSPH and the hospital and medical school, but the PHA Division of Maternal and Child Health succeeded in reaching this goal, while also weaving in the surviving community health threads from the EHD. The division was underwritten by the Children's Bureau, which from its creation in 1912 until the mid-1960s was the single most important agency leading the development and implementation of federal maternal and child health policy. Under SS Title V, the Children's Bureau administered federal matching grants for maternal and child health and disabled children's services, which became the largest category of clinical services administered by state and local health departments. Congress consistently increased appropriations for these programs, which grew from $19 million in 1950 to more than $87 million by 1966–1967. During this period, federal aid to maternal and child health (including handicapped children) was second only to hospital construction among federal health grants to states.[46]

Some historians and analysts have cast the 1950s as a period of declension and crisis in public health, characterized by declining federal, state, and local support for general health services as well as formidable new challenges in the areas of chronic diseases and medical care administration. Furthermore, they allege that Congress reduced the autonomy of health departments by favoring appropriations for categorical programs rather than increasing general public health grants. To be sure, many public health professionals, whether in leadership or on the front lines, exhibited signs of demoralization and malaise. Yet a closer analysis of patterns in public health training, employment, spending, and programming yields a more complicated but positive picture. For the major public health disciplines of mental hygiene and maternal and

TABLE 4.3

Federal and State Contributions to Public Health Spending, 1935, 1950, and 1964
(in Millions of US Dollars)

	1935			1950			1964		
	Federal	State/Local	Total	Federal	State/Local	Total	Federal	State/Local	Total
Maternal/child health[1]	0	7	7	20	10	30	59	151	209
School health	0	10	10	0	31	31	0	160	160
Other public health	7	112	119	68	291	359	224	395	619
Total	7	119	136	88	332	420	283	706	988

Source: Congress and the Nation 1945–1964 (Congressional Quarterly, 1965), 1114.
[1] Includes programs for physically disabled children.

child health, the 1950s was a decade of remarkable growth and innovation, at Johns Hopkins and nationally.[47]

In 1950, the congressional appropriation for PHS grants to states for general public health work was already at an all-time high. President Harry Truman unsuccessfully proposed to nearly double the amount to strengthen existing public health services and extend coverage to unserved areas. Although the appropriation plateaued at the 1950 level for several more years, by 1960 it had increased past the level that Truman had requested. Meanwhile, total federal public health spending (excluding facilities construction, medical research, and medical care programs) increased from $7 million in 1935 to $88 million in 1950 and had reached $283 million by 1964 (table 4.3). Total state and local spending for public health also rose substantially, roughly tripling from 1935 to 1950 and then doubling again by 1964, but the federal share of funds steadily mounted throughout the period. Two of the fastest-growing federal public health agencies were the US Children's Bureau and the National Institute of Mental Health (NIMH), which both provided essential support for corresponding Johns Hopkins medical and public health departments (table 4.4).[48]

Elaine Tyler May has observed that "procreation during the cold war era took on almost mythic proportions" because "the fundamental principle of postwar parenthood [was that] children were a 'defense—and impregnable bulwark' against the terrors of the age." In this context, maternal and child health achieved new political, economic, and social significance. Birthrates among American women had declined by nearly one-third between 1920 and 1940, but with the postwar baby boom, the birthrate first topped 4 million in 1954 and remained at that level for the next decade. By 1960, the birthrate had reached a twentieth-century high of 3.6 births per woman, and over one-third of Americans were under age 18. As postwar rates of hospital insurance rose

TABLE 4.4
Federal Funding for Public Health Programs, 1950–1964 (in Millions of US Dollars)

	1950	1955	1960	1964
Grants to states				
General	14.1	13.1	24.7	14.0
Maternal and child health	11.2	11.9	17.4	27.3
Crippled children	7.6	10.6	17.1	27.7
Venereal disease	12.4	3.0	6.4	5.9
Tuberculosis	6.8	6.0	5.3	2.9
Environmental sanitation	1.0	3.7	2.7	4.5
Mental health	3.3	2.3	4.9	6.7
Cancer	3.2	2.2	2.2	3.4
Heart disease	1.8	1.1	2.9	6.1
Alaska	1.3	1.2	0	0
Chronic diseases	0	0	0	11.6
Radiological health	0	0	0	1.8
PHS grants to states (excluding construction)	62.7	55.1	83.6	111.9
Hill–Burton hospital construction	57.1	74.6	143.4	152.0
Non–Hill–Burton construction	0	0	46.8	90.0
PHS grants to states (all sources)	119.8	129.7	273.8	353.9
Communicable Disease Center	7.5	4.6	8.7	8.4
Vocational rehabilitation	24.7	25.6	48.6	87.6
Total	152	159.9	331.1	449.9

Source: Annual Reports of the Federal Security Administration (1950) and the Department of Health, Education, and Welfare (1955, 1960, 1964).

rapidly, hospital deliveries became the norm and communities mobilized to raise Hill–Burton matching funds to build new general hospitals with modern new pediatric and obstetrical units as well as special children's hospitals. Pediatrics as a medical specialty achieved new status by guiding anxious parents striving to raise healthy, well-adjusted children, and funding increased for medical research on children's diseases such as polio, leukemia, sickle cell anemia, and birth defects.[49]

Beginning in 1939, universities and health agencies could apply for SS Title V grants without matching requirements to support special projects in maternal and child health, including training, research, and hospitalization of premature infants and women with complications of pregnancy. Congress doubled appropriations for these grants in 1946 in response to the positive results achieved by the wartime Emergency Maternity and Infant Care program, and the increased funding enabled schools of public health to launch new research and training programs. In 1947, JHSPH received one of the four inaugural Title V training grants awarded to the schools of public health at Johns Hopkins, Harvard, University of California–Berkeley, and University of North Carolina.[50]

As the school's enrollment steadily rose, the EHD could no longer meet students' need for field training sites. In 1939, Parran and Farrand had expressed disappointment that the EHD was "less useful than anticipated in giving practical training in public health administration." The report observed critically, "We were impressed at Johns Hopkins, as at Harvard, by the inadequacy of the opportunity for practical training in public health administration offered by these Schools. It is a most difficult task, yet one of the most essential in public health teaching." Paul A. Harper, head of the Division Maternal and Child Hygiene, would make great strides in expanding practice placement opportunities for all JHSPH students.[51]

In the medical school, Pediatrics chair Robert Cooke became Harper's strategic ally in fostering joint teaching programs. Cooke rebuilt his department to establish Pediatrics as a champion of underprivileged and developmentally disabled children. He also revamped the residency program and encouraged residents to embrace careers in public health as well as scientific and clinical paths. Cooke and Harper built an advanced doctoral training program in Maternal and Child Health (MCH), and Harper established research and teaching agreements with the health departments of Baltimore City and the surrounding counties of Baltimore, Anne Arundel, Calvert, Carroll, and Montgomery. MCH students also did field placements in the Maryland Department of Health under the supervision of Edward Davens, chief of the Bureau of Maternal and Child Health. Collaboration with a broad range of health agencies became a permanent hallmark of the program, and a 1975 self-study noted that city, county, state, and national health program administrators "actively participate[d] in the instructional activities of the Department" by teaching courses and supervising fieldwork.[52]

To complement the growing number of clinical programs such as MCH, mental hygiene, and audiology and speech, Stebbins made it a top priority for PHA to establish a Division of Public Health Nursing, headed by Ruth Benson Freeman from 1950 to 1971. Students and faculty collaborated extensively with Freeman, who began her career as a visiting public health nurse in New York City, and then taught at New York University and the University of Minnesota School of Public Health before serving as administrator of nursing services for the American Red Cross during the critical period from 1946 to 1950. Among many leadership and consulting positions, Freeman served as president of the National League for Nursing and the National Health Council, as well as a member of the PHS Public Health Nursing study section. In APHA, she served on the executive board, governing council, and *American Journal of Public Health* editorial board. Freeman frequently advised agencies such as the US Air Force, WHO, NIH, and Rockefeller Foundation Division of Medical and Natural Sciences.[53]

After Freeman's arrival, the Division of Mental Hygiene applied for NIMH training grants for psychiatric education and nursing education, and the division began to enroll more nurses. Many had worked in the EHD and contributed to the school's studies of maternal and child health and mental hygiene. By 1952, the majority of public health administration courses dealt with clinical medical care programs in nursing, maternal and child health, mental hygiene, and venereal disease. Freeman observed that such programs reflected an increasing "emphasis on health problems that require individualized rather than mass treatment [and] necessitated the use of a multi-disciplinary professional group in planning and effectuation of health programs." She complained to Stebbins in 1952 that "none of the courses currently given provide a satisfactory orientation" to fields such as nursing, social work, nutrition, or health education, so she developed a new course, "Non-Medical Professional Services in Health Agencies." These fields were dominated by nonphysicians and women who graduated from the practice-oriented state schools, not Johns Hopkins, whose Department of Biochemistry produced cutting-edge research on nutrition but did not train nutritionists for schools and public health agencies. Freeman and Stebbins also worked together to create a joint orientation course that acquainted public health administrators, hospital administrators, and public health nurses with recent developments in TB, VD, mental health, and maternal and child health, presenting them as a related whole.[54]

Freeman collaborated with Marcia Mann Cooper (ScD 1947) in the Division of Mental Hygiene, who also promoted interdisciplinary research and training. Cooper directed the EHD Mothers Advisory Service, which brought psychiatrists, public health nurses, and medical social workers together to offer practical childrearing advice and support mothers in addressing their children's behavior problems. Child guidance clinics using interdisciplinary teams had their roots in the diagnostic outpatient clinics established for mentally disturbed juveniles at the turn of the twentieth century in cities such as Boston, Chicago, and Philadelphia. By 1930, there were more than 200 child guidance clinics registered with the National Committee for Mental Hygiene.[55]

The Mothers Advisory Service received referrals from local physicians and all the childcare agencies in Baltimore City as well as many across the state. By the 1950s, the Mothers Advisory Service was one of the few remaining threads of the school's relationship with the EHD, and Cooper moved into assisting clinics and social agencies in evaluating children with special needs and placing them for foster care and adoption. Cooper's multidisciplinary team from the Division of Mental Hygiene, Baltimore City Schools, the School Health Division of the City Health Department, and the Johns Hopkins Hospital departments of Child Psychiatry, Neurology, and Otology also helped coordinate the medical and educational needs of children with brain injury or communication handicaps, including screenings for participation in experimental classes.[56]

Ruth Freeman and Marcia Cooper challenged gender and disciplinary barriers in the physician-centric culture of Hopkins to fulfill the Parran–Farrand Report's charge to provide unified training to all types of public health workers. With the growth of local outreach programs like the Mothers Advisory Service, maternal and child health services became the largest clinical component of most public health departments. Although still grounded in pediatrics and obstetrics, maternal and child health had broadened to include other clinical specialties involved in the care of handicapped children. Public health nurses remained central to the field, but social workers played an increasingly critical role.[57]

Along with research units like the Mothers Advisory Service, visiting professors and speakers were another facet of the school's relationships with the outside world. Stebbins seemed to know everyone in the world of public health, and he enlivened the school with a steady parade of prominent public health figures. In 1954–1955, for example, JHSPH hosted public lectures by Ernst Leopold Abramson, director of the National Institute of Public Health in Sweden; the microbiologist René J. Dubos of the Rockefeller Institute for Medical Research; geneticist Boris Ephurssi of the University of Paris; and APHA executive secretary Reginald Atwater. Students could interact with visiting lecturers such as Jerome Cornfield of the NIH Office of Biometry; Joseph A. Bell, chief of epidemiology for the NIH Laboratory of Infectious Diseases; and Marcelino Pascua, director of Health Statistics for the WHO.[58]

By the early 1960s, Hygiene graduates from the Reed and Stebbins era headed the national health agencies of India, Thailand, Venezuela, El Salvador, and Puerto Rico. They directed the PHS divisions of Nursing, Venereal Disease, and International Health as well as the CDC sections on Epidemiology, Health Services Training, and Parasitology and Mycology. At NIH, they headed the Tropical Diseases Laboratory and the institutes devoted to allergy and infectious diseases, heart disease, and mental health. In foundations, they served as associate director of the Rockefeller Division of Medicine and Natural Sciences, Asia representative for the Population Council, and director of the National Foundation's Division of Congenital Malformations. JHSPH alumni led the Pennsylvania Department of Health and the bureaus of medical rehabilitation and heart disease in New York State, the chronic disease section in Missouri, the VD control and handicapped children's divisions in South Carolina, and the Bureau of Vector Control in California.[59]

The Social Determinants of Health and Developmental Disabilities

Domestic and international programs to improve maternal and child health during the twentieth century shared many important features but also highlighted differences in resources, national attitudes toward gender and professional roles, and patterns of health system organization. The early public health campaigns in the American South and Latin America were disease focused and did not specifically target young children. The New Deal made some advances in improving maternal and infant mortality rates, particularly through health department programs to provide contraceptive, prenatal, and well-child services and to educate midwives on safe delivery and neonatal care. The golden age of child health in the United States began in the late 1930s with the development of effective antibiotics, followed by the introduction of the DPT vaccine in 1942 by Pearl Kendrick (ScD 1932) and Grace Eldering (ScD 1942) and the success of the 1954 Salk polio vaccine trials. Before World War II, many North American maternal and child health programs had been closely allied with family planning and social work, but the three fields subsequently developed into increasingly separate specialties. Developing countries would not undertake broad pediatric immunization campaigns for several decades, and immunization rates remain dismally low in some areas even today. For example, a 2011 study by JHSPH researchers found that in Sierra Leone, 31 percent of the population has never received measles vaccination; in Madagascar, the figure is 21 percent.[60]

US infant mortality had declined significantly during the 1930s and 1940s, but the rates for deaths during the first 24 hours of life had remained virtually unchanged. Virginia Apgar (MPH 1959) came to JHSPH to work with Harper on the problem of perinatal mortality. Apgar, a professor of anesthesiology at the Columbia University College of Physicians and Surgeons, was an expert in obstetrical anesthesiology who had attended over 17,000 births. In the early 1950s, she had developed and applied the Apgar score (table 4.5), calculated by adding subscores for five physiological measures, to evaluate the condition of newborn infants and determine the need for resuscitation. The Apgar score also served as a standard for comparing the effects on newborns of different types of maternal pain management and delivery practices. Her coursework in biostatistics sharpened quantitative skills that were essential for her scoring studies.[61]

During her year in the MPH maternal and child health track, Apgar led a seminar on perinatal problems, particularly the causes, diagnosis, and management of fetal asphyxia, a common cause of death. She emphasized that "the highest death rate during viable human life occurs from the onset of labor to two days after birth." Among surviving infants, delivery complications caused serious and often unknown levels of tissue damage to the brain, heart, lungs, kidneys, liver, and endocrine glands. Apgar urged public health officials to join in "a concerted effort to correct the errors in the conduct of labor and delivery and the immediate care of the newborn infant." Not until 1968 would MCH offer an advanced course in Growth and Development of the Fetus and Newborn, taught by Pediatrics faculty. In the 1970s, a course in Neonatal and Infant Health Care was introduced as part of the JHSPH nurse–midwifery curriculum.[62]

After conducting thousands of evaluations of newborns, Apgar had gained significant experience with congenital defects, and at Hopkins she began to explore further their connections with conditions of pregnancy, such as hydramnios (excessive volume of amniotic fluid), which was associated with certain types of birth defects. The School of Hygiene also taught her more about the incidence of birth defects and the public health approach to preventing and managing them on a population basis. In her subsequent research, she correlated infants' Apgar scores with cases of congenital disabilities to investigate how they might be prevented or ameliorated through early identification of potential risks. After graduating in 1959, Apgar accepted a position with the National Foundation–March of Dimes as the first chief of its new Division of Congenital Malformations, where she became an early authority on teratology, the study of birth defects. Only one year before Apgar died in 1974, the Department of Epidemiology appointed her a lecturer in medical genetics.[63]

Apgar came to JHSPH at the high tide of research on the relationships among maternal factors during pregnancy, labor, and delivery; premature birth and fetal loss; and congenital and developmental disabilities. Joint Medicine–Hygiene research on maternal and child health focused on two main areas: identifying and reducing the risks associated with pregnancy, labor, and delivery and comparing normal versus abnormal mental and physical development in children from birth onward. This research built on the statistical and methodological foundation of the earlier EHD studies of the physical and mental health of mothers and children. Using the extensive data from the EHD

TABLE 4.5
Apgar Score

	0	1	2
Heart rate	Absent	<100 per minute	100–140 per minute
Respiration	Absent	Irregular	Strong, crying
Reflex	Absent	Weak	Grimace, sneeze
Muscle tone	Flaccid	Some flexion	Strong flexion
Color	Blue	Extremities blue	Pink

Source: "Obstetric Anesthesia and a Scorecard for Newborns, 1949–1958," Virginia Apgar Papers, National Library of Medicine Profiles in Science (http://profiles.nlm.nih.gov/ps/retrieve/Narrative /CP/p-nid/181, accessed June 16, 2013).

Family Studies, JHSPH faculty published a series of journal articles that constitute an important early contribution to biostatistics and population studies of disease (appendix B). The EHD data were also used in longitudinal studies of chronic disease and disability by prominent non-Hopkins researchers such as Jean Downes and Selwyn D. Collins of the NIH Division of Public Health Methods.[64]

One of the most influential yet unacknowledged concepts advanced in these articles is that the family is an essential unit of public health research, an idea championed by Wade Hampton Frost. He wrote that epidemiology must pursue "a more systematic, detailed and critical study of the relation of morbidity and mortality not to the broad conditions, but to the intimate details of the community, domestic and individual life." Drawing on the EHD Family Studies, biostatistician Margaret Merrell noted in 1952 that "the variety of structural patterns that we recognize as families, and the alteration of these patterns with the flow of time, make the problem [of defining and classifying the family unit] difficult, particularly in follow-up studies such as those involved in chronic disease." Moreover, the variation among the members of each family further complicated "the job of selecting appropriate measurements and classification for individuals." Given these difficulties, most epidemiological studies analyzed disease rates among individuals without attempting to link the data by family unit. Merrell noted that even in studies of secondary attack rates of infectious diseases among family members of infected individuals, "the family is only a selecting and primary sorting mechanism [so that] both classification and analysis are on an individual basis."[65]

Yet since community epidemics were often actually "the summation of little family epidemics," Merrell argued that analysis by family units, despite its challenges, was "far more illuminating" and went "to the heart of the epidemic problem." The specific research aims of family studies would require varying criteria for family membership, such as "common shelter and provision of food regardless of relationship, blood relations who have a common dwelling unit, the group covered by a medical insurance plan, or, as in genetic studies, certain blood relations regardless of place of residence or even whether living or dead." Thus, Merrell's flexible definition of family contrasted with the standard cultural norm of the 1950s nuclear family, composed of a married couple (a male breadwinner and housewife) and their children.[66]

The families who were the subjects of this intensive research in PHA were also the clients of an expanding public health and social services system. As noted in chapter 2, Baltimore during the 1950s was undergoing profound demographic and economic shifts. Many of the archival photographs depicting the Mother's Advisory Service and the maternal and child health clinics of the EHD show white students and faculty observing or caring for African-

American women and children. With only token numbers of black students and no black faculty appointed until 1963, JHSPH had become a white institution in a majority-black neighborhood.[67]

Early health services researchers analyzed data from private prepaid group plans such as the United Mine Workers and Kaiser-Permanente and from public plans such as the Health Insurance Plan of Greater New York. Unlike these better-known examples, the cooperative research conducted by Johns Hopkins and the BCHD on the Baltimore City Medical Care Program emphasized the urban roots of health services research as a public policy response of city and state governments to postwar demographic and economic changes such as suburbanization and the resulting concentration of inner-city poverty. The Baltimore studies also revealed the politically and racially charged nature of the attempts to control costs and change physician behavior yet also deliver better patient care.[68]

Early twentieth-century explanations of the causes of fetal and neonatal mortality as well as serious abnormalities in surviving infants had focused on brain damage caused by obstetrical trauma during delivery. At midcentury, investigators emphasized fetal asphyxia and anoxia as well as the role of maternal factors such as rubella, Rh factor, bleeding, and toxemia (preeclampsia). Many congenital neurological conditions, such as cerebral palsy and epilepsy, were thought to be hereditary, and little was known about the distribution of birth defects in the population or their long-term effects on development. Scientific racism remained influential, and many medical researchers attributed the higher reported rates of mental retardation and behavioral disorders among black children to biological racial inferiority.[69]

The work of PHA faculty to measure and ameliorate the health effects of urban poverty dovetailed with some of the earliest and most comprehensive studies conducted on the origins of developmental disabilities by epidemiologist Abraham M. Lilienfeld, biostatistician Rowland V. Rider (ScD 1947), pediatricians Paul A. Harper and Hilda Knobloch in the PHA Division of Maternal and Child Health, and psychiatrists Benjamin Pasamanick and Paul V. Lemkau in the PHA Division of Mental Hygiene. Taken together, these studies must be considered among the school's most far-reaching contributions to public health research. JHSPH research on the relationships among pregnancy complications, premature birth, and child development shared three characteristics. The studies used innovative methodology that helped to establish the etiology and incidence of several poorly understood congenital conditions. Carefully planned, large-scale case-control studies highlighted race and socioeconomic status as critical factors in both initial damage to the fetus or infant and in the child's subsequent development. Finally, in both their publications and advisory roles to health officials and policymakers, JHSPH faculty emphasized the broad preventive applications of their research for policy and practice.

After finishing an MPH at Hopkins in 1949, Lilienfeld had worked under Morton Levin in the New York State Department of Health to establish an innovative program of epidemiological and medical research, professional training, and clinical services for cerebral palsy. The New York State survey constituted the first epidemiological study of cerebral palsy in the world. It was also one of the earliest to use record linkage, a technique developed by JHSPH in the EHD, to unite different types of birth, clinical, and epidemiological data to deepen the understanding of a disease. Lilienfeld and E. Parkhurst reported in 1951 that cerebral palsy was positively associated with certain abnormal events during pregnancy and parturition, which also resulted in higher rates of stillbirth and neonatal death. Lilienfeld and Pasamanick had worked together on establishing the record-linking portion of the study, and in 1950, they both left New York to join the JHSPH faculty in PHA.[70]

Lilienfeld, Pasamanick, and Pasamanick's doctoral student Martha E. Rogers (ScD 1952), a registered nurse and NIMH fellow, posited a "continuum of reproductive casualty" extending from conception through the perinatal period that encompassed all forms of fetal death and disability. Lilienfeld's team was among the first group of researchers to explore in large, case-controlled studies how complications of pregnancy affected the viability of the fetus in utero and during and immediately after delivery. The studies differentiated between genetic and nongenetic factors (maternal, environmental, socioeconomic, and iatrogenic) and emphasized that certain maternal complications more frequently resulted in premature birth, which in turn was associated with congenital defects and behavioral disorders. Whereas previous public health efforts had been primarily directed at reducing maternal and infant mortality, Lilienfeld and his coauthors called for a new public health emphasis on the causes and prevention of maternal and fetal morbidity, since they were "also related to certain neuropsychiatric disorders [including epilepsy, cerebral palsy, mental retardation, and behavioral problems] which are in themselves important public health problems."[71]

Whereas Lilienfeld focused on complications during the prenatal and perinatal period, Pasamanick and his wife Hilda Knobloch investigated the long-term behavioral effects of maternal and birth complications by examining infants and young children, with special attention to the role of the family's race and socioeconomic status. In his early research on black infants in New Haven, Connecticut, and New York City's Harlem neighborhood, Pasamanick had disputed theories of racial inferiority and concluded that lower birth weights and poorer nutrition explained higher rates of mental retardation among black children.[72]

Race affected the collection and interpretation of data, sometimes in surprising ways. Lilienfeld and Pasamanick had expected the rates of prematurity and neonatal abnormalities to be higher among cases than controls, but this was only true for white infants, while rates for black infants were nearly as high among controls as cases. Because far fewer black women gave birth in hospitals, they had a selectively higher proportion of abnormal pregnancies and deliveries among those for whom hospital records were available. School segregation actually facilitated the selection of controls in the retrospective study of maternal and fetal precursors of behavior problems in children who had been referred to the Baltimore City Public Schools Division of Special Services. Each child with behavior problems was matched with "another child of the same sex in the same class [who had not been referred, which] resulted in automatic matching by race, economic status, and age due to segregation and school districting."[73]

The disadvantages of racial discrimination and dire poverty faced by most inner-city East Baltimore residents were borne out in JHSPH research, with consequential implications for public health policy and practice. By correlating data from birth certificates, hospital records, and census tracts, Pasamanick, Knobloch, and Lilienfeld found that the rate of maternal complications among 803 women who gave birth in Baltimore hospitals was 5 percent among whites in the highest economic quintile, 15 percent among whites in the lowest economic quintile, and 51 percent among nonwhites. In an analysis of more than 42,000 live births to mothers in Baltimore hospitals during 1950 and 1951, Rider, Tayback, and Knobloch found that 11.4 percent of black infants were born prematurely, compared to only 6.8 percent of white infants. Among babies born to mothers over age 30, both the overall rates of prematurity and the racial disparity within those rates were even greater—9.4 percent for white infants and 21.8 percent for black infants. Black rates of premature birth were also "strikingly greater than those in the lowest socioeconomic white groups," which led the authors to hypothesize that "Negro socioeconomic status is lower than that in even the lowest white groups" and therefore "prematurity rates increase exponentially below certain economic thresholds." Nearly six decades later, this observation would be strongly confirmed by JHSPH studies of fetal loss and premature birth among women in the developing world, published in the *Lancet* in 2013.[74]

At the conclusion of their 1956 article on precursors of neuropsychiatric disorders, Lilienfeld, Pasamanick, and Rogers emphasized that their findings "above all indicate areas where preventive measures may serve to decrease the enormous weight of individual and social loss and suffering." During the 1950s, state and local health departments began to incorporate the care of mentally and physically handicapped children more fully into maternal and child health programs. About 30 percent of children served by handicapped children's agencies had congenital malformations, the largest single diagnostic category.[75]

The pregnancy and prematurity research at Hopkins strongly advocated for two main methods for preventing infant mortality and childhood disability: prenatal care for mothers and developmental screening for infants and pre-school children. To make "hard scientific results available to pediatric practi-tioners and public health workers," Harper summarized the group's findings in a seminal textbook, *Preventive Pediatrics, Child Health and Development* (1962), which outlined the process of healthy mental and physical development, guidelines for nutrition, the evolution of communication skills in children, and the recommended schedule of immunizations. He also identified signs of devel-opmental problems and discussed developmental delays, epilepsy, and cerebral palsy. Public health services for children, including those with mental and physical handicaps, received extensive attention. Harper presented the topic in the context of the family and social environment, which represented a new em-phasis in maternal and child health services in the early 1960s.[76]

The Baltimore studies of the developmental consequences of maternal com-plications and premature birth continued and expanded the school's earlier research in the EHD on the relationship between population health and socio-economic characteristics, such as Miriam Brailey's work to measure and im-prove racial disparities in rates of childhood TB. In the United States and Canada, the growing numbers of doctors, hospitals, and research institutes that accompanied the medicalization of childbirth had the potential to either undermine or enhance population-based approaches to maternal and child health, which had traditionally been grounded in the disciplines of pediatrics, obstetrics, and public health nursing. Not until the mid-1960s would Great Society federal health programs reemphasize the mutual dependence of socio-economic and health status and the interconnected nature of social welfare and maternal and child health. In developing countries with limited health care infrastructure and fewer trained health professionals, government pro-grams to deliver medical, public health, and social welfare services remained more unified.[77]

After the divisions of Maternal and Child Health and of Mental Hygiene were granted departmental status in 1962, they continued to build on their landmark studies of developmental disability and to use this evidence to shape the first federal policies aimed at aiding families caring for mentally and physi-cally handicapped children. The National Association for Retarded Children (NARC)—renamed the Association for Retarded Citizens in 1981—awarded its first research professorship to Robert Cooke, who led the Johns Hopkins Department of Pediatrics to emphasize the prevention and treatment of developmental disabilities. NARC appointed Cooke the first chair of its Research Advisory Committee, and in 1959, the Joseph P. Kennedy Jr. Foundation awarded him a 10-year, $1.275 million grant to fund interdisciplinary research on mental retardation, build new laboratories, and promote new innovations. Cooke built close relationships with the Kennedy family, particularly Sargent and Eunice Shriver, and was appointed to the health care transition team when John F. Kennedy took office in 1961. The Joseph P. Kennedy Jr. Foundation also funded Abe Lilienfeld's research on Down syndrome (known as mongolism until Asian researchers protested against the term as a racial slur in the mid-1960s), which resulted in a major case-control study among Baltimore children and the publication in 1969 of the first monograph on the epidemiology of the condition.[78]

As Cooke, Harper, and Lemkau worked to increase the scope and reach of services for developmentally and physically disabled children, divisions among the three chairs reflected disciplinary and political splits over which medical specialties and federal agencies should have primary responsibility for such services. Psychiatrists on state boards of mental health had traditionally overseen institutions for children with developmental disabilities, but the psychoanalysts who came to dominate the profession believed such children were incapable of benefiting from psychotherapy. As developmental disabilities historian Edward Shorter has noted, "The analysts had breathtakingly erroneous notions of the causes of [mental retardation], believing it to be the result of faulty parent–child dynamics, of 'refrigerator mothers' and the like." During an era when few doctors chose to specialize in developmental disabilities, which were considered a hopeless and incurable condition that inevitably led to institutionalization, Cooke and Lemkau both dedicated themselves to bettering the quality of care and public programs then available for developmentally disabled children, while Harper helped to ensure that pediatricians were trained to recognize early signs of developmental problems in infants and young children.[79]

Pediatricians believed that their specialty should take the lead in caring for mentally handicapped children, but it was the outspoken Cooke rather than the soft-spoken Harper who clashed with psychiatrists on this issue. In Cooke's own department, Leo Kanner, the first self-described child psychiatrist, upheld psychiatry's role in evaluating and treating children with delayed mental and emotional development. Harper and Lemkau had been active in reforming the Maryland Department of Health, and Lemkau had also chaired one of the earliest NIMH reviews of program development in mental retardation. While Lemkau was critical of the psychoanalysts' abandonment of the field, he wanted progressive mental hygienists to oversee care for mentally disabled children within state health departments.

During the 1960s, Lemkau led the JHSPH Department of Mental Hygiene to develop an active research and training program in the epidemiology of developmental disabilities, and in 1965, the department began a contract with the city of Baltimore "to provide qualified and adequate psychiatric services for the conduct of the City Health Department's full-time mental hygiene clinic for children in the Eastern Health District." Lemkau's first-generation research and teaching on the "continuum of casualty" applied a life course framework to understanding the impact of physiological, social, and environmental factors on children's development, behavior, and life chances. This rich vein of inquiry would blossom further in the 1980s under Sheppard Kellam's chairmanship, with the establishment of the Prevention Research Center in 1983 and the development of the Good Behavior Game, an intensive long-term intervention in collaboration with Baltimore City Public Schools.[80]

Harper and Lemkau opposed Cooke on the issue of creating a new institute for studying children's diseases within the NIH. Harper and Congressman John Fogarty were among those who wanted children's health research to remain based in the Children's Bureau, but Cooke felt that the Bureau's personnel had "neither the interest nor the capacities to develop intensive research programs of a basic nature in the biological or behavioral aspects of human development." Lemkau, with close ties to the NIMH, shared the agency's desire to retain its oversight of research on intellectual disability. When Cooke, supported by the rest of President Kennedy's task force on health, proposed to establish a new child health institute within the NIH, he ran afoul of director James Shannon. Shannon had been loyal to the categorical disease model of the agency's early years and resisted the creation of age-based institutes, and US Secretary of Health, Education and Welfare (HEW) Abraham Ribicoff was also uninterested in a child health institute. With persistent lobbying, Cooke and the Kennedys won over Fogarty and his influential colleague Senator Lister Hill, and the National Institute of Child Health and Human Development (NICHD) was established and funded in 1963.[81]

The School of Hygiene's studies of the complex relationship between complications of pregnancy, premature birth, abnormal neonatal conditions, and developmental disabilities were part of the foundational developmental research that was instrumental in convincing Congress to amend the Social Security Act in 1963 and 1965. These maternal and child health amendments authorized federal grants to enable states to provide comprehensive maternity care to high-risk mothers; to develop high-quality, comprehensive health services for preschool and school-age children; and to broaden maternal and child health programs to serve children with handicapping conditions. As chair of the APHA Maternal and Child Health Section's Committee on Legislation, Harper testified in 1962 in support of the proposed amendments to SS Title V, emphasizing the crucial role of prenatal care in preventing infant mortality, developmental disability, and a wide range of congenital health problems. Harper's Baltimore studies of infant mortality had proven that "the mother who does not get prenatal care is twice as likely to lose her baby as is the mother who gets adequate prenatal care." Harper also contended that federal funds for handicapped children's programs "purchase more service and results per dollar than any other Federal money spent for medical care."[82]

The provisions of SS Title V lay the groundwork for a national maternal and child health services network. These programs were characterized by a strong federal role in funding and setting priorities, state administration and provision of mandatory matching funds, statewide health planning to meet federal guidelines, and local delivery of services. The expansion of the scope and budgets for federal maternal and child health programs during the 1960s had three major effects: (1) It was a major step in the evolution of SS Title V into a national health system for low-income mothers and children, (2) it transformed public health practice by significantly expanding maternal and child health services at the state and local levels, and (3) it benefited schools of public health by providing additional support for maternal and child health research and training, with a heightened emphasis on public health nursing. These federal programs would provide fundamental support for the new departments of Mental Hygiene and Maternal and Child Health that grew out of the extensive JHSPH research in these areas.[83]

Conclusion

During the EHD's first decade, Huntington Williams had worked with Thomas Parran, Lowell Reed, Wade Frost, and Allen Freeman to develop the EHD as a model for public health departments nationwide. Reed and Ernest Stebbins had moved to expand and deepen the relationships among the BCHD, the Johns Hopkins Medical Institutions, and the local health care system. But in the shifting postwar political climate of the Red Scare and conservative efforts to roll back the New Deal, JHSPH leaders began to seek more fertile fields in which to plant the seeds of cooperation between public health and medicine, at home and abroad. The PHA divisions of Maternal and Child Health, Mental Hygiene, and Public Health Nursing preserved some measure of cooperation with the BCHD and enjoyed a remarkably synergistic teaching and research collaboration with the medical school and hospital. They also promoted the diversification and expansion of field training opportunities for public health, medical, and nursing students.

The maternal and child health program in particular was broadly interdisciplinary and successfully fostered a population perspective, even in the most medicalized fields such as genetic diseases and premature birth. Stebbins, Harper, and many of their public health peers were convinced that curbing population growth was essential for transcending the limits of public health, especially in the world's poorest, most unstable areas. By the mid-1960s, reproductive health and family planning would become the dominant focus of Harper's Department of Maternal and Child Health, which he accordingly renamed Population and Family Health.

Stebbins believed that his cherished Department of Public Health Administration surely held the key to solving the problems confronting the school. The future of public health lay in providing the leadership, data, and methods for the broad-scale planning of government health services, using the latest computing technology and statistical expertise as well as in-depth social and economic analysis. These convictions would guide the school into the 1960s and inform the founding of four new cornerstones for the future, the departments of International Health, Population Dynamics, Behavioral Sciences, and Medical Care and Hospitals.

Public health's entry into clinical settings advanced the goals of providing continuity of care for patients and improving the quality and availability of medical and public health services. These developments highlighted the social and economic determinants of health as well as the value of systematic organization, planning, and evaluation of health care from the institutional to the international levels. Such concepts would form the basis of a new public health field, health services research, toward which Stebbins had been guiding JHSPH since his arrival in 1946.

CHAPTER FIVE

Rethinking the Public Health Curriculum

Even in the midst of rapid growth in external funding for sponsored research, the School of Hygiene and Public Health had been running an ever-growing deficit since the end of the war, because enrollments were increasing while endowment income and general operating funds from the university were not. JHSPH's finances differed from schools of public health at state universities, which were supported by appropriations from state legislatures. These funds were relatively stable, if not always generous, during the postwar period of significant growth in public higher education. Only a small portion of JHSPH receipts came from tuition, even though the price doubled from $600 in 1950 to $1,200 by 1954. By 1955–1956, the university's entire deficit was in the Medical Institutions, which focused scrutiny on the duplication of departments between Hygiene and Medicine.[1]

As university administrators struggled to solve the School of Hygiene's financial woes, the faculty was divided over educational priorities. Could the school maintain its traditional commitment to the basic science of public health and also make room for the growing number of applied fields within public health administration?

During the 1950s, the school's attempted curriculum reforms coalesced around three main issues: (1) the School of Hygiene's role in teaching a model of continuous medical care across the full spectrum of prevention, treatment, and rehabilitation; (2) basic science teaching in the Master of Public Health and Doctor of Science programs (the school would not award its first PhD until 1965); and (3) whether the MPH should be reformed, lengthened, or abolished to allow an exclusive focus on the doctoral degrees. These questions shaped the 1956–1957 deliberations of the Committee to Review the Educational Objectives of the School of Hygiene and Public Health, chaired by Thomas Turner.

Throughout these discussions, the pros and cons of a closer relationship with the medical school loomed large. The Turner Committee's interim report revealed a rancorous split between a contingent of basic science faculty who viewed a formal alliance with the medical school as the best path to recovering and enhancing the school's illustrious research tradition versus faculty both inside and outside the basic sciences who viewed JHSPH's independence as paramount to ensuring the quality of teaching and research programs.

Teaching Preventive Medicine

The Department of Preventive Medicine had been founded in 1939 at the Johns Hopkins School of Medicine with a Rockefeller grant in an effort to strengthen public health teaching for medical undergraduates. But its chair, Perrin H. Long, showed open disdain for public health. Ignoring the guidelines proposed by Rockefeller officials, he had insisted on separating instruction in preventive medicine from that in public health, which he called "unattractive to medical students because it is frequently remote from the clinical point of view [and] frequently concerned with the applied techniques and methods which are useful in a professional Public Health practice, but which are remote from the intellectual interests of the students." Long also objected to "the presence of foreign students and others [from the School of Hygiene] whose educational foundation has not been too firm."[2]

Long claimed that physicians had already had plenty of exposure to preventive measures in the military and declared, "In the department of preventive medicine our first aim should be to make good doctors of these men and I propose to allot the first nine months of their time to doing just that thing. . . . To project him from the army into the organized teaching leading to an MPH would be unwise and . . . if the money is given to the department of preventive medicine it will be used to develop individuals interested in preventive medicine and not in the methodology of public health." Not surprisingly, the department at Hopkins did not long outlive the initial 10-year Rockefeller grant, which was not renewed. Long's prowess as a clinical researcher attracted other offers, and he left to head the Department of Medicine at the Downstate Medical Center of the State University of New York.[3]

In 1952, the Hopkins medical faculty voted to dissolve the Department of Preventive Medicine as a separate department; instead, the School of Hygiene would teach concepts of public health and preventive medicine to medical students in the required biostatistics course and more indirectly in certain basic science courses that were contracted to Hygiene faculty, including bacteriology, immunology, and pathology.[4]

A frequent theme in the Committee on Preventive Medicine's deliberations and those of preventive medicine faculty nationally had been that preventive medicine instruction required clinical material, a group of asymptomatic patients who would enable students to learn to detect early signs of illness and apply preventive measures. The committee insisted that the absence of such patients "constitutes a real handicap to the teaching program of the School" and urged the development of a program to improve the facilities for "teaching and research in the prevention, diagnosis and treatment of disease which shall include: (a) The provision of a selected group of individuals for whom total medical care is provided, (b) Reorganization of the outpatient services to meet the needs of the three medical institutions [the hospital, medical school, and School of Hygiene], (c) Provision of facilities for convalescent care and rehabilitation."[5]

The JHSPH Advisory Board emphasized the need to implement these recommendations, particularly the reorganization of the outpatient services jointly by the three medical institutions, since the EHD clinics were no longer open to provide field training to JHSPH students. To accomplish this goal, the School of Hygiene appointed a Committee on Teaching Public Health to Medical Students, chaired by William B. Cochran and also including Paul Harper, Paul Lemkau, Philip Sartwell, Ernest Stebbins, Thomas Turner, and Wilson Wing. In May 1953, the committee issued what became known as the Cochran Report, which drew on new objectives issued by the Association of American Medical Colleges. Just prior to this, Stebbins had been working with Maryland state health officer Robert H. Riley and APHA secretary Reginald Atwater to launch the American Board of Preventive Medicine and Public Health, first approved by the AMA Section on Prevention and Industrial Medicine and Public Health in 1948.[6]

In the context of the dramatic postwar growth of private health insurance coverage; the unprecedented influx of public funding for medical services, facilities, and research; and the widespread (although not unchallenged) acceptance of the concept that public health was essential to the nation's defense and economic welfare, the Cochran Report revamped the criteria for what the modern physician should know. The report's authors asserted that "the objectives of public health and clinical medicine are coming closer together; all of this points to a joint endeavor for teaching and research in health supervision."

New MD graduates should understand community health needs and the objectives of government and nonprofit agencies such as health departments, hospitals, and voluntary organizations. They should also understand health protection through environmental sanitation and control of health hazards; communicable disease control; programs to promote the health of special groups such as infants, schoolchildren, pregnant women, and industrial workers; provision of medical services for the indigent; utilization of auxiliary services such as nursing, rehabilitation, and medical social service; and the community-based control of problems such as cancer, heart disease, diabetes, hypertension, alcoholism, and mental disorders via screening programs and the delivery of health services to populations with limited access to medical care.[7]

But the Cochran Report warned that "this growth in clinical services [in public health] has serious disadvantages in that it serves to fractionate the care of the patient, who goes to one physician in a public health clinic when he is well, and to another physician when he is ill. The individual patient will be better served if all of his medical care in health and in illness is under the supervision of a single physician or a group of physicians, provided that these physicians develop the same competence and enthusiasm for health supervision that they already give to the care of illness." Medical schools and the medical profession should ensure that "the training of all physicians does lay the foundation for competence in health supervision," which would be valuable whether graduates chose careers in private practice or public health, since "approximately half of the time of internists, pediatricians and obstetricians is occupied with problems of health supervision rather than with organic disease."[8]

The Cochran Report's challenges were ably met by Paul Harper, who fulfilled the original charge to the Department of Preventive Medicine and proved that public health principles could be successfully integrated into clinical instruction for both medical and public health students. In 1949, Harper had begun working with a group of families "who would provide a laboratory for study of the factors in family and community life which influence health and disease." Initially, Harper's division partnered with the Department of Pediatrics to provide care for a pilot group of indigent children who were already eligible for the Medical Care Program but whose families met certain selection criteria: residence in the EHD for at least five years, married two-parent families with new or expected infants, eligible for ward service at Johns Hopkins or Sinai hospitals, and currently without a family physician. Harper developed this pilot program into the Home and Office Care program, the first clinical service to be established for the sole use of a School of Hygiene department.

Approved by the JHH Medical Board in spring 1951, the Home and Office Care Program emphasized research and teaching in problems of growth and development and began operating at the Johns Hopkins Hospital in January 1952, with 90 percent of visits in the clinic and 10 percent in homes. By 1953, a small staff of physicians, public health nurses, and a medical social worker provided medical and public health services to 115 children in 50 families. The Home and Office Care Program was a site for clinical experience as well as a source of real-world case material for Hopkins medical and public health students. In 1952–1953, the program provided field experience to 39 Hygiene students and 16 second-year medical students, and 10 MPH students in the Maternal and Child Health track gained advanced training in clinical pediatrics while serving as part-time instructors and caring for patients for six months. In addition, 75 fourth-year medical students in the maternal and child health seminar examined case records from the program.[9] Harper, like Alexander Langmuir, saw important parallels between epidemiology and clinical medicine. Both were, in Langmuir's mind, "collective sciences depending on a synthesis of knowledge derived from all medical sciences." Even though the methods of observation and data collection were different, the intellectual processes of drawing conclusions were nearly identical. Epidemiological syndromes could be "as specific and distinctive as clinical syndromes." Hundreds of thousands of clinical diagnoses were made every day, each affecting a single person, while epidemiological diagnoses were much rarer but involved vast numbers of people and often huge amounts of money.[10]

Like the original plan for the EHD, the Home and Office Care Program hoped to select families "that will have stability and will be representative of problems encountered in medical and public health practice." But where the EHD's families had been subject to intense scrutiny and frequent intrusions from Hygiene faculty and students, Harper and Stebbins emphasized the goal of making "our contacts with these families as natural as possible—to see them when they need service." Drawing on experience with both the Medical Care Program, which by definition served indigent patients, and the EHD, whose population had grown increasingly poor, black, and migratory, Stebbins and Harper eschewed the traditional reliance of urban teaching hospitals on large indigent populations to provide clinical material. They stipulated that "not more than 1/3 of these families should be from the indigent group since indigent families often have economic and social difficulties which make for instability and which over-shadow the medical problems."[11] Both the heightened priority on clinical teaching and the shifting urban landscape had undermined the Rockefeller Foundation's earlier emphasis on community field epidemiology, and the School of Hygiene now shifted toward clinical epidemiology.

The Cochran Committee identified programs such as Home and Office Care (subsequently renamed Family Care) as "probably the most significant development in departments of preventive medicine at the present time" because they enabled students to see patients in home and office settings, "to see them as members of family groups, and to become acquainted with some of the social and environmental factors which influence the patient's reaction to illness and which complicate the problem of providing good medical care." Medical students would be introduced to the Family Care Program by caring for a pregnant woman or newborn child. Citing the Health Insurance Plan in New York and the Baltimore City Medical Care Program, the committee estimated that to support the teaching and research needs in preventive medicine and public health, the Family Care Program would need to enroll a total of 800 families or 3,000 individuals, half over age 16 and half under. Similar comprehensive care teaching clinics had been established at the University of North Carolina and Boston University with the assistance of the Commonwealth Fund. Stebbins wrote the Fund's president, Lester Evans, to request support for Harper and the Family Care Program. "Our need to expand this program and to put it on a firmer foundation is accentuated by our new responsibilities for the teaching of medical students as a result of a decision of the Medical School to discontinue its Department of Preventive Medicine. This gives us a great opportunity to emphasize health supervision of family groups in the teaching of medical and public health students."[12]

At the beginning of the 1950s, required preventive medicine and public health courses had occupied 40 hours in the fourth year of the Hopkins MD curriculum. In response to the Cochran Report, the curriculum was reconfigured in 1953–1954 with a course in biostatistics the first year and in epidemiology the second, as well as a fourth-year seminar, Community Health Organization, which provided "a general orientation in public health" with attention to "specific disease problems and major public health activities of governmental and voluntary health agencies." But some medical faculty criticized the Family Care Program's pedagogical relevance for medical students. Barry Wood, just before he was named Vice-President of the Johns Hopkins Medical Institutions, had published a 1953 broadside attack in the *Journal of Laboratory and Clinical Medicine* against medical education reform that threatened the primacy of basic science by incorporating the social and psychological aspects of disease. Wood denounced such initiatives, charging that they taught "students less about the science of medicine and more about the practical aspects of home care and office practice." Stebbins had objected to Evans, "Nothing could be farther from our intent. We see a family care program as an opportunity to study and to teach the developing field of knowledge about the patient who has no unusual disease but who is subject to stresses that effect [*sic*] his health and who is seeking guidance and health supervision."[13]

The Family Care Program did not receive the philanthropic funding that Harper and Stebbins had tried so hard to secure, and Harper would shift his focus to international family planning in the early 1960s. By then, the public health requirements for medical students would be whittled down from 17 hours in 1954 to a single three-hour course by 1963, Field Work in Social Medicine, which would use field trips rather than clinical experience with patients to illustrate "the interrelationship of medical and social problems and the services of various community agencies." The MD curriculum would, however, evolve to require just over one-quarter of the coursework to deal with chronic diseases, significantly higher than at other medical schools. Abe Lilienfeld's Department of Chronic Diseases was actively involved in teaching these courses, which would finally succeed in incorporating concepts of continuous care into the medical curriculum, since preventive and follow-up care was critical to the management of chronic disease patients. Lilienfeld also taught medical students epidemiology. Otherwise, the battles over teaching public health to medical students ended with both sides generally withdrawing to their respective campuses.[14]

Teaching Basic Science

As the size, complexity, and expense of standard laboratory equipment grew, the school was desperately short of lab space and was admitting MPH students "to the maximum capacity of the physical facilities of the institution," which affected the quality as well as quantity of students. As the school's leaders recognized the need to reform the MPH program, the Doctor and Master of Science in Hygiene programs were declining in popularity. From 1945 to 1949, Johns Hopkins granted an average of only four ScD degrees per year, the lowest number in the school's history. W. W. Cort, chair of Parasitology, explained the effects of tightening budgets on his department's students to Stebbins in March 1950: "We are having just as difficult a time this year making ends meet as we had last. Some of our old equipment is wearing out and has to be replaced. The greatest difficulty we have is financing the research of our ScD students. We try to choose inexpensive problems, but most of them need animals and some special equipment. It is hard to see how we can get along next year without an increase."[15]

In contrast to the MPH and DrPH students, the science programs were intended to prepare nonphysicians for scientific careers in public health research. Admissions requirements included a bachelor's degree with preparation in mathematics, physics, biology, and chemistry. Students completed two years of coursework in their area of specialty, with a written exam and a thesis for the ScM. To be accepted into the doctoral program, candidates had to demonstrate reading knowledge of two foreign languages and pass an oral examination by a faculty committee during the second year. The ScD candidate then completed a third year of coursework and comprehensive written exam in his or her specialty as well as a dissertation based on an original investigation and oral presentation before the committee. To help attract quality ScD candidates, the School of Hygiene convinced the university to establish five fellowships beginning in the 1950–1951 academic year, with additional fellowships provided by agencies such as the US International Cooperation Administration, WHO, and US Air Force. This enabled the enrollment of ScD students to rise from 27 in 1948–1949 to 43 by 1952–1953.[16]

But the faculty's uneven level of engagement with even the most advanced, research-oriented students marred the program. In December 1954, Turner told Stebbins, "I am becoming more and more concerned about the character of our final oral examinations for ScD candidates," which he described as "at the best incredibly dull and at the worst downright sadistic." By the 1950s, the majority of ScD students were in Parasitology, but attracting good students in other disciplines continued to be problematic. In 1956, the ScD Committee recommended shortening the name to "Doctor of Science," because "the 'in Hygiene' scares away students." In the era of William Welch, "hygiene" had connoted the high-grade science of the German institutes of hygiene; with the rise of Madison Avenue mass advertising, "hygiene" was more likely to be associated with mouthwash and sanitary napkins. Turner judged that the School's basic science graduate program had "gone along without conspicuous failure and without distinction."[17]

To address the growing sense of ennui surrounding the Doctor of Science program, David E. Davis and Fred Bang in Pathobiology and Paul Lemkau in the PHA Division of Mental Hygiene began discussing a new interdisciplinary course that would incorporate principles from parasitology, vertebrate ecology, and the behavioral sciences. They invited biochemist Roger Herriott to participate, and in the spring of 1954, Herriott sent a proposal to Turner for a joint basic science course, The Biology of Infectious Agents. The course would help "MPH and science students alike" to "integrate the various similarities and differences in life cycles [of infectious agents]." Content would emphasize common developmental stages and concepts, including host range specificity, mode of entry and exit from the host, degree of parasitism, reservoirs of infection, and modes of replication, distribution, and activation as well as mechanisms of immunity and resistance. Faculty from the Departments of Microbiology, Pathobiology, Biochemistry, and Epidemiology would jointly teach the course, which

Herriott proposed as a substitute for the current course in virology offered by the Department of Microbiology.[18]

Turner replied with a barrage of objections. He could not conceive of the virology course being replaced by "a purely discussion course" that "would be wasteful of time," yet allow students to "play a very passive role indeed." He stressed the Department of Microbiology's obligation to provide high-quality training in virology and asserted that the MPH general microbiology course did in fact teach "the fundamentals of the host–parasite relationship" and its bearing on prevention and control. Although he conceded the appeal of "the idea of joint courses or integrated courses for MPH students," in practice they had "not been outstandingly successful," with the notable exception of the course in biostatistics and epidemiology. To avoid duplication and seek areas of collaboration, Turner suggested a review of all the courses offered by the "numerous other groups in the School that are interested in microbiological problems, particularly in the virus field."[19]

Bang, Herriott, Lemkau, and other faculty in their departments developed the course anyway, on the premise that biology was the common emphasis of Microbiology, Pathobiology, and Biochemistry and "because public health is concerned with the problems of groups of humans." The course stressed "the properties of groups of biological units and how they respond to changes"; it was designed to "focus the students' attention on group problems in biology and how the study of animal or simple systems permit the careful examination of hypotheses which then may serve as a guide in the study of humans." The course's sections included Genetic Composition, Growth and Aging of Populations, Behavior of Human and Vertebrate Animal Populations (with lectures on mental hygiene and anthropology), and Relation of Infectious Agents.[20]

Instead of using marbles to simulate disease outbreaks in human populations, as in the Reed–Frost model, students would learn about human population dynamics and the interactions of disease and environmental factors by studying animal populations. Lemkau, who taught the behavioral component, declared in his division's annual report that "active teaching participation in Pathobiology I signaled behavior study as a recognized basic science in the School." Lemkau's labs discussed social class distribution and differences in access to treatment for schizophrenia as well as the effect of sensory stress on psychological test performance. His colleague Marcia Cooper used children's drawings to demonstrate normal and deviant development.[21]

Manfred Mayer questioned the basic premise of both Bang's concept of Pathobiology and the course's "Growth and Aging of Populations" section that the growth of bacteria, protozoa, and animal populations could serve as a model for understanding human population dynamics. He protested, "The broad manner in which the population concept is introduced throughout this outline has only limited application and real meaning in terms of practical health problems." Mayer, a nationally known immunologist, also objected to the "grossly inadequate" attention given to infectious agents in public health and concluded, "It would be appalling to abandon Microbiology 2 [Principles of Public Health Microbiology] and substitute the proposed course." Carl Lamanna, who also taught several introductory microbiology courses, was much more sanguine and favored creating an interdepartmental course, since the mere existence of departments did not require "that instruction be organized on a similar parochial basis."[22]

Microbiology 2 did remain in the curriculum, but the course description was substantially revised and its credits were reduced from 12 to nine hours per week. After the faculty voted in 1957 to replace Microbiology with Public Health Biology as the MPH science requirement, Turner surmised that "perhaps graduate instruction in these areas for the general public health student is no longer indicated, except on an elective basis." He had gradually concluded that the basic science disciplines of microbiology, physiology, and biochemistry should be considered "preclinical" fields to be combined with those in medicine and taught to medical undergraduates and specialized doctoral students in Hygiene.[23]

Lemkau wanted MPH students to continue to engage in basic science coursework but wrote Turner that Hygiene faculty needed to stop teaching only what they knew, be willing to transcend disciplinary boundaries, and "continuously [extend] ourselves to deal with the issues that press from the field." As an example, he cited prenatal exposure to rubella, histoplasmosis, tuberculosis, meningococcal meningitis, and the encephalitides, which greatly increased the risk of future behavioral disorders. "By confining teaching to the laboratory character of the organisms concerned, this important application of microbiology to the life of the person in his environment is missed." Discussing socioenvironmental factors in disease "would perhaps give the student more feeling of relationship between the laboratory and the world; it seems to me he [the student] is complaining about this separation."[24]

Biochemistry had been the first department to arrive at Turner's conclusion that the basic sciences would be better off focusing on students specializing in lab science and dispensing with MPH candidates. Biochemistry 1 had never been a requirement, but during the 1930s and 1940s, the department's signature offering had been Experimental Methods in Nutrition. The course taught students to perform lab experiments on rat models for dietary diseases in humans, but it was dropped in 1954, by which time the department's courses catered solely to advanced students interested in modern biochemical research methods such as spectrophotometry, electrophoresis, immiscible solvent partition, isotopic tracer techniques, and fluorimetry. Roger Herriott, chair of Biochemistry from 1948 to 1975, introduced the first JHSPH courses on the properties of DNA, and he broadened the department's horizons to explore the biochemistry of viruses and proteolytic enzymes, including the role viruses played in spreading infection by injecting bacteria with their DNA. Yet such courses were beyond the interests and abilities of most MPH students, whose curriculum now included no elective courses in biochemistry.[25]

Bacon F. Chow, associate professor of biochemistry, highlighted the public health importance of "nutrition *in utero*, the nutritional requirements of the aged and recent concepts on the nutrients essential to prevent and combat metabolic diseases." Lemkau seconded the relevance of nutrition to the health of pregnant women and unborn children but questioned the department's traditionally narrow focus on the effects of vitamin deficiency: "Biochemistry, at least in this country, should spend more time on the findings on brain physiology and chemistry and their relation to behavior than on nutrition per se." Hygiene faculty seemed to agree that the old ways of teaching basic science to MPH students were inadequate. They were sharply divided, however, on whether basic science should remain a core requirement and, if so, how the laboratory disciplines could best be integrated with the broadening range of public health knowledge and practice.[26]

The Committee to Review the Educational Objectives of the School of Hygiene and Public Health

Due to the high level of interest generated by the theme of the 1955 annual APHA conference, "Where Are We Going in Public Health?" the AHPA executive board convened a task force in 1956 to conduct "a critical examination of the role of the American Public Health Association in facilitating attainment of the objectives of tomorrow's public health program." Health departments were extending their boundaries to include personal health and rehabilitation services, civil defense, mental health, and chronic diseases, and the list kept growing. Meanwhile, the Committee to Review the Educational Objectives of the School of Hygiene and Public Health was deliberating at Hopkins, the latest in a series of self-study committees to dissect and diagnose the growing pains of the Johns Hopkins Medical Institutions.

The Commonwealth Fund underwrote the MPH component of the review and had also sponsored a comprehensive study of the MD program two years earlier, led by John Whitehorn, chair of Psychiatry. The Hygiene committee met weekly throughout the 1956–1957 academic year and included seven department chairs (Thomas Turner, William G. Cochran, Ernest L. Stebbins, Abel Wolman, Philip E. Sartwell, Frederik B. Bang, and Roger M. Herriott), the heads of the two largest PHA divisions (Paul A. Harper and

Paul V. Lemkau), and university vice-president Barry Wood. All were full professors in JHSPH.[27]

In a report issued in early 1957, the APHA task force challenged schools of public health to modernize their curricula to reflect changing demands. The top priority was more effective recruitment and selection of personnel for training in public health, which required increased funding for fellowships. Public health curricula needed to be broadened to encompass new areas of responsibility and functions, with "increased content from the fields of social and behavioral sciences, administration, economics, and communications." The task force also urged schools to provide more adequate field training facilities and to develop continuing education programs to update public health personnel on current practices. These recommendations built on those first put forth in the 1939 Parran–Farrand Report and the subsequent work of the APHA Committee on Professional Education.[28]

Thomas Turner and Barry Wood, vice-president of the Medical Institutions, charged that the MPH was not a true graduate degree worthy of Johns Hopkins because it did not require comprehensive exams or a thesis. Despite the fact that the MPH at Johns Hopkins, unlike the growing number of schools of public health at state universities, required an MD and previous public health field experience, Turner called it "a cheaply earned degree" that attracted "a few good students, a large group of mediocre students, and too many who are poor by any academic standards [and absorbed] an undue amount of faculty energy."

Turner and some other faculty advocated lengthening the MPH to two years and requiring a thesis and written exam or eliminating the MPH entirely to concentrate on the DrPH program. Either way, training a smaller, more select group would, Turner hoped, return to the school's "original concept of the over-riding importance of research as an educational way of life." Despite these proposed changes, the MPH remained the backbone of the school's teaching program with essentially the same requirements: one year of coursework and at least three months of field experience (either prior to admission or before graduation). What did change was the MPH curriculum, with major implications for all JHSPH programs.[29]

As Turner prepared to chair the internal review of the School of Hygiene, he expressed his general feelings toward schools of public health in a letter to his friend Basil O'Connor. He complained that "so-called health educators write and talk a good deal of tripe. Certainly the stuff that is taught in most of the public health schools is not only drivel, but it is mighty dull to boot. However, I have recently been made Chairman of a committee which is charged with the job of trying to take a good hard fresh look at our School of Public Health and our graduate education program in general. So I shall, of necessity, be interested in the general problem of health education." Turner formulated the committee's mission as two questions: "(1) if we had no public health schools today, would it be worth starting one and, (2) assuming that one was to be started, what kind of product would you attempt to turn out."[30]

Based on the Turner Committee's deliberations and research, including consultations with 18 prominent public health leaders from outside JHSPH, Turner issued an interim report in December 1956 for comment by the faculty. Its recommendations included revising the MPH schedule and increasing the academic year from 32 to 36 weeks. The requirements for biostatistics, epidemiology, and public health administration were unchanged, but microbiology was, for the first time in the school's history, replaced by a new interdisciplinary course, Public Health Biology. The traditional sanitary engineering requirement was now taught jointly with Environmental Medicine faculty and renamed Environmental Hygiene. Over half of the 35 electives were offered in the Department of PHA, whereas only six were offered in basic sciences.[31]

Reactions to the proposed new MPH course schedule were mixed. Manfred Mayer remarked that "there exists confusion in regard to the respective roles of research and teaching in the activities in this School." He felt that the MPH curriculum should emphasize "present day public health practice" rather than the latest advances, with "a clear and concise understanding of the basic fundamental concepts prevailing today in the various scientific disciplines contingent upon public health." Mayer had "purposely limited instruction in many areas of immunology" and saved "hot" research topics such as the detailed mechanisms of anaphylaxis or complement action for specialized elective courses. Like Turner, he saw research in biology and medicine as a whole that "should not be divided into categories or compartments depending on school affiliation within the University." Rather, teaching was "the justification for the existence of each of these schools as a separate organization."[32]

The interim report's first conclusion was its most controversial: "The medical sciences constitute the core of public health and preventive medicine. The School of Hygiene, therefore, should draw closer to the School of Medicine and the Hospital, particularly in view of the increasing importance of such problems as cardiac, mental and malignant diseases." Most Hygiene faculty members rejected a merger, and some, such as parasitologist Lloyd Rozeboom, felt that even pursuing closer ties with the medical school would endanger the unique public health emphasis and character of the school, particularly its attempts to incorporate the social and behavioral sciences. Rozeboom confessed his uneasiness about "close physical and administrative associations with the medical school[, which] results from my conviction that this eventually will lead to dimming of the public health objectives, and submergence of the School of Hygiene group into the medical science research program of the medical

school. Public health will not be served by imitation or duplication of the research and teaching programs of either the medical or [liberal arts and sci-
ences] schools."[33]

Although Turner conferred with several members of the APHA task force,
Ruth Freeman was its only representative from Hopkins, and her comments to
Turner's committee reflected the APHA position that public health degree
programs should be independent from medical schools. Freeman criticized "the
extraordinary burden that has been placed on students in the past in terms of
hours of work required outside of class," which left "very little time for delib-
erative thought on the part of the students during their first weeks at school."
Likewise, Paul Harper objected that the MPH curriculum allowed "little
opportunity for independent work or thought. The shortage of time makes it
almost impossible to learn by doing, and most of the 'clinical' courses are taught
without benefit of clinical experience."

Freeman and JHSPH alumni both advocated shortening the laboratory
portion of the microbiology requirement, which one-third of students had
criticized as "too detailed, too mechanical and too unproductive in developing
the student's thinking." Stebbins observed that newer schools of public health,
by reducing emphasis on the basic sciences, had been able to "more fully develop certain areas such as the behavioral sciences, sociology, and some phases
of administration to a higher level than we have been able to do here at Hopkins." Freeman was, moreover, "disturbed that we still provide no opportunity
to discuss the broad problems and philosophy of public health, or to talk
through the 'why' of what they are doing in the first quarter." Young health
officers had reported that "they haven't yet had much opportunity to grasp the
long range significance and human importance of what they are doing," and
alumni likewise expressed a longing for "more orientation in history, theory,
principles, and philosophy of public health."[34]

Johns Hopkins was the first school of public health to introduce specialty
MPH tracks, but its curriculum had also long been criticized as overly narrow. E. B. Wilson, chair of Vital Statistics at the Harvard School of Public
Health, had written Reed in 1941 that even the DrPH should guarantee "a
wide acquaintance with the public health field," but he chided, "as I read
your latest catalog I should say that in the second year you practically didn't
make any effort to broaden the knowledge of the candidate in the general
public health field but forced him to specialize in some one department and
in the things that the head of the department thought to be germane to that
specialization."[35]

Over a decade later, the external review of the hospital administration
program had urged more specialization and fewer core courses. Freeman, however, alleged that creating specialized tracks resulted in "much duplication,

particularly when guest speakers provide the main substance of the instruction." Microbiologist Carl Lamanna agreed that specialization often served faculty more than students: "For the most part, our public health students come to school to learn the 'how,' that is, they are concerned and will be concerned with the solution of practical problems." He feared that the faculty would, however, continue to expect the curriculum to accommodate their individual research interests, and he urged his colleagues to instead adapt themselves to the needs of students. "There is great danger," Lamanna noted, "that the academic life removes the faculty from a true appreciation of the headaches and heartaches met with by the public health worker in the field."[36]

The MPH curriculum was struggling under the burden of what John C. Whitehorn, chair of Psychiatry in the medical school, termed "instructional elephantiasis" that had resulted from the simultaneous vast growth of traditional scientific medical knowledge and awareness of the role of modern social, economic, and behavioral factors in determining health and well-being. With the proliferation of specialized tracks on top of the core curriculum, Hygiene students risked becoming "jacks of all trades but masters of none," with less opportunity than their predecessors to engage their fellow students in or outside of class. One way to relieve the pressure in the crammed one-year MPH program was to replace it with a two-year DrPH degree that only admitted MDs and focused on training health officers. But Kenneth L. Zierler, who taught environmental medicine MPH courses, questioned whether most MD applicants would be willing to sacrifice an additional two years for training or were necessarily more competent or suited for research than non-MDs. At the faculty meeting to discuss the interim report, Zierler unintentionally "drew blood" with his observation that "the report implied elimination of many foreign students," most of whom were in the MPH program. Mayer observed that the report's proposition to focus on producing elite public health leaders who would undergo longer, more in-depth training in research "would be as unrealistic as the proposition that Annapolis should train only Admirals."[37]

Not surprisingly, Stebbins challenged numerous assumptions in the interim report, which he reminded Turner was "a document that was primarily for discussion within the family" and should not be shared with the medical school. Stebbins was particularly critical of Turner's statements that most recent major changes in public health had "been sparked by scientists" and that "public health officials are creatures of this revolution, not masters of it. Schools of Public Health, including the School of Hygiene, have not been greatly influential in giving direction to these far-reaching developments." Stebbins countered with a list of visionary public health leaders who had created the NIH, reformed and modernized the New York State Health Department, and drafted major new legislation with the PHS and Children's Bureau.

He also praised the JHSPH faculty who had helped to develop "the modern concept of public health," reform Maryland's public health system, and train public health leaders worldwide.[38]

Conclusion

The response to the interim report underlined the fact that JHSPH had always been a hybrid of graduate, postgraduate, and professional school. The Turner Report essentially recommended jettisoning the school's traditional professional degree, the MPH, to concentrate on highly specialized graduate and postgraduate training for MDs. But the proposals to emphasize the DrPH with a strengthened research emphasis and to exclude applicants without an MD from all but the Master of Science program could have a potentially fatal impact on the school's finances. Since the MPH drew the largest number of students but required no thesis, eliminating it would simultaneously shrink enrollment (and thus tuition revenues) while increasing the number of students requiring research supervision. Ultimately, financial considerations in the other Medical Institutions, the university, and the halls of Congress were the most important factor in deciding the fate of the MPH and the departmental balance of power in the School of Hygiene.

CHAPTER SIX

The Postwar Geopolitics of American Public Health

World War II had two interlocking consequences for public health: the elevation of national defense and foreign policy as rationales for shoring up public health education, research, and services. While Miriam Brailey was under fire in Baltimore for refusing to sign Maryland's loyalty oath, events on the other side of the world drew America further into the Cold War. In 1949, the Soviet Union tested its first nuclear weapon and China underwent its Communist Revolution, followed in 1950 by the USSR and China backing North Korea's invasion of South Korea. President Harry S. Truman had been the first president to take a public stand on behalf of both civil rights and national health insurance, which nearly cost him the 1948 election. In his second term, Truman was forced to subordinate domestic reform to foreign policy concerns, especially after he deployed US troops in 1950 to defend Korea south of the 38th parallel against the North Korean invasion backed by China and the Soviet Union. The 1952 presidential election ended the 20-year Democratic dominance of the White House. The winner was Republican candidate Dwight D. Eisenhower, the general who had led the D-Day invasion of Normandy during World War II and was also the brother of Milton S. Eisenhower, who succeeded Lowell Reed as president of Johns Hopkins University in 1956.[1]

Although the Cold War dampened dissent and bolstered conservative arguments against social reform, it also provided a powerful rationale for public health spending. During the two postwar decades, the full-time staff of the PHS (including the Communicable Disease Center and NIH) exceeded 34,000, more than double its prewar size. Between 1948 and 1960, annual appropriations for the PHS quadrupled to $840 million. Some of this increase was due to the expansion of the NIH and the Hill–Burton hospital construction program, but the rest of the PHS budget also enjoyed a healthy expansion.[2]

Public health's new status as a primary tool of US diplomacy was signified in the establishment of the WHO in 1948 and President Truman's Point Four program to provide US technical assistance to developing countries, including disease control measures against malaria, TB, and other major epidemics. Assistant Secretary of State Adolf A. Berle Jr. told the Pan American Sanitary Bureau in 1943, "The fate of world powers really hangs on [public health] work, and as it progresses, it is plain that the future of the American continents hinge both on the content and the quality of that work. If the public health problems in South America are ever thoroughly solved, we may have that last chance of the world to create a huge area in which nations, without a background of hatred, can begin to achieve their destinies."[3]

Johns Hopkins exemplified in spades the many ways that the Cold War intensified the military's relationship with schools of public health and how the US–Soviet rivalry became a new justification for the public health mission, even in agencies and schools that were far removed from international health. Every aspect of JHSPH—its research, its students, and its relationships with the outside world—adapted to the new realities in a country constantly looking over its shoulder for potential threats, yet fervently hoping for peace.

Public Health for National Defense

Schools of public health benefited from the wave of returning veterans who enrolled or joined their faculties. Public health agencies gave hiring preference to veterans, who had acquired deep practical experience in developing innovative methods under difficult conditions overseas. Veterans and active duty personnel were instrumental in shaping the strategy and tactics of the many new international health agencies created within the PHS, the State Department, and the United Nations (UN). The 1950s saw a dramatic growth in the size of both the State Department's overseas technical aid programs and the US military. In response to the concerns of the United States and its Western allies in the North Atlantic Treaty Organization (NATO) that the Soviet Union might launch an offensive in Western Europe, the United States increased the number of divisions in the region from one to five to strengthen NATO's ground, air, and naval forces. The Air Force claimed the largest share of the military budget increase, since the Eisenhower administration implemented a New Look policy that deemphasized conventional ground forces and depended heavily on a commanding lead in American air power and nuclear superiority. The Army Reorganization Act of 1950 created a dedicated Army Medical Service to serve military health needs.[4]

At Hopkins during the 1950s, military agencies sponsored 20 to 30 percent of enrolled students, and Ernest Stebbins noted in 1956 that Department of Defense representatives had urged schools of public health to partner with them to meet the urgent need to train more medical officers. In 1957, the Association of Schools of Public Health invited the Army to send its officers to civilian schools to "meet the specialized requirements in military preventive medicine" with instruction in topics such as handling mass casualties and devastation from total warfare, problems of tropical and arctic preventive medicine, treatment of injury and trauma, and adapting epidemiological methods for military use. W. L. Treuting of Tulane told US Army Surgeon General Silas B. Hays, "Students from the armed forces have been outstanding contributors to the level of the student body of the Schools of Public Health."[5]

The military was a source of income as well as ingenuity for schools of public health. The Department of Defense sponsored faculty research as well as military officer training. At Johns Hopkins, for example, federal defense contracts in 1955–1956 represented two-thirds of external funding for the Department of Biochemistry and one-third for Environmental Medicine. Departmental expenditures under government contracts more than tripled from $53,000 in 1945–1946 to $180,000 by 1957–1958, and the total during that period for the whole school exceeded $1 million. During the relatively lean years of 1952–1953 and 1953–1954, government contracts represented roughly one-quarter of all external funding.[6]

The PHS had been an important partner for JHSPH since the beginning; during the 1950s, it eclipsed both Rockefeller and the NFIP as the school's most important funder. In 1946, the PHS formalized the Malaria Control in War Areas program on a permanent basis as the CDC. Its founder, PHS Bureau of State Services director Joseph Mountin, envisioned the CDC as "a large, well equipped and broadly staffed agency with the primary function of aiding the states in the control of communicable diseases." Mountin's second-in-command was Justin Andrews (introduced in chapter 1), who served as the CDC's deputy director from 1946 until he was named director in 1951. To head the newly formed CDC Epidemiology Section, Andrews recruited Alexander Langmuir, who remained on the JHSPH faculty as a lecturer.[7]

During the 1950s, nearly every aspect of American politics and culture was colored by fears of atomic attack and the global spread of totalitarianism under the aegis of the Soviet Union. As hostility grew between the United States and the Soviet bloc, public officials issued strident warnings of the potential dangers of nuclear, biological, and chemical warfare on US soil. Communicable disease epidemics were fading in frequency and severity, while these new threats seemed even more terrible than the ravages of polio or diphtheria. Epidemiologists were in very short supply, but Langmuir secured additional funding to train a new force of CDC epidemiologists by emphasizing the Cold War threat of biological warfare and the strategic need to maintain close relationships with state and local health authorities in the event of a national emergency. He named the program the Epidemic Intelligence Service (EIS), cashing in on the spy-versus-spy cachet of the Central Intelligence Agency, recently created in 1947.

As the founding father of EIS, Langmuir defined and instituted modern methods of disease surveillance that proved invaluable for guiding national health policy and the allocation of public health resources. For example, the mass malaria eradication campaign in the southern United States, from which the CDC was created, had been in full swing for nearly a decade before epidemiological investigations in 1947 revealed that a high percentage of reported cases were unsubstantiated by lab tests. Although malaria had undoubtedly been endemic into the 1930s, it had already disappeared before the DDT spraying program had gotten under way, largely in the absence of planned public health measures. As Langmuir later noted, "This experience was a major factor emphasizing the necessity of a more current and comprehensive system of surveillance," which proved to be crucial to responding to public health crises such as the 1957 Asian flu pandemic. Langmuir created an interstate tracking system for epidemiological data, by which the CDC could constantly receive current information from states on the incidence of communicable diseases. Such knowledge enabled the CDC to provide immediate support when disease rates began to spiral, including national planning and management to prevent and control the spread of epidemics.[8]

On arriving at the CDC, Langmuir had been immediately faced with conflict between his agency and the newly expanded NIH. The NIH and its predecessor, the PHS Hygienic Laboratory, had a long and storied history of providing assistance in controlling epidemics, including Wade Hampton Frost's work on polio and the 1918 influenza pandemic. For this reason, the NIH was reluctant to give up this responsibility, even though the CDC's congressional charter charged the new agency with serving the states in the control of communicable disease, including responding to state and local requests for aid during epidemics. When Langmuir pressed NIH officials on whether they would accept responsibility for answering all epidemic aid requests, they replied, "Certainly not. Only the interesting ones."[9]

Langmuir was in almost constant telephone contact about new disease outbreaks with his former JHSPH colleague Martin Frobisher at the National Microbiological Institute. Langmuir remembered that when his staff received a request for assistance, "State health officers were astounded to find bright, young, responsive epidemiologists in their offices the next morning, or even sometimes the same day that they called. Each epidemic aid call was an adventure and a training experience, even the false alarms." Langmuir's dedication to providing prompt assistance to states won the transfer of the epidemic aid function from the NIH to the CDC, although the two agencies continued to send out joint epidemiological teams. D. A. Henderson (MPH 1960), later appointed JHSPH dean in 1977, was one of the adventurous epidemiologists who came to work for Langmuir. The excitement of aid calls made epidemiology more competitive with clinical practice, which Henderson thought was boring by comparison.[10]

Langmuir and Andrews brought in Philip Sartwell, John Hume, and Abe Lilienfeld from JHSPH to teach the first EIS orientation course in 1950. The team chose the case-study method developed by Frost and Maxcy at Hopkins as "the best way to prepare officers for epidemiologic investigation in the field." Once the course was established, junior officers served as instructors, many of whom went on to teach epidemiology in schools around the country. Of the more than 1,000 officers who entered the EIS between 1951 and 1980, 278 joined university faculties, 206 worked for federal health agencies, and 61 worked for state or local health agencies. Another 100 worked in the global smallpox eradication campaign under Henderson. Thus, the JHSPH Department of Epidemiology played an important early role, directly and indirectly, in developing the CDC training program to become the nation's largest producer of epidemiologists. In turn, a significant number of EIS alumni went on to become JHSPH deans, department chairs, and faculty.[11]

Through the 1950s, training and other cooperative programs between federal agencies and state and local health departments enjoyed steady expansion. The PHS teamed with state and local agencies in activities that ranged from mobile health units in Alaska to community mental health. The CDC was the backbone of these efforts, and by 1955, the agency offered 176 courses annually across the country for over 3,700 employees in all fields. CDC officers also worked in state and local health departments to promote new federally funded immunization campaigns.[12]

The Cold War also shaped the evolution of the aviation medicine residency, another public health training program with strong roots at JHSPH. The same year that the school's faculty assisted in founding the EIS, Turner drew on his Army background to help Stebbins found the Department of Environmental Medicine. Like the syphilis control program, Environmental Medicine was a joint venture with Medicine that further enhanced basic science collaborations and strengthened JHSPH science degree programs. The department was the first formal joint Medicine–Hygiene department and, as the *American Journal of Public Health* reported, it would be the first to combine "research comparing individual illness and community disease." Anna Baetjer had excellent qualifications in environmental and lung physiology as well as in-depth experience with the military as both a consultant and trainer of military medical officers. Stebbins and Turner could have built on her impressive gains during and after the war in industrial health and in Baltimore's crusade against lead paint poisoning, but the school's leadership once again passed over Baetjer as a candidate for department chair.[13]

Stebbins and Turner instead decided to branch out into the wide-open field of aviation medicine. They offered the position of chair to Joseph L. Lilienthal, an expert in the physiology of respiration and neuromuscular function. Lilienthal had spent the war studying oxygenation of the blood and carbon monoxide poisoning in pilots at the Naval School of Aviation Medicine in Pensacola, Florida, and had then come to Hopkins to head the Division of Physiology in the Department of Medicine, whose faculty now held joint appointments in Environmental Medicine.[14]

JHSPH was among the first sites for the aviation medicine residency program established by the US Air Force and American Board of Preventive Medicine. Lilienthal served on the NRC Committee on Aviation Medicine and, with Stebbins, cofounded an MPH aviation medicine track that prepared physicians to manage "the medical, environmental, and operational problems involved with high speed, high altitude flight aboard jet aircraft, [such as] heart and lung function, high altitude and hyperbaric physiology, [and] accident investigation and crash safety." Flight surgeons provided medical support for military operations in all terrain, weather, and altitude and also supported the Air Force's humanitarian and disaster response missions in areas hit by floods, hurricanes, and earthquakes. Stebbins observed that "the extremely rapid development of air transportation has created new and fascinating problems," such as the major industrial health challenge posed by nearly 1 million licensed US pilots. After the space race began, aviation medicine evolved into aerospace medicine. Environmental Medicine faculty member Richard L. Riley would apply his air hygiene research to develop air purification systems for NASA's space capsules.[15]

Beginning in 1952, first-year aviation medicine residents enrolled as MPH students at the schools of public health at Hopkins, Harvard, or the University of California–Berkeley, then spent the second year at the School of Aerospace Medicine at Brooks Air Force Base, Texas. The third and final year, residents were stationed at Air Force bases around the country for supervised experience in aviation medical practice. Each year, eight flight surgeons entered the aviation medicine MPH track at Johns Hopkins. Created in the ashes of the Department of Preventive Medicine, the aviation medicine program was a forerunner of the General Preventive Medicine Residency founded at JHSPH in 1962.[16]

Meanwhile, on the floor of the US Senate, Joseph McCarthy's most outrageous and headline-grabbing accusations of communist infiltration were leveled at agencies with essential national security roles such as the US Army, State Department, and Veterans Administration (VA). If Miriam Brailey suffered for her personal and intellectual convictions, Joseph Lilienthal was a victim of guilt by association. At the Perry Point VA Hospital outside Baltimore, Lilienthal collaborated with famed psychiatrist W. Horsley Gantt, cofounder of the Psychophysiological Laboratory at Perry Point. Lilienthal's Hygiene doctoral students were "most enthusiastic" about their sessions with Gantt, a frequent visiting lecturer.[17]

Gantt, while living in Russia in the 1920s as a staff member of the American Relief Administration, had studied under Russian psychiatrist Ivan Petrovich Pavlov. In 1929, Gantt joined the Johns Hopkins medical faculty in physiology and founded the Pavlovian Laboratory, building on Pavlov's work on conditioned reflexes and psychiatry to understand more fully the connections between physiological functions and behavior. Gantt actively promoted the exchange of ideas between American and Russian scientists, and during the war, he had been associated with the National Council of American–Soviet Friendship, which was placed on the House Un-American Activities Committee's list of disloyal organizations.[18]

McCarthyism was in full swing in 1953, when Eldon Bailey, the VA's national director of security, led an investigation of Gantt, resulting in his temporary suspension from Perry Point. In 1954, McCarthy's Senate colleagues had finally voted to censure him, describing his behavior as "contrary to senatorial traditions." But the investigations of suspected communist sympathizers continued apace, and in July 1955, an investigator for the Senate Subcommittee on Federal Employee Security pushed Lilienthal to confess wrongdoing even though Perry Point administrators had refused to relinquish his personnel file. Afterward, Lilienthal wrote in a heated letter to JHSPH dean emeritus Lowell Reed, "It was a little breath-taking to hear the point of view now being expressed by these people." Lilienthal placed the blame for allowing the loyalty investigations to continue squarely on Surgeon General Leonard Scheele, whom Lilienthal hoped would "take a lamb out behind his 20 story brick outhouse [possibly a reference to the NIH Clinical Center Building in Bethesda, Maryland, completed in 1953], sacrifice it, examine its entrails and read the auguries properly. If he does perhaps he can stiffen his spine and straighten out the real mess in Washington." In November 1955, just months after Lilienthal was exonerated of charges that he had harbored Communist sympathies, he died of a sudden heart attack at age 44. W. F. Hamilton, president of the American Physiological Society, paid tribute to Lilienthal's "forceful rebellion to conditions that frustrated the advancement of science."[19]

Throughout the era of McCarthyism and long afterward, the domestic anticommunism attacks on government involvement in health services created an environment of suspicion that undermined public confidence in public health in some quarters, even as the great public health victories of polio and penicillin were grabbing national headlines. Public health agencies from the local to the federal level had to be extremely cautious about their public statements, hiring decisions, and programming. Health departments' relationships with lawmakers, other government units, the medical profession, and community stakeholders suffered as well. In such a context, many public health leaders saw little advantage and great risk in proposals to move beyond public health's traditional duties: environmental sanitation, communicable disease control (but not treatment), and educating the public about personal health and hygiene.

Two of the most politically acceptable avenues for the expansion of public health's authority were in civil defense and contributing to the health mission of the armed forces. As the example of aviation medicine proved, public health methods were easily adapted to a variety of military applications. JHSPH faculty studied the effects of high temperature and other environmental factors on human performance and examined the comparative physiology of parasites to assist the Navy in developing antiparasitic drugs. The largest sponsors of defense contracts at JHSPH were the Atomic Energy Commission (AEC), the Office of Naval Research, and the Air Research and Development Command. Immediately after the Soviet *Sputnik* flight in October 1957, the director of the Security Division of the AEC notified all universities with research contracts that Soviet bloc nationals could still visit US universities but were prohibited from entering areas, projects, or activities sponsored by AEC contracts.[20]

One instructive example of the school's defense contract research was a study by microbiologist Carl Lamanna of type C botulinal neurotoxin for potential military use as an antidote to protect soldiers. *Clostridium botulinum*, the bacteria that causes botulism, is a potential biological weapon since it secretes toxic proteins that block neuromuscular transmission, causing severe muscular weakness and paralysis. Type A is also used today for therapeutic medical and cosmetic procedures and is manufactured commercially as Botox.

Lamanna and research associate Wayne I. Jensen used mice to test the toxicity and measure of protection offered by a toxoid (an inactivated toxic bacterial protein that still stimulates antibodies) from type C *C. botulinum*. Even though conventional mouse testing had deemed the toxoid safe, it produced an "unexpected pathologic response" when injected into various experimental animals, who slowly developed a harmful cellular reaction. Testing in Rhesus monkeys, rabbits, and guinea pigs produced extreme muscular weakness and "an acute condition terminating in death within a few days," suggesting the existence of a second toxin distinct from the known neurotoxin.[21]

Lamanna and Jensen also analyzed the procedures for producing and testing the toxoid. While they were evaluating whether type C *C. botulinum* also produced disease-causing agents in experimental animals, the control animals caged with the toxoid-injected animals also became sick after three weeks and exhibited "gross pathological lesions" in the lungs, which the researchers believed might suggest that the infected control animals had produced a specific antibody to the toxoid (in fact, the histologic lesions merely indicated the production of toxins, not proof of immune response via production of antibodies). JHSPH researchers thus saved the lives of unknown thousands of military personnel by demonstrating that type C botulinal toxoid, intended to protect US troops against biological warfare, was both infectious and seriously toxic.[22]

Epidemiological and environmental studies of the polar regions were another aspect of military research at JHSPH. In 1949, the PHS established an Arctic Health Research Center in Anchorage to improve the overall health of Alaskans and reduce the world's highest incidence of TB among the Eskimo population. The PHS also coordinated with the Naval Arctic Research Laboratory at Point Barrow on defense-related projects for preserving the health of troops in potential battle environments. One of the case studies for the required MPH public health administration course involved developing a plan for preventive medical service for a military unit sent to the Arctic. The US Navy's Operation Deepfreeze scientific research program in Antarctica included studies by pathobiologist William J. L. Sladen (ScD 1957) of penguins and other marine life, based on public health concepts of population biology and epidemiology. He banded over 6,000 Antarctic sea birds to track their population growth and migration and, with his wife Brenda Sladen, studied the population dynamics, diseases, and behavior of the Alaskan fur seal. To complement their atomic and arctic interests, Hygiene faculty collaborated frequently with the US Army Medical Research and Development Command, which JHSPH dean John Hume later wrote had "proved to be of mutual benefit and has led to the development of new methodologies and information which will prove to be extremely useful to the entire scientific community."[23]

Public health's traditional emphasis on prophylaxis and preparedness made it a natural standard-bearer for civil defense, which also provided a welcome justification for pursuing many longstanding public health goals. In July 1954, the Department of Health, Education and Welfare assigned responsibility for the public health aspects of civil defense to the PHS, whose commissioned officers could be swiftly mobilized and deployed to areas stricken by enemy attacks or subsequent communicable disease outbreaks "during periods of stress and disorganization." The PHS was charged with planning and coordinating efforts to restore essential community health facilities during a national emergency, although it was expressly restricted from treating casualties.[24]

Since emergency public health services were essential to civil defense, recruitment and training of public health workers gained new urgency. John B. Hozier of the Office of the Surgeon General's Emergency Health Planning Unit made a plea for boosting the ranks of public health specialists to protect America's 165 million citizens from the effects of biological, chemical, nuclear, and radiological attacks, especially the 70 million inhabitants of critical target areas who might be driven from their homes. "The task of training the numbers needed for public health civil defense," Hozier declared, "is greater than the capacity of any state or, for that matter, of any single federal agency." Civil defense necessitated close cooperation between the PHS and other national agencies, including the Federal Civil Defense Administration, Atomic Energy Commission, Walter Reed Army Institute of Research, and Army Chemical Corps.[25]

The PHS also strengthened and expanded its collaborative programs with state and local health departments, which often benefited non–civil defense activities as well. For example, to minimize the effects of a biological or chemical attack, civil defense personnel needed to provide an early warning and implement control measures promptly. Hozier cautioned that "the extreme vulnerability of water distribution systems to attack by saboteurs is generally realized. Every house connection and every fire hydrant is a possible point of entry of a contaminant." The PHS worked with public health departments to develop procedures to more rapidly and accurately detect, identify, and control disease-producing and poisonous agents used in biological weapons. Such research could have important applications for environmental health goals such as monitoring the effects of air and water pollution or protecting workers and consumers from the hazards of toxic chemicals. At JHSPH, federal agencies with civil defense responsibilities funded the work of Anna Baetjer on environmental toxicology, Joseph Lilienthal and Richard L. Riley on lung function and airborne pathogens, and Cornelius Krusé and Abel Wolman on the dangers of radiation exposure.[26]

The threat of either conventional or biochemical warfare also warranted additional research in communicable disease control, which Hozier noted was "in the direct interest of survival during disasters. The needs of civil defense demand that communicable disease research look at the exotic diseases, as well as the common diseases, that may well be revived under emergency conditions. In general, the same principles apply to the control of diseases whether or not the causative agent is introduced by enemy action." Attacks that used disease-causing pathogens could be foiled if the nature and extent of exposure was discovered before the end of the incubation period, but existing lab procedures were often laborious and time-consuming, particularly for viral and rickettsial diseases, which could require weeks to identify. More research was also indicated to develop new compounds that could disinfect or neutralize contaminated areas and on methods for their safe and effective use. Finally, mental hygiene research could shed light on the anticipated behavior and needs of an evacuated population under severe stress, enabling public health officials "to offer protection to panicked and disorganized populations." To imagine the implications of the dire situations envisioned by Hozier, one only had to watch the latest science fiction movie portraying global catastrophe after an alien invasion, nuclear apocalypse, or the rampage of a technology-spawned monster.[27]

Training the Global Health Workforce

Alongside the expansion of defense-related public health programs, the Roosevelt and Truman administrations also stimulated American schools of public health to develop foreign research and training programs along the lines of those established by the Rockefeller Foundation at Johns Hopkins and Harvard. One of the earliest of these collaborations had begun in 1932, when the Rockefeller IHD had provided support to establish both the EHD in Baltimore and JHSPH's Indian counterpart, the All India Institute of Hygiene and Public Health in Calcutta. The All India Institute was the first school of public health in Southeast and South Asia, and the IHD sent John Black Grant to serve as director from 1939 to 1945. In keeping with Wickliffe Rose's vision of an international network of schools of public health, the EHD was an integral part of Rockefeller's template for establishing schools overseas. The high volume of foreign and domestic visitors at times interfered with the EHD's day-to-day operations.[28]

The largest source of foreign visitors to the EHD was Rockefeller Foundation fellows from Latin America. As part of his Latin American "Good Neighbor" policy, President Roosevelt established the Office of Inter-American Affairs, directed by Nelson Rockefeller. Between 1940 and 1950, the Office of Inter-American Affairs brought nearly 1,200 health professionals and scientists (mostly physicians and sanitary engineers) from 18 Latin American countries to study at Johns Hopkins and other US schools, with fellowships funded by the PHS, the Rockefeller Foundation, and the Commonwealth Fund. Latin American public health professionals were largely trained at Johns Hopkins and Harvard, such as the founders of Chile's first school of public health. Among them was Abraham Horwitz, who earned an MPH in 1944 and served as the first director of the University of Chile School of Public Health. Horwitz helped to develop the Chilean National Health Service and to eradicate small-pox in Chile. As director-general of the Pan American Health Organization from 1958 to 1975, he was one of the school's most influential alumni and shaped research and policy on nutrition, health policy and financing, zoonotic diseases, and infectious disease epidemiology, especially malaria and polio. JHSPH alumni also established the first schools of public health in many Latin American countries and served as ministers of health of Costa Rica, Brazil, Puerto Rico, El Salvador, and Venezuela.[29]

Despite the later failure of the school's partnership with the city health department, the EHD may have had a more lasting influence on public health outside the United States than within it. In 1947, just as the fourth EHD census was causing headaches for Huntington Williams, a documentary film crew arrived to shoot what amounted to an elaborate recruiting advertisement for the Johns Hopkins School of Hygiene and Public Health. The US State Department Information Agency produced *Journey into Medicine* as a propaganda film to educate foreign audiences about the achievements of the American medical and public health systems. The plot follows "Mike," a recent medical graduate, through an internship at Columbia Presbyterian Hospital, a pediatric residency at Cornell University's New York Hospital, and an MPH at Johns Hopkins. JHSPH and the EHD served as the stand-in for all of American public health.

The film's climactic event is a diphtheria outbreak in East Baltimore. In a war room scene, Mike and a team of JHSPH faculty and BCHD officials plot the cases on a map of the EHD, where public health nurses go door to door to rally the community to line up their children for shots of antitoxin. The film could have been called *Journey into Public Health*, since, after helping to quell the epidemic, Mike concludes that he belongs on the front lines of public health rather than treating individual patients in private practice. Mike's onscreen conversion to public health was so convincing that the *American Journal of Public Health* called the film "particularly effective for third and fourth year medical students who are at the period when they are seeking to decide in which field of medicine they can be of maximum service and derive the greatest personal satisfactions."[30]

Journey into Medicine was written and directed by top Hollywood filmmakers and earned an Academy Award nomination for best documentary feature. The State Department translated the movie into multiple languages, including Cambodian, and showed it to audiences worldwide. Professional organizations such as the APHA and the International Congress of Pediatrics hosted screenings at their annual conferences. *Journey into Medicine* captured on film the Hopkins model of public health training and research at the height of the EHD's success. The film symbolized the allure of a public health career in the 1940s and 1950s, when academic, professional, and government organizations joined forces to recruit more health professionals into a field that was deemed essential to the nation's welfare and defense.[31]

Journey into Medicine was also used to recruit US-trained foreign health professionals, who were critical in waging the global war against malaria, TB, and other epidemic diseases. Before the war, most foreign public health students in the United States were sponsored by the Rockefeller IHD, but after the division's merger with the medical sciences program in 1951, the Rockefeller fellowship program dwindled. WHO and the US State Department became the leading sponsors, and students' interests and geographic origins broadened as the proportion of foreign students rose from about one-fifth of enrollments in the late 1930s to about one-third during the postwar decades. The chartering of the WHO in 1948 marked the beginning of an idealistic new era for the promotion of public health around the globe. By 1961, WHO had sponsored 10,000 trainees worldwide, which brought the first students from the Middle East, Asia, and India to JHSPH in significant numbers.[32]

Dean Stebbins was among the key proponents of foreign exchange programs for public health education. His experiences responding to the health and humanitarian crises generated by World War II had earned him an appointment to the WHO expert advisory panel on public health administration. As a member, Stebbins was instrumental in guiding planning for new public health agencies around the globe. In a report he coauthored on the postwar reorganization of health administration in Italy, Stebbins recommended a national unification of government health and medical services under a Ministry of Health. Under a regional system of local public health centers, population units of 10,000 to 50,000 could receive basic preventive services and public health supervision and medical care. The national Ministry of Health would ensure the continuity of inpatient and outpatient care from the national to local levels, including social insurance organizations. The Ministry of Health would also regulate provincial health officers under civil service guidelines and ensure adequate salaries. Echoing the Parran–Farrand Report, Stebbins emphasized that the government should provide training facilities for physicians to learn administrative and technical skills and should establish schools of public health, directed not by scientists but by administrators with "broad training and experience in public health administration."[33]

At midcentury, however, most US schools of public health were ill-prepared to train either foreign or American students in the methods and knowledge required for building foreign public health systems from the ground up.

International health was covered in fewer than three pages in the 1950 first edition of the textbook *Principles of Public Health Administration*. And international students were not always well suited or prepared for study in American universities. As early as 1943, Reed had expressed concern that some foreign students were coming to Hopkins without a clear understanding of the difference between public health and medicine and had no real intention of doing public health work. Foreign students were often first admitted as special students and then transferred to degree programs after they had demonstrated the ability to meet graduate-level admissions requirements. They were also more likely to encounter academic difficulties due to language and cultural barriers, less rigorous medical training in poor countries with fewer resources, and the uncertainties inherent in admitting students from distant countries, sight unseen, at the behest of the Rockefeller Foundation. At a 1952 meeting of the Association of Schools of Public Health, public health deans complained to officials from WHO and US-based agencies that international students were still arriving with "no better preparation in language and little if any improvement in provision of credentials at the outset."[34]

Some observers also questioned the relevance of US-centered curricula for international students. A case in point was the Office of Inter-American Affairs fellowship program. In 1955, the US Department of State joined the Office of Inter-American Affairs with two other divisions to form the International Cooperation Administration (ICA). By the end of the 1950s, ICA's Office of Public Health oversaw cooperative health programs in 36 countries with a budget of $80 million and a staff of more than 300 public health workers from the United States. Likewise, the total WHO budget had doubled to $26 million, and the United Nations Children's Fund (UNICEF) assisted maternal and child health and infectious disease control projects in 71 countries and territories, including the BCG vaccination of nearly 120 million children against TB as well as smaller programs to combat yaws, leprosy, and trachoma.[35]

By the end of the 1950s, the ICA had concluded that Latin American health professionals should be trained in their home countries instead of being brought to the United States, although foreign public health institutions sometimes pushed back against American proposals to end exchange programs. Henry van Zile Hyde, who had directed the international health units of the Office of Inter-American Affairs, PHS, and ICA, complained to public health deans at a 1961 ASPH meeting that "we have continued to bring foreigners here and seem to have stopped institution building abroad." Eugene Campbell, the current director of ICA's Office of Health, pointedly asked the deans, "How much do the schools of public health really identify with the U.S. role in world health? Sometimes we get the feeling that they believe they are being put upon in getting foreign students, and at other times we get quite the opposite impression."[36]

At Johns Hopkins, South Asia was by far the school's leading source of foreign public health graduates after World War II. Between 1945 and 1980, nearly 100 Indian and another 30 Pakistani students earned degrees (most were physicians with MPHs), and many returned as senior academic faculty, administrators in the Ministry of Health, or researchers and regional officers in WHO or the UN Population Division. For example, Kishore Chandra Patnaik (DrPH 1950) wrote his Hopkins doctoral thesis in public health administration on "The Organization and Administration of an Official District as a 'Field Training Area' (Practice Field) with a School of Public Health in India." Patnaik carried the EHD model back to the All India Institute and went on to serve as an epidemiology officer in India's Central Bureau of Health Intelligence. South Asian JHSPH graduates also influenced their country's governments to formulate and implement population policies designed to accelerate modernization and economic growth by attempting to significantly lower death, disease, and fertility rates.[37]

Fueled by the incentive of WHO traineeships, many in the postwar wave of international students chose JHSPH for its reputation as the leading American center of syphilis research. The Division of Venereal Diseases' clinical research on penicillin in early syphilis, together with the Department of Bacteriology's work on the disease's immunological aspects, would significantly influence postwar international VD control efforts. The penicillin trials provided incomparable experience to young researchers like Tsun Tung (ScD 1941), an instructor in Bacteriology who left Hopkins in 1944 to direct China's penicillin production project. After John Hume took over in 1947 as director of the VD control MPH program, it shifted from training PHS officers to work in the American South to preparing foreign physicians to work in the WHO global VD control campaign. In 1949, the WHO Expert Committee on Venereal Diseases urged foreign health officials to avail themselves of "control methods recently developed in the United States, particularly penicillin treatments of syphilis and evaluation of their effectiveness for national and international programs." The WHO Syphilis Study Commission also sent physicians from Europe, India, and South America on three-month stays at Hopkins and other leading programs in the United States.[38]

One foreign physician whose JHSPH training led directly into a key role in WHO's global campaign against VD was Huan-Ying Li (MPH 1952). Her native China was being torn apart by World War II, and despite her interest in studying bacteriology and physiology, laboratory facilities there were very limited. As all Chinese medical graduates were required to do, Li completed a one-year internship as an army medical officer in the Kuomintang, the nationalist

Chinese party led by Chiang Kai-shek. Li had never heard of Johns Hopkins until her father visited Baltimore as part of a Chinese government delegation assigned to learn about the B&O Railroad as a model for postwar reconstruction. The B&O officials urged him to consider sending his physician daughter to Johns Hopkins, but instead of studying clinical medicine, she chose to work in the School of Hygiene with Thomas Turner. When her father brought her to meet Dr. Turner for the first time, the 26-year-old Li handed him her blue booklet with all her transcripts and grades from the US-recognized Tong Ji Medical School, and Turner agreed to admit her (see photo gallery).[39]

After her army internship in obstetrics, gynecology, and pediatrics, she had told her classmates, "I'm not so much interested in people." It was *groups* of people who interested her, and she fell in love with epidemiology at Johns Hopkins. Her teacher was Alex Langmuir, soon-to-be head of the Epidemic Intelligence Service at the CDC. As Turner's research associate, she assisted in his research to determine the most effective type and dosage of penicillin against *Treponema pallidum*, a spirochete bacterium with subspecies that cause treponemal diseases such as syphilis, bejel, pinta, and yaws. Many evenings, she walked in to campus and up to the lab to make the daily *Treponema* counts, using oil immersion to increase the resolution of the microscope.[40]

Despite his busy schedule, Turner made time to visit Li in Johns Hopkins Hospital when she had to have an emergency appendectomy. But what most impressed Li about Turner was his faith in her ability to do independent scientific research. "In China," she commented, "it's all tradition, all about following the teacher. But that's not science. You must have an inquisitive mind and ask yourself, what can I contribute other than what others have done?" Turner would give Li a tough research question and let her figure it out on her own.[41]

Li shared a lab with Robert Nelson, and her intimate knowledge of the TPI test and the wide range of sophisticated immunological tests used at Hopkins became the springboard for her global health career fighting the major scourges of yaws, syphilis, and leprosy. In 1950, WHO asked Turner to head the global campaign against yaws, a severe tropical disease that was most common in rural areas of the developing world. He dispatched Li to work for the campaign in Indonesia. After interviewing for the job in Geneva, she soon found herself out in the field supervising Indonesian public health workers on the island of Java. Everything she had learned at Johns Hopkins came together when she had to oppose a German WHO consultant who wanted to inject patients with penicillin at five times the recommended dosage, using the same syringe in different patients. She wrote to the WHO official in Geneva who had given her the job to make her case that the German doctor's procedure was medically unsound, especially since it also increased the risk of hepatitis infection. When the letter arrived from WHO that confirmed Li's objections, her

German colleague remarked, "Chinese chairs are not comfortable." Li took the comparison to the traditional straight-back wooden chair and flipped it back at him, saying, "We Chinese, we keep our backs straight."[42]

In 1950, yaws infected more than 20 million people worldwide, with over half the cases in Asia; by 1955, the WHO campaign had been "dramatically successful," particularly in Indonesia, where Li had worked for three years, and in Thailand. After spending another three years with WHO's VD campaign in Burma, Li returned in 1959 to Beijing to join the faculty of the Institute of Dermatology at the Chinese Academy of Medical Sciences. At that time, the Chinese government was intent on eradicating VD, and Li was assigned to supervise the TPI test's application in China. The test was extremely complicated and expensive, at a cost of $100 US dollars per test run, and she tried unsuccessfully to convince her superiors that the test "didn't suit our country." Nonetheless, she loyally advised the national TPI testing program, and in 1963, she would publish the definitive article in Chinese on using the TPI test to diagnose syphilis.[43]

After growing bored with syphilis, which was relatively easy to diagnose and treat, Li spent a decade in rural eastern China (during Chairman Mao Zedong's Cultural Revolution), where she worked to improve the health of farmers. Based since 1979 at the Beijing Tropical Medicine Research Institute, she has remained active into her 90s. With the advanced knowledge gained during a nine-month WHO Fellowship to visit the world's most prominent leprosy research centers in the United States, England, and Asia, Li had conducted seminal research on the use of multidrug therapy to control leprosy, once a lifetime sentence of suffering and isolation for hundreds of thousands of Chinese patients. She has also trained scores of Chinese scientists and health professionals in multidrug therapy methods for leprosy control that were applied systematically across the country beginning in the early 1980s. The modern prevalence rates of leprosy reached their height in China in the 1960s, at more than two cases per 10,000 population; by 1998, the rate had been drastically reduced to 0.05/10,000.[44]

Another JHSPH graduate who made great contributions to fighting leprosy was the Belgian Catholic missionary Michel Lechat (MPH 1963, DrPH 1966), whose leprosarium in the Belgian Congo was the setting for the 1960 Graham Greene novel *A Burnt-Out Case*. After the book's publication, Lechat's notoriety interfered with his daily work, and he came to Hopkins to earn a doctorate in epidemiology. After Lechat took a course on queuing theory from Charles Flagle (profiled in chapter 8), the two collaborated on devising optimum methods of screening for leprosy in areas with high rates of infection but inadequate laboratory facilities. Lechat led in developing the epidemiometric model of leprosy, which uses computerized mathematical simulations to analyze the impact of long-term treatment of leprosy under different regimens, and applying operations research principles to leprosy treatment. He served as president of both the International Leprosy Association and the International Leprosy Union. JHSPH's complementary strengths in operations research and international health would form the basis for an intensive research program in health systems that led in conducting planning and evaluation for health services and workforces around the world.[45]

The longstanding partnership between the Rockefeller International Health Division and Johns Hopkins yielded a lasting East–West partnership in graduate public health education, public health practice, and population research. China had been a major source of international JHSPH graduates, but Huan-Ying Li was the last Chinese student to attend Johns Hopkins before Mao Zedong's Communist Revolution closed exchange opportunities in the United States. During the 1950s, China and Latin America were eclipsed by India as the largest source of foreign students at JHSPH.

Showdown

In medical schools at most universities, including Johns Hopkins, the preclinical basic science departments had withered during the 1930s and 1940s, while the full-time clinical staff had grown along with rapid medical advances and new areas of specialization. In addition to training Li and many other international students, Turner made basic science teaching a central part of efforts to restructure both medical and public health education at Hopkins and led a university-wide push to substantially enlarge the basic science faculty and promote cooperation among Hygiene, Medicine, and Homewood. Turner's success in strengthening basic science as an interdivisional bridge was all the more remarkable, given that his primary appointment was in Hygiene, and both he and the school had remained committed to infectious disease as Medicine moved toward chronic disease.

The medical faculty hoped to raise $5 million in endowed support for additional basic science positions and another $5 million to construct a new Basic Sciences Building, planning for which highlighted growing tensions between Medicine and Hygiene. Since its construction in 1947 next to the Welch Medical Library across Monument Street from the Hygiene building, the shared New Hunterian Laboratory building had been intended to relieve the intense need for more spacious and modern accommodations for the burgeoning basic science research programs in both schools. In September 1956, the PHS appointed Turner to the newly created National Advisory Council on Health Research Facilities, which reviewed construction grant applications for $90 million earmarked under Hill–Burton over three years.[46]

In December, just as the Turner Committee issued its interim report to the JHSPH faculty, the PHS approved the School of Medicine's $1.86 million request for a new Basic Sciences Building. Although Bang and Herriott were members of the architectural planning committee, their departments of Pathobiology and Biochemistry were not allocated space in the new building. One month after the PHS grant announcement, the Medical Planning and Development Committee and the Medicine and Hygiene advisory boards agreed on a cost-cutting plan whereby Medicine would house and administer four joint basic science departments—Microbiology, Physiology (which absorbed Environmental Medicine), Pharmacology, and a new endowed Department of Biophysics—with both schools contributing to their budgets. JHSPH seemed to gain space only when departments left the Hygiene Building: just as the Department of Preventive Medicine had vacated the seventh and eighth floors in 1951, Microbiology now prepared to move across Monument Street to the Basic Sciences Building, which completed Turner's efforts throughout the 1950s to merge his department with the School of Medicine.[47]

The year 1957 was one of reckoning for the School of Hygiene. In January, Turner was offered the deanship at Downstate Medical Center of the State University of New York and was on the short list for an executive position in the American Cancer Society. Wood knew that the Johns Hopkins University trustees and administration were considering eliminating the school or downgrading it to become a medical school department, and he wrote ominously to Keith Spalding in the Office of the President, "It is possible that certain things may happen in the School of Hygiene within the next few months which will make Dr. Turner want to reconsider the New York State offer." Meanwhile, Wood reported proudly to the Board of Trustees in spring 1957 that the School of Medicine was improving basic science teaching and had received a five-year $250,000 PHS grant for basic science fellowships. The medical school's deficit had disappeared, due in no small part due to Turner's efforts, along with a combined $6.1 million from the Ford and Rockefeller foundations for the revised medical education program, as well as a new income stream from establishing a private outpatient services program.[48]

Instead of leaving for New York, Turner stayed at Hopkins to become the new Dean of Medicine and took Manfred Mayer, David Bodian, and several other JHSPH science faculty members with him. Despite Turner's efforts over the years, neither Mayer nor Bodian had been promoted to full professor. Although the School of Hygiene made Bodian an eleventh-hour offer of a raise and full professorship in Epidemiology, he declined in order to accept the chairmanship of the Department of Anatomy, his first home at Hopkins. Mayer and his students would go on to lead the field of complement research at the molecular level in the 1960s and 1970s, and he was elected president of the American Association of Immunologists in 1979.[49]

Although Turner and Wood still held joint appointments in Hygiene, John Black Grant of the Rockefeller Foundation wrote after a visit to Baltimore, "Stebbins feels that Barry Wood is prejudiced in favor of the Medical School as against Public Health." Morale in the School of Hygiene suffered as more faculty left. In 1957, Biostatistics chair William G. Cochran accepted Harvard's offer to lead a new Department of Statistics. He was followed by two other senior faculty members, which left Biostatistics with "a skeleton staff which will be further reduced next year unless prompt action is taken." The doyenne of biostatistics, Margaret Merrell, had planned to retire but stayed on as interim chair during 1957–1958. She wrote Stebbins, "It may be hard for anyone outside the field to realize the extreme shortage of persons with the qualifications we require and we are probably handicapped in this competitive area by the loss of prestige accompanying the simultaneous resignations of three senior members of the staff." Cochran's successor, Jerome Cornfield, stayed only two years, and Biostatistics remained without a chair for another year until 1960, when Allyn Winthrop Kimball was named chair of Biostatistics, and another full professor, David B. Duncan, also joined the department.[50]

In 1958, Wood wrote Evans that "the central issue which all schools of public health now face [is] whether they should continue to exist as separate schools. This view has arisen primarily as a result of the increasing emphasis upon preventive medicine which of necessity breaks the conventional boundaries between clinical medicine and public health." Turner, Wood, and the Hygiene basic science faculty wanted to uphold the traditional primacy of laboratory research, and most but not all advocated closer cooperation with the medical school. Turner, Wood, and John C. Bugher, director of the Rockefeller Foundation's Division of Medical Education and Public Health, actually favored merging the two schools entirely and downsizing the School of Hygiene into a single medical school Department of Preventive Medicine and Public Health.[51]

To gauge the effect of confining all types of public health instruction inside a medical school department, one could look to Harvard, whose school of public health did not become fully independent of the medical school until 1946 (until then the two schools had shared a complex administrative relationship and a dean, David L. Edsall). Up to that point, the Harvard School of Public Health had received $3.7 million from the Rockefeller Foundation, which Edsall had used primarily to strengthen preventive medicine instruction in the medical school. According to Alan Gregg, director of the Rockefeller Division of Medical Sciences, Edsall had done "very little that is affirmative or tangible" for the public health departments. Gregg candidly told Harvard president James B. Conant that "in the view of the Public Health men in this country you scarcely have a school. Have you a teacher under 60 whose work is primarily in that school and who has a wide reputation in the Public Health field?" Gregg charged that Harvard Medical School's relationship with its School of Public Health had been one of "suffocation, patronage, [and] petty rivalries."[52]

As the School of Hygiene and Public Health labored to avoid the fate of being absorbed into the medical school, the basic science bridge between Medicine and Hygiene crumbled within a few years after Turner was appointed dean of Medicine. One after another, prominent scientists rejected offers to chair the joint science departments, and by 1961, the departments of Microbiology, Pharmacology, Physiology, and Biophysics had all dissolved their affiliations with Hygiene. Environmental Medicine was reincarnated as a small Hygiene department in 1961 under the chairmanship of Joseph Lilienthal's longtime colleague Richard Riley—as in 1950, Anna Baetjer was passed over.[53]

The School after Turner and *Sputnik*

In the fall of 1957, as faculty in JHSPH watched their colleagues leave and their school's prestige dim, Americans stared incredulously as the Soviet satellite *Sputnik I* streaked across the October night sky. *Sputnik*, the first spacecraft to orbit the Earth, was a slap in the face to American technological and military superiority, and the following July, Congress passed legislation to create the National Aeronautics and Space Administration. In the late 1950s, federal spending on defense and scientific research grew apace as the US–Soviet rivalry heated up in the wake of protests during Vice-President Richard M. Nixon's 1958 tour of Latin America, followed by the Berlin and Cuban Missile crises early in John F. Kennedy's presidency.[54]

The US government, the largest contributor to the PAHO, WHO, and UNICEF, also increased support for international health. Proponents of disease eradication, who followed Fred Soper and fomented his ideas with evangelistic zeal, argued that judicious application of technical methods such as DDT and chloroquine could greatly improve health conditions prior to economic development and that morbidity and mortality must be sufficiently reduced in order for the health of workers and consumers to reach a level to support sustained growth. These assumptions were fundamental in President Truman's Point Four program, which created the postwar US technical assistance programs in health, agriculture, and engineering within the framework of using foreign aid to contain communism.

The WHO global malaria eradication campaign, launched in 1955 under its new Director-General, Marcolino G. Candau (MPH 1941), achieved its greatest successes in Asia. In India, where malaria had caused an estimated 1 million deaths annually, the number of recorded cases fell from 75 million in 1951 to 50,000 in 1961. Such statistics led champions of international public health to claim that disease control measures modeled on the global malaria eradication campaign represented the best value per aid dollar invested. Timothy D. Baker (MPH 1954), who played a key role in the late 1950s malaria eradication campaigns in India and Ceylon (later Sri Lanka), remembered that "we were seduced by Fred Soper's success in northeast Brazil in truly eradicating the most efficient mosquito vector, *Anopheles gambiae*."[55]

At the 1959 APHA conference, Myron E. Wegman (MPH 1938), dean of public health at the University of Michigan, spoke eagerly of "the extraordinary opportunity we have for promoting peace through understanding among nations and among health workers. Ours is the advantage of having a common language which can often surmount the obstacles of the Tower of Babel." Addressing the APHA again in 1961, Wegman declared, "Nowhere can health be more effective than as an avenue for peace." International health represented a welcome source of renewed optimism and pride for an American public health profession that was still adapting to the domestic challenges of controlling chronic disease and administering government medical programs. By going abroad to address the most widespread health problems in developing countries—sanitation, water supply, and control of communicable disease— public health found itself back on familiar ground.[56]

Public health interventions had the potential to achieve rapid, dramatic results on a mass basis; they also had great propaganda value against communism and social unrest and served to legitimize local governments and their US allies. As global health historian Randall Packard has observed, "The apparent speed with which malaria could be brought under control with DDT, together with its short term effects on other household pests, made malaria control particularly attractive for those who saw tropical disease control as an instrument for 'winning hearts and minds' in the war against communist expansion."[57]

But in their tendency to target a specific disease as an enemy to be conquered apart from the other needs or opinions of human hosts, the mass campaigns against malaria, yaws, and TB reflected the vertical organization and cultural biases of the US military and the prewar public health initiatives in the American South, Latin America, and the European colonies of Asia and Africa. "One-shot" methods such as spraying homes with DDT and single injections with penicillin or BCG vaccine made it seem unnecessary to work closely with local populations. American field workers sincerely believed that they were helping the inhabitants of developing countries to build up their governmental health services and spread the benefits of modern medical technology. But such efforts sidestepped the need to reform caste- and class-based health systems. The enduring inadequacies of rural health infrastructures in developing countries prevented many postwar international health programs from sustaining their successes beyond the initial "attack" phase.[58]

At the same time, American technical assistance in general came under increasing criticism, notably in the scathing 1958 novel *The Ugly American*, which decried the linguistic and cultural incompetence of the American contingent in Vietnam. A National Research Council Division of Medical Sciences report contended that research on tropical medicine since 1945 had been "limited in scope and neither planned nor coordinated to achieve specific objectives—despite the fact that year after year the United States was spending increasingly larger amounts of money for the support and development of health projects in the tropics and contiguous areas." The NRC report's authors argued that agencies such as the ICA and PHS were still "unnecessarily constrained by ambiguity of authority" and made a strong case for granting them the freedom to conduct international health research on its own merits, regardless of its applications back home.[59]

Although the School of Hygiene was nearly a casualty of the continual struggles for power, funding, and space between it and the School of Medicine, Stebbins allied with Senator Hubert H. Humphrey, a Minnesota Democrat, to help to pass two major federal programs, one domestic and one international, that initiated a longstanding collaboration between Humphrey and the Association of Schools of Public Health. The two bills rescued JHSPH from the brink of fiscal disaster by using national defense concerns to stimulate funding for public health research and training.

The first was federal legislation to assist schools of public health, which Humphrey introduced in May 1955 as the Emergency Public Health Training Act. Echoing Alex Langmuir's justification for founding the EIS, Humphrey proclaimed, "The training of personnel to protect the public against disease is as essential a part of public responsibility as is the training of personnel for the military forces to protect our Nation against a military aggressor." The bill passed in 1956 and was later redrafted by the quintessential advocate of federal health funding, Senator Lister Hill of Alabama. As ASPH presidents, Stebbins and Hugh Leavell of Harvard led the lobbying push to pass the Hill–Rhodes Public Health Professional Training Act, authorized in 1958 on a two-year emergency basis and then renewed every five years from 1960 until the program ended in 1978.[60]

Humphrey served on the Senate Foreign Relations Committee with John F. Kennedy; both men had presidential ambitions and wanted to make their mark in foreign policy. The Democrats on the committee, along with Senate majority leader Lyndon B. Johnson, wanted to shift the main emphasis of US foreign aid from military assistance to long-term development. In a 1959 speech,

Humphrey declared that "we must grasp and keep the initiative as the peace-maker, and not let [Soviet premier Nikita] Khruschev run away with it." Humphrey called for a "dramatic, worldwide 'Health for Peace' program, with vastly expanded international medical research." At his urging, Congress funded an intensive study of WHO research and pledged "substantial support to any sound program that may emerge from the proposed study, subject to participation by a number of other member states." Humphrey also conducted a series of hearings on the role of the US government in international medical research and issued the findings in 1961. The report called for increased support for research and better evaluation methods, greater attention to long-range planning, and more efficient cooperation between the PHS, ICA, nongovernmental organizations (NGOs), and schools of medicine and public health.[61]

International health organizations responded with a series of steps to bolster research and promote evaluation of existing programs. The PHS, WHO, and PAHO signed international cooperative research agreements, and the International Health Research Act of 1960 authorized the use of federal funds for evaluation studies by consultants to international health agencies. The 1960 legislation reinvigorated both intramural and extramural planning, research, and training programs under an array of federal agencies, which would support an international health research boom across JHSPH. The International Health Research Act also stipulated that research activities conducted outside the United States must benefit the health of Americans. This reversed the pattern of the previous two decades, where the disease control techniques developed in the American South were applied overseas during World War II and in the early WHO global health campaigns.[62]

Together, funding from the International Health Research Act and Hill–Rhodes solved the financial crisis at JHSPH and underwrote the expansion of public health enrollments nationally. In 1960, for the first time in years, no Johns Hopkins unit, including Hygiene, posted a deficit. Hopkins initially received $200,000 per year from the Hill–Rhodes program, a sum that, the JHU Board of Trustees noted approvingly, "assures relative stability in the financing of the School of Hygiene and Public Health for at least five years and hopefully will permit an attack on the School's greatest problem—lagging academic salaries." By 1970, JHSPH was receiving nearly half a million annually from Hill–Rhodes, which supported a sixfold increase in master's students between 1957 and 1977 (table 6.1). Hill–Rhodes helped all schools of public health, and 60 percent of public health graduates received traineeships during the program's 20-year span. At the doctoral level, NIH training and research grants accelerated growth until doctoral students once again outnumbered master's students, as they had in the school's early years.[63]

TABLE 6.1
JHSPH Enrollments and Hill–Rhodes Federal Aid, Selected Years

	1956–1957	1966–1967	1976–1977
Master's	49	121	320
Doctoral	43	135	337
Hill–Rhodes traineeships	0	$274,870	$513,493

Despite the financial stability and expansion that Hill–Rhodes and other federal programs provided to schools of public health, their growth was dwarfed in comparison to that of medical schools. Thomas Turner had gained top-notch grant-making experience while on the leadership team at JHSPH and as an adviser to national programs on syphilis and polio, and he adroitly applied this experience after he left JHSPH to assume the helm of the School of Medicine in 1957. The medical school's jaw-dropping expansion under Turner was underwritten by two main sources: NIH grants for research and construction, as well as a steady parade of grateful patients and other private donors who more than quadrupled the endowment between 1945 and 1965.

Conclusion

When Ernest Stebbins had arrived at JHSPH in 1946, the world had been his oyster. With the war concluded, his opportunities to use his skills and notoriety to lead a public health renaissance had seemed limitless. Instead, his first decade as dean had been sobering in many respects, filled with challenges beyond his control—Huntington Williams's recalcitrance, the Rockefeller Foundation's decision to retreat from its longstanding commitment to schools of public health, and the schism and desertions that followed Turner's report. Stebbins could not have guessed that his choices would be so constrained by the transgressions of boundaries on a map, whether in Korea, Berlin, or East Baltimore. Stebbins, who had witnessed the victory over polio at close range in the school's laboratories and the NFIP's committee meetings, suffered himself from post-polio syndrome, and the pain had begun to infringe on his ability to work long hours. He would eventually resort to using a cane.

During the 1950s, the locus of collaboration between Hygiene and Medicine had shifted from infectious disease toward noncommunicable disease and health services administration, including public health nursing, financing, and operations research. After 1957, JHSPH maintained its science programs in Biochemistry and Pathobiology, but by the time the dust had settled in the early 1960s, JHSPH had lost most of its basic science faculty in physiology, immunology, and microbiology and ended the joint program of teaching public health to medical students.

Despite these setbacks, Stebbins had emerged victorious on several important fronts. If 1957 had been a bear year for the school, 1959 was equally bullish. Although Turner and Stebbins had clashed while they were both in Hygiene, Turner's departure to the medical school actually fostered significant new collaboration between the two schools, such as the Department of Chronic Diseases headed by Abe Lilienfeld. Stebbins was now free to expand the school's programmatic scope to include a wider range of disciplinary methods, particularly the social and behavioral sciences. The majority of the school's growth during the 1960s would originate outside the school's traditional strengths in the basic sciences of bacteriology, immunology, and physiology, and two new departments, International Health and Population Dynamics, would involve long-term projects in South Asia, where the school had yet to establish a foothold. Stebbins recruited a new assistant dean, Timothy D. Baker, who garnered an ICA grant in 1961 to establish the world's first academic unit devoted to international health. Paul Harper embarked on a new stage of his career when the Rockefeller Foundation sent him to West Pakistan as a member of a committee to plan the country's family planning program, which became the basis for the Department of Population Dynamics. Stebbins initiated discussions with the Rockefeller Foundation and the PHS to establish a major new radiation control program, realized as the Department of Radiological Science. A young EIS officer named Donald A. Henderson enrolled with the MPH class of 1960. From 1966 to 1977, Henderson would direct the WHO campaign against smallpox, the first disease to be successfully eradicated worldwide, and then return to JHSPH as dean. Each of these new initiatives were examples of the ways that the Cold War stimulated the growth of both domestic and international health programs that provided a major new income stream for Johns Hopkins and all schools of public health.

CHAPTER SEVEN

Missionaries and Mercenaries

The protean nature of postwar public health brought together both wide-eyed optimists who expected public health to change the world and hardnosed realists who saw it as part of the first line of defense against communist aggression. In 1963, Visvanathan Rajagopalan wrote to his former Hopkins engineering professor Abel Wolman and eloquently summarized the immense challenges India faced to supply its large, dispersed population with clean water. "Today, even if by some magic all the money is made available, the problem would not be solved until the right type of leaders in the profession needed to implement the programme are available. More than mere technical proficiency, faith in the work and a religious zeal to carry it out seem essential in this profession." Rajagopalan sounded themes that are central to understanding the history of postwar international health: the high expectations for Western aid and technology to solve mass-scale health problems, as well as the importance of training public health personnel from both the United States and abroad who not only possessed scientific knowledge but were deeply committed to adapting it to local conditions and priorities. The ideal public health worker had to have the mind of a mercenary and the heart of a missionary.[1]

The first APHA annual meeting to focus on international health was held in 1959, and its theme, "Public Health Is One World," anticipated the later conceptual transition from international to global health. William H. Foege, director of the Communicable Disease Center's smallpox eradication program and CDC director from 1977 to 1983, wrote in 2012,

> It was possible in the past to see international health as something physically removed—the object of our endeavors. The term 'international' suggested a dichotomy between 'national' [in the United States] and the rest of the world. In truth, every place on earth is both local and global. The change [from international to global health] suggests a unity to health where we are all in this together and where everything affects everything else. It was never possible to adequately protect the health of citizens in one country without being involved with health everywhere.[2]

This sea change in perspective was only just beginning as APHA delegates listened while Gaylord Anderson, public health dean at the University of Minnesota, acknowledged the sins of past international health campaigns and laid out the requirements for a better future. Anderson deemed it "essential that in each country the [international health] program be adapted to the mores, to the customs, to the culture of these people. It is essential that we avoid the temptation to try to superimpose upon them something that appears to be useful simply because we [in the United States] have found it to be good."[3]

Chapters 7, 8, and 9 survey the creation and development of the Johns Hopkins School of Hygiene and Public Health's international and domestic programs in maternal and child health, family planning, and health services research, all of which were embodied in the new concept of primary health care. These chapters grapple with the question leveled at JHSPH back in 1938: why did JHSPH invest so much energy and resources in saving lives on the opposite side of the globe while seeming to sidestep the urgent health problems at its East Baltimore doorstep? In the 1960s, the school would embrace social and behavioral science methods that were crucial for understanding the social and economic determinants of health, as well as for building the cultural competency necessary to improve both health outcomes and data collection. JHSPH faculty and students would, however, find themselves swept up in rapid social and political change at home and abroad, proving undeniably that all public health was both local and global.

The First Division of International Health

In 1959, the ASPH met in Minneapolis to hear a proposal by Eugene Campbell, director of the ICA's health division, for a new academic international health consulting and training program. Its purpose would be to conduct systematic studies of economic, social, and political factors in public health and advise on the best methods for adapting US public health technology for use in underdeveloped countries. ICA's health experts had concluded that American public health interests were "too narrow, too restricted, and too oriented to domestic concerns to attack effectively the broad range of pressing health problems which occur in underdeveloped countries and which desperately require solution if economic development programs are to prove successful." American public health workers were seriously ignorant of social, cultural, political, and economic conditions in developing countries, and even faculty in the 11 US schools of public health were frequently unfamiliar with the home countries of their foreign students, who comprised approximately 20 to 25 percent of current enrollments. Curricula remained primarily oriented toward domestic issues, and international health activities were "sporadic and uncoordinated," which was a disservice to the 400 foreign students that ICA sponsored in the United States annually.[4]

Continuing education for new and veteran international health workers was an important goal, since ICA employed over 300 public health fieldworkers, with about 60 new workers going out each year. Better staff orientation was needed to improve the performance of US workers and acclimate them more rapidly to their foreign assignments. Campbell criticized US personnel with specialized backgrounds for having "an excessively limited view of their role in serving the purpose of the ICA program" and failing to act on "opportunities to draw on, or cooperate with, others in the program." Over the course of their assignments, international health workers also lost touch with recent developments in their fields, particularly those who had been overseas longest. These outmoded workers not only reduced the effectiveness of ICA programs but also had difficulty returning to the US public health workforce. Without effective continuing education, these workers might create "a separate class of public health workers [in ICA] with a generally lower level of technical competence than that of their colleagues working in the U.S."[5]

The public health deans, led by Jack Snyder of Harvard, bristled at Campbell's criticisms of their schools and voted against applying for the grant because they were suspicious of probable federal constraints on academic freedom, and some schools had found ICA difficult to work with. But Harvard was also content to pass on the opportunity since its international health activities had received substantial private funding from Rockefeller and other foundations. Despite Hopkins' own ups and downs with ICA in the JHSPH faculty exchange program with the University of the Philippines throughout the 1950s, assistant dean Tim Baker had come to Hopkins from the agency and knew what to expect. On the return flight to Baltimore, Baker told Stebbins that he thought Hopkins should apply for the grant to found a division of international health, and Stebbins gladly agreed. As Baker recalled, "That's where the money was."[6]

Stebbins and Baker worked closely with Campbell to develop a clear sense of purpose for a training center and reservoir of expertise that could serve federal agencies abroad and still meet academic standards. Campbell called JHSPH "the logical choice for this proposal," given its longstanding experience in public and international health, proven working relationships with government agencies, proximity to Washington, and "the initiative it has shown in this specific area." The proposed Division of International Health would "provide tremendous insight and impetus to ICA's health activities carried out by other schools and organizations" and would be a "single center in the U.S. to which qualified international public health workers are drawn by the documentary resources, the stimulus of comprehensive research programs, and the presence of leaders in the field." Snyder later urged ICA to "utilize the services of the various faculties of the American universities which can further its objectives in international health rather than to concentrate on the development of a single international school of public health under the aegis of ICA. The host countries and their health problems are so many and diverse that a single school cannot alone mobilize the resources which are so vitally needed."[7]

In April 1961, JHSPH received a five-year grant of $250,000 to establish the world's first academic unit focused on international health. The Division of International Health would function as "the principal academic base of ICA's health work" and would conduct a comparative study of international health curricula in the United States and abroad. It would also design research to improve the agency's international health programs, particularly for training American and foreign personnel, and serve as a clearinghouse and reference service. WHO pledged its cooperation, and the PHS provided additional funding for the Division of International Health.[8]

The process of negotiating the contract with ICA indicated a number of obstacles that the new division would have to overcome. P. Stewart Macaulay, executive vice president of Johns Hopkins, and H. Ridgely Warfield, director of the Johns Hopkins Institute for Cooperative Research, told Stebbins that "$50,000 a year is totally inadequate for the establishment of the kind of program envisioned in the contract." Macaulay was "staggered by the apparent unlimited scope of the program which you are expected to undertake," and he urged Stebbins "very definitely to limit its scope to reasonable proportions." He also objected to the contract's instructions for the division to undertake "comprehensive studies of the social, economic, historic and political factors influencing the development and administration of health programs in various countries representing the differing regions of the world," which sounded to Macaulay "like a multimillion dollar undertaking rather than a quarter of a million dollar project. . . . I am not at all optimistic that the project is feasible as it has been presented in the draft contract." Warfield warned that "the ICA Office of Public Health and the Public Health Service will be prone to exert a considerable amount of direction."[9]

In 1962, the original contract with ICA was amended with the new US Agency for International Development (USAID) as the granting agency. The five-year contract amount was nearly doubled, and a new responsibility was added for health manpower planning research "in each of five less-developed countries of different levels of economic development in various parts of the world." The contract stipulated that "the Grantee will not publish without consulting A.I.D." and the agency did in fact refuse to allow Tim Baker to release the division's first annual progress report. In keeping with the Kennedy administration's new civil rights policies, the contract also included a clause barring discrimination on the basis of "race, creed, color, or national origin" (but not sex).[10]

JHSPH faculty would teach US and international students in both formal degree programs and a new two-month health planning course for foreign senior officials. The State Department press release emphasized that the new Division of International Health in the Johns Hopkins Department of Public Administration would focus on "the trainee's needs and the needs of his country in order to tailor a postgraduate experience with greater local value." But Stebbins intended that the division's primary teaching function would be "preparing U.S. candidates for international work [with] both I.C.A. and W.H.O. closely involved." Stebbins felt that "most foreign candidates should go to regional schools in their own areas," especially for field training. He also wanted to follow up with foreign students "to help them back into their own local working environment." In 1962, Baker and Stebbins founded a preventive medicine residency, which Baker advised ICA officials could be used to "recruit a high caliber of young men in a training position where they might be persuaded of the advantages of international health as a career." Approximately one-third of the residents went into international health.[11]

In 1961, Stebbins recruited John Hume to return as assistant dean and to take over as chair of PHA. Hume, who succeeded Stebbins as dean in 1967, was the descendent of three generations of missionaries in India. His uncle, Edward Hicks Hume, founded the Yale Mission Hospital and Hunan Medical College in Changsha, China, and wrote the book *Doctors East, Doctors West*. Hume had directed the JHSPH venereal disease control program from 1947 to 1955 and then had spent the past six years as medical director of the ICA mission in India. The search for a director of the new international health division was already in full swing, with Stebbins and Baker deliberating among a "who's who" list of major figures in public health, most of whom were JHSPH alumni.[12]

Abel Wolman was a giant in international health who could have conceivably steered the division toward addressing the problem of waterborne and diarrheal diseases, which at that time caused 500 million disabling illnesses and 5 million infant deaths annually worldwide. Wolman maintained that "the greatest problem of environmental hygiene is the international rather than local control of environmental infection. . . . In the world at large, the adequacy of the water supply, in volume and in quality, still remains the greatest single area of environmental hygiene." But Stebbins and both his assistant deans were PHA faculty who were not primarily interested in the urgent developing world problems of water supply and sanitation.[13]

Despite JHSPH's established presence in Latin America and the Philippines, the mainland of East Asia was the home of over 40 percent of the school's international graduates between 1950 and 1981, and another 15 percent of foreign alumni were from India and Pakistan. The cumulative experiences of students and faculty, the direction of US foreign aid policy under John F. Kennedy and Lyndon B. Johnson, and the magnetic pull of the movement to curb world population growth would all point the compass of the school's overseas activities toward South Asia.[14]

The Pull of South Asia

USAID was born during the heady optimism of John F. Kennedy's first year as president. As a senator, Kennedy had cosponsored the Kennedy–Cooper Bill for economic development aid to India as a stepping stone toward his 1960 presidential bid, and India emerged as the centerpiece of his foreign economic development policy. Shortly after his inauguration, Kennedy declared a "Decade of Development" with the optimistic goal of enabling at least a dozen poor countries to achieve self-sustaining growth by 1970. Kennedy and his advisers broke with what they viewed as the Eisenhower administration's narrow, opportunistic emphasis on winning friends and promoting military alliances and focused instead on nation building and economic modernization to foster long-term stability and growth. Kennedy brokered the formation of the Alliance for Progress to promote democracy and an indigenous New Deal in Latin America, but over the course of his presidency, he accorded the greatest attention to the needs of India and Southeast Asia as a strategic counterbalance to communist China.[15]

After Kennedy's assassination in November 1963, his successor Lyndon Johnson continued to make India a top priority and told Indian Planning Minister Asoka Mehta and Ambassador Braj K. Nehru in 1966 that there was "no area or people in which we were more interested or more concerned about." Between 1966 and 1975, the top recipient of US foreign aid was Vietnam, with $19.7 billion, and India and Pakistan together received $5.8 billion. These countries sent the highest numbers of high-level health officials to Johns Hopkins for the Senior International Health Planners course, a USAID-funded program developed by Tim Baker. The two-month course taught the essentials of national health planning to many of the US advisers and foreign personnel who went on to build the infrastructure for health services and professional training programs in these countries (table 7.1 lists a representative sample of students from 1969). US foreign aid during those years totaled $5.4 billion to the Republic of Korea, whose government Baker would assist in developing the health services and manpower portion of its Second Five-Year Plan in 1966. Of the total net $70.4 billion in US foreign aid from 1966 to 1975, the Far East and Pacific received half and the Near East and South Asia received one-quarter, which closely corresponded to the proportion of students from those countries who enrolled at JHSPH.[16]

The composition of the Hopkins Board of Trustees also reflected these geopolitical developments and further reinforced the university's intimate ties with the international policy and finance elite. The Hopkins board included

TABLE 7.1
Students Enrolled in the 1969 Senior International Health Planners Course at JHSPH

Sponsor	Title	Agency	Country
WHO	Deputy director of public health services	Ministry of Health	Israel
WHO	Planning department official	Ministry of Health	Iran
WHO	Deputy director of medical services	Ministry of Health	Swaziland
WHO	Senior adviser, International Relations Office	Ministry of Health and Social Welfare	Poland
WHO	Assistant undersecretary	Ministry of Health	Sudan
WHO	Director, Statistics Division	Ministry of Health	Ethiopia
USAID	Regional chief health officer (American)	USAID	South Vietnam
USAID	Two senior officials, Health Planning Division	Ministry of Health	South Vietnam
USAID	Chief	Directorate of Nutrition	Indonesia
USAID	Director	Maluku Provincial Health Services	Indonesia
Self-funded	Director	Norwegian Save the Children Project	Algeria

Source: "Preliminary List of Senior Health Planners, 1969," Abel Wolman papers, series 9, box 8, "Survey of Health Planning 1969" binder, JHU Hamburger Archives.
Note: Twenty-one degree-seeking JHSPH students were enrolled, for a total of 33 students.

former Secretary of State Christian A. Herter; Paul H. Nitze, Kennedy's assistant secretary of defense for International Security Affairs; and Eugene R. Black, president of the World Bank from 1949 to 1961 and Johnson's adviser on Far Eastern affairs. Lincoln Gordon, Kennedy's ambassador to Brazil, would become president of Johns Hopkins in 1967.[17] In his examination of the transformation of demographic knowledge during the first two postwar decades, global development historian John Sharpless emphasizes the importance of "complex linkages between government economic planners, foreign policy experts, corporate leaders, professional demographers, and the directors of major philanthropic foundations. These linkages provided a network for the reworking of demographic knowledge to make it more 'user-friendly' to policymakers and created a political climate in which such a profound shift in policy was possible." The Johns Hopkins School of Hygiene and Public Health was among the foremost academic institutions that played a crucial role in the international network of demography, philanthropy, and foreign policy. This network had been developing since before World War II, but the Vietnam War would act as a catalyst for new growth, particularly after Robert S. McNamara, secretary of defense and architect of the US strategy in Vietnam under both Kennedy and Johnson, was appointed to lead the World Bank in 1968.[18]

While serving as president of the Population Association of America in 1942, Lowell Reed had proposed that the biological sciences at Johns Hopkins should devise "an approach to the population problem, with particular emphasis on those forces that influence human reproduction." India, with one of the world's largest populations and highest birthrates as well as a strong health reform tradition, was the first target of the postwar movement to curb global population growth. In 1951, Reed had urged the Rockefeller Foundation to recast its overarching mission to focus on "the world problem of population growth and the attainment of adequate usable resources" through coordinated support for programs in health, agriculture, education, social sciences, and humanities, with the unifying theme of human ecology.[19]

The Rockefeller Foundation followed Reed's advice and also declared its intention to withdraw from graduate public health education. Instead, Rockefeller began to support population researchers such as Indian demographer Chidambara Chandrasekaran (MPH 1948). In 1938, as a doctoral student in statistics at the University of London, Chandrasekaran had heard Raymond Pearl's visiting lectures on the Baltimore Birth Control Clinic, later published as a chapter in *The Natural History of Population* (1939). Chandrasekaran, a Rockefeller Foundation fellow, took advanced biostatistics courses with Rowland V. Rider, Lowell Reed, and Margaret Merrell. His arrival in Baltimore coincided with the fourth EHD census, and although there is no evidence that he participated, he was certainly exposed to its methodology. Chandrasekaran would take the methods he learned in Baltimore—the comprehensive fertility questionnaire developed by Pearl at the Baltimore Birth Control Clinic; the advanced sampling techniques taught by Reed, Merrill, and Rider; and the EHD principles for training interviewers and ensuring accurate data collection—and apply them to conduct field research with far-reaching implications for demography and the development of India's population policy.[20]

By 1956, six faculty members in the departments of Biostatistics and Pathobiology taught courses dealing with the concept of populations from the perspectives of demography, vertebrate ecology, and international health. Maternal and child health were noticeably absent, however. As postwar public health programs ground into gear, American and developing world health professionals encountered one another on a sustained, widespread basis for the first time, just as American graduate and professional training programs desegregated and began admitting African Americans and Latinos in greater numbers. At US schools of public health, foreign physicians, nurses, and sanitary engineers learned powerful new tools for fighting disease while also challenging their American counterparts to rethink Western notions of public health.[21]

National policymakers in the PHS and the State Department began to increase training opportunities for health professionals of all races, religions, and nationalities in the belief that their disease-fighting prowess could help promote economic growth in poor, underresourced regions, whether in the American South or the developing world. In spring 1948, these worlds met in Baltimore at a dinner party hosted by African-American physician Maceo Williams (profiled in chapter 1) for six JHSPH students and their spouses who had been sponsored by the government of India, including Chandrasekaran. Given that India had just won independence from Britain through the efforts of civil rights leader Mohandas K. Gandhi, the dinner conversation must have been lively.[22]

At the fall 1948 APHA meeting, Chandrasekaran met Sushila Nayar (DrPH 1950), who had served as personal physician to Gandhi and his family. Chandrasekaran urged her to apply to JHSPH to prepare for a future position as national health minister. Nayar had come to the United States on a UN fellowship to observe maternal and child health programs. She had been Gandhi's disciple since she was five years old. As a young woman, she had accompanied him on preaching tours across India, had gone to jail with him, and had nursed his supporters during their imprisonment. In 1945, Gandhi appointed Nayar medical director of the Kustruba Gandhi National Memorial Trust Fund, which he established in his wife's honor to advance the medical, social, economic, and educational welfare of India's rural women and children. Nayar organized rural medical centers affiliated with the nearest hospitals, where she trained women and girls to provide both preventive and curative care. After

Gandhi was assassinated in 1948, Nayar went on a US speaking tour to promote his ideas about peace and nonviolence but complained to an American journalist, "What's the matter with reporters who would rather write about my sari than about my message?"[23]

At Hopkins, she took time off from the lecture circuit and her duties as a Gandhian civil rights leader and international spokesperson for the Women's International League for Peace and Freedom to write her doctoral thesis in maternal and child health. Nayar was the first JHSPH doctoral graduate in Maternal and Child Health, and one of the first in the United States. Her adviser was Paul Harper, a pediatrician whose outlook on population dynamics flowed directly from his concern for the health and welfare of the hundreds of families under his care in the EHD and the Family Care Clinic that he established at Johns Hopkins Hospital in 1950. Nayar worked closely with the Maryland State Health Department Division of Maternal and Child Health to analyze maternal deaths and confirmed that postpartum bleeding was the leading cause of maternal death in Maryland. Today, postpartum bleeding remains the leading cause of maternal death in the developing world, responsible for an estimated 125,000 deaths each year.[24]

In the mid-twentieth century, few American physicians appreciated the health benefits for both mothers and infants of spacing births several years apart. On the basis of 35,188 obstetrical cases, Nicholson J. Eastman, chief of obstetrics at Johns Hopkins Hospital, concluded in 1944 that child spacing had no advantage to the babies or their mothers.[25] Nayar and her fellow Indian students at JHSPH influenced their American colleagues to pay closer attention to the health consequences of frequent childbearing for both mothers and infants. Chandrasekaran recalled in his autobiography, "My stepmother's demise opened my eyes to the lot of Indian women. Unending household chores coupled with frequent childbearing sapped their energy resulting frequently in their untimely death." Satya Swaroop (MPH 1948), chief statistical officer of the Punjab Public Health Department, analyzed the Punjab's "pitiably low figures of longevity," particularly among women, and advocated taking measures to make "reproduction an easy and risk-free process by all possible means." He also emphasized the importance of general social improvement for women, which would convey the double benefit of reducing both maternal and infant mortality. Swaroop went on to serve as chief of the WHO Statistical Studies Section.[26]

While he was in the United States, Chandrasekaran had collaborated with American statistician W. Edwards Deming to develop a technique known as the Chandra–Deming formula to estimate birth and death rates more accurately in areas with incomplete vital statistics by comparing the existing system with the results of a scientifically sampled household survey. At the International Union for the Scientific Study of Population conference in 1961, Ansley Coale, one of the main proponents of demographic transition theory, would help to promote the Chandra–Deming formula by citing its utility for determining accurate estimates of population change. Variations of this method are now widely used to estimate birth and death rates in developing countries.[27]

The UN Population Division recruited Chandrasekaran and sent him to Bangalore to direct the UN–Government of India's Mysore Population Study. The Mysore Population Study further refined the Chandra–Deming formula and pioneered in using interviews to collect detailed information on knowledge, attitudes, and practices (known as KAP surveys) regarding fertility and family planning, including contraceptive use, and demonstrated that such data could be used to analyze fertility determinants. The study of India's large and diverse Mysore State also became a model for evaluating the completeness of birth and death registration and other demographic data in developing countries. Finally, the study's finding that the population was growing faster than previously estimated guided India's first Five-Year Plan and helped to convince Prime Minister Jawaharlal Nehru and other senior officials to place greater emphasis on a formal policy to slow population growth.[28]

At the UN, Chandrasekaran also prepared a working paper that analyzed the interaction of social, economic, and demographic factors in population growth, which formed one of the bases for the landmark synthesis of world population data, *The Determinants and Consequences of Population Trends* (1953). Chandrasekaran supervised the project, assisted by Margaret Bright, a University of Wisconsin–trained demographer in the UN Department of Social Affairs, and the two spent three weeks in Baltimore at the Welch Medical Library to prepare the section on mortality. The eminent Irene Taeuber said of the accomplishment, "One who has struggled with world literature for two decades can only bow humbly to those who achieved monumental coverage with minimal errors and integrated the massive citations and notes into a significant report. No scholar concerned with the planning or guidance of [population] research can long maintain self-respect without a well-thumbed copy." Demographers still consider the study to be the definitive account of relationships between population and socioeconomic development, and it has been periodically revised in the series now called *World Populations*.[29]

With the Chandra–Deming formula, the Mysore Study, and the first major survey of world population trends under his belt, Chandrasekaran returned in 1954 to the All India Institute as chair of Biostatistics and then worked with Bright again in Bombay at the UN Regional Demographic Training and Research Centre (later renamed the International Institute of Population Sciences). Chandrasekaran directed the center from 1959 to 1964, which was a frequent waystation for demographers, including Frank Notestein, Irene B.

Taeuber, Dorothy S. Thomas, and Henry S. Shryock Jr. The US–India relationships among Hopkins, the All India Institute, the Rockefeller Foundation, the Population Council, and the UN Population Division had thus produced a Hopkins-trained Indian demographer who adopted biostatistics and public health methods to become India's leading population analyst and a key shaper of government population policy. When the PHA Division of Chronic Disease recruited Bright to Johns Hopkins in 1959, she in turn brought the insights of international population dynamics and sociology to bear in the arena of public health.[30]

Along with Chandrasekaran, Swaroop, and Nayar, another child-spacing advocate and key figure in the Hopkins–India network was Carl E. Taylor, who first met Nayar in the late 1940s in Fatehgarh, Punjab, where he directed the Presbyterian Mission's Memorial Hospital. Like John Black Grant and many other early international health leaders at Hopkins, Taylor and many members of his field research staff were missionaries or children of missionaries. Taylor was both and had grown up in Indian jungles, traveling from one village to the next by oxcart and living in tents. As a boy, he had held the retractor while his father performed surgery under the trees. In 1949, Taylor conducted the first health survey of Nepal, where he operated on babies with cleft lips and palates, thereby sparing them from the ostracism of a society that at that time believed the defect was caused by evil spirits.[31]

Although Taylor was profoundly shaped by his missionary background, he remarked in an interview that "I didn't wear it on my sleeve."[32] Henry van Zile Hyde, speaking at Yale in 1955, observed that

> the medical missionary is a forerunner in spirit, more than technique, of the official international programs in health. Where can we derive more immediate satisfaction of our moral urge than in the field of health, sharing our resources in order to solve the massive immediate human problem touching every man? . . . The emergence of man toward health constitutes a fact of our times within our own sphere of responsibility that is very truly affecting the future of mankind. India will never again be what it was yesterday, nor will Brazil, nor Mexico, nor Haiti, nor Indonesia, nor any country in the so-called underdeveloped belt.[33]

While Taylor was earning a doctorate in public health at Harvard, his adviser, John E. Gordon, had hired him as assistant director of the Khanna Study of Population Problems in the Rural Punjab. Fluent in Hindi and Punjabi, Taylor facilitated cooperation with the Indian government and the Christian Medical College in Ludhiana, where he joined the faculty from 1953 to 1956 and established the Department of Preventive Medicine.[34]

From 1953 to 1960, the Rockefeller Foundation had awarded over $1 million to Gordon and Taylor's classmate John B. Wyon at the Harvard School of Public Health to conduct a landmark demographic study involving monthly home visits in 11 villages containing over 16,000 people. Gordon and Wyon published their research in 39 journal articles as well as a monograph, *The Khanna Study: Population Problems in the Rural Punjab* (1971). The book's generally positive published reviews acknowledged that the study's contributions lay less in proving the efficacy of birth control programs (which the authors admitted had little effect on fertility rates in the Khanna region) than in the novel, in-depth application of epidemiological methods to study population dynamics as affected by births, deaths, and migration. The Khanna Study would serve as an important template for subsequent population health research, including Taylor's.[35]

Taylor credited the Khanna Study for its contributions to understanding why villagers were cautious about family planning and for identifying five enduring principles for future family planning strategies in rural areas of developing countries: reducing child mortality, promoting community education, encouraging social and material progress that recognized the economic value of children, providing incentives for delayed marriage and small families, and ensuring supplies of effective contraceptives that met each couple's needs and preferences. The APHA International Health Section later praised the Khanna Study as "one of the world's pioneering studies in community epidemiology" and established the Gordon–Wyon Award in 2006 to recognize excellence in community-oriented public health, epidemiology, and practice.[36]

The Khanna Study, the EHD surveys, and Chandrasekaran's study in India's Mysore State were among the largest and most intensive demographic surveys to date. They used punch cards to process the large data sets on IBM computers, as Johns Hopkins had done in the EHD since the late 1940s. The Mysore and Khanna studies were some of the earliest scientific, large-scale surveys of knowledge, attitudes, and practice in family planning, but Khanna also constituted the first controlled field trial of a contraceptive program and one of the first such programs in a rural developing country.[37]

During the 1950s, Taylor published two of the earliest popular US articles on birth control and medicine in India in the *Atlantic Monthly*. In "Will India Accept Birth Control?" (1952), Taylor highlighted India's high birthrate as "in itself an important cause of death. Starting at puberty, most Indian women have babies as fast as is biologically possible [, averaging] six or seven children in addition to uncounted miscarriages and abortions. Only three or four babies survive to adulthood; [and] one fifth to one fourth die before they are one year of age, and 45 per cent before they are five." Such figures led Taylor to conclude, "No other single health measure would so significantly improve maternal and child health in India as adequate family planning."[38]

In 1956, Taylor joined the faculty of the Harvard School of Public Health, where he urged his colleagues to explore "the direct deleterious effects on mothers of frequent births under conditions of poor obstetric practice, the results of crowded housing, lack of facilities for medical, educational and social benefits, and the mental health problems resulting from families having more children than they can adequately care for." In 1962, Taylor would come to Johns Hopkins and Nayar would be appointed India's minister of health, where she acted as an essential advocate for Taylor's studies of the connections among reproductive health, nutrition, and primary health services.[39]

Hopkins' strong ties to ICA in India made Taylor a natural choice to direct the new Division of International Health. One of Taylor's strongest supporters was Hugh R. Leavell, assistant dean of public health at Harvard, who had worked alongside Taylor to improve methods for training Indian health workers. Stebbins, Hume, and Baker had met Taylor while he was on sabbatical from Harvard, administering an ICA program to train medical graduates to establish departments of preventive medicine and public health in Indian medical schools. Taylor had also known John Black Grant, whose son James P. Grant was deputy director of ICA and had supported Hopkins' proposal to establish the Division of International Health.[40]

In the 1960s and 1970s, Taylor and other JHSPH faculty guarded against ethnocentrism and sought to gain broad acceptance for their findings by pursuing two main goals in international research and training programs: first, a holistic approach to public health that integrated reproductive health services into strengthened systems of primary care and, second, innovation in public health research methods. Both of these goals would be realized in Taylor's use of extensive randomized controlled field trials to evaluate multiple approaches to interrelated problems in nutrition, diarrheal diseases, maternal and child health, and family planning in the Narangwal Studies in northern Punjab, India. Another source of innovation was the application of operations research principles in the studies of health workforce needs in a range of countries, conducted by Taylor with senior International Health faculty Timothy Baker and William Reinke.

The Johns Hopkins Center for Medical Training and Research

Taylor's research at Narangwal joined two other South Asian field sites that JHSPH established in the early 1960s: the Johns Hopkins Center for Medical Research and Training (CMRT) in Calcutta, India, and Paul Harper's population research center in Lahore, West Pakistan. Although the NIH was overwhelmingly focused on domestic research, the International Health Research

Act provided $5 million annually under two NIH divisions: the tropical medicine program of the National Institute of Allergy and Infectious Diseases (NIAID) and the broader international health program in the NIH Office of International Health. The directors of both these units, as well as the medical director of the NIH Laboratory of Infectious Disease, were JHSPH alumni. All would be closely involved in funding and guiding the CMRT in Calcutta, established by Frederik B. Bang in the Department of Pathobiology.[41]

The CMRT began as an effort to revive tropical medicine, which had languished at Johns Hopkins since its heyday in the 1940s. In 1959, Fred Bang and Tom McGowan in Pathobiology founded a new tropical medicine program with medical school faculty members A. McGehee Harvey and Leighton Cluff in the Department of Medicine Division of Infectious Diseases and Immunology. In October 1960, Baker, Stebbins, McGowan, and Cluff joined officials from four other universities (California–Berkeley, Tulane, Maryland, and Louisiana State) with tropical medicine programs to meet with NIH director James Shannon, and all five institutions subsequently expanded their activities to establish International Centers for Medical Research and Training. Shannon, a highly regarded physiologist, had played a leading role in the NRC's malaria research program during World War II and was the first chair of the NIH Malaria Study Section. Research on malaria and other tropical diseases remained a high priority during his tenure from 1955 to 1968. Shannon also worked closely with Rhode Island Congressman John E. Fogarty, a champion of NIH and international health research, who chaired the House Appropriations Subcommittee on Labor, Health, Education, and Welfare.[42]

The NIH program required grantees to establish a long-term cooperative agreement with an overseas institution, to define research according to the needs of the selected country, and to conduct onsite field training for foreign health research personnel. Over time, training was deemphasized, and the program shifted its focus to assisting foreign countries in building institutions that could conduct their own training and research activities. Pathobiology had been instrumental in the JHSPH exchange program with the University of the Philippines, and the department's foreign alumni returned to establish new research units in their home countries. An Iranian, Chamseddine Mofidi (MPH 1951), founded the malaria program at the University of Tehran, which became the Department of Pathobiology in 1966 when the university established Iran's first school of public health, directed by Mofidi. Aklilu Lemma (ScD 1964), who wrote his thesis on schistosomiasis, founded the Institute of Pathobiology at Haile Selassie University in Addis Ababa, Ethiopia. Lemma (see the photo gallery) made a critical discovery after he observed large numbers of dead snails in areas downstream from where the endod (soapberry) plant was used as a detergent for washing clothes. He developed an endod-derived pesticide that could be used to kill the snail vector that caused schistosomiasis, without harming mammals or plants. The plant was affordable and widely available in areas where the disease was endemic: Africa, South America, and Asia.[43]

The Department of Pathobiology and the medical school Division of Infectious Diseases and Immunology devised a joint tropical medicine program that included public health, clinical, and biological aspects. Although Bang had previously worked with the US Army Tropical Medical Research Unit in the Philippines and Bangkok, Thailand, he was fascinated with India, and he, McGowan, and Cluff chose the country for its acute health needs, available scientific talent, and the ready acceptance of English. They found the best lab and clinical facilities and professional staff in Calcutta at the All India Institute of Hygiene and Public Health and the Calcutta School of Tropical Medicine, which featured excellent health centers in rural and urban settings. In partnership with these institutions, a $1.9 million NIH grant established the Johns Hopkins Center for Medical Research and Training in February 1961. John Hume's experience in India proved helpful in problem solving with Indian officials and in gaining the initial trust of Indian researchers and clinicians.[44]

Although Bang's CMRT in Calcutta and Taylor's research site in northern India were geographically separated by nearly a day's air travel, they were connected in several ways. Taylor had obtained NIH funding in the late 1950s to establish a leprosy research project with Mukta Sen at the All India Institute. After Taylor affiliated with Hopkins, he and Bang mapped the rates of leprosy in the villages of West Bengal and traveled together to meet with national health officials in India, Nepal, and Bangladesh to negotiate research and training agreements for Hopkins. Taylor served on the Coordinating Committee for the CMRT at Hopkins, and he called Fred Bang his "strongest supporter" among the JHSPH department chairs, many of whom were initially suspicious that Taylor's division might compete with their own overseas research programs. Of all Hygiene faculty, Bang best understood Taylor's depth of experience related to Indian village life and its value for grounding the school's teaching and field research programs.[45]

Calcutta had urgent health problems and was home to several of India's research institutes, but the city offered few teachers or investigators who were well trained in public health. Stebbins had remarked in 1961 that "requirements for degrees—and everybody wants a degree—impose serious obstacles to what might be the wisest course [for training foreign students]. Research training in Calcutta under NIH support ought to overcome this problem." In the initial discussions about founding CMRT, the All India Institute wanted to send both its faculty and students to Baltimore. Bang and Stebbins, however, were concerned about the cost and administrative burden of an exchange relationship, as well as the ability of Indian applicants to fulfill admissions and degree requirements. They intended for CMRT's training program to be based in Calcutta with degrees awarded through the All India Institute, and Bang had reserved the right to select the doctoral students from India who would work with Hopkins CMRT faculty. In reality, Bang later acknowledged that the center was primarily oriented toward research, not training, so he eventually dropped "training" from its title.[46]

Cholera was among the first targets of CMRT research, which would prove to have a major impact on the global standards for managing the disease. Calcutta's Infectious Diseases Hospital had admitted 8,000 cholera cases in 1959, most during the summer, and was deemed the best site in the country for clinical research in infectious tropical diseases. Charles C. Carpenter, a Johns Hopkins Hospital resident, and R. Bradley Sack (ScD 1968), a postdoctoral fellow, came to the CMRT in late 1962 to study cholera at the hospital. They estimated that untreated cases could be fatal in more than 50 percent of patients.

During a cholera epidemic the following spring, they conducted bacteriological, serological, and metabolic studies with A. Mondal, the hospital's chief physician. With the standard treatment of intravenous (IV) glucose followed several hours later by saline and alkali therapy, most deaths were caused by shock, metabolic acidosis, and uremia. Carpenter and Sack found that these conditions could be better managed by providing alkali sooner to counteract acidosis. As soon as the patient's blood pressure was restored by administering IV isotonic saline, additional saline and sodium lactate was given to replace fluids and electrolytes. The results of controlled studies overwhelmingly favored the new alkali replacement therapy, which became the standard cholera treatment at the hospital. Carpenter and Sack were also able to reduce the duration of diarrhea in cholera patients by adding tetracycline to fluid and electrolyte replacement, which helped control dehydration more quickly and shortened the length of hospitalization to approximately three days. The early research on cholera achieved the CMRT's goal of conducting scientific studies of local diseases and applying the results to improve health on a broad scale.[47]

Tom McGowan, the CMRT's first local administrator, left at the end of 1962, frustrated with the difficulties of dealing with Indian officials as well as American researchers. McGowan felt that Bang did not delegate adequate authority to him, which hampered his relations with others. Harvey Fischman (MPH 1964, DrPH 1965), a veterinarian and Pathobiology doctoral candidate, succeeded McGowan. Three weeks after his arrival, Fischman wrote to Bang, "My feeling is that the time is ripe to begin to lay plans for expansion of this program in as many directions as possible. The field is fertile, the ground work has been laid and if we supply the proper people in projects of marked interest to the Indians, there will be very little problem in making them move." B. K. Aikat, director of Pathology and Bacteriology at the Institute of Postgraduate Medical Education and Research, and R. N. Chaudhuri, director of the Calcutta School of Tropical Medicine, were eager to collaborate and welcomed more investigators at their institutions, and the CMRT did establish collaborative programs in virology research with Aikat and in zoological research with the University of Calcutta. But internecine conflict threatened the Hopkins CMRT enterprise.

Bang's "comprehensive, expansive approach" to research differed from the "specific, problem-oriented clinical approach of the School of Medicine." The medical school wanted to focus on specific endemic diseases, while Bang reserved the right to allow individual researchers to explore their special interests. Although all agreed that the research projects should be sustainable after the original investigators left India, this was often difficult in practice, especially with a two-year limit on residency imposed by the Indian government. Fischman warned Bang of the need to strengthen existing programs before starting new ones and urged him to hire a virologist and a parasitologist to continue research begun in these areas.[48]

Charles Carpenter headed the medical cholera program and proposed to administer it separately from the other JHSPH programs. He preferred that a physician with clinical experience administer the cholera program, which reflected ongoing tensions between the schools of Hygiene and Medicine, as chapter 6 has shown. At a March 1963 executive committee meeting, Bang worried that the cholera program's narrower clinical focus might stifle the CMRT's breadth of scientific inquiry. He requested and got an additional JHSPH representative, John Hume, to even the representation on the executive committee. Public health historian Elizabeth Fee writes of Bang, "Quick to grasp new ideas, and voracious in absorbing new fields of knowledge, Bang could be impatient with details, and he often sent researchers to India without much careful planning. The investigators therefore frequently arrived in India with undefined roles and unclear job descriptions. The School of Medicine, aghast at this administrative abandon, focused on slowly and carefully planning its cholera program." Fischman urged Bang to clarify the virology program's basic aims and its specific importance to India.[49]

While he continued to search for Fischman's replacement, Carpenter took over as interim administrator, and Bang feared that the cholera program would dominate the larger mission of CMRT. When NIH director James Shannon visited CMRT in fall 1963, he praised the cholera program, which most closely followed the NIH model of a categorical disease program. Shannon advocated increasing the number of senior American researchers and also emphasized the need for long-term projects with an institutional base that would allow them to continue after the departure of individual researchers. In 1964, NIH renewed the CMRT grant at $500,000 per year for five years.[50]

Along with cholera, CMRT researchers also made important contributions to the treatment and control of leprosy. John H. Hanks, director of the Leonard Wood Memorial Leprosy Research Lab in the Department of Pathobiology, conducted leprosy research with Carl Taylor in Punjab and CMRT in West Bengal. They developed field lab methods to study transmission and host resistance, and Hanks helped set up the leprosy lab in the All India Institute. The lab confirmed the existence of a carrier state and developed two tests using skin biopsies for detecting infection. The CMRT lab also developed a skin test antigen, lepromin, that was standardized and used worldwide by WHO. Hanks contributed major scientific knowledge toward the in vivo cultivation of the leprosy bacillus and tissue culture techniques generally. He succeeded in growing rat leprosy, but researchers have never been able to grow human leprosy in cell culture. In 1964, McGowan and Bang began administering Taylor's leprosy program through CMRT and transferred the research studies from the Punjab to West Bengal, which had a high prevalence of the disease.[51]

Despite these successes, Bang complained that the word *medical* in the name of the Center for Medical Research and Training shortchanged the center's emphasis on the connections between public health and local ecology. Pathobiologist Charles Southwick decided to apply for Smithsonian funding for the CMRT ecology program so that his group would not "feel the need to justify ecological work in medical terms," but despite such concerns, most JHSPH investigators felt free to examine complex relationships among people, pathogens, vectors, and the endlessly fascinating local environment. Gerhard Schad had done arctic research before coming to Calcutta, where he studied hookworm ecology and life cycle and found that, although transmission occurred only during monsoon season, larvae could survive in the lungs of humans during the dry season. Rozeboom studied filariasis, which was spreading in Southeast Asia due to rapid urbanization and inadequate sanitation. Wilhelm Kloene headed a four-village comparative long-range study of respiratory viruses in rural areas. Since many domestic animals lived in close contact with humans, they shared respiratory and other infections. A study of 200 children over two years took monthly cultures to determine the prevalence of respiratory viruses and found that maternal antibodies had little effect, since 16 percent of young children tested positive. Moreover, the seasonal distribution during and after the monsoon season differed greatly from the winter prevalence in the temperate zone. Finally, a groundbreaking study determined that in tropical areas, acute respiratory viruses were usually more common (representing 40 percent of illnesses) than diarrheal diseases (which represented 25 percent).[52]

CMRT promoted the flowering of relationships with Indian colleagues, but Americans frequently got lost in the thickets of Indian officialdom. The Hopkins researchers lived in housing that was luxurious by Indian standards and also enjoyed access to local athletic and country clubs and touring the surrounding area. But the Americans chafed at taxes, import licenses, and the customs difficulties that tied up important medical equipment and supplies because local officials were unaware of the high-level agreements governing the CMRT. Reliance on overseas suppliers was a drawback of bringing Western medical technology to developing countries, and resulting delays in treatment sometimes caused serious or fatal complications in patients.

Moreover, back in Baltimore, the JHSPH admissions committee had rejected several Indian government officials who had applied to the DrPH program. Nowshir Kaikobad Jungalwalla (MPH 1949), director of the All India Institute, reminded Bang in 1963 that in the original discussions about establishing CMRT, one goal was to develop a "faculty to faculty relationship between the two teaching institutions." Jungalwalla wanted Hopkins faculty to participate in the faculty activities of the All India Institute and for his faculty to be given appointments at JHSPH. He wrote Bang, "This relationship between the two institutions should be on a broad basis and . . . not merely be confined to research programmes." Despite the limitations of NIH funding, Jungalwalla emphasized that "the ultimate objective, which should be brought in now and given urgent attention, is the development of an Institute to Institute relationship between the All India Institute of Hygiene and Public Health and the Johns Hopkins School of Hygiene and Public Health."[53]

Bang replied that Jungalwalla was "perfectly correct" that the original conversations had included provisions for faculty exchange but that the PHS had changed its policy to exclude "training procedures and exchange of people not having to do with research. Thus we must look for separate support for this kind of thing." He explained that the NIH grant did not give the School of Hygiene the authority or funding to bring all interested parties to Baltimore, but after continued pressure from Jungalwalla and others, Hopkins secured private funding for travel expenses. Internal conflicts among medical and political groups in Calcutta also adversely affected the CMRT's relationship with the central government. Bang complained, "It is impossible to operate in India and not do something that someone is against. The mere fact that both Indians and Americans speak the same language by no means produces universal understanding."[54]

Along with the tensions with Jungalwalla, Bang worried that CMRT would not be able to recruit additional personnel unless he could "improve our housing arrangements and the supply of essential items such as powdered milk and baby food." In the early 1960s, CMRT's four American staff and their families were living in a boarding house and rented apartments in conditions that were, according to Bang, "unsatisfactory and seriously threaten the development of the plan." Although the center already had significant NIH support for research, Bang applied for USAID funding specifically so CMRT could be eligible for Public Law (P.L.) 480 grants to construct research facilities and obtain basic supplies.[55]

The Agricultural Trade Development and Assistance Act of 1954, known as P.L. 480, was another of Hubert Humphrey's gifts to the school. As a US senator from the grain-belt state of Minnesota, Humphrey had sponsored P.L. 480 as a way to stabilize farm prices by enabling the US Department of Agriculture to buy an enormous surplus of agricultural commodities from farmers. The State Department then either gave or sold the wheat, corn, soybeans, and other food products as part of the US foreign aid program. Developing nations facing food shortages could buy American surpluses with local currencies at below-market prices to feed their hungry citizens—India, which faced a severe famine in the mid-1960s, had bought approximately 600 million tons of food through P.L. 480 by 1970. Dubbed "Food for Peace," P.L. 480 was politically brilliant because it married the liberal objective of increasing humanitarian foreign aid with the hardnosed capitalist goal of maintaining farm prices in the United States and opening new markets abroad. It was one of the most unassailable bipartisan programs ever devised. Revenue generated by the P.L. 480 program was deposited in a special account within the purchasing country, which the State Department had to spend on local development projects or other expenses for the country's embassy. This created a nearly endless supply of supplemental funds to support local expenditures for USAID-funded projects. On a smaller scale, P.L. 480 also funded the NIH Scientific Activities Overseas program, which by 1972 spent US$25.5 million annually. Throughout the 1960s and 1970s, JHSPH's three South Asian centers received substantial support in the form of local currency expenditures from P.L. 480, which joined the USAID and NIH grant programs that became mainstays of JHSPH external funding.[56]

In 1965, Dean Stebbins alerted JHU President Milton Eisenhower that Congress was considering a bill that would authorize the use of P.L. 480 funds to promote and expand universities' participation in the US foreign assistance program, which passed as the 1966 Food for Peace Act (it is worth noting that, in deference to powerful southern state interests, cotton and tobacco were among the seven principal commodities shipped to developing countries under P.L. 480). To conduct research and training programs abroad, universities had previously relied on short-term contracts with USAID, the first of which had been with Johns Hopkins to establish the Division of International Health. In addition to the act's provisions to encourage developing countries to pursue agricultural reforms to build self-sufficiency, the 1966 amendments enabled schools of public health to maintain permanent staffs abroad to conduct research, train graduate students and local personnel, and provide technical assistance, including institutional development in connection with foreign aid projects. Although all US universities were eligible, those best positioned to take advantage of the program were schools with large faculties and existing connections to international research. Brad Sack, who later succeeded Bang as principal investigator for CMRT, noted that Harvard, Hopkins, and the London School of Hygiene and Tropical Medicine were the main schools of public health during this period that committed to sending their faculty to live overseas for long periods, which Sack called "invaluable" for supporting high-quality international health research.[57]

Bang observed in 1965 that the CMRT program was "the biggest and best challenge I have met." By 1967, with the funding boost from the amended P.L. 480 program, CMRT's professional staff had grown from four to 12 Americans as well as five Indians. During its 15-year life span, CMRT trained and employed over 80 researchers from India and the United States, who published over 400 articles in Indian, American, and international journals. Research spanned cholera rehydration therapy, respiratory diseases, hookworm and urban filariasis, leprosy, zoonotic diseases, and the role of nutrition in infection.[58]

The P.L. 480 program even became the subject of a class problem for the Senior International Health Planners course. Just as the small groups of students were putting the finishing touches on their comprehensive health plans for their assigned countries, course director William Reinke issued a simulated bulletin that the P.L. 480 grain shipment to India had been contaminated, and rumors were starting that caused families to stop feeding the bad wheat to their children, which affected their nutritional status and also disrupted the family planning program because of rumors that the bad wheat was causing bleeding among women. Students had to react and adapt their health plans, which revealed cultural differences among the international students. Those from India wanted to form a committee to investigate and solve the problem, while the Middle Eastern students decided to simply disregard the bulletin, since they reasoned that "if we reacted to every rumor that gets circulated in our part of the world, we'd go crazy."[59]

USAID and P.L. 480 funding helped to displace the strong, mutually reinforcing relationship between the armed forces and schools of public health that had begun during World War II and flourished during the 1950s. The advent of international health programs placed the schools on a tangential path of indirect rather than direct influence in military affairs. As the number of students increased who received Hill–Rhodes scholarships or were planning to serve in foreign health programs, the proportion of military officers at JHSPH declined, especially once American deployments to Vietnam accelerated after the Gulf of Tonkin Resolution in August 1964. The atmosphere on the Hopkins campus, like campuses everywhere, became less hospitable to students on military scholarships, although they continued as always to congregate around Anna Baetjer, who had been teaching occupational health and physiology to medical officers since World War II.

W. Henry Mosley (MPH 1965), who joined the CDC's Epidemic Intelligence Service in 1961, remembered that by the mid-1960s, even the EIS's approach to public health was "not at all" influenced by a military way of thinking. "None of us ever wore uniforms, including Alex Langmuir and D. A. Henderson and all that. . . . [E]ssentially we didn't feel like it was military at all except we had some privileges of the military. But there was no sense of military mentality. And it was very separate from things like Fort Detrick, [Maryland, outside Baltimore,] which was doing all the military research and all that." At both the CDC and the School of Hygiene, the approach to public health became less militaristic—less vertical—and looked outward to communities and populations.[60]

Population Bombs, IUDs, and Other Incendiary Devices

In the 1960s, "population control" became the next frontier for international health (at this time, *population control* was the term used by both supporters and opponents of family planning programs administered at the national or population level. In the twenty-first century, *population control* is used pejoratively by critics of these programs). The movements to limit the developing world's population growth and to ameliorate its health problems overlapped considerably. Admittedly, proponents of family planning and international health occupied distinct camps that were often in tension over which should receive top priority, but their coterminous intellectual memberships received support from many of the same philanthropies, US federal agencies, and international organizations. At JHSPH, faculty and alumni in International Health worked to integrate family planning within a range of reproductive health and primary care services. In the Division of Population Dynamics in the Department of Public Health Administration, Paul Harper's cooperative research in Pakistan was more vertically organized, with both the division and the government working to promote stand-alone family planning programs.

In 1959, Dean Stebbins sent Harper to accompany Marshall C. Balfour (MPH 1948) of the Population Council to assist the government of Pakistan in formulating a national family planning program. Pakistan was a strategic choice, with a population of 105 million and a birthrate of 50 per 1,000 population, one of the highest in the world. The Population Council and the Rockefeller

Foundation provided $250,000 over five years for a program to add contraception to existing health services in urban areas, aimed at reaching at least 10 percent of the population of reproductive age. The program also proposed to train 1,200 doctors, nurses, and health visitors in family planning methods each year at four provincial training institutes.

With additional funding from the Ford Foundation and Pakistan's government, Harper founded the West Pakistan Population Research and Evaluation Center (WEPREC) in 1961. The family planning training program was based in the capital city of Lahore, and Harper's research was based at the rural health center in Lulliani, a nearby village of 12,000. Harper's work seemed destined for success, given the strong support of Pakistan's president Ayub Khan for the national family planning program, which Khan backed with commitment of $7 million over the next five years.[61]

At Hopkins, Harper established a specialization in population in the Division of Maternal and Child Health, which became a department in 1962, the first in a series of administrative transitions that reflected the growing importance of population-level family planning as a major domestic and international health policy issue. Yet the initiative to establish a formal Division of Population Dynamics at JHSPH in 1964 came from two demographers, Margaret Bright in Chronic Diseases and Helen Abbey in Biostatistics, who vetted the idea with Frank Notestein at the Population Council. They conceived the division as a demographic research center, and Bright arranged for Irene Taeuber of the Office of Population Research at Princeton University to come to Baltimore as a visiting professor to help establish the program.[62]

Stebbins and Harper, however, moved to base the division in Maternal and Child Health. Harper explained that his department was the logical administrative home for the new division "because of the close relationship between maternal child health work and family planning work in those countries with active governmental programs, [and] the fact that the majority of physicians in family planning agencies have medical training which would normally place them as maternal and child health majors." Harper also stressed the value of training in population and fertility regulation as a core field for all public health students. In August 1965, Harper changed his department's name from Maternal and Child Health to Population and Family Health, which moved into the new South Wing of the Hygiene Building. The department consisted of two divisions: Population Dynamics, headed by Harper, and Maternal and Child Health, headed by Donald A. Cornely (the school's domestic work in family planning and maternal and child health during this period is discussed in chapters 8 and 9).[63]

On June 10, 1963, and February 9, 1964, big-city newspapers across the United States published letters signed by Stebbins and other prominent international health figures, such as John B. Wyon and George C. Shattuck of Harvard. The letters appeared in two full-page advertisements sponsored by Hugh Moore, author of the 1954 alarmist pamphlet *The Population Bomb* (also the title of Paul R. Ehrlich's 1968 bestselling book). The first letter urged President Kennedy to approve "a greatly accelerated program for limiting world population," while the second called on President Johnson to inaugurate "substantially increased programs of research [on world population growth] within the National Institutes of Health" and USAID.[64]

Despite some disagreement about methods and priorities, proponents of population control were united in the belief that rapid population growth was a serious threat to US and world security. They lobbied Congress to support US-led global population control efforts. Albert B. Sabin, chair of the NRC advisory committee on tropical medicine, identified population control as not just the next frontier for international health but as insurance against Armageddon:

> Competent analysts have indicated that the extraordinary increase in population, which is greatest in the economically depressed areas, threatens to nullify all efforts to improve the living standards of the people, whose misery and despair constitutes the greatest threat to world stability and peace. Accordingly there are many who believe that the continued acquisition and application of knowledge designed to prolong life and to eliminate the miseries and handicaps of disease, without comparable *concurrent* activities directed at fertility control, will in effect, before long, result in the even greater miseries of hunger, poverty and war, and thereby create the greatest potential threat to human survival in all parts of the world.[65]

Sabin and his contemporaries believed that lowering birthrates in the poor nations of Asia, Africa, and South America would help to stabilize conflict-prone regions. In this worldview, family planning programs complemented US military strategies for hemming in a Soviet-led communist bloc that sought to leverage political unrest to foment revolutions around the globe.[66]

Against the backdrop of growing concern in the industrialized West over the potential geopolitical consequences of rapid population growth in the developing world, Paul Harper opened his 1964 proposal for a Division of Population Dynamics at Hopkins with the statement, "Many informed persons believe that the need for controlling population growth is the world's most important problem, not even excepting the need to control atomic weapons." In June 1965, Harper organized a five-day conference at JHSPH on population dynamics for senior USAID staff and representatives from American universities, foundations, and private agencies. The conference produced the first official guidelines for USAID population programs, which were distributed to all USAID Missions and personnel. Speakers included leading population experts from the Population Council, USAID, and academic population research centers. Harper and Minoru Muramatso published the proceedings as the field's first textbook, *Population Dynamics* (1965).[67]

Marshall C. Balfour, the senior Asia representative of the Population Council who had accompanied Harper on his initial trip to Pakistan, outlined the elements for successful family planning programs in developing countries. Existing models of the WHO campaigns against communicable disease loomed large at the conference—they presented both encouraging records of success to emulate and standards to compete against. Balfour argued that developing countries could more easily afford population control than malaria eradication. He also contended that the training methods for disease campaigns were unsuitable for population control, and no new methods had yet been developed. Balfour emphasized the imperative need to involve top-level government officials, since "the basic problem in the developing countries is one of organization and administration. Census data, special surveys, the improvement of vital statistics, pilot projects and training of personnel, all play a part in evolving policies and programs." All of these activities would, he predicted, also serve to strengthen the public health infrastructure. But even as Balfour spoke, the WHO malaria eradication campaign, launched with great fanfare in 1955, was struggling to deliver on its optimistic promises to eliminate recurring expenses for malaria control and treatment within a decade.[68]

Immediately after the USAID population conference, the Ford Foundation granted $800,000 to Johns Hopkins to establish the Division of Population Dynamics. The division received an additional $1.2 million in matching grants, three-quarters from a training grant from the NICHD and the remainder from USAID, the Population Council, and the Rockefeller Foundation. The original 1961 USAID grant that had established the Division of International Health was amended in 1964 to include Population Dynamics, which gave faculty in the two divisions joint appointments and supported their involvement in training students as well as overseas research and consultation. The Division of Population Dynamics offered opportunities for study in three population-related fields: demography, physiology of reproduction, and public health administration. Joint programs of study were available through the Homewood departments of Biology, Political Economy, and Social Relations and the School of Medicine departments of Gynecology and Obstetrics, Human Genetics, and Pharmacology and Experimental Therapeutics.[69]

The USAID population conference demonstrated that academics in the fields of public health, economics, and demography were the greatest sources of influence on the decision of President Johnson and Congress to endorse population control as official US policy in 1965. Johnson shifted the calculus of US policy firmly toward restricting population growth when he reckoned that "less than five dollars invested in population control is worth a hundred dollars invested in economic growth."[70]

One of the most important advocates of limiting world population growth was Oxford-trained historian Phyllis Piotrow (PhD 1971), then legislative assistant to George S. McGovern, the liberal US senator from South Dakota and later a Democratic presidential candidate. In April 1965, Piotrow became the founding executive director of the Population Crisis Committee, co-founded by Moore, which played a major role in raising public and political support for population programs. She was one of the first doctoral students in Harper's Division of Population Dynamics, and while still at JHSPH, she worked closely with Reimert Ravenholt to write the first legislation to fund USAID population programs. Her dissertation, published in 1972 as *World Population Crisis: The United States Response*, was acclaimed as the definitive history of the development of US government policies and programs on international population growth and family planning. Piotrow became a leading advocate for extending the use of the birth control pill in the developing world and joined the JHSPH Population Dynamics faculty in 1978 as the first director of the Population Information Program. In 1988, she established the Center for Communication Programs, which has since provided global leadership as a source of technical, financial, field, and training assistance for more than 100 reproductive health communication and other health-related programs in developing countries.[71]

Piotrow's committee, as well as the Ford Foundation, Population Council, and International Planned Parenthood Federation, was instrumental in convincing President Johnson to urge Congress to "give a new and daring direction to our foreign aid programs designed to make a maximum attack on hunger and disease and ignorance in those countries that are determined to help themselves, and to help those nations that are trying to control population growth." The International Health Act of 1966 reorganized the international health functions of the departments of state and HEW and included a two-thirds increase in funding for USAID health programs (including family planning) for 1966–1967 to over $150 million (this was still only 6 percent of the $2.5 billion total USAID budget). Johnson's chief justification for these new policies was his conviction that "population growth now consumes about two-thirds of economic growth in the less developed world. As death rates are steadily driven down, the individual miracle of birth becomes a collective tragedy of want."[72]

When Johnson met in 1966 with Indian Planning Minister Asoka Mehta and Ambassador B. K. Nehru, they agreed to "work tactfully and pragmatically for the development of an indigenous Asian counterweight to China." Since India contained more than half the noncommunist population of Asia,

Johnson hoped that aiding economic development in India would enable the United States to avoid the much costlier option of increasing direct military aid to the region. This strategy, combined with the Indian national government's early commitment to reducing the country's birthrates, ensured that India received the greatest proportion of family planning funding from USAID.[73]

USAID's new priorities were reflected in a revised budget subcategory, "Population Dynamics and Public Health," for which the India Mission's funding rose from $388,000 in 1965 to $1.9 million by 1967. India's First Five-Year Plan in 1951 had identified malaria as "the most important public health problem in India and its control should therefore be assigned topmost priority in any national planning." With the new cooperation of USAID, the Fourth Five-Year Plan gave the strongest support yet for family planning, backed by a commitment of $200 million to achieve a reduction of the birthrate from 40 to 25 per thousand population by 1971.[74]

As the flood of population control funding continued, Harper's research extended its international reach. In 1967, the Ford Foundation awarded the division $380,000 over three years to establish a family planning program in Nigeria in cooperation with the University of Lagos Medical School, which built on the existing relationship that had developed through the JHSPH Division of International Health's Nigerian Health Manpower Study. Following the 1968 visit to Pakistan of a UN/WHO advisory mission on family planning that included Chidambara Chandrasekaran, the government of Pakistan requested major assistance for its family planning program from the UN and its constituent organizations. In August 1970, Pakistan signed an agreement with the newly created UN Fund for Population Activities (UNFPA), where Chandrasekaran was chief of Population Policies and Programmes. By the end of 1970, the UNFPA was supporting 20 projects in Africa, Asia, Latin America, and the Middle East with a total budget of $9 million.[75]

In 1969, Ford provided nearly $1 million over six years to support endowed professorships for the Division of Population Dynamics at JHSPH. Although qualified faculty were in short supply and high demand, Harper recruited a group of outstanding faculty—John Kantner, Melvin Zelnik, John Biggers, Ismail Sirageldin, and Zenas Sykes. When Harper had initially proposed in 1965 to appoint foreign nationals to one-third of the NIH trainee positions, Donald Harting, acting director of NICHD, pointedly replied, "I must reiterate that the purpose for which the funds are awarded is to increase the number of domestic research workers. Foreign nationals are included only in the exceptional situation where they can make a contribution to the domestic training effort." But training developing-world professionals in population control methods was a key objective of USAID, the Ford Foundation, and other overseas-oriented organizations; by the mid-1970s, about half of the students in the Department of Population Dynamics were foreign.[76]

Given the enormous federal and private support for population control programs, whether for US-based training and research at universities such as Johns Hopkins or through the national governments of countries such as India and Pakistan, what were the actual results? During India's first three Five-Year Plans through 1966, health programs overall had been given relatively low priority and funding by the Indian government, with only 5 percent of the total national budget allocated to health. During the 1950s, India had established over 4,000 traditional family planning clinics that provided complete medical and contraceptive services at reduced or no cost, but they had reached only a small fraction of the population. By 1965, only 0.7 percent of married fertile couples were estimated to be using condoms "regularly and effectively," even though the government provided them free of charge. The 1967 USAID Country Assistance Program for India noted that coordinating the provision of contraceptive services to large groups of women "must be repeated thousands of times to reach the present estimated target population of 71 million fertile married couples and bring the desired reduction in birthrates. In a country such as India this objective poses a most horrendous organizational, educational and administrative challenge."[77]

Pakistan's family planning program likewise struggled to gain acceptance for traditional contraceptives such as diaphragms, condoms, and spermicidal foam. Between 1962 and 1964, John C. Cobb, the medical director of Harper's research project in West Pakistan, oversaw the testing of a new method, the intrauterine device (IUD), which Harper praised as "a major breakthrough, since the I.U.D. is the one contraceptive technic which does not require repeated action by the users, is nearly one hundred percent effective, and is removable." Based on the results of the IUD trials by Cobb's group and many others, the Population Council threw $2.5 million into manufacturing and global distribution of the plastic Lippes Loop IUD. Envir Adil, appointed in 1964 as Pakistan's family planning commissioner, worked with Harper to secure government approval in Pakistan's 1965–1970 Five-Year Plan for the use of IUDs nationwide, with a 10-fold budget increase for family planning. By 1968, family planning ranked as the third largest employer in Pakistan, after railroads and the army.[78]

Pakistan, India, Taiwan, South Korea, and other poor, populous countries pursued the rapid, nationwide adoption of the IUD in in the 1960s before it had received US Food and Drug Administration (FDA) approval in the United States. This raised serious questions about the ethics of state-sanctioned population control, which threatened to displace voluntary clinic and hospital-based family planning services. India's Department of Family Planning was overseen by the national Ministry of Health, led by Sushila Nayar beginning in 1962. From the beginning, Nayar defended her authority over family planning as subordinate to protecting the nation's health, and she continually resisted in-country experts of the Ford Foundation, USAID, and others in the "crowd of Americans" in Delhi who wanted to wage a no-holds-barred campaign to reduce birthrates. Nayar wanted to expand family planning services within a medical model centered on providing comprehensive health care, and she pressured state health ministers to enforce the policy that required sterilization operations, whether vasectomies or tubal ligations, to be performed only by trained doctors. In early 1964, Nayar sent a group of Indian national and state health officials on a two-month US tour, including a week in Baltimore at the School of Hygiene, to learn about the development of US health services and schools of public health. With support from the Ford Foundation, the Indian Ministry of Health set up demonstration districts in five states to provide basic health services. The Ministry also established a school of public health in New Delhi to train health officers for the demonstration districts, each of which would serve 2 million people.[79]

Nayar faced opposition from within the Indian government and her own unit, including India's first director of family planning, B. L. Raina. In 1963, Raina shifted his country's emphasis away from "a somewhat passive clinical approach" and toward mass education and extension services, which sought to persuade large numbers of men and women who were not currently using contraception to limit their family size. This policy was reinforced as a condition of the central subsidies to Indian states that supported from 75 to 100 percent of the costs of family planning programs. By 1965, nearly 1 million vasectomies had been performed in India, more than in the preceding 10 years combined.[80]

Yet American and Indian population control advocates leveled increasingly strident criticisms that India's program was not going far enough. In India, widespread use of the IUD was preceded by a wave of vasectomies performed in temporary camp hospitals, which demonstrated the potential of mobile units to deliver a one-time outpatient procedure on an unprecedented mass basis. The largest number of vasectomies had been performed in Madras, where officials had introduced incentive payments. The payments pushed the boundary between voluntary and involuntary sterilization, especially among the extremely poor, for whom the incentive payment might represent a large percentage of their annual income.

Even *Time* magazine criticized Nayar for her Gandhian belief in *brahmacharya*, or abstinence to cultivate the virtue of self-control, even though she was "the official most responsible for selling the urgency of contraceptives."

Time cheered when she stepped down as health minister in 1967, calling her a "backward-looking spinster who had never shown any enthusiasm for birth control programs and, in fact, sometimes did not even bother to spend her department's allocated budget." It was true that Nayar had opposed adopting the IUD before it had been clinically tested in India, but she accepted the device once the Indian Council of Medical Research approved the use of the Lippes Loop IUD in 1965. At the beginning of Family Planning Week, *Time* had reported, "the grey-haired spinster waved a delicate, S-shaped twist of plastic at her audience of newsmen in New Delhi last week and announced triumphantly: 'It's foolproof.'" It was also extremely cheap to manufacture, at only a penny per unit. The Indian government paid to advertise the message "A small family is a happy family. Plan your family the 'loop' way" on tens of thousands of billboards and in slideshows at intermission in 5,000 movie theaters across India.[81]

The national government and USAID began a cooperative population control program that promoted IUD insertions on a rapid mass basis via temporary "loop camps." The camp hospitals, like the network of rural medical centers that Nayar had worked to expand since the 1940s, targeted the rural 80 percent of India's large, scattered population with least access to traditional health services. The hospitals were run by women doctors and also pioneered in training female nurses, midwives, and health visitors. Yet the premium on efficiency and cost-effectiveness at the camp hospitals could easily undermine basic medical standards such as ensuring sterile conditions and screening at-risk patients via medical histories and thorough examinations.[82]

Just as the malaria eradication campaign had emphasized vector control with DDT as the universal ideal method, so the family planning campaigns in India, Pakistan, and other developing countries relied heavily on the IUD as "the cheapest most effective and most convenient device available." In 1965, India set the astronomical goal of implanting 29 million IUDs within the next five years. The budget for family planning services had mushroomed from the rupee equivalent of less than $1 million in the First Five-Year Plan (1951–1956), to $27 million in the Third Five-Year Plan (1961–1966), to $200 million in the Fourth Five-Year Plan (1969–1974). The USAID family planning program in India "anticipated that [the] advantages [of the IUD] can be impressed upon a sizeable portion of the public," but critics including Nayar and Taylor opposed exclusive reliance on the IUD, especially if it meant that nonphysicians with little or no training would be inserting them.[83]

India had nowhere near the necessary number of trained health professionals, and its rural health infrastructure was utterly insufficient to handle the inevitable percentage of follow-up cases for bleeding, cramping, or expulsion of the device. Taylor objected that "the search for any one ideal contraceptive is unrealistic" since "each method has a threshold of inconvenience and cost which determines the level of motivation needed for effective use. Individual differences in motivation and physiology will obviously be met best by a varied assortment of methods." The IUD's more serious side effects included ectopic pregnancy, pelvic inflammatory disease, and perforated uterus. In both Pakistan and India, the government had rushed into promoting the campaign before adequately training personnel, printing instruction manuals, or ensuring the availability of patient counseling or follow-up care. Such inferior quality treatment caused women to magnify the hazards of the IUD among their friends and relatives, leading many to have them removed even when they did not experience complications.[84]

In 1966, a group of India's cabinet members took advantage of the impending crisis on the border with Pakistan and the election of a vocally pro-family planning prime minister, Indira Gandhi. The cabinet members renamed Nayar's department the Ministry of Health and Family Planning and attempted to establish a semi-independent family planning program. Before Nayar stepped down in 1967, she reluctantly accepted the policy of setting numerical targets for the number of sterilizations and IUD insertions in each state. She refused to the end, however, to adopt a national program to pay cash incentives to all those who accepted these procedures, which individual states had already been doing to varying degrees. Her successor, demographer Sripati Chandrasekhar, made the policy official within a few months after he took office. In contrast to Nayar's emphasis on voluntary family planning within comprehensive health services, he favored compulsory sterilization of men with more than two children, with fines for violators.[85]

Like neighboring India, Pakistan's national government was increasing its commitment to reducing birthrates as official policy. The catalyst for establishing the JHSPH Division of Population Dynamics had been Harper's West Pakistan Population Research and Evaluation Center. As part of Pakistan's National Research Institute of Family Planning, the center had guided the "mass movement of family planning" from 1965 to 1970, on which the national government had spent $60 million (about $410 million in 2015). The program was intended to lower Pakistan's fertility rate by promoting the voluntary adoption of first traditional methods and then the IUD recommended by Harper's research team. After Harper retired in 1970, the Division of Population Dynamics became a full department, and W. Henry Mosley (MPH 1965) was named chair in 1971.[86]

As an MPH student, Mosley had taken Helen Abbey's demography course, which "really got me interested in population studies when I went to Bangladesh." Mosley also learned from his classmate H. A. H. Mashaal (MPH 1965), an Egyptian WHO epidemiologist stationed in West Pakistan who had 20 years of experience doing population-based malaria surveillance. From 1965 to 1971, Mosley headed the epidemiology division of the Pakistan–SEATO Cholera Research Laboratory, which in 1978 became the International Centre for Diarrhoeal Disease Research, Bangladesh (ICDDR,B). For more than 40 years, ICDDR,B, located in Dhaka, has been a research and training base for many JHSPH faculty working on cholera vaccine research and geographic information systems.

Mosley expanded the scope of the cholera vaccine research to undertake one of the most massive and detailed studies to date of population in South Asia. From 1965 to 1969, the field staff of 800 made daily visits to participating households in the Matlab District to ensure that no one who was vaccinated was afflicted with cholera. Mosley followed Mashaal's procedure of enumerating and keeping record books on every house, which facilitated the study of population growth based on a variety of demographic data, including rates of neonatal mortality, abortion, stillbirths, infanticide, and contraceptive use. The survey revealed only a 2 to 3 percent rate of contraceptive use and no change in birthrates despite Pakistan's intensive national family planning program. Mosley showed his confidential report to the USAID office in Karachi, with data to show that the majority of women who had accepted IUDs were having them removed due to side effects or because they could collect a payment multiple times for each insertion. The mission director threatened Mosley with deportation, advising him to mind his own business and stick to cholera research.[87]

In January 1969, USAID sponsored an international family planning conference in Dacca, East Pakistan, to trumpet the success of Pakistan's population control program to the world in conjunction with President Ayub Khan's celebration of his country's "decade of development," which had included significant industrialization, modernization of agriculture, and expansion of the educational system. President Johnson visited Karachi to compliment Pakistan on its economic progress, and Robert McNamara, president of the World Bank, called Pakistan "one of the greatest successes in development in the world." During the conference, a general strike was in progress against Khan's regime, but Mosley arranged to take a field trip to nearby Matlab with three Volkswagen minibuses full of top population officials from the Ford Foundation, NIH, and CDC, ostensibly to show them the field study in operation. During the trip, Mosley shared his data on the failure of Pakistan's family planning program and the ineffectiveness of the standard cholera vaccine. While the group was eating lunch on the grounds beside the canal, a group of several hundred young Bengali men with black armbands attacked a large family planning poster and dragged it into the canal, shouting and yelling. The terrified officials returned to the conference in Dacca, and within a few months,

President Khan's government had collapsed. Chapter 12 continues the narrative of Mosley's leadership of the Department of Population Dynamics from 1971 to 1977.[88]

The Narangwal Study

As the examples of the difficulties encountered by JHSPH programs in India and Pakistan have shown, USAID's population program was frequently not integrated with the agency's larger economic development mission nor attuned to the unique factors that influenced population growth in each country or locally from region to region. Demographer Kingsley Davis branded such policies as just another vertical approach that used high-tech methods to "treat" high birthrates as if they were a disease. Disease eradication campaigns, despite debates over their methods, were fueled by a universal agreement that death should be avoided, whereas the ideology of family planning often directly clashed with the social mores and religious beliefs in many developing countries, especially among poor, rural populations. The goal of curbing population growth was based on a Western capitalist model that took for granted the survival of most children into adulthood. This model also discounted the value of children in the family economy of developing societies, where offspring were an essential labor source and later served as caregivers for aging parents.[89]

In the JHSPH Department of International Health, Carl Taylor set out to address such criticisms and improve population health in rural areas of the developing world by creating a new research model for primary health care. After he joined the Harvard School of Public Health faculty, Taylor had discussed the prospect of expanding Harvard's research on population change with William M. Schmidt, chair of Maternal and Child Health. Schmidt had told him that "unless there is widespread, continuing improvement in the conditions under which people live, reproductive patterns are not likely to be markedly influenced by planned parenthood programs." Throughout his career, Taylor's research was informed by "obsessive attention to involving Government of India officials and educators," with the goal of producing practical results that were "rapidly and directly meaningful in improving the quality of life of Indian villagers."[90]

When Taylor decided to leave Harvard in 1962 to become the founding director of the Division of International Health at Johns Hopkins, he had just been awarded a five-year USAID startup grant to establish the Narangwal Rural Health Research Center as a research and training base in the villages surrounding Narangwal, about 30 miles (52 kilometers) west of Khanna in the Ludhiana district of Punjab. Harvard's dean, Jack Snyder, warned him that "the Punjab belongs to Harvard," since the Khanna Study had been based there. But after some wrangling with the Harvard administration, Taylor brought the USAID grant with him. Additional funding came from P.L. 480 grants. Taylor would preserve Khanna's rigorous epidemiological standards at Narangwal as he carved out a unique interdisciplinary role for public health in population research. The Khanna Study's orientation toward improving the quality and results of health services in rural India had much in common with the health services research in the Office of Health Care Programs in Baltimore and Columbia, Maryland (discussed in chapter 9).[91]

The official USAID Country Assistance Program document for India justified continuing the efforts to reduce high child mortality rates "in order to gain receptivity for family planning," but Sushila Nayar's priorities as Minister of Health were the reverse, to use family planning to reduce maternal morbidity and mortality via child spacing. Nayar's support was critical to establishing Taylor's research base in India on a firm footing. She proposed the topic of Taylor's study of nutrition and infection in weaning-age children, and she chaired the first four Narangwal Conferences, held under tents to convene 50 or 60 senior national and state health officials and medical educators from the seven teaching health centers that collaborated in the study. Taylor reported that he had traced "multiple major improvements in the organization of rural health centers and the training of doctors directly to the continuing associations in these conferences."[92]

Tim Baker observed that while "Abel Wolman was interested in cities, Carl Taylor was interested in villages." His commitment to village life shows in his description of his family's new home in Narangwal, where he credited his wife Mary with doing "a superlative job of redesigning and decorating one of the most disreputable houses in the village. It is on the banks of the village Toba or tank where drainage accumulates, it also is bordered by the Harijan area and a vacant field which is the prime latrine area of this section. . . . [T]he sad state of our surroundings makes our own little home seem even more of a jewel." Baker used to debate with Taylor over whether it was better to spend $1,000 to provide health services in the remote villages when the same service could be provided for $10 in the cities. "And Carl Taylor would say, invest in the remote villages."[93]

Taylor refused to give in to the philosophy that rural people should be urged leave the only life they had ever known, just because infrastructure was cheaper to build in cities. In the United States during the 1960s, federal housing and mortgage policies were subsidizing the depopulation of cities to enable an affluent group of Americans to enjoy the benefits of good schools, large yards, and low crime rates. Just as strongly as any US suburbanite, Taylor felt that Indian villagers had a fundamental right to live in the open spaces and verdant jungles where he had lived and walked since childhood with his missionary family. He wrote, "If better health, nutrition, education, and social amenities can be provided in the villages of the world, there is some chance that the flow of people to the crowded cities might be reduced. The intrinsic beauty of ancient civilization may be enhanced where it is most viable—in the villages."[94]

Taylor, therefore, saw family planning as integrally related to the overriding goal of providing basic health services at the village level. He also emphasized both the ethical and practical importance of sensitivity to patients' cultural and personal preferences, and he believed that the long-term success of family planning programs depended on first providing good-quality health services and building a foundation of trust between patients and providers. Taylor elucidated the principles he pursued at Narangwal in his 1968 article, "Five Stages in a Practical Population Policy." The first stage was to respond to existing demand, since Taylor had found that merely publicizing the availability of family planning services caused about 10 to 15 percent of women to come forward (at this time, family planning programs in India and elsewhere were overwhelmingly aimed at women, and only in the 1990s would population researchers begin to give more attention to involving men). The second stage involved providing quality technical service and convenient administrative organization, since "the quality and tone of clinical and followup services can set the preconditions for longterm success." Taylor pointed to the relatively greater success of IUD programs in Taiwan, Korea, Singapore, and Hong Kong, where "considerable supporting health services were already available."[95]

After the basic family planning services had been established, Taylor recommended that in the third stage, the goal should be to "improve family planning motivation by caring for the health of mothers and children. This is especially important among the most needy. Much of the initial rapid acceptance of family planning derives from the pressure of health problems, but parental concern is not limited to high parity women." Taylor stated unequivocally that "developing a practical population policy requires a decision on the basic issue of *whether it is reasonable to try to lower the birth rate without concomitantly working on the death rate.*" Exclusive emphasis on population control without working to expand and improve basic health services was "a shortsighted policy which will work only in a stage one situation." Taylor's sentiments were echoed by WHO director-general Marcolino Candau, who lamented that "foreign aid from both government and private foundation sources has, in fact, shifted funding from health to population programs."[96]

Among the Khanna Study's most important insights was that in countries with high infant and child mortality rates, the largest proportion of deaths occurred between ages one month and two years, whereas in developed countries, most deaths occurred in the first month. With Gordon and Wyon, Taylor was among the first to recognize the relationship between malnutrition and susceptibility to infection in young children. They described the weaning syndrome as a particularly serious health threat whereby a child already suffering from malnourishment due to weaning practices of going directly from breastfeeding to an adult diet experienced a normally nonlethal infection such as measles or diarrhea. This contributed to further protein loss and malnutrition, which then caused "increased susceptibility to common infections and a spiraling deterioration" of more infections and malnutrition, resulting finally in death or serious interference with mental and physical development. Taylor observed, "This syndrome responds dramatically to better nutrition, immunization, early treatment, better home environment, and the diverse benefits of enlightened mothering. Such changes follow general economic development, although they are accelerated by health education and public health programs." He identified the paradox that "prevention of the weaning syndrome appears to be one of the main immediate causes of the world's population crisis, but it also appears to be essential to population limitation among the low parity women who are most important demographically. This stage of linking family planning to child [health] care may be a transitory but necessary stage through which programs must pass." Taylor's own subsequent research would advocate a permanent and fundamental connection between family planning and maternal and child health.[97]

By directly connecting economic development, improved health services, and child survival as incentives for family planning, population control programs could lay the groundwork for the fourth and fifth stages, which involved educating families to alter their long-term outlook on their material future. As economic development increased average income and wealth, financial considerations would exert more influence on decisions to limit family size. From the early 1960s on, Taylor had stressed the need for research on the role of sociocultural factors in population control, such as encouraging the education of women and the postponement of marriage. In the 1960s and early 1970s, very few researchers studied the influence of or interaction among such factors as age at marriage, proportion of fertile women in the overall population, or the effects of breastfeeding on fertility, but JHSPH faculty promoted awareness of the social and cultural context of family planning and its implications for maternal and child health.[98]

In this respect, they contrasted with the sexism and general insensitivity for which USAID family planning programs were sometimes criticized. In a hearing on the USAID appropriations bill in 1969, a woman described the program in her developing country as "to say the least, repulsive. It was run by men, who were telling women what to do, it was not a part of a health education program or community clinic of any kind, nor did it include the family physician or doctors in the villages that they were working in, and it was not a program that was conducive to results in that area."[99]

In light of such criticisms, one of Narangwal's major contributions was to confirm the value and effectiveness of nurse midwives and other community health workers. These paraprofessional health workers, who were nearly all women, came online in developing countries at the same time that nurse practitioner programs were on the rise at Hopkins and across the United States. Both trends were shaped by a combination of expanding demand for health care and a growing appreciation of the role that gender and cultural attitudes played in patient outcomes. Nurses led in both devising and applying methods for improving health outcomes in organized health systems. The growing scope and complexity of nurses' roles in clinical practice and the planning of government health services in the United States and abroad were evident in the heavy involvement of JHSPH nurse faculty in clinical teaching, advising students, planning field experiences, and consulting with health agencies and Hygiene faculty. Ruth Freeman, head of the PHA Division of Public Health Nursing, characterized the teaching responsibilities of nurse faculty as "heavy as compared with other faculty." International Health was a frequent requestor of nurse consultants, who were required for all country-level health workforce surveys.[100]

The expansion of national health systems brought to the fore the issue of how to maximize available human resources with limited numbers of trained health professionals. Before coming to Hopkins, Taylor had conducted a survey of Indian physicians to determine what factors determined their attitudes toward rural practice. He concluded that attracting physicians to rural areas was a "losing battle" and that most rural health problems in developing countries did not require a physician, particularly with the aid of appropriate technology, such as oral rehydration therapy. Domestically as well as abroad, health care administrators and policymakers continued to assume that physicians would lead teams of health professionals, whether in ministries of health, health departments, or hospitals. Bill Reinke, who worked closely with Taylor and Tim Baker on health manpower studies in a variety of countries, recalled that their research "raised questions about the total reorientation of job descriptions, and the organization and management of [health] services." Reinke observed that doctors were not trained or interested in administrative management and were "very much not oriented toward the organization. It's the individual patient, and even [an] individual patient's gallbladder, or an individual patient's heart or whatever." The question of whether nonphysicians could lead was "the biggest battle, particularly internationally." Reinke, whose background in industrial management had taught him to determine what qualifications, experience, and training were needed for each position within an organization to ensure its optimal functioning, concluded that the maldistribution and shortages of health workers was "very much an operations research type of problem."[101]

In 1967, Taylor's Division of International Health became a full department. By 1969, the USAID Office of Population Programs had begun to recognize the advantages of a more nuanced strategy for reducing birthrates in developing nations. The USAID population division awarded a substantial grant to JHSPH that enabled Taylor to initiate a major research project at Narangwal to evaluate the integration of family planning with the expansion of rural health services, a new policy emphasis of the Indian Ministry of Health. The project would attempt to provide quantitative evidence to demonstrate "important causal linkages between family planning and child [health] care and child survival." Taylor proposed to use "sophisticated data collection and detailed multifactorial analysis" to identify a feasible, cost-effective package of maternal and child health services that integrated family planning. The three goals of the project were to test the effectiveness of using integrated health services to increase the utilization of family planning, to demonstrate the new approach "under difficult conditions . . . in the least developed districts" of Punjab and Bihar, and to develop mass training methods to equip the large numbers of health personnel needed to offer the integrated services on a widespread basis, which would rely heavily on auxiliary nurse midwives. In summary, Taylor wanted to develop and test the ideal method of providing quality village health services "within realistic resource limitations." The grant also provided stable support for JHSPH doctoral students and preventive medicine residents working in both India and Nigeria.[102]

Almost from the beginning, Taylor encountered increasing bureaucratic obstacles and funding cuts from the Indian government, where disenchantment with family planning was beginning to set in due in large part to the collapse of the IUD insertion program. In 1969, he wrote to Sripati Chandrasekhar, Nayar's successor as India's Minister of Health, Family Planning, and Urban Development, "I find myself embarrassed now by the fact that I have been critical of certain aspects of the family planning program. [Commissioner of Family Planning] Deepak Bhatia greeted me the other day by saying, 'Here comes the leader of the dissidents.' I just want you to know that I am completely shifting my stand. . . . Everything I am saying these days is to stress the positive achievements and point out how we can build solidly for program improvements on what has been done."[103]

Taylor was less conciliatory during appropriations hearings for USAID in 1971, when he told the House Committee on Foreign Affairs, "I have learned that the initial rush of desperate women [for contraceptive services] does not represent the majority and that the problem is not simple. I shudder as I see overly evangelistic recent converts to the population cause produce antagonism by aggressive pressure on uncertain politicians in developing countries." Taylor described his research at Narangwal that measured "the impact of different packages of minimal health services on family planning utilization. As our results come in, we will no longer have to guess how necessary maternal care is to family planning acceptance or whether child care increases the confidence of parents that children can survive and therefore they can safely limit numbers." Hopkins researchers tested similar programs in urban and rural Nigeria, Chile, and the Philippines.[104]

In Pakistan, however, USAID's top-down, vertical approach prevailed. As an adviser to Pakistan's national family planning program, Paul Harper had helped gain widespread acceptance for the IUD as a cheap and effective form of contraception well suited for campaigns in developing countries. At JHSPH, Harper had pursued a broader vision for a department that housed both domestic and foreign activities in maternal and child health, demography, and family planning. Since the USAID research grant for the West Pakistan Population Research and Evaluation Center represented only a minority of the funding for the Department of Population and Family Health, Harper was freer in Baltimore than in Pakistan to pursue a diverse research and training program with grants from the Ford Foundation and NICHD. His lasting contribution to Hopkins was to establish a well-funded, truly interdisciplinary department that brought together demographers, biostatisticians, public health administrators, physicians, nurses, social scientists, and basic scientists who trained a force of well-rounded graduates in the constituent disciplines of population dynamics. Harper's original plan for the department would not survive his retirement, however, especially given the increasingly balkanized structure of federal grant programs in domestic health and welfare, as well as international health and population programs.

Conclusion

Since all three of the school's main international research units were based in South Asia, the 1971 Bangladeshi War for independence from Pakistan was the first in a series of international crises with long-term repercussions for faculty across JHSPH. Because the United States supported Pakistan instead of India, the war caused further deterioration of the already strained Indo–American relationship. After Nixon's historic visit to China in February 1972, the United States shifted its attention away from India as a counterweight to the Soviet Union. The Narangwal Project was terminated in 1974 when the Indian government refused to approve the long-term visas for the Hopkins faculty living there.

In addition to the upheavals in South Asia, the Vietnam War undermined the credibility of USAID and foreign aid generally. Congress defeated Nixon's foreign aid proposals in 1971 and 1972, and an alliance of antiwar liberals and antiwaste conservatives gutted USAID in 1973 and imposed severe administrative restrictions. Under the Foreign Assistance Act of 1973, USAID shifted its focus away from providing technical assistance and toward improving living standards and meeting "basic human needs," including nutrition, health, and education. US foreign development policy increasingly pursued multilateral aid through international agencies instead of bilateral programs such as US-AID's work in India. Shocks to the global food and energy markets also curtailed available support from the P.L. 480 program, from which JHSPH had received $685,000 in 1968–1969 (8 percent of the entire budget, including 58 percent of International Health expenditures). Congress significantly altered foreign food aid programs after the United States and Soviet Union experienced grain shortfalls, and after 1971, purchasing countries were required to pay in dollars instead of local currency, eliminating the supply of unexpended rupees for JHSPH projects in India. The P.L. 480 program saw further cutbacks after the Organization of Oil Exporting Countries (OPEC) quadrupled oil prices in late 1973 and the world economy entered a period of rapid inflation.[105]

TABLE 7.2
Population Funding at JHSPH, 1967–1973

Funding Source	Total	Total (in 2015)
USAID	$5,209,058	$32 million
US Department of Health, Education and Welfare	$2,894,200	$17.8 million
Ford Foundation	$1,675,370	$10.3 million
Other	$420,645	$2.6 million
University	$337,107	$2.1 million
Rockefeller Foundation	$214,000	$1.3 million
Population Council	$117,245	$720,000
Total	$10,867,625	$66.9 million

Source: "Background Data for A.I.D. Site Visit Committee on Johns Hopkins 211-d Institutional Support Grant," Mar. 28–29, 1972, Records of the Office of the President, Series 13, box 10, "President's Office 1971–72 Hygiene—AID" folder.

TABLE 7.3
Budgets of JHSPH Departments with South Asian Research Centers, 1970–1980

	1970	1975	1980	% Federal
International Health	$841,000	$925,000	$770,000	56
Population Dynamics	$752,000	$1,250,000	$3,300,000	84
Pathobiology	$1,345,401	$1,900,000	$1,920,000	68

Source: JHU Treasurer's Reports.

By 1977, Senator Charles H. Percy expressed concern "that AID, without the forced turnover of the Peace Corps, is increasingly becoming a way of life for a lot of people abroad." As an example of how USAID field staff lived in separate enclaves, Percy cited a "huge hotel in New Delhi with bowling alleys and everything else just for our AID personnel. Then the program was cancelled and we had a white elephant on our hands." Echoing the criticisms of *The Ugly American* two decades before, Percy called USAID "an entrenched bureaucracy that sort of feeds on itself. Those people are really living in a style of life that they could never afford back here and they are just hanging on to these jobs." Carl Taylor termed the 1970s "long years of minimal support for U.S. involvement in international health."[106]

Massive political shifts during the late 1960s and 1970s resulted in several reorganizations of both USAID and HEW, which disrupted foreign and domestic maternal and child health programs. Family planning programs, however, largely escaped the fiscal and administrative turmoil. In both USAID and the stateside War on Poverty, the goal of reducing birthrates was dominant in antipoverty programs. Whereas the public health programs of both the Children's Bureau and USAID underwent decentralization and defunding, population and family planning programs remained separately administered and financed and thus better protected. From 1967 to 1973, the two universities receiving the most USAID funding were the University of North Carolina and Johns Hopkins (table 7.2). A comparison of the budget trajectory of the three JHSPH departments with overseas USAID projects shows that International Health, where three-quarters of faculty salaries were funded by USAID grants, was much harder hit by the agency's defunding (table 7.3). USAID supported only 6 percent of faculty in Population Dynamics, which in the 1970s was largely funded by NIH, as was Pathobiology's Center for Medical Research and Training.[107]

In the decades ahead, the Department of International Health focused its attention increasingly on other issues facing low- and middle-income countries while family planning became primarily the purview of the Department of Population Dynamics.

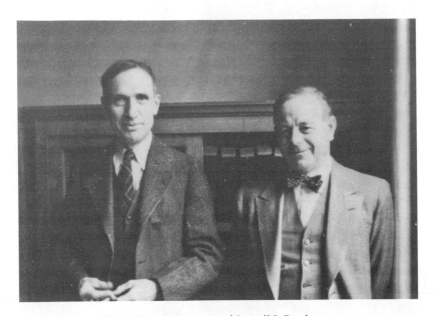

1. JHSPH deans Wade Hampton Frost and Lowell J. Reed, c. 1937.

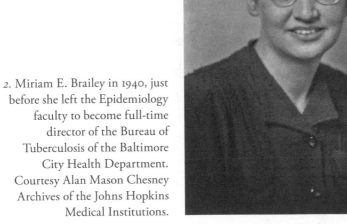

2. Miriam E. Brailey in 1940, just
before she left the Epidemiology
faculty to become full-time
director of the Bureau of
Tuberculosis of the Baltimore
City Health Department.
Courtesy Alan Mason Chesney
Archives of the Johns Hopkins
Medical Institutions.

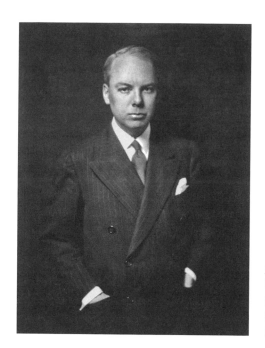

3. Thomas B. Turner, chair of Bacteriology/Microbiology, 1939 to 1957. Courtesy Alan Mason Chesney Archives of the Johns Hopkins Medical Institutions.

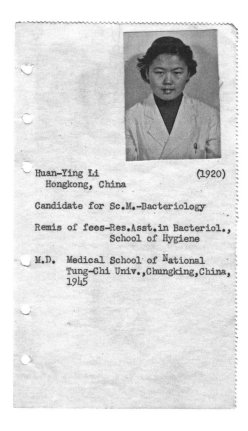

Huan-Ying Li   (1920)
Hongkong, China

Candidate for Sc.M.-Bacteriology

Remis of fees-Res.Asst.in Bacteriol.,
            School of Hygiene

M.D. Medical School of National
      Tung-Chi Univ.,Chungking,China,
      1945

4. Turner's student Huan-Ying Li, 1948. Li went on to lead in introducing multidrug therapy to control leprosy in China. Courtesy Alan Mason Chesney Archives of the Johns Hopkins Medical Institutions.

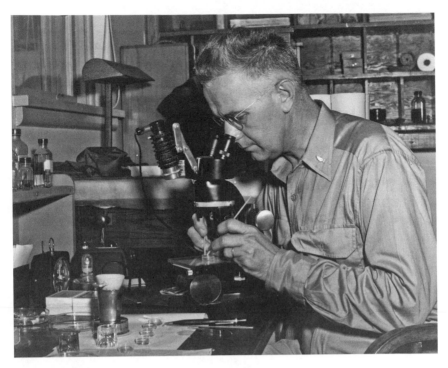

5. Malariologist Lloyd Rozeboom during World War II.

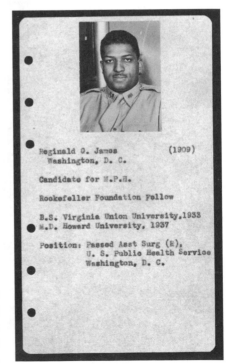

Reginald G. James   (1909)
Washington, D. C.

Candidate for M.P.H.

Rockefeller Foundation Fellow

B.S. Virginia Union University, 1933
M.D. Howard University, 1937

Position: Passed Asst Surg (R),
          U. S. Public Health Service
          Washington, D. C.

6. Reginald G. James in his US Public Health Service uniform as a student at JHSPH, 1945. Courtesy Alan Mason Chesney Archives of the Johns Hopkins Medical Institutions.

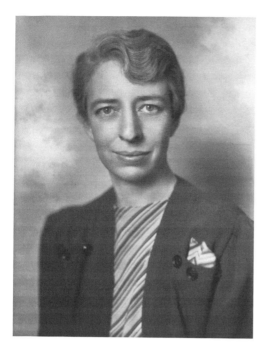

7. Margaret Merrell, c. 1945, when she was chief statistician for the PHS clinical trials of penicillin treatment of early syphilis. Courtesy Alan Mason Chesney Archives of the Johns Hopkins Medical Institutions.

8. Ernest L. Stebbins in 1946, shortly after coming to JHSPH from the New York City Health Department. Courtesy Alan Mason Chesney Archives of the Johns Hopkins Medical Institutions.

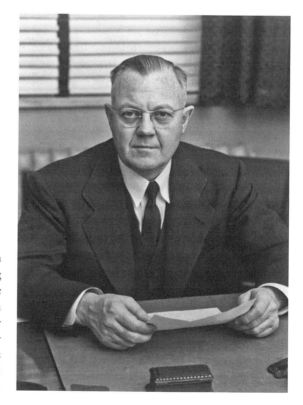

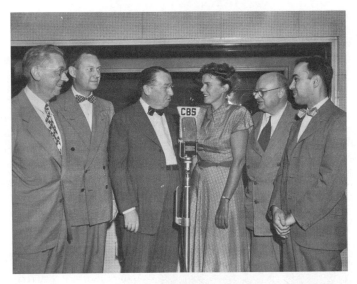

9. Howard Howe, David Bodian, and Isabel Morgan in the Department of Epidemiology under the leadership of Kenneth F. Maxcy from 1939 to 1954 conducted groundbreaking research on the pathology and epidemiology of polio that laid the foundation for Jonas Salk's vaccine. JHSPH established the Center for Research on Poliomyelitis and Virus Diseases in 1941 as the school's first research center and the first at a US university to focus on polio. Pictured in 1948 at the first International Poliomyelitis Conference in New York are Howard Howe; Raymond Bieter; Basil O'Connor, president of the National Foundation for Infantile Paralysis; Isabel Morgan; Watson Davis; and David Bodian, who helped oversee the national vaccine trial in 1954. Courtesy of the Alan Mason Chesney Archives of the Johns Hopkins Medical Institutions.

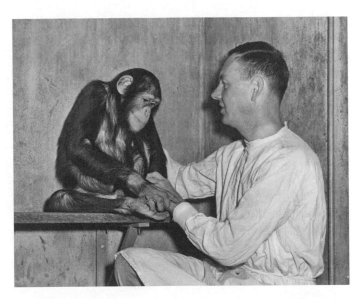

10. Howard Howe and Yogi the chimpanzee at the polio research lab, c. 1950. Courtesy of the Alan Mason Chesney Archives of the Johns Hopkins Medical Institutions.

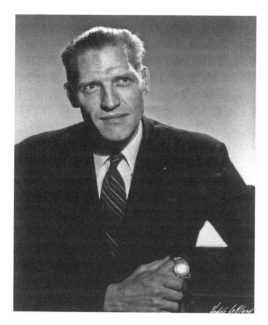

11. Paul Lemkau, c. 1955. Lemkau founded the Division of Mental Hygiene (now the Department of Mental Health) in 1941. He chaired the 1969 World Mental Health Assembly and conducted surveys of mental health in Japan, Yugoslavia, Italy, Venezuela, Mexico, and other Latin American countries. Courtesy Alan Mason Chesney Archives of the Johns Hopkins Medical Institutions.

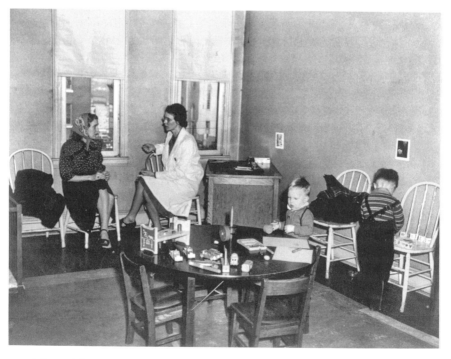

12. Marcia Mann Cooper (in white coat, c. 1950) in the Department of Mental Hygiene directed the Mother's Advisory Service, which provided child guidance advice to Baltimore mothers.

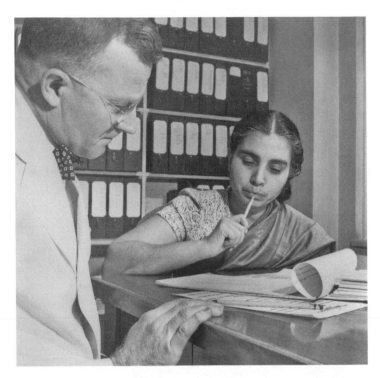

13. Paul Harper and Sushila Nayar, 1950. Courtesy Alan Mason Chesney Archives of the Johns Hopkins Medical Institutions.

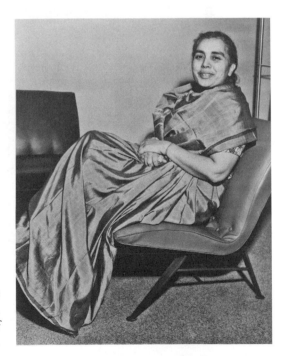

14. Sushila Nayar, India's Minister of Health, 1962. Courtesy of the Library of Congress.

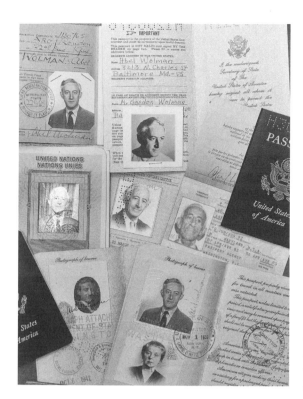

15. Abel Wolman's passports. Courtesy of Special Collections, The Johns Hopkins University.

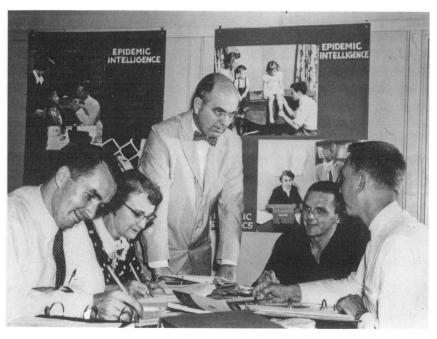

16. Alexander Langmuir and an early class of Epidemic Intelligence Service officers, mid-1950s. Courtesy of the David J. Sencer CDC Museum.

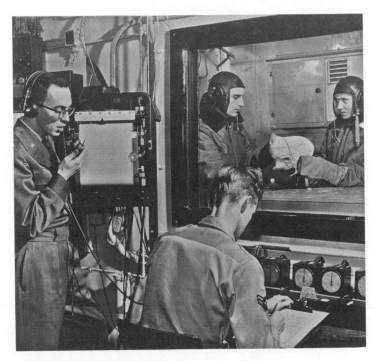

17. Aviation medicine residents observe and experience the physiological effects of Arctic flight conditions at the US Air Force School of Aviation Medicine at Randolph Field, Texas, c. 1952. Johns Hopkins was among the three schools of public health selected to provide the first year of training for the two-year aviation medicine residency program established in 1950. Courtesy of the US Air Force Office of History.

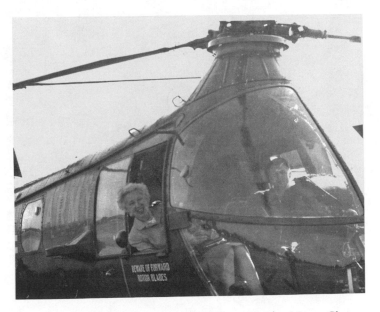

18. Anna Baetjer in an Army helicopter, c. 1955. Courtesy Alan Mason Chesney Archives of the Johns Hopkins Medical Institutions.

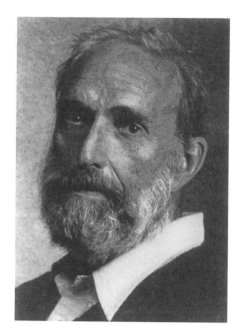

19. Frederik Bang, chair of Pathobiology from 1953 to 1981, c. 1979. Courtesy Alan Mason Chesney Archives of the Johns Hopkins Medical Institutions.

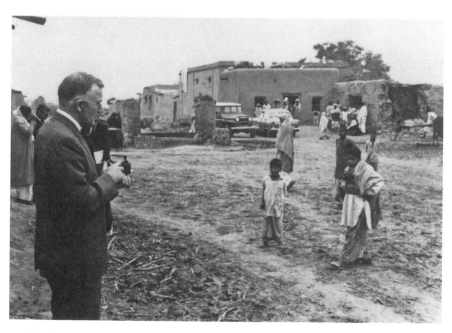

20. Paul Harper on his first visit to Pakistan, 1959. Courtesy Alan Mason Chesney Archives of the Johns Hopkins Medical Institutions.

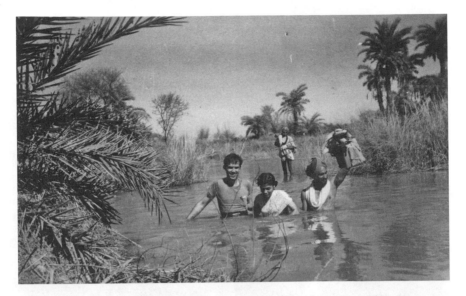

21. Carl Taylor in the field in India, late 1950s. Courtesy Alan Mason Chesney Archives of the Johns Hopkins Medical Institutions.

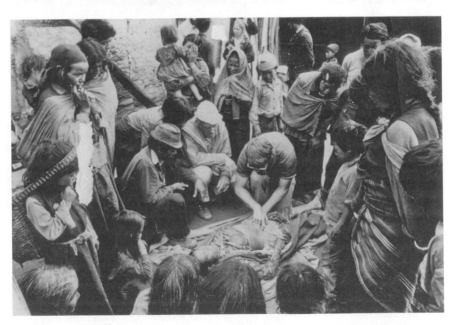

22. Carl Taylor examines a patient in Nepal, c. 1960. Courtesy Alan Mason Chesney Archives of the Johns Hopkins Medical Institutions.

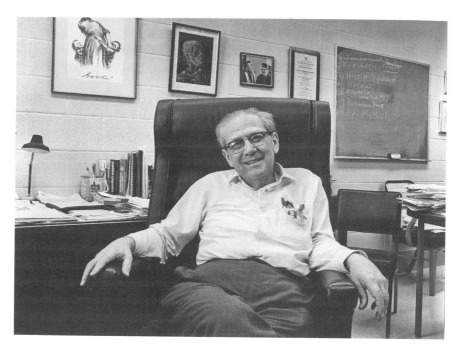

23. Abraham M. Lilienfeld, Chair of Chronic Disease 1961–1970 and of Epidemiology 1970–1974. Courtesy of the Alan Mason Chesney Archives of the Johns Hopkins Medical Institutions.

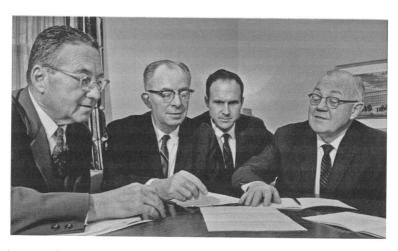

24. Assistant deans Harry Chant, John H. Hume, and Timothy D. Baker and Dean Ernest L. Stebbins, 1963. Courtesy of the *Baltimore Sun*.

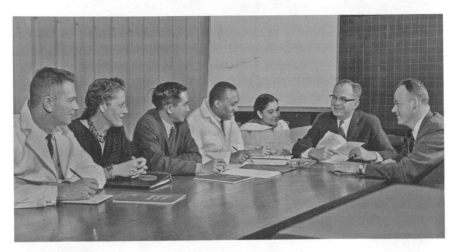

25. Associate Dean John Hume with JHSPH students, 1963. Courtesy of the *Baltimore Sun*.

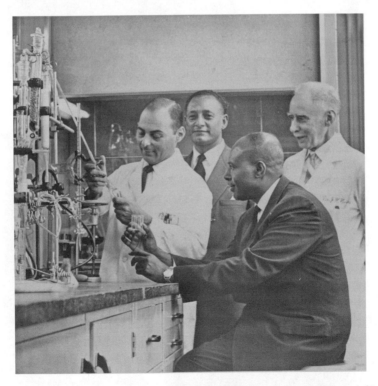

26. Leprologist John H. Hanks (far right) with Aklilu Lemma (second from left) and other Pathobiology students, 1963. Courtesy of the *Baltimore Sun*.

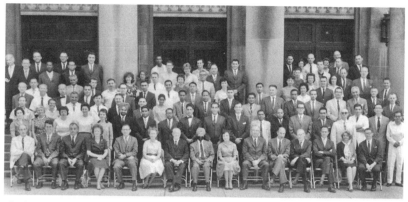

1. Dr. Young	35. Mr. Dinowitz	69. Miss Holden
2. Dr. Hall	36. Dr. F. Hall	70. Miss Marcus
3. Dr. Alexiou	37. Dr. Mashaal	71. Mr. Lennox
4. Miss Edmands	38. Mr. Chi-Jen Lee	72. Miss Cunningham
5. Dr. Mayers	39. Dr. McLaughlin	73. Dr. Magee
6. Dr. Freeman	40. Dr. Krager	74. Dr. Soo Hwa Lee
7. Dr. Stebbins	41. Dr. Thapa	75. Miss Hetherington
8. Dr. Singh	42. Dr. Pardoko	76. Miss. J. Gay
9. Dr. Abbey	43. Dr. Justiniano	77. Dr. Goggin
10. Dr. Hume	44. Dr. El-Dadah	78. Mr. E. Cooper
11. Dr. Flagle	45. Dr. Giri	79. Dr. Gey
12. Dr. Lemkau	46. Dr. Rayson	80. Mr. Chandler
13. Dr. Baker	47. Mr. Sebsibe-Abebe	81. Dr. Thomson
14. Miss Forman	48. Dr. Bello	82. Mr. Lukin
15. Dr. Klarman	49. Dr. Reynolds	83. Dr. Sobiesk
16. Dr. Pena de Grimaldo	50. Dr. Mehra	84. Dr. Bellerive
17. Mrs. Meyer	51. Dr. Coppege	85. D . Blackburn
18. Miss Janèt Hale	52. Dr. D. Ferguson	86. Dr. Mahapatra
19. Mrs. Kimbro	53. Mr. Dresser	87. Dr. Soopikian
20. Miss Murphy	54. Dr. Webb	88. Mr. Yilma Mekuria
21. Dr. Thind	55. Dr. Rogier	89. Dr. McElwain
22. Dr. Hossain	56. Dr. Kassira	90. Miss J. Smith
23. Dr. Khan	57. Mr. Hitchcock	91. Miss DeBella
24. Dr. Amini	58. Dr. Nobrega	92. Dr. Gordon
25. Dr. Ahmad	59. Mr. Vargas Mena	93. Dr. Masi
26. Dr. Raafat	60. Mr. Sylk	94. Dr. Vicens
27. Dr. Maqbool	61. Dr. Yi	95. Dr. Jane K. Meyer
28. Dr. Robinson	62. Dr. Andrews	96. Dr. Fischman
29. Mr. Gonzalez-Valdivieso	63. Dr. Meng	97. Dr. Kolbye
30. Dr. Gaitan	64. Dr. Kyung Ja Kim	98. Miss Hewitt
31. Dr. Kern	65. Dr. DeHart	99. Mr. Imre
32. Dr. Lopez-Muniz	66. Dr. E. Ferguson	100. Mr. W. Cooper
33. Dr. Chong	67. Dr. Tewari	101. Mr. Christensen
34. Dr. Bux	68. Mr. Boyd	

27. JHSPH faculty and students, 1965. Courtesy Alan Mason Chesney Archives of the Johns Hopkins Medical Institutions.

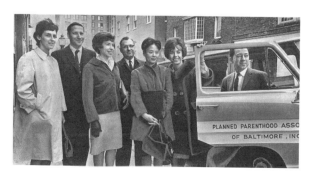

28. JHSPH students in 1966 attend classes on contraceptive methods at the Baltimore offices of Planned Parenthood on Charles Street, which served as the training center for the national Planned Parenthood Association. Courtesy of the *Baltimore Sun.*

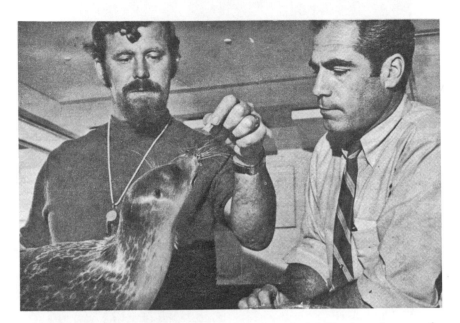

29. Ray Harmon, a research assistant in Pathobiology, feeds Miko the seal as part of marine biologist Carleton Ray's research on the population biology of polar marine animals, 1969. Courtesy of the *Baltimore Sun*.

30. Poster from the Maryland Iron-Fortified Infant Formula program, c. 1970, which became a model for the federal Women, Infants and Children (WIC) nutrition program. Courtesy of Dr. David M. Paige.

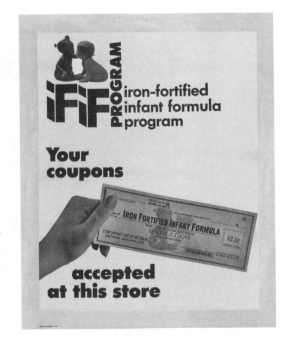

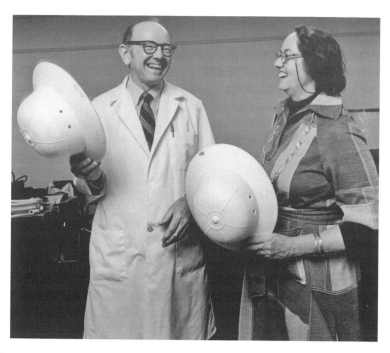

31. Roger M. Herriott, chair of Biochemistry from 1948 to 1975, and Edyth Schoenrich, associate dean for Academic Affairs and professor of health services administration, c. 1976.

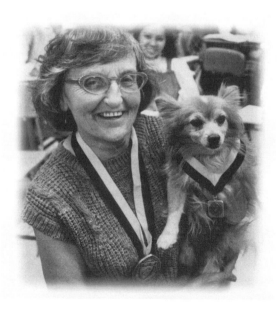

32. Legendary biostatistics teacher Helen Abbey and her dog Pepe, who accompanied her to every class, with their Ernest Stebbins medals, 1985. Courtesy Alan Mason Chesney Archives of the Johns Hopkins Medical Institutions.

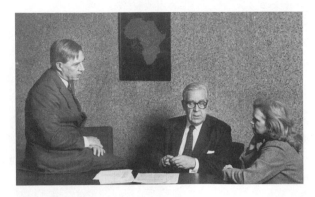

33. D. A. Henderson, Halfdan T. Mahler, and Karen Davis at WHO headquarters in Geneva, 1985. Henderson was dean of JHSPH from 1977 to 1990; Mahler was director-general of WHO from 1973 to 1988; Davis was chair of Health Policy and Management from 1983 to 1992.

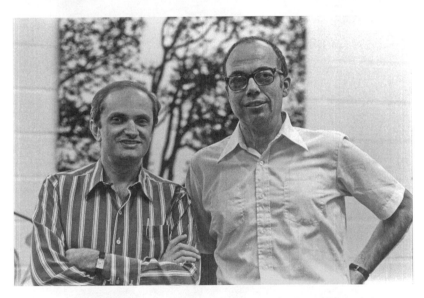

34. Moyses Szklo and Leon Gordis, c. 1980. Szklo and Gordis established the Summer Institute in Epidemiology at JHSPH in 1983, which has taught more than 10,000 students as of 2016.

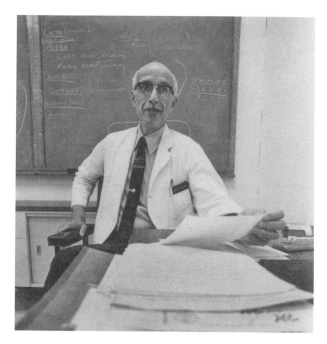

35. George W. Comstock, director of the Johns Hopkins Training Center for Public
Health Research, c. 1975. Courtesy Alan Mason Chesney Archives of the Johns
Hopkins Medical Institutions.

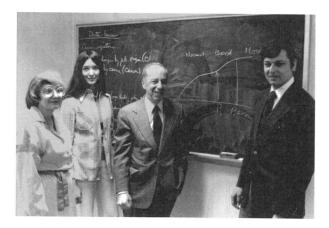

36. Pearl German, Laura Morlock, Sam Shapiro, and Donald Steinwachs at the
Health Services Research and Development Center, c. 1975.

CHAPTER EIGHT

The Social Sciences, Urban Health, and the Great Society

In the mid-1960s, the Institute for Sex Research in Bloomington, Indiana, commonly known as the Kinsey Institute, hosted a week-long seminar for officers in the CDC Venereal Disease Branch. Ernest Stebbins had dispatched Margaret Bright, a former UN demographer and expert on survey design and interviewing techniques, to assist senior Kinsey researchers, who instructed CDC officers on how to take sexual case histories as a tool for controlling venereal disease. Bright remembered, "The Kinsey mode of interviewing is the best that I've ever seen. [The Kinsey researchers] interviewed all of us. And they start out by telling you, don't answer the question if you can't answer it truthfully." Using a keyboard with about 60 numbered keys that corresponded to questions, "they knew what every question was on that board. And they [could] skip around with you to make the interview flow more readily. And then at the end, when there was any lull, they could ask one of the questions that hadn't been punched down. It was really a classy kind of thing." After the day of instruction concluded, evenings were spent watching movies from the Kinsey Institute's extensive archives and trading stories with the likes of William H. Masters and Virginia E. Johnson, who would become famous with the publication of *Human Sexual Response* in 1966.[1]

This chapter examines the School of Hygiene and Public Health's growth from the early 1960s until 1967 in the local context of the relationship between Johns Hopkins University and Baltimore. The city's public health problems were a common denominator for the school's programs in the social sciences, public health nursing and administration, maternal and child health, family planning, and the planning and evaluation of health services. The next chapter addresses these themes from 1968 through the 1970s.

Social and Behavioral Sciences Drive the School's Growth

Bright's involvement in the inaugural CDC workshop at the Kinsey Institute highlighted the rise of social and behavioral sciences methods within public health. Practitioners looked to sociology and other new disciplinary tools to augment and guide more accurately the traditional "magic bullets" for controlling infectious disease, such as penicillin. By 1960, VD rates were rising rapidly again after more than two decades of decline, and the House Appropriations Committee held hearings and demanded that the PHS devise a plan to eradicate syphilis (this was, after all, at the height of the WHO's malaria eradication campaign and shortly before the WHO launched its smallpox eradication campaign in 1966). In a report issued in late 1961, a national task force chaired by New York City Health Commissioner Leona Baumgartner recommended that the surgeon general inaugurate behavioral science research to correct the "critical lack of knowledge" regarding the social, cultural, and psychological aspects of sexual behavior related to the spread of VD infection. Yet such concepts were unfamiliar to many in the CDC's Venereal Disease Branch. Raymond Forer, a sociology professor at Emory University, was the branch's first chief of Behavioral Science Activities who set out to "to gain acceptance for a new discipline" within the agency. It was Forer who had requested the assistance of the Kinsey Institute to train CDC officers in what would today be termed *cultural competency*, particularly effective methods of persuading individuals to share sensitive information to be used in casefinding and partner notification.[2]

The partnership among JHSPH, the CDC, and the Kinsey Institute was also an example of the medicalization of "social diseases" that were transformed from objects of moral condemnation to targets of public health concern. At the same time that Congress was tilting at the windmill of syphilis, JHSPH and the Baltimore City Health Department were establishing one of the nation's first public alcoholism clinics. While Abraham M. Schneidmuhl, director of the mental health clinic in the EHD, was working with Marcia Cooper's Mothers Advisory Service, he had discovered that many of the children's problems were connected to their parents' alcoholism. In 1960, Schneidmuhl joined the Mental Hygiene faculty and founded an alcoholism clinic with support from the city and state health departments. A psychologist and medical social worker provided weekly group counseling for alcoholic TB patients. The clinic was advertised on local jazz and R&B radio stations, and it quickly attracted patients of both sexes and all age, racial, and social groups.[3]

Schneidmuhl worked with his MPH classmate Wallace Mandell (MPH 1959) to establish the EHD alcoholism clinic on a firm footing. The two psychiatrists saw a major need for programs to train qualified staff to administer drug and alcohol treatment programs, and Mandell helped formalize a curriculum for a six-month alcoholism counselors training program, which grew rapidly. After Mandell left Baltimore to help establish community mental health programs in the Texas Department of Health, he continued to consult with Schneidmuhl and further expanded the program by obtaining an NIMH training grant. But when Mandell approached the Johns Hopkins Hospital about hosting the training program, hospital officials replied that "we train doctors."[4]

Schneidmuhl and Mandell were among the academic researchers and public health educators who replaced the temperance movement's former cultural authority by framing habitual heavy drinking as a new disease, alcoholism, that struck victims with susceptible physiological and psychological traits, whom they labeled alcoholics. After Prohibition ended in 1933, levels of social drinking had increased along with what psychiatrists, sociologists, social workers, and other experts labeled "excessive, pathological drinking." During the 1940s, the founding of the Yale Center for Studies on Alcoholism, directed by biostatistician and physiologist E. M. Jellinek, and the National Committee for Education on Alcoholism, headed by publicist Marty Mann, signaled an era of increased public awareness and funding for alcoholism as a problem that could be solved by scientific research and therapeutic intervention.[5]

The alcoholic beverage and tobacco industries embraced this paradigm, which isolated alcoholism and respiratory problems as individual aberrations from the otherwise benign, even beneficial, rituals of social drinking and smoking depicted in advertisements and enjoyed by millions of Americans. In 1954, the tobacco industry created the Council on Tobacco Research. In 1969, the US Brewers Association enlisted Thomas Turner, former chair of the JHSPH Department of Microbiology and dean of the School of Medicine from 1957 to 1968, to establish the Medical Advisory Group (MAG, forerunner of the Alcoholic Beverage Medical Research Foundation). The MAG advised the association's members and conducted research on the positive and negative health effects of alcohol consumption. Key to both industries' support for research on alcohol and tobacco use was their contention that their products were not in themselves addictive, and most consumers could use them responsibly without harming their health. Accordingly, the Carling Brewing Company, which produced 800,000 barrels of beer annually, hosted the weekly alcoholism treatment seminar that Schneidmuhl established in May 1964.[6]

In academics generally and in public health particularly, the 1960s marked the rising legitimacy and influence of social and behavioral sciences. From the federal to the local level, public health agencies accorded increased funding and attention to preventing and treating mental illness, as well as initiated new programs that decriminalized substance abuse and treated it as a form of mental illness. In schools of public health, social epidemiology methods that were originally developed to address problems such as sexually transmitted disease and narcotics addiction accrued important broader implications for risk factor epidemiology and behavioral interventions to improve individual health outcomes. The social and behavioral sciences evolved to become a core discipline that, alongside biostatistics and epidemiology, could be used to study any public health problem.

Sociology was also useful for understanding the factors that drove the epidemiology of chronic diseases. Bright was the first of many sociologists recruited by Abe Lilienfeld, head of the Public Health Administration Division of Chronic Diseases. The second was Mary A. Monk, who specialized in the epidemiology of mental illness and was among the first to apply a public health framework to study suicide. She developed a standard child behavior inventory to facilitate epidemiological research on abnormal or deviant behavior. Lilienfeld viewed social and behavioral sciences as basic tools for understanding all types of chronic disease and the aging process. Two sociologists who influenced him were F. Stuart Chapin (who developed the case-control study) and Harold F. Dorn of the NIH Division of Public Health Methods, as well as social science–minded epidemiologists such as John E. Gordon at Harvard. Bright remembered that Lilienfeld told the small group of early Chronic Disease faculty to welcome collaboration with every department because "the whole school was ours."[7]

In the early 1960s, the school's few sociologists were spread out among multiple departments. Bright recalled the risks and challenges of working in interdisciplinary public health in an era when boundaries were clearly drawn between academic departments. "We [sociologists] were working with people that had completely different training than us, [which] was sort of hazardous." Bright had to determine "how to keep your integrity as a sociologist and demographer like I was, and still work in a school of public health. And you get tremendously diluted because you have to learn about public health, but they needed you for a certain point of view and since you were really a minority, they wanted you to bend towards them." While some of her colleagues dropped or muted their disciplinary identity and began to call themselves social epidemiologists, Bright "never ceased to call myself a sociologist and a demographer."[8]

Compared to other schools of public health, JHSPH had been slow to develop new social or behavioral science courses. While Johns Hopkins had continued to require microbiology until 1957, most MPH programs had already reduced their emphasis on traditional laboratory sciences in favor of applied fields, including behavioral sciences, sociology, and public health administration. An American Public Health Association task force had recommended expanding the public health curriculum to increase content from social and behavioral sciences as well as administration, economics, and communications. Ruth Freeman, head of the PHA Division of Public Health Nursing, had served on the task force and urged Stebbins (who was both JHSPH dean and chair of PHA) to apply these recommendations, exclaiming that she wanted Johns Hopkins to be "ahead of the parade instead of behind it!"[9]

In 1960, JHSPH formally recognized the importance of social and behavioral sciences by proposing to establish a new Department of Behavioral Sciences. Throughout the decade, JHSPH welcomed more sociologists, psychologists, economists, and demographers who contributed to public health research on family planning, community mental health programs, social and cultural factors in the etiology of chronic diseases and aging, comparative animal behavior, and international health manpower planning. By 1963, 10 courses in six departments featured social and behavioral science content, including the economic and political aspects of financing and organizing health services. The most fundamental such course, Behavioral Science Perspectives in Public Health, introduced methods in anthropology, sociology, and psychology as applied to "socially-induced pathology in the individual." As a wave of concern over the deteriorating morals of America's youth washed over the media and popular culture, JHSPH students discussed case studies on the problems of "mental deficiency, neglect, delinquency, illegitimacy, abortion, and birth control."[10]

In 1964, Lilienfeld teamed with James S. Coleman, chair of the Department of Social Relations on the Homewood liberal arts and sciences campus, to establish a joint PhD program in sociology and public health that would "prepare persons whose disciplinary identification will be as sociologists, but who will have systematic training and research experience in an area of public health," such as population dynamics and ecology, epidemiology, public health administration, animal social behavior, or sociology of mental health. The first PhD in the new joint sociology and public health program was awarded to Clyde E. Martin (PhD 1966), one of the principal instructors at the CDC interviewing workshop. Martin was Alfred Kinsey's coauthor on his two landmark volumes on male and female sexuality, and they had demonstrated "the power of the full [sexual] history, thoughtfully elicited and analyzed" as a valuable tool for all types of sexually transmitted disease epidemiology, which transformed the CDC's standard casefinding procedures. The survey design and interviewing techniques first developed by behavioral scientists, including rigorous methods of data collection and analysis, would become integral to public health research.[11]

Martin wrote his dissertation with Lilienfeld on the epidemiology of cervical cancer, which was among the earliest in-depth studies of the relationship between cervical cancer and sexual history as well as racial, ethnic, religious, and other cultural factors. Martin identified age at first coitus and marital instability as two key epidemiological factors. "Unstable marriage," he wrote, "is known to be associated with unstable sexual relationships, and with illegitimacy, venereal infection, prostitution, and emotional problems—all of which appear in various studies as correlates of the cancer." Martin remained in Baltimore to work for the National Institute of Child Health and Human Development, and his work on cervical cancer helped to establish its etiology as a sexually transmitted disease.[12]

Lemkau and his close ally Paul Harper, head of the Division of Maternal and Child Health, had lobbied Stebbins for years to elevate their divisions to independent departments. Yet the departmental proposal for Behavioral Sciences in the school's 1960 long-range plan had not even mentioned the existing Division of Mental Hygiene. This may have been because Lemkau, although he held a joint appointment in the medical school, had little interest in collaborating with somatic psychiatrists, and his division had never been oriented toward clinical or basic science research—the traditional Welchian gold standards. His catalog statement for Mental Hygiene omitted the biological causes and drug treatments for mental disorders; instead, these conditions were "closely related to cultural, sociologic, and family environment . . . as well as to the impact of experiences at different periods of development of the central nervous system and personality."[13]

Nonetheless, Lemkau was able to leverage the social science zeitgeist to increase federal funding for doctoral and postdoctoral mental health training. He declared in 1961,

> The facts [from community mental health surveys] speak loudly of the association between social welfare and psychiatry, between social welfare planning and psychiatric planning. From a therapeutic viewpoint, no modern psychiatrist imagines that psychiatric illness is cured by absolutely individual treatment. . . . 'A sound mind in a sound body' is no longer an adequate aim. Social psychiatry is more than a fad, and the aim must now be 'a sound mind in a sound body, a sound family and a sound community' if it is adequately to express present health notions.

Lemkau and his successor as chair, Ernest Gruenberg, both emphasized the fundamentally social nature of mental health and illness, and they also influenced the NIMH to offer specialty training fellowships in fields such as cultural anthropology, sociology, and social psychology, which they defined as basic sciences for mental health and psychiatry.[14]

In recognition of Lemkau's success in attracting NIMH funding, and with the school overall on more stable financial footing thanks to the Hill–Rhodes program, the JHSPH Advisory Board approved the creation of four new departments in 1962: Mental Hygiene, Maternal and Child Health, Chronic Diseases, and Radiological Science (discussed in chapter 10). The school added three more departments in 1967: International Health; Behavioral Sciences, which emphasized a sociological approach to understanding population health; and Medical Care and Hospitals, which applied social, statistical, and economic analyses to improve the quality and efficiency of health services on a system-wide level. Except for Radiological Science, social and behavioral sciences were central to the missions of six of the seven new JHSPH departments established during the 1960s.

The disciplinary growth of social and behavioral sciences played out against the backdrop of the School of Hygiene's physical expansion and East Baltimore's visible deterioration. Things did not start out that way. In 1939, the Baltimore City Health Department proudly announced a new alliance with JHSPH "for the conduct of special research studies in and adjacent to the slum clearance projects of the City Housing Authority which happened to be located within the Eastern Health District." The studies were intended to provide "a critical evaluation of the effects of slum clearance and the rehabilitation of blighted areas on the health and welfare of a city like Baltimore." The very first slum clearance project had been St. John's Court on Fallsway, exactly a mile from the JHSPH campus, and the BCHD annual report published a photograph of the slum before its demolition with the caption "A Slum That Is No More."[15]

In the 1940s, JHSPH leaders had envisioned a united Johns Hopkins Medical Institutions that could foster expanded access to health services and could also pioneer in creating innovative new educational programs. Abel Wolman had emerged as a convincing advocate for modern urban planning and environmental protection, particularly of water resources. His Ecology of Housing course at JHSPH dealt with the "health, social and economic implications" of housing and its relationships to public health and government programs in welfare, enforcement of housing codes, public housing, slum clearance and rehabilitation, and urban planning. In 1947, Wolman had issued a prescient warning that "deteriorating environment flanking the whole [Johns Hopkins medical campus] will become increasingly objectionable from the standpoint of student, staff and patient use."[16]

In the 1940s, JHSPH had helped establish and administer the government-funded low-income medical care programs for both the state of Maryland and city of Baltimore. In the 1950s, Paul Harper's Home and Office Care program had evolved to become a central part of the school's research and teaching in public health administration and maternal and child health. Johns Hopkins Hospital was the institutional anchor in Baltimore for all these programs serving low-income residents, which became the basis for the university's successful appeals for large philanthropic and government grants. In each proposal, Johns Hopkins Hospital and the schools of medicine and public health had promised to be innovators in the delivery and organization of health services and to lead the way in state-of-the-art research and training programs, all of which would serve as models to guide the rest of the country.

In the 1960s, this pattern continued on the largest scale yet. As the city of Baltimore's housing and infrastructure crumbled around the East Baltimore campus, Johns Hopkins launched an unprecedented building boom. The university enlisted a local developer to spearhead a series of new projects that were under construction by 1960: apartments for married house staff and students, a shopping center, a doctors' office building with apartments, and even a new Sheraton Hotel. At Johns Hopkins Hospital, the Children's Medical and Surgical Center was completed in 1964 to replace the woefully outdated Harriet Lane Home for pediatric patients.[17]

As JHSPH research activities had grown throughout the 1950s, the school had resorted to housing new programs in an old fraternity house and other off-campus buildings scattered around the neighborhood, which had rendered impossible "the highly desirable interrelationship of the faculty and staff of the different units." JHSPH joined the transformation of the medical campus when it began construction on two nine-story wings, completed in 1964 and 1968 at a total cost of $4.5 million. The new wings added 82,000 square feet to the existing 112,000 square feet in the school's original 1926 main building and north wing. But the full-throttle pace of programmatic expansion meant that departments had outgrown the additional space even before the buildings were completed, and the school had to rent an additional 20,000 square feet of outside space. Obsolete wet laboratories from the heyday of polio and syphilis research occupied fully half the space in the original main building, which was also not air-conditioned.[18]

Still, even partially relieving the school's longstanding space crunch enabled JHSPH leaders to double enrollment and move forward with new ventures. The modern facilities housed the newly established departments of Medical Care and Hospitals, Behavioral Sciences, and International Health, and they provided space for the departments of Biostatistics, Epidemiology, Maternal and Child Health, Mental Hygiene, Pathobiology, and Public Health Administration, as well as the new WHO World Schistosomiasis Research Center. Three departments received top priority for funding and space in the new building: Radiological Science, International Health, and Public Health Administration. All involved various aspects of comprehensive health planning and drew upon synergistic relationships between federal agencies and private foundations to generate support for academic research in public health that complemented emergent national policy goals.[19]

In 1969, the year after JHSPH opened its new $4.5 million eight-story Behavioral Sciences Wing, the school's 10-year planning document proposed to add 100 faculty positions by 1978–1979, with 22 in Behavioral Sciences, the largest increase of any department. This wild-eyed optimism for the future of Behavioral Sciences flowed from the charisma and vision of founding chair Sol Levine, a then-steady torrent of federal grant money, and the expectation that the department would lead the way in promoting interdepartmental research and turning out large numbers of doctoral students.[20]

The dramatic growth of Johns Hopkins in East Baltimore reflected—and sometimes anticipated—national trends. By 1972, of the 102 academic medical centers in the United States, 89 were located in central cities with populations greater than 250,000; the vast majority exceeded 1 million. The social and behavioral sciences nourished the academic flowering of JHSPH, while Hill–Burton and federal urban renewal programs financed construction across the medical campus. Congress amended the Housing Act, originally passed in 1949 to provide "a decent home and a suitable living environment for every American family," to extend urban renewal grant eligibility to universities (in 1959) and hospitals (in 1961) *without* any requirement to include residential housing in their redevelopment projects. From 1969 to the present, Johns Hopkins and other private teaching hospitals have benefited from Section 242 of the Housing and Urban Development Act of 1968, which changed existing policy to allow the Federal Housing Authority (FHA) to guarantee mortgage insurance for construction loans to nonprofit hospitals, whether private or public. As of January 2010, FHA had guaranteed $15.7 billion worth of hospital mortgages. Thus, federal housing and urban renewal policy, first drafted with the goal of benefiting residential redevelopment, including better health and sanitation, became a tool for slum clearance to make way for institutional and business development, particularly where higher education and health care interests were combined.[21]

Public Health Nursing and the Politics of Family Planning

In the go-go 1960s, public health professionals and federal policymakers elevated family planning to the center of the domestic and foreign social welfare agenda. The expansion of both the domestic health care sector and USAID programs in family planning and international health also helped drive a rapid increase in demand for trained nurses. The status of the nursing profession was further buoyed by the passage of Medicare–Medicaid in 1965, as well as other Great Society legislation to broaden health care access and address special health needs. As American involvement in the Vietnam War escalated, military and civilian federal agencies attempted to address the nursing shortage within the framework of Johnson's War on Poverty at home and abroad. The domestic programs emphasized the needs of poor, disproportionately minority inner-city dwellers with the stated goal of "maximum feasible participation of the poor," while the foreign aid programs adopted a more top-down approach to poverty in the largely rural developing world. Both fronts of the War on Poverty placed nurses at the center of policy debates over the respective roles of race, health, and fertility as factors in economic development.

Despite the fact nurses were the single largest segment of the public health workforce, most schools of public health did not require a public health nursing course. Writing to her friend and colleague Martha Eliot, chair of Harvard's Department of Maternal and Child Health, Ruth Freeman criticized the schools for their "almost apologetic attitude toward the public health practice content as compared with medical research and practice content. A proliferation of courses and dearth of synthesis." JHSPH had not included nursing in its departmental structure or degree programs until 1950 and only admitted nurses on an exceptional, case-by-case basis. Margaret Gene Arnstein, who in 1934 became the school's first nurse graduate, was recognized with a Lasker Award in 1955 for her work with the PHS Nursing Service and went on to head the Yale School of Nursing from 1967 to 1971. Freeman, as head of the PHA Division of Public Health Nursing, had worked to increase the number of qualified nurse applicants to JHSPH, but their number sharply decreased after 1957, when the Committee to Review the Educational Objectives of the School of Hygiene and Public Health had recommended emphasizing doctoral programs and limiting the MPH to physicians except in special cases.[22]

Freeman did not take this development lying down and mobilized outside pressure to change the policy. Stebbins and assistant dean Tim Baker had "caught hell from the nurses" at the 1960 annual meeting of the New York State Health Department, where both men had previously worked as district health officers before coming to Johns Hopkins. Stebbins was a member of the Joint Committee on the Study of Education for Public Health, which met in September 1961 and lamented that the field of public health administration, including schools of public health generally, had "lost ground in regard to leadership and status." The group discussed a list of worries that the profession was failing to attract top nurses or to take initiative in new fields, was "letting intolerable situations persist with minimum resistance," and was losing "logical responsibilities such as medical care, psychiatric services, sanitation and water to other governmental agencies who are less timid in accepting new or bigger tasks." Within a few short years, the surge in federal funding for programs to improve maternal and child health and to expand the health care workforce would support JHSPH initiatives that would substantially address all these concerns and elevate the status of nurse students and faculty.[23]

Freeman subsequently credited Stebbins and the JHSPH admissions committee for taking "a strong stand in favor of a multi-discipline student group." She identified psychiatric public health nursing as an important growth area and recommended enrolling more nurses and adding a nurse to the Mental Hygiene faculty. Freeman and Lemkau recruited Betty Cuthbert (MPH 1959), then serving as coordinator of behavioral sciences at the Johns Hopkins Hospital School of Nursing. After joining Mental Hygiene in 1961, Cuthbert led efforts to integrate training in psychiatric and public health nursing among the Johns Hopkins Hospital, School of Medicine, and School of Hygiene. From 1958 to 1963, the full-time enrollment of nurses doubled to 13, including four doctoral students.[24]

Freeman also took steps to stimulate nursing research to a level consistent with other units of the school and to address the need for additional nurse faculty to advise the increasing number of nurse doctoral students. Unlike some schools of public health, Hopkins had no separate Department of Public Health Nursing, but nurses in the departments of Maternal and Child Health, Mental Hygiene, International Health, and Epidemiology ensured that nurses were involved in diverse teaching and research activities while developing specialized competence within the faculty. In 1964, Freeman received a five-year PHS Nursing Faculty Research Development grant, which fostered an environment for the active pursuit of research that encouraged departments to include nurses as consultants and to undertake projects focused on public health nursing. The grant also funded a nursing research faculty member, released faculty time for research planning, and provided travel funds to strengthen field study centers such as the Richmond City Health Department Instructive Visiting Nurse Association. Freeman established the School of Hygiene Nurse Faculty Council to evaluate, strengthen, and set goals for nursing in the school and to coordinate departmental goals and programs involving nursing.[25]

Of all public health fields, maternal and child health provided the greatest opportunities for nurses with public health degrees. In 1962, the Maternal and Child Health Section of the APHA predicted, "The postwar baby boom will, within the next several years, be converted into the phase of young prolific parenthood, with the consequence that demands for maternal and child care will be tremendously increased." The first half of the prediction about "young prolific parenthood" failed to materialize, since the parents of the Baby Boomers proved to be a demographic anomaly. The smaller Generation X, born between 1961 and 1981, was the result of adult Boomers returning to their grandparents' trends toward marrying later or not at all, reduced birthrates, and higher divorce rates. But the demand for government-sponsored maternal and child health services increased for other reasons related to the changing politics of race, poverty, and reproduction.[26]

White and nonwhite birthrates in the United States had been roughly equal before World War II but the white birthrate began to fall faster than the nonwhite rate during the 1940s and 1950s, in part as a result of federal and state maternal and child health programs that reduced the higher incidence of complications and stillbirths among poor black women. The proportion of blacks receiving federal Aid to Families with Dependent Children (AFDC) also increased for two reasons. During the Great Migration of African Americans out of the rural South, their numbers increased in urban areas and in nonsouthern states, both places where it was easier to apply for and meet eligibility requirements for AFDC. Second, postwar economic prosperity lifted a larger percentage of whites than blacks out of poverty, which meant that, by the 1960s, AFDC served a higher percentage of black clients than when the program had been established under SS in 1935.[27]

Just as civil rights protests were successfully exposing the vast inequities resulting from racism and as President Johnson was launching the War on Poverty under a new agency, the Office of Economic Opportunity, Assistant Secretary of Labor Daniel P. Moynihan sparked national controversy with his report, *The Negro Family: The Case for National Action*. Moynihan was a respected sociologist who cowrote Johnson's landmark June 1965 speech at Howard University that outlined the most ambitious civil rights agenda in US history, in which Johnson explicitly blamed centuries of white racism and discrimination for the current monumental social problems faced by African Americans. To emphasize the need for reform, the 1965 Moynihan Report focused on the black matriarchal family, which Moynihan identified as the basis of a modern culture of poverty among inner-city blacks that had roots extending back to slavery. Moynihan cited the disproportionately high number of single female-headed households and illegitimate births to support his contention that "at the heart of the deterioration of the fabric of Negro society is the deterioration of the Negro family."[28]

Moynihan drew upon the scholarship by sociologists and physicians on the plight of the black family, which they argued was a natural consequence of 350 years of intense oppression under slavery and Jim Crow segregation. For example, a study of rural Mississippi black children by Hildrus A. Poindexter, dean of the Howard University Medical School, had concluded that "the worth while racial potentialities of Negro infants born and reared in rural southern environment are not sufficiently well developed at chronological maturity to make them either a local community asset or prepare them for respectable social adjustment elsewhere." Moreover, Poindexter claimed that "very few of the rural Negroes born and reared in the southern states become healthy adults." Although the Moynihan Report highlighted the negative consequences for black families of centuries of white racism and mistreatment, the report was harshly criticized by both New Left liberals and black power advocates, whose nationalist rhetoric emphasized black self-worth, the uniqueness and value of black family life and culture, and the capacity of African Americans to endure and triumph over harsh circumstances. Yet the report also helped to make the urban black family a cause célèbre and the target of a new wave of federal health and welfare programs. Moynihan, whose ideas appealed to a broad swath of Washington policymakers, served as adviser on urban affairs to President Richard M. Nixon.[29]

Moynihan had wanted the War on Poverty to provide poor families with full employment, a guaranteed minimum family income, adoption services, and birth control, yet only the last measure actually became federal policy. Advocates of population control argued that grinding poverty, whether in the city streets of Baltimore, the agrarian South, or the hinterlands of the developing world, was caused by an imbalance between large family size and limited material resources and economic opportunity. University of North Carolina sociologist Rupert Vance wrote in 1962 that high birthrates made the poverty of Appalachia "self-renewing" and that its people could "no longer allow themselves the luxury that the American people are now enjoying in the midst of the new prosperity—that is the enjoyment of the 'baby boom.'"[30]

At the opening of the 1960s, while Paul Harper was guiding the development of Pakistan's national family planning program, Maryland women remained largely isolated from birth control information and services. The state Department of Public Welfare forbade its social workers to answer their clients' questions about controlling fertility. In the United States, middle- and upper-class white women, particularly those who were married, could request their private physicians to fit them with a diaphragm, the main form of contraception that women could control before the advent of birth control pills. White married women also requested the majority of hospital abortions.[31]

In 1919, JHSPH had hosted a lecture on "Motherhood" by J. Whitridge Williams, chief of obstetrics at Johns Hopkins Hospital. Williams urged the capacity crowd of white Baltimore women to do their patriotic duty by bearing at least three children. He warned the audience that failure to do so was to sell their birthright to immigrants and was tantamount to race suicide. The school's values in the realm of sexuality had changed significantly by the 1950s, when Mental Hygiene students were encouraged to study topics that dealt with sexual behavior or attitudes and enabled students to test "the extent of tolerance for studies in more or less sensitive areas." In 1957, Baltimore City Public Schools officials consented to a study on the management of out-of-wedlock pregnancy in a school system, which uncovered "a previously unrecognized lack of communication between school and health authorities that frequently resulted in the young pregnant girls, a high-risk group, receiving inadequate prenatal care."[32]

During the 40 years between 1920 and 1960, Baltimore's black population grew steadily and the proportion of children under age 20 increased from 30 to 44 percent. By 1960, Baltimore City's total population was over 40 percent black, which ranked the city alongside Washington, DC, and Wilmington, Delaware, among major US cities with the largest percentage black populations. In 1961, African-American first-graders outnumbered their white counterparts in Baltimore City public schools for the first time, and the number of births to black women exceeded the number to white women. Of more than 73,000 annual home visits from Baltimore City Health Department nurses, 70 percent were to African Americans, the majority for maternal and child health.[33]

In 1960, Planned Parenthood of Maryland (whose board included significant numbers of JHSPH faculty) orchestrated a letter-writing campaign by civic, business, and religious leaders to change the state's policy, which cleared the way for public maternal health clinics to begin providing family planning services. The BCHD first offered contraceptives in postnatal clinics in early 1964, and Maryland's county maternal health clinics followed in 1966. The next year, Baltimore City deputy health commissioner Matthew Tayback (ScD 1953) oversaw the opening of a family planning clinic in Northwest Baltimore that distributed birth control pills to sexually active teens who obtained parental permission. Under the direction of Laurie Schwab Zabin, the state became a model for Planned Parenthood's national strategy. JHSPH students took courses at the Baltimore Planned Parenthood office on Charles Street (see photo gallery), which launched a family planning training program for the Planned Parenthood Federation of America.[34]

Tayback, a lecturer in Biostatistics who served as Baltimore's Assistant Health Commissioner for Research and Planning from 1953 to 1969, was a highly astute observer of government health services in an urban context. Tayback found that during the 1950s, attendance at the BCHD's free prenatal clinics had increased by 133 percent, to one of every four live births by 1960, yet nonwhite infant mortality had risen a tragic 70 percent during the same period. On the basis of work by Tayback and other JHSPH faculty on the social and economic determinants of health, Stebbins secured a $100,000 five-year grant from the Kellogg Foundation in 1957 to support more systematic studies of how community health administration could improve the quality of urban health services. The Kellogg grant was renewed for another five years in 1962 to conduct an in-depth analysis of the Baltimore City Medical Care Program to determine the effectiveness of methods used to control drug costs, the reasons why indigent residents of distant counties chose to be hospitalized in Baltimore City hospitals, and factors in physicians' participation or nonparticipation in the indigent care program, such as size of practices and levels of experience and training. These studies helped form the basis of what would become a signature JHSPH strength in health services research.[35]

As these events unfolded, Margaret Bright drafted a 1966 proposal for a community-based family planning program in Baltimore City that outlined guiding principles for the school's family planning training and research. Suburbanization and the concentration of poverty in central urban neighborhoods were major factors in Baltimore's changing racial composition. According to Bright's demographic study of nearly 6,000 Baltimore families, many better-educated residents, both black and white, had moved beyond the city limits. Those who remained were highly mobile, especially women of childbearing age, and Bright correctly predicted that the city's "constantly shifting population" would move even more frequently in the future, making it increasingly difficult to maintain contact and accurate records for public health and family planning programs. Bright also documented the increase in out-of-wedlock births, which by 1965 had reached 40 percent of black and 6 percent of white live births, even though the total birthrate for both races had declined to the lowest level since World War II. By such measures as single-parent households, illegitimacy, and change of address, JHSPH's research on the epidemiology of black Baltimore families had emphasized the instability of poverty to explain the disproportionately high numbers of black women and children caught in the "continuum of reproductive casualty."[36]

As a sociologist, Bright had been directly influenced by Moynihan, and she even attempted to recruit him to the JHSPH faculty in Behavioral Sciences. Although he did not accept the offer, Moynihan later served as US ambassador to India from 1973 to 1975 and intervened with government officials on behalf of JHSPH faculty. Moynihan and Bright both assumed that nearly all illegitimate children were unwanted, and their proposals took at face value the cultural norms that, in 1965, consigned mother and child alike to dismal fates. As Bright observed in her report, "There is no single thing that brings more stigma to a woman in our society, and reduces her opportunity chances, more than does bearing an illegitimate child."[37]

In keeping with War on Poverty rhetoric, Bright named reducing illegitimacy as the goal with the greatest potential "to remove inequalities in our society." In her proposal, Bright urged the outspoken targeting of specific groups, citing as a model the public health campaign against venereal disease, which "had to get over this delicacy of approach in order to get the job done. . . . Public controversy on this point will be a very healthy indication that we are on the way to facing the problem realistically." The groups that warranted "concentrated effort" and government funding were mothers of illegitimate children, mothers in their teens, and mothers of more than four children, all of whom in Baltimore City included disproportionate numbers of black women. Women in these three categories were also "easily identified," since most births were in hospitals where mothers could be "reached at the time of delivery" with family planning information and services, a strategy that had also been tested and proven successful in developing countries. Borrowing from the public health lexicon, Bright acknowledged that a program targeted toward women who had already had at least one child was "not a primary prevention program" that would completely prevent all illegitimate births, and she looked ahead to the eventual development of school-based programs.[38]

Bright, Stebbins, Harper, Carl Taylor, Henry Mosley, John Hume, and, later, John Kantner, Melvin Zelnik, Laurie Zabin, and Phyllis Piotrow were among those at JHSPH who influenced the new federal health programs to explicitly connect limiting fertility with preventing both disease and poverty. In some government-sponsored and community nonprofit clinics, contraceptives were offered alongside prenatal and postnatal care to promote child spacing as a method of promoting healthier mothers and babies. Other clinics offered only birth control without general health services to conserve funding and reach as many women as possible. After the Johnson administration embraced population control as a tool for promoting political stability at home and abroad, Congress amended SS to mandate federal support for family planning in 1967. Later that year, it also earmarked $35 million of USAID's budget for family planning, 10 times the previous year's figure. In 1970, Congress passed the Family Planning Services and Population Research Act, which established grants to support expanding domestic family planning clinics, training service providers, conducting research, and engaging in community education and outreach. The program provided access to contraceptive services, supplies, and information, giving priority to low-income clients. To meet the considerable staffing needs of new government reproductive health and family planning programs, the PHS Division of Public Health Nursing supported university-based pre- and postdoctoral fellowships to train professional nurses in specialized clinical practice, and the Children's Bureau began funding short courses in the care of premature infants for nurses in state health departments.[39]

When Reimert Ravenholt, head of USAID's population program, lectured annually to JHSPH students in the introduction to international health course, he always promoted the "next big thing" in family planning, such as colored condoms. But in the Department of Population and Family Health, Don Cornely and Paul Harper's strong opposition to abortion had set them at odds with population control "supply siders" such as Ravenholt, who considered abortion one among many acceptable forms of birth control. Margaret Bright remembered lecturing in one of Harper's courses on fertility control in Japan, which had been achieved in large part through legalized abortion. Harper "turned livid," since he did not want to foster a pro-abortion perspective among the students. In this, Harper and Cornely were in agreement with Population Council leaders such as Frank Notestein, who warned the organization's staff to "constantly and firmly take the anti-abortion stance" to counter criticisms that they were "against life."[40]

After Harper retired in 1970 and the US Supreme Court ruled in favor of legalizing abortion in the 1973 *Roe v. Wade* decision, interest in abortion as an aspect of research, teaching, and public policy grew among JHSPH students and faculty. John Kantner served as chair of Population Dynamics from 1978 to 1985, between Mosley's two terms. Whereas Harper, Cornely, and Mosley had all held MDs, Kantner was a sociologist and demographer known for his extensive research with Melvin Zelnik on sex, contraception, and pregnancy among unmarried American teenaged women. Kantner had served on the faculties of Punjab University in Pakistan and the University of Indonesia, as well as on the staffs of the Population Council and Ford Foundation.[41]

Population Dynamics students frequently sought the advice and mentoring of Hopkins pediatrician Janet Hardy, whose work with the Collaborative Perinatal Project had honed her sensitivity to the implications of racism and poverty for the health of inner-city families. Hardy held several leadership roles in the Baltimore City Health Department and became intimately involved in the community health issues that most concerned East Baltimore residents. From 1976 to 1985, Hardy served as the founding director of the Johns Hopkins Adolescent Pregnancy and Parenting program. Two of Hardy's students from JHSPH, Irvin M. Cushner (MPH 1971) and Laurie Schwab Zabin (PhD 1979), became national leaders in the family planning movement who together founded the Alan Guttmacher Institute in 1972.[42]

Zabin had first met Alan F. Guttmacher in the 1950s, when she was his obstetrics patient at Johns Hopkins, and she became his close friend and collaborator. In 1963, Ernest Stebbins had endorsed Guttmacher's book *Planning Your Family: The Complete Guide to Contraception and Fertility* as the "most complete and authentic information concerning family planning that I have ever seen. It is written with great understanding of the problems of sexual relationships and of the need for family planning. I am confident that if widely read it will be an important factor in the improvement of physical and mental health and human well being." Yet he told the book's editor that he "would prefer that the phrase sexual revolution not be used in the title. I don't believe that there has been a sexual revolution. It seems to me that there has been an all too slow recognition for better understanding of sexual relations and of the importance of contraception in the improvement of relationships between husband and wife. I am afraid that term might be misinterpreted and might detract in some measure from the value of the book."[43]

Despite Stebbins's misgivings, the sexual revolution proceeded apace. In the late 1960s, Zabin had directed the Neighborhood Family Planning Center under the auspices of the Baltimore Community Action Agency (funded by the federal Office of Economic Opportunity) and Planned Parenthood. In 1975, she enrolled in the PhD program in Population Dynamics and used Kantner and Zelnik's data on teen pregnancy and contraception to do a life table analysis of young mothers. She concluded that 50 percent of teen pregnancies had occurred within six months of becoming sexually active, and 20 percent had occurred in the first month. These findings made national headlines and energized efforts to establish school-based contraceptive clinics as a public health intervention that transformed the previous laissez-faire approach to family planning in the United States. After graduating in 1979, Zabin joined the Gynecology–Obstetrics faculty with a joint appointment in Population Dynamics and continued to work closely with Hardy.[44]

In 1981, Hardy and Zabin initiated an afterschool medical clinic that provided sex education and contraception to East Baltimore junior and senior high school students and reported a 15 percent drop in teen pregnancy after three years. Using data from Hardy's Johns Hopkins Collaborative Perinatal Study, Hardy and Zabin's further research revealed that "women who had delivered their first child as an adolescent were at significant risk for pregnancy complications and perinatal mortality and that surviving children were at substantial health and developmental risk." They applied these observations to implement three sequential intervention programs for pregnant and parenting adolescents, designed to improve maternal pregnancy and health outcomes, maternal educational attainment and knowledge of family planning, and child health and development. In collaboration with Baltimore City schools, the interventions were also designed to lower teen pregnancy rates among selected middle and high school students.

Finally, Hardy and Zabin conducted a comparative study of prenatal and obstetrical care for low-income black teen mothers who received care in a traditional setting in Johns Hopkins Hospital versus those in a multidisciplinary program that provided "high quality medical and obstetrical care, an emphasis on nutrition, nursing service which links prenatal clinic sessions with outpatient and inpatient care, social work to provide psychosocial support and services, education to prevent further unintended pregnancy, a team approach, an approach sensitive to development and cognitive levels, and access to consultation for specific medical problems." Mothers in the multidisciplinary program had lower rates of maternal complications and cesarean sections, and their babies had fewer neonatal complications and nearly half the incidence of low birth weight as babies born to mothers in the control group. Thus, Hardy and Zabin built on the earlier pregnancy, prematurity, and development research at JHSPH to establish teen pregnancy as the earliest point on the continuum of reproductive casualty.[45]

Nursing faculty in the departments of International Health, Epidemiology, Population Dynamics, Maternal and Child Health, and Public Health Administration were crucial to the school's work in reproductive and child health. One example was Jean Galkin in Epidemiology, who studied the relationship of medical care utilization to age, sex, race, marital status, and diagnosis among patients of three Johns Hopkins Hospital clinics. She left in 1964 to become dean of nursing at American University. Another was Elizabeth Edmands in Maternal and Child Health, who was an important contributor to the school's pregnancy and prematurity research, studied black Baltimore women's use of contraceptives, conducted a survey of nursing schools' curricula on population problems and family planning, and served on Baltimore City advisory committees for the health department and public schools.[46]

Alongside the large volume of charity care provided by the Johns Hopkins Hospital inpatient and outpatient programs, the expansion of JHSPH research and training in both family planning and public health nursing maintained the school's distinctive emphasis on population health. Faculty such as Tayback, Bright, Freeman, Cuthbert, and Edmands all played important roles in addressing urgent community health needs through Baltimore City's public schools and health department clinics. Yet the clientele of these community health programs that supported research and teaching at Johns Hopkins was increasingly all black. The school, its international student diversity notwithstanding, had virtually no African-American faculty and few black students or staff and so became a white bastion in a majority-black neighborhood. Because the NIH and USAID grants specified cooperation with foreign nationals in host countries, the school's field sites in India and Pakistan were more inclusive than the research and training programs on the home Baltimore campus.

Health Services Research and the Urban Sociology of Health

In the midst of growing social upheaval during the 1960s, Baltimore's dinner clubs played an integral role in the social life of the city and the School of Hygiene. JHSPH faculty belonged to the Maryland Medical Reunion, founded in 1881 by Baltimore's leading physicians, and the Caduceus Club, established by Hopkins medical and public health faculty in 1923. According to Thomas Turner, a star of the dinner club scene, "In a category all its own was the 14 West Hamilton Street Club, which played an innocent but nevertheless significant role in the affairs of The Johns Hopkins Medical Institutions. Founded in the early 1920s, its membership was limited to 100 men drawn mainly from the professional life of Baltimore," including lawyers, architects, writers, "and other self-styled intellectuals." In this intimate, confidential, and privileged setting, "institutional policies were aired, prospective professors evaluated, and the affairs of town and gown subjected to a kind of integration." But only a very limited kind; the elite dinner clubs, like Baltimore's private beach and swimming clubs, continued to restrict their membership to white Protestants, even after the civil rights movement outlawed segregation in the public sphere.[47]

In 1962, Dean Ernest Stebbins, Associate Dean John Hume, and the president and director of Johns Hopkins Hospital, Russell A. Nelson, invited the director of the hospital's Operations Research division, Charles Flagle, to dine at the West Hamilton Street Club. The three administrators told Flagle about their plans to reorient the Department of Public Health Administration to focus on the economics, sociology, and behavioral aspects of public health. Novel analytical and statistical methods were a key component of PHA's community health administration studies, and Stebbins and Hume offered joint appointments to Flagle and his operations research group, who were based in the School of Engineering. Flagle introduced the first Hygiene courses in health services research, and his students learned to apply advanced statistical and industrial management techniques to solve the practical problems of health care administration and to implement planning and evaluation studies for large, complex health systems.[48]

Operations research at JHSPH had originated in collaborations between the School of Engineering and the Johns Hopkins Hospital to improve the quality and efficiency of staffing and patient care on a systematic basis. In 1951, the US Army established its Operations Research Office (ORO) at Hopkins, and its annual allocation from the Department of Defense topped $4 million within five years. The ORO was administered in the School of Engineering's Department of Industrial Engineering, led by dean and department chair Robert H. Roy. After Lowell Reed became president of Johns Hopkins in 1953, he was concerned that the university was losing control of the off-campus research institutes that had proliferated during and after the war. Operated under government contracts, many institutes conducted highly classified activities that were largely unknown to the rest of the university community, and Reed called the institute directors together to explain the scope of their work to the deans. He invited the group to explore new ways to collaborate, and

Russell Nelson began to work closely with the ORO's director, Ellis A. Johnson, to streamline the operations of the Johns Hopkins Hospital.[49]

Nelson recognized similarities between the military problems of organization and supply that operations research had been developed to solve and those of a hospital, which also had to deploy scarce resources to meet critical but constantly shifting demands. Like many hospitals, Johns Hopkins faced a severe nursing shortage that forced the temporary closure of wards, further exacerbated by an annual turnover rate of nearly 100 percent. Its outpatient clinics were also massively overcrowded, and patients arrived en masse early in the morning and often waited throughout the day. In 1956, Nelson had hired Flagle, then an assistant professor of industrial engineering, to direct its new operations research unit. Flagle had worked as an operations analyst at ORO while completing his doctoral thesis in engineering, and he soon applied his knowledge of stochastic processes to solve the hospital's two most challenging problems: maintaining adequate nurse staffing and relieving the congestion in the outpatient clinics.[50]

Hospitals had begun to establish intensive care and other specialized units around 1950, as lifesaving medical technology grew more sophisticated and required special infrastructure, but hospitals lagged in changing their staffing policies to accommodate the increased patient monitoring that new drug and surgical therapies required of nurses. Flagle and his team observed one of the Medical Service wards around the clock to classify inpatients by their severity of illness and corresponding need for nursing care, and then developed mathematical algorithms to determine the number of staff hours required for critically ill, moderately ill, and nearly self-sufficient patients. This allowed the director of nursing services to rationally predict staffing needs and allocate personnel to each unit accordingly, which greatly improved patient care and staff morale. Flagle recalled how gratifying it was for him and his staff "to see the daily number of intensive care patients, arriving randomly and independently into what was in effect an infinite channel queue, closely follow a Poisson distribution just as the math said it should." Johns Hopkins Hospital was one of the first to adopt the principle of progressive patient care, which separated patients not only by type of illness but also by their required levels of care and stage of recovery. By using nursing staff and ward space more efficiently, hospitals could increase their admissions while also improving both the cost and quality of care.[51]

Of all the outpatient clinics, pediatrics was the most crowded and chaotic. Several hundred young patients arrived every day, first thing in the morning, and each had to wait repeatedly to pass through a series of gauntlets before eventually being examined by a clinician. An initial evaluation directed them to quarantine or the appropriate clinic subdivision, then the business office evaluated their eligibility for charity care, then a cashier processed their payment, and finally an aide took their temperature and weighed them before taking them to an examining room. Flagle's team saw that the clinic was set up like an automobile assembly line, with each task performed in a single channel, but the randomly variable needs of patients required multiple parallel channels. Based on his recommendations, all the clinic staff were trained to perform all the types of tasks so that they could be done in any order and some steps could be combined, and three entry points were set up to replace the single admissions desk. The system drastically reduced wait times and overcrowding. Another patient-flow study in the ophthalmology clinic resulted in instituting scheduled appointments at regular intervals and training nurse specialists to perform the patient preparation tasks of refraction and a visual fields test.[52]

In 1958, Stebbins reincarnated the defunct hospital administration program by convincing the Kellogg Foundation to award JHSPH another five-year grant of $100,000 for a study of community health administration in cooperation with the ORO. To lead it, Stebbins invited Flagle, who taught in the School of Engineering's new interdisciplinary Business and Industrial Management graduate program alongside several Hygiene faculty. With the new connections among the hospital and schools of Hygiene and Engineering, Hygiene students expressed increasing interest in operations research courses and participating in Flagle's hospital studies.[53]

Under the 1946 Hill–Burton Act, the PHS provided technical assistance and developed guidelines for designing, constructing, and managing hospitals and health facilities. In 1949, Hill–Burton was amended to include an extramural research program to address growing concerns that federal aid to hospital construction was causing an oversupply of beds and unnecessary hospitalization in some areas while others remained in need, and that the new hospitals were struggling to operate efficiently due to a shortage of nurses and administrative personnel. Assistant Surgeon General Jack R. Haldeman oversaw the PHS Hospital and Health Facilities Study Section and expanded its initial focus on physical infrastructure to encompass planning and evaluating community health care needs and coordinating existing services into regional systems. The work of the Operations Research Unit attracted Haldeman's attention, and Flagle was appointed as a member in 1958. The following year, Flagle joined the American Hospital Association Council on Education and Research and later served on the first editorial board of the council's journal, *Health Services Research*.[54]

The macro aspects of health services research required pooling voluminous data from hospitals, nursing homes, physicians' offices, and public health clinics, as well as developing uniform definitions of care and coding practices. In 1955, the Commission on Professional and Hospital Activities had promoted the establishment of a national hospital discharge database, but national data were still largely incomplete for community health indicators such as rates of prenatal care or immunization for communicable disease. Tayback and his coauthor Helen Wallace charged that "this lack of medical intelligence represents a serious deficiency in the administration of public health."[55]

To remedy this and other knowledge gaps, as well as address the criticism that the Hill–Burton hospital construction program had never lived up to its promise to improve the distribution and financing of health services as well as facilities, Congress approved two programs as amendments to the Hill–Burton Act. The 1961 Community Health Services and Facilities Act provided federal support for research on "improved ways of delivering needed health services, with special attention to the needs of the chronically ill and aged." The 1964 Health Facilities Areawide Planning Act offered federal matching grants for projects that developed and carried out comprehensive regional or metropolitan plans to coordinate existing and proposed health facilities and services. These acts represented a philosophical shift from addressing shortages to improving quality of care. They both placed a priority on improving efficiency and access in the health care system, which established a federal commitment to health services research to drive and implement national health policy goals.[56]

During its first decade, the PHS Hospital Facilities Study Section had been guided by salaried government physicians who thought "in terms of improving the system" on such matters as staffing problems and standards for architectural design and construction. Flagle recalled, "So many things that we did early on to cope with shortages" enabled community hospitals to use existing beds and hospital staff so much more efficiently that the issues "just melted away as major problems." The study section was renamed Health Services Research in 1959, after the arrival of a group of politically liberal academic physicians who advocated national health insurance. Philip R. Lee at the University of Minnesota and Cecil G. Sheps and Kerr L. White at the University of North Carolina concerned themselves with the total system and were bothered by the "fiefdoms" in hospitals that allocated control of beds by medical or surgical specialty, which often resulted in inefficient use of bed space that drove up costs. The study section soon recognized that the growing dominance of American medicine by specialist physicians would have far-reaching consequences across the health care spectrum, not just in bed usage patterns.[57]

Flagle observed, "Academic entrepreneurial politicians were actively invading the territory and actually, through their domination of the [Health Services Research] study section, they guided the flow of a lot of research money into health services research." The study section began to award the majority of Hill–Burton research grants to universities instead of hospitals, which helped to shift the balance of power within the Johns Hopkins Medical Institutions. When Flagle was still director of the hospital's Operations Research Unit, he had taken a stack of federal grant proposals to Thomas Turner, dean of the medical school, who "turned livid before he got past the first page," Flagle recounted. "When he saw that the hospital was the sponsor of this grant and the umpty-hundred thousand dollars would go to the hospital, which would dole it out to the people on our projects, it was then and there he told me that there was a binding agreement that the hospital will not apply for federal grants, that this will be the privilege of the School of Medicine." Although Russell Nelson and many others in the hospital and medical school were dismissive of the School of Hygiene, Flagle accepted Stebbins's invitation to cast his lot with public health by transferring his primary appointment from the School of Engineering.[58]

Just after Flagle and his operations research group joined the Department of Public Health Administration, Stebbins and Hume helped to recruit two new faculty members who would complement Flagle's analytical strengths and advance the mission of developing new ways to improve the cost-effectiveness and quality of health care systems. At Flagle's suggestion, Hume and Stebbins recruited Kerr White to head the new PHA Division of Medical Care and Hospitals in 1965. The division finally fulfilled Lowell Reed's original 1947 plan to establish a division of medical care at JHSPH that would "concern itself with the problems of the social and economic factors in disease and disability" and offer interdisciplinary courses that explored the intersections of medicine, public health, and sociology.[59]

The other new arrival was Donald A. Cornely (MPH 1958) recruited by Paul Harper, chair of Population and Family Health. After Harper launched the new Division of Population Dynamics, he tapped his former student to direct the Division of Maternal and Child Health, which became a separate department in 1971. Like Harper, Cornely was a pediatrician and JHSPH alumnus. As head of Maternal and Child Health from 1965 to 1989, Cornely emphasized research on family planning program evaluation as well as teen pregnancy prevention, issues that were also central to the Department of Population Dynamics in the 1970s and 1980s. He was well positioned to influence national maternal and child health policy, since he served on the advisory board of the PHS Maternal and Child Health/Crippled Children grants program from 1964 to 1970 and was chair from 1967 to 1970. During the same period, Cornely was the founding chair of the American Academy of Pediatrics Section on Public Health Pediatrics and was active in APHA as a member of the governing council and the Maternal and Child Health Section Committee for Public Medical Care for Children. Before coming to Hopkins, Cornely had served on the faculties of the University of Pennsylvania School of Medicine (1952–1962) and University of Pittsburgh Graduate School of Public Health (1962–1965) and headed the Maternal and Child Health Division of the Philadelphia Department of Public Health (1958–1962). He also directed the American Academy of Pediatrics Pediatric Research, Education and Practice Study from 1963 to 1965.[60]

In a 1962 *Journal of Pediatrics* article titled "Urban Medical Blight," Cornely had published one of the early calls to improve pediatric care for inner-city children. After his return to JHSPH, he worked to carry out this goal in Baltimore in collaboration with the chairs of Public Health Administration (John Hume), Mental Hygiene (Paul Lemkau), Population and Family Health (Paul Harper), and Pediatrics (Robert Cooke), who comprised one-quarter of the membership of the Medical Care Committee for the Maryland State Board of Health. This committee had been established in 1945 to advise the state Medical Care Program. With funding from the Board of Health and the federal Children and Youth Projects program, Cooke and Harper established the Johns Hopkins Comprehensive Child Care Center (CCCC) in 1966, which became one of the models for the Head Start Child Development Act of 1969.[61]

Cooke had been instrumental in initiating and planning Head Start with Sargent Shriver, who directed the flagship War on Poverty agency, the Office of Economic Opportunity. The CCCC, like the EHD once had, reached out to neighborhood families and offered a broad range of services in one location that also facilitated research. The CCCC replaced the hospital-based Home and Office Care Clinic as a clinical training site for students in Pediatrics and Maternal and Child Health. Research compared outcomes between the CCCC and a standard maternal and child care clinic housed in the same building, using data from several census tracts near the hospital.[62]

In studies conducted over a 20-year period, epidemiologist and pediatrician Leon Gordis, with JHSPH colleague Abe Lilienfeld and Hopkins pediatrician Romeo Rodriguez, demonstrated the effectiveness of the CCCC and other federally funded comprehensive care programs in dramatically reducing rates of rheumatic fever among inner-city Baltimore children. Their initial research in the early 1960s showed that both initial and recurrent attack rates were more than twice as frequent in blacks as in whites, which supported the observation that the disease tended to cluster in predominantly black, low-income urban neighborhoods and was relatively rare in suburban areas. By comparing the findings from the 1960–1964 period to those from 1968–1970, the investigators found that the rates in black Baltimore children had dropped dramatically, while the rates in whites had stayed the same. Importantly, the incidence of rheumatic fever in census tracts that were eligible for comprehensive care decreased 60 percent, whereas ineligible census tracts showed virtually no change.[63]

To further confirm that the change was the result of comprehensive care programs and not other social and economic factors, the Hopkins study examined the clinical records and determined that the entire decline in rheumatic fever was due to cases where patients had shown clinically overt acute pharyngitis that induced their parents to seek the newly available quality health care, rather than cases with subclinical symptoms. These findings were borne out by other studies in other cities, as well as by hospital discharge data, which showed the rate of discharges for rheumatic fever declined from 14 per 100,000 in 1965, the year that legislation was enacted for the comprehensive pediatric care programs, to only one case per 100,000 by 1981. Gordis concluded that federal comprehensive care programs had eliminated both racial disparities in rheumatic fever and the disease itself.[64]

Maryland's Medical Care Program to reimburse physicians and hospitals for providing inpatient and outpatient care to low-income patients had grown from a budget of $1 million in 1948 to $7.5 million in 1961 and then more than tripled to $26 million by 1966, with virtually no federal assistance. After the passage of Medicaid in 1965, community organizers launched campaigns to encourage East Baltimore residents to exercise their rights to care, and participation continued to rise. By 1971, the state would spend $90 million for the program, with an additional $5.6 million from Medicaid.[65]

But rising enrollments were not the only factor behind the surging costs of both state medical care programs and Medicaid, which were also driven by the treatment-oriented structure and priorities of the health system. Medicaid, as JHSPH professor of international health Robert D. Wright observed, "was designed for operation by a bunch of medical fire fighters who only went into action when they saw a blaze. Little if any thought was given to prevention." Like Wickliffe Rose, coauthor of the 1915 Welch–Rose Report that had established the original plan for JHSPH, Wright argued that broader application of public health and preventive medicine would greatly reduce the demand for the services of doctors and allied health professionals. Such calculations, however, did not account for the maldistribution of physicians and health facilities *within* a geographic area or the ways that their locations were determined by the effects of political and economic disempowerment.[66]

Many of the issues surrounding the health status of poor and underserved populations raised by the school's work with the CCCC and Medicaid in Maryland were tackled by Kerr White, whose Division of Medical Care and Hospitals became an independent department in 1967. Research and training were devoted to improving the efficiency and effectiveness of personal health services. The physician-oriented department included a hospital administration track and oversaw the general preventive medicine residency. Medical Care and Hospitals faculty surveyed the myriad macro-level relationships among the health care workforce, service providers, finance systems, and public and private agencies as well as the micro-level factors affecting physician behavior and patient attitudes in clinical practice.[67]

Despite the rapid increase in funding to cover the cost of treating poor Marylanders, of whom the vast majority were Baltimore residents, many downtown hospitals followed the national trend of relocating to the suburbs. Johns Hopkins Hospital had been founded with the mandate to provide for "the indigent sick of this city and its environs, without regard to sex, age, or color, who may require surgical or medical treatment." In 1966, the hospital's leaders charged the Health Care Programs Working Committee with evaluating whether the hospital should leave East Baltimore, but both practical and ideological considerations moored the hospital to its historic site. David Everheart and Barbara Starfield (MPH 1963) from the Medical Care and Hospitals faculty served on the committee, and both they and committee chair Robert M. Heyssel advocated for strengthening the hospital's outpatient programs to both improve service to the community and provide educational and research opportunities for the Medical Institutions. The hospital's trustees, moreover, decided that they had invested too much in recent capital improvements for a move to be feasible. Yet over the past decade, those improvements had breached the community's faith, creating serious obstacles to research, education, and patient care at Johns Hopkins. In the late 1950s, 1,355 African-American households had been forced to vacate for the Medical Institutions' Broadway urban renewal project but were promised new homes in the redeveloped neighborhood. The hospital and the city reneged and instead built the 10-story Reed Hall (named for JHSPH dean Lowell Reed and completed in 1957) and three-story housing for Hopkins medical and public health students and residents. This housing, known as "the compound," was surrounded by a gated, barbed-wire fence that was deeply resented by community residents, summarized by one observer as "Civilization here, savagery there."[68]

One of the first students to work with White at the intersection of race, poverty, health care access, and public policy was Jack Wennberg (MPH 1966). Wennberg had already attracted national media attention as a postdoctoral fellow in the Johns Hopkins Department of Medicine, where he led a Johns Hopkins Hospital study published in *JAMA* on the drug Orabilex. In 1963, the 29-year-old Wennberg had written to the FDA three times to request action on his report that Orabilex, an X-ray contrast medium used to visualize gallstones, caused kidney complications that may have resulted in as many as 100 deaths around the United States. The drug might have remained on the market indefinitely if Wennberg had not appealed to Senator Hubert Humphrey, head of a drug policy investigation subcommittee, who also enlisted the White House. The manufacturer finally withdrew the drug in January 1964 after President Johnson threatened to call a meeting with FDA officials. Wennberg called the Orabilex study representative "in a microscopic way [of] the whole problem of drug control."[69]

In summer 1966, Tayback arranged for Wennberg to conduct a study for the Maryland State Health Department that functioned as a medical care audit on a sample of more than 300 welfare patients in 19 private Baltimore City nursing homes. Medical records indicated that admissions exams were often incomplete or not performed at all, and more than two-thirds of the patients had not had standard procedures such as urinalysis and blood counts. Wennberg found that in the five facilities with the lowest rates of completed admission medical exams, one in five welfare patients died within 28 days of admission, which indicated that hospitals, physicians, and the Department of Public Welfare were sending acutely ill, poor, elderly patients to nursing homes where they would not receive appropriate medical care.[70]

Maryland state health commissioner William J. Peeples called the study "damning to both doctors and nursing homes." Wennberg's report noted that although nursing homes were expected to provide long-term care of the chronically ill, some were in effect operating as acute hospitals, even though nursing homes lacked the medically required professional staff, facilities and supporting emergency services found in a general hospital. Wennberg exclaimed, "That contemporary medical institutions exist into which a patient may enter and die without recorded evidence of a referral or an admission diagnosis is indeed extraordinary. . . . It seems clear that the referring hospitals are in some instances using the nursing homes as resources for the management of terminal patients." Wennberg's study called for major changes in the management of medical affairs and admission policy within nursing homes, as well as raised questions concerning the role of hospitals, community physicians, and the Department of Public Welfare in placing patients in nursing homes.[71]

Conclusion

During the 1960s, the Johns Hopkins Medical Institutions received major support from foundations as well as new federal grant programs to support maternal and child health services and the War on Poverty. In the context of growing activism among civil rights groups and community action programs, these initiatives attempted to counter the effects of substandard living conditions and lack of access to primary care in poor neighborhoods such as East Baltimore. Health services research not only aimed to address socioeconomic factors in the provision of clinical care but also introduced powerful new methodologies that originated outside public health in disciplines such as systems engineering and industrial management.

The unprecedented growth of Johns Hopkins and its peers was driven not only by federal research and construction funding but also by the expansion of the health care sector, which increased from only 4.3 percent of national gross domestic product in 1950 to 7 percent by 1970, and now, in 2015, stands at 18 percent. Johns Hopkins and other large academic medical centers became the top employers in cities such as Baltimore that were rapidly losing their population and industrial economic anchors. Therefore, the School of Hygiene and Public Health was developing its understanding of the socioeconomic determinants of health just as those indicators were worsening for more and more Baltimore residents, while the general population was enjoying greater access to health insurance and services than ever before. This tension would stimulate the continued growth of the social sciences and health services research at JHSPH. The tumultuous 1960s also sowed the seeds for the emergence of bioethics as a core field of inquiry and for faculty to more openly embrace advocacy on policy issues ranging from national health insurance to injury control to environmental justice.[72]

CHAPTER NINE

Surviving the Seventies

As associate dean since 1961, John Hume had played a pivotal role in establishing and expanding the school's foreign programs in International Health, Population Dynamics, and Pathobiology. As chair of Public Health Administration, he had also presided over the dramatic growth of domestic programs in medical care and hospital administration as well as social and behavioral sciences. Ernest Stebbins had selected Hume as his heir apparent, but when Stebbins announced that he would step down as dean in 1967, faculty were divided over whether the school should pursue new directions or remain on the course that Stebbins and Hume had set.[1]

Hume was a consummate public health insider with decades of career experience in both domestic and global public health. But during the 1960s, the heads of federal agencies scoffed at the once-mighty US Public Health Service as stodgy and hidebound. Key officials in the Kennedy and Johnson administrations increasingly ignored the PHS and circumvented the surgeon general to pass health reforms they considered "revolutionary." Ironically, Stebbins had helped set in motion the long slide in the power of the PHS. He had co-chaired the congressional committee that first proposed in 1947 to reorganize the Federal Security Agency as a cabinet-level Department of Health, Education and Security. Although the plan did not pass during the Truman administration due to partisan politics, Congress approved the creation of the Department of Health, Education and Welfare shortly after President Dwight D. Eisenhower took office in 1953. This new structure had the potential to interfere with the surgeon general's direct access to the president, if the surgeon general was at odds with HEW. In the 1960s, HEW Assistant Secretary Wilbur Cohen convinced President Kennedy to oust Surgeon General Leroy Burney, who had been a great friend to his alma mater, JHSPH. Cohen viewed him as a "competent man but a reactionary," in part because Burney had been appointed by Eisenhower, a Republican president. During the 1960s, Cohen would strip the office of most of its authority.[2]

The Johnson administration acted to disempower further the relatively apolitical PHS by removing some of its existing responsibilities and denying it any new roles. For example, the omnibus 1964 Economic Opportunity Act vested authority for funding and administering community health programs in impoverished neighborhoods in a new agency, the Office of Economic Opportunity (OEO), which would be beset by a severe political backlash against the OEO's stated philosophy of "maximum feasible participation of the poor." The 1965 Medicare/Medicaid Amendments to the Social Security Act represented another major expansion of the federal health bureaucracy beyond the PHS.[3]

At JHSPH, the committee to select a new dean was equally divided between Hume and Philip R. Lee, a Johnson administration hotshot. Lee had served as director of health services in the USAID's Office of Human Resources and Social Development and was currently Assistant Secretary for Health and Scientific Affairs at HEW, where he was among those circumventing the PHS. Lee's former colleague at USAID, Malcolm Merrill, called Lee "a man of broad vision" who had done a "phenomenal job" at USAID, yet his unorthodox operating style had "stirred things up" and irritated "bureaucratic types." Lee had stressed prevention far above treatment in foreign aid programs and was "much concerned with medical education and manpower issues."[4]

Merrill suggested that Lee would be a "more exciting dean" but characterized Hume as "a real pro, sound, substantial," who might be "more consistently constructive over the long haul." Charles Smith, who had recently worked with Hume on a national training committee, likewise characterized Hume as "safe and generally progressive hands" but felt that Lee might be "a better choice for the next generation," and he had "no doubt that the School would break new ground under him." According to Smith, Lee was "not part of the establishment" and had "an extremely keen mind" that would enable the school to make "larger and faster gains."[5]

The search committee's decision was made for it when Lee declined to become a candidate for the deanship and subsequently replaced the surgeon general as head of the PHS when HEW was reorganized in 1968. As JHSPH dean, John Hume upheld Stebbins's priorities, emphasizing the expansion of health services research and the integration of the social and behavioral sciences into the public health curriculum. But Hume could not have foreseen the coming decade of challenges that crested one after another, many of which were amplified by national and international crises.[6]

Chapters 9 through 12 deal with JHSPH during the decade of Hume's deanship from 1967 to 1977. Growing public opposition to the Vietnam War, followed by the withdrawal of US troops and the fall of Saigon in 1975, translated into isolationism in Congress. In the 1970s, foreign aid funding declined at the same time that population control was displacing public health as a priority within USAID. Détente between the United States and Soviet Union eased anxieties about potential nuclear or biological attacks, and national defense lost its power as a justification for public health spending. With the development and widespread use of vaccines, antibiotics, and other powerful new therapeutics, schools of medicine and public health sharply curtailed their teaching and research in infectious disease, where public health had achieved its greatest successes to date. These trends channeled federal investment in public health into domestic programs with broad bipartisan support. The resulting initiatives focused on solving public health problems that were making headlines and the nightly news, including hunger, drug addiction, the "health manpower crisis," the skyrocketing cost of health care, the health hazards of pollution and other environmental exposures, and questions surrounding the safety and efficacy of prescription drugs and medical procedures.

1968 and Everything After

The connections among urban sociology, health services research, and public health administration were further reinforced by the events of the late 1960s, when the southern civil rights movement moved into northern cities, while black power activists worked to secure for their communities the Great Society promises of ending poverty and broadening health care access. African Americans were growing angrier by the day in the face of racial discrimination, unemployment, dilapidated housing, and harsh police tactics in inner-city neighborhoods, all of which stood in stark contrast to the greatest level of affluence in American history. Summer riots had erupted in a series of cities, most violently in the Los Angeles neighborhood of Watts in 1965 and in Detroit and Newark in 1967. Yet Baltimore remained calm.[7]

As the Johns Hopkins Medical Institutions (JHMI) considered expanding their role in addressing community health needs, the university contemplated how it should exercise leadership to solve urban problems nationally and in Baltimore, such as creating an urban studies center to coordinate existing teaching and research programs among 16 departments. In a 1967 talk to Hygiene faculty on "Hopkins' contribution to urban society," JHU president Lincoln Gordon credited the contributions of Abel Wolman (water and sewer supply and urban planning), Paul Lemkau (mental health services and epidemiology), and Cornelius Kruse (rodent control and air pollution) but acknowledged that they had been "on an individual basis [with] no institutional commitment." Gordon warned of the current critical situation in the neighborhood surrounding the East Baltimore campus, in which "Hopkins must assert greater leadership," and asked, "Is there more Hopkins could be doing in urban affairs through the School of Hygiene and Public Health?" These discussions laid the foundation for Johns Hopkins to establish two interdisciplinary centers in 1968 that addressed urban issues, both located in East Baltimore: the Office of Health Care Programs, focused on health care access under the auspices of JHMI, and the Johns Hopkins Center for Urban Affairs, a broader, university-wide urban policy institute.[8]

JHU provost William Bevan strongly urged the school to "involve itself as much in domestic programs as in foreign programs, looking at the 'new' problems that we are facing in modern urban society along with working at the old problems in new settings overseas." But in a special summer 1967 issue of the *Johns Hopkins Magazine* to commemorate the school's 50th anniversary, the focus was entirely on the school's foreign programs. The issue's cover, titled "The War against Suffering," featured a haunting graphic of a brown-skinned, dark-eyed child, emblematic of the developing-world suffering that the School of Hygiene and Public Health had done so much to alleviate. The articles extolled the school's truly path-breaking work in fighting parasitic diseases, planning the national health systems for countries across four continents, and conducting field epidemiology studies in Chad and Turkey. Not one word of the 44-page issue mentioned the school's considerable work in Baltimore over the past half-century or current efforts to address local health problems.[9]

At the same time that plans at Hopkins were coalescing for the Office of Health Care Programs, a group of elite scientists and physicians was discussing a national institute devoted to health and biomedical planning. Alexander Hollander, head of the Biology Division of the Oak Ridge National Laboratory, and Frederick Seitz, president of the National Academy of Sciences, met on December 13 and 14, 1967, with representatives of several major research universities, including Kerr White and Allyn Kimball of Johns Hopkins. Their deliberations resulted in the National Center for Health Services Research and Development, established in the PHS Health Services and Mental Health Administration in 1968. The center's budget provided funding to establish academic centers at several universities, including Johns Hopkins under the

Office of Health Care Programs, which received approval from the Board of Trustees on April 1, 1968.[10]

One of the early planning meetings to develop the national health services research center was held at the National Academy of Sciences in Washington, DC, on April 4, 1968, the day that civil rights icon Martin Luther King Jr. was assassinated in Memphis, Tennessee. Up to this point, Baltimore had not witnessed any major civil unrest. Two days passed peacefully, but early on the evening of Sunday, April 6, a crowd gathered in East Baltimore and began smashing windows and setting fires to businesses on Gay Street, about a mile from the JHSPH campus. Baltimore was one of more than 130 American cities and towns where crowds took to the streets in fear and frustration after King's assassination. The 1968 riots that originated in East Baltimore took 43 lives, caused 3,500 injuries, resulted in 25,000 arrests, and inflicted $12 million in property damage—second only to the destruction in Washington, DC, estimated at $15 million. The violence following King's assassination constituted the largest national occurrence of social unrest since the Civil War.[11]

When Assistant Dean Tim Baker got a phone call warning him that "they're going down the streets smashing windows of cars," he knew the riots had started. A frightened student called and asked him to come into East Baltimore and pick her up, but Baker refused. She lived in married student housing, and he told her, "You've got a perfectly good husband who can protect you, and it would be crazy to try and come in at this point. You'd be exposed to more danger. The compound will be safe." David Paige (MPH 1969), who was then a second-year resident at Johns Hopkins Hospital, had finished his on-call shift and was driving home with his wife. As they drove down Madison Street on Sunday afternoon, their car was stoned. "We were devastated that the riots were breaking out. It was just the unraveling of our world and society and everything we dreamt about. You know, we wanted to hang up a sign, 'We're with you.' "[12]

JHSPH students and faculty responded to the riots with intense emotion and commitment to healing the devastated city. In oral history interviews more than 40 years later, many described the riots as one of the most unforgettable events they had ever witnessed. In the fall of 1968, James Longcope (ScM 1969), a Navy medical officer who had treated soldiers in Vietnam, taught a course on the "Phenomenology of Violence" at the Freedom School established by Response, a group of white residents committed to social change in Baltimore. Future US Senator Barbara Mikulski, then a social worker in the Baltimore City Department of Social Services, also taught in the Freedom School. JHSPH faculty members Matthew Tayback and Cornelius Krusé appeared on an episode of the local Baltimore TV program *One City, Indivisible*, a cooperative effort between Johns Hopkins University and WJZ-TV. As its inaugural episode, the one-hour program featured "Rats, Rats? Rats!" as the first urban social problem to be documented and dealt with. The series was conceived as a way to encourage Baltimore residents across the city to unite to solve common problems and reverse the divisions that threatened the city's very survival.[13]

On March 31, 1968, Lyndon Johnson declined to accept the Democratic nomination for reelection. In November, Vice President Hubert Humphrey suffered a razor-thin loss to Richard M. Nixon, who ran on a law-and-order platform and rode a wave of anti-Democratic sentiment into the White House. Both Johnson's withdrawal and Humphrey's loss were blamed on Vietnam and the breakdown of civil order at home, most visibly during the riots in April and at the Democratic National Convention in Chicago that August. As a US senator and Johnson's right hand, Humphrey had been a great friend to JHSPH, and his defeat was a serious blow for the school. Humphrey and JHSPH both responded to the changing political winds by redoubling their efforts in support of domestic health programs. The school's existing strengths in three areas—planning and evaluating government medical care programs, reproductive and child health, and substance abuse prevention and treatment—corresponded to policy areas championed by Humphrey and other liberal Democrats and moderate Republicans.

Although the university had already begun planning the Center for Urban Affairs, Office of Health Care Programs, and Health Services Research and Development Center three years before the riots, the violence and destruction during 1968 added urgency to national and local efforts to mount a concerted response to the racial, economic, and public policy challenges facing urban communities. Of the domestic policy trinity of housing, education, and health care, the last seemed to offer the brightest possibilities for improvement, perhaps because health care had the strongest political lobby in Congress and the longest and most successful record of productive public–private partnerships. In addition, disease among the poor more directly threatened the well-being of the nonpoor than did ignorance or substandard housing.[14]

Russell Nelson's successor as director of Johns Hopkins Hospital, Robert M. Heyssel, was cognizant of the growing problems and risks faced by big-city hospitals. Less than two months after the riots, he called the hospital's ambulatory care clinics "a Social Action program more than a Medical Program. It is clear that what we do in East Baltimore should be related as far as is possible to what the people in East Baltimore would like to see us do, not what Hopkins believes is best." Addressing the Health Care Programs Working Committee, Heyssel cited Chicago, New York, and Nashville as examples of cities where medical schools had developed community ambulatory care plans, and he recommended meeting with East Baltimore community leaders and representatives of city, state, and federal agencies to discuss local needs, financing, and ways to ensure compatibility with other nonmedical approaches. Finally, he proposed "a detailed study of the present ambulatory care operation at Hopkins proper . . . specifically aimed at professional activities and quality of medical care," which could draw on the Johns Hopkins Comprehensive Child Care Center as a model. In December 1968, the Board of Trustees of the University and Hospital approved plans to develop outpatient health care programs and to reorganize the Johns Hopkins Hospital outpatient department, with the goals of improving service to the community and providing educational and research opportunities for JHMI. Heyssel was named director of the Office of Health Care Programs.[15]

In 1969, the Ford Foundation awarded a $500,000 development grant to enable the Center for Urban Affairs to expand the university's course offerings on urban issues, conduct research, evaluate existing programs, and act as a consultant to city government. Through the center, President Gordon wanted Johns Hopkins to "make significant contributions to the improvement of life in urban America." Given JHSPH's major involvement in urban health reform and the recent creation of a new department devoted to the application of social and behavioral science methods to evaluating and improving health services, it was natural that the center's director, Sol Levine, and research director, Margaret Bright, were both JHSPH faculty in the Department of Behavioral Sciences. Levine appeared on the *One City, Indivisible* television series to discuss the state's role in the problems of metropolitan Baltimore with Marvin Mandel, Maryland's newly elected governor, and Homer Favor, director of the Urban Study Center at Morgan State College.[16]

Eugene M. Feinblatt was appointed co-director of the center with an appointment in Public Health Administration. As Mayor Tommy D'Alesandro's assistant, Feinblatt had played a major role in minimizing violence and keeping shaken residents calm. From 1963 to 1969, he had chaired the Baltimore Department of Housing and Community Development and drafted legislation that created the Baltimore City Urban Renewal and Housing Commission, which he was later appointed to lead and oversee the redevelopment of the Inner Harbor and expansion of subsidized housing. Feinblatt and Levine met frequently with community residents and activists to hear their concerns and attempt to devise solutions.[17]

At the end of 1969, the Commonwealth Fund, Carnegie Foundation, and Rockefeller Foundation announced their commitment to providing $800,000 over three years to support the Office of Health Care Programs, which would "coordinate and lead an institution-wide commitment at Johns Hopkins to help improve the nation's systems and arrangements for providing medical services and care." The office was touted as "a new chapter in the University's leadership in medical education" that would fulfill the medical school's "promise that *health care will emerge at Johns Hopkins as a field of study comparable in importance and quality to the School's distinguished work in the biomedical and clinical sciences."* The philanthropies expected their investment in the Office of Health Care Programs to "have a profound influence on the advancement of all of medical education, and on the improvement of the organization and delivery of health care in communities across the country."[18]

To address the health care needs in the neighborhood immediately surrounding the medical campus, the Office of Health Care Program's two main initiatives were the East Baltimore Medical Plan, a prepaid comprehensive health care program, and the East Baltimore Health Center, run by Hopkins medical and public health faculty and students. At the same time, the office established another prepaid comprehensive health plan in the mostly white planned community of Columbia, Maryland. In early 1971, Nixon announced a plan modeled on the Columbia Health Plan, which provided members' families with unlimited medical treatment for $51 per month.[19]

President Gordon praised "the cooperative spirit [that has] developed among the School of Medicine, the School of Hygiene and Public Health, and the Hospital." He emphasized to the foundations that the university's leadership viewed the Office of Health Care Programs "not merely as a new kind of service opportunity with considerable merit as such, but also and mainly as an innovative educational, research, and operational program with strong potential for *application beyond Baltimore and Columbia.*"[20]

The East Baltimore prepaid group practice program, directed by Torrey C. Brown, involved the cooperation of 13 different government agencies, "all with different guidelines, administrative rules, etc.—a herculean task." The federal agencies were Medicare (Social Security Administration), Medicaid (which also involved the city of Baltimore and state of Maryland departments of health, as well as the corresponding departments of welfare), the Children's Bureau, Office of Economic Opportunity, PHS Bureau of Comprehensive Health Services, the National Center for Health Services Research and Development, and Housing and Urban Development's Model Cities program. Community representatives created the East Baltimore Community Corporation to provide guidance in designing and implementing the East Baltimore health plan. But Heyssel, echoing concerns once voiced by Huntington Williams about the advisability of publicly administered health services, noted that local physicians were "to the right of the AMA on the question of prepayment and group practice, and [they] have given us considerable difficulty and are continuing to do so."[21]

The difficulty of launching the East Baltimore plan was compounded by a major state-level reorganization of some of the plan's main sponsors. On July 1, 1969, the Maryland state departments of health and mental hygiene were combined into a single cabinet-level agency, and the state's Medicaid program was transferred from the state Health Department to an office under the direct control of state Secretary of Health Neil Solomon. Solomon and Tayback, who had been appointed assistant secretary, took on the challenge of shaping up Maryland's often-criticized and financially troubled Medicaid program. Maryland's top two health officials were both JHSPH faculty members, and they spearheaded comprehensive planning for state indigent care programs that aimed to upgrade the quality of care in Medicaid and services for the mentally disabled.[22]

In response to Jack Wennberg's 1966 report on nursing home abuses, Solomon also appointed Tayback to lead a major reform effort to improve conditions in nursing homes, which were still unlicensed, yet received substantial state as well as Medicaid funding (after stepping down as secretary of health, Solomon would have his medical license revoked in 1993 for unethical behavior in his medical practice). Tayback helped to create the Bureau of Licensure and Enforcement to identify deficiencies and enforce compliance via inspection visits by a sanitarian and nurse, and he also pushed to professionalize nursing home administration by establishing a professional board of examiners. By 1971, the state's nursing home regulations were among the most comprehensive in the nation, and Tayback reported that "substantial progress has been made in areas of sanitation, environmental health and life safety," and every licensed Maryland nursing home had been brought up to state fire codes. In 1974, he was named the first director of the Division on Aging, charged with developing Maryland's comprehensive, coordinated system of health, social, and community services for senior citizens. Throughout his career in city and state health agencies, Tayback remained a member of the Biostatistics faculty at JHSPH.[23]

In addition to overseeing the East Baltimore and Columbia health plans, the Office of Health Care Programs also administered the Health Services Research and Development Center. To spearhead data collection and analysis for the community health programs, Malcolm L. Peterson was appointed as the center's director in July 1969. Kerr White chaired the advisory board, with representatives from each of the medical institutions, and the majority of faculty affiliates were in the JHSPH departments that dealt with health services research. The center was involved in developing the overall program in East Baltimore and the record and information systems for the Columbia program. After Peterson stepped down to become dean of the new School of Health Services (discussed below), Sam Shapiro served as director of the Health Services Research and Development Center from 1973 to 1982.[24]

Shapiro had headed the Natality Analysis Branch of the PHS National Office of Vital Statistics and had come to Hopkins from the Health Insurance Plan of Greater New York, where he was director of research and statistics. At

HIP, Shapiro directed the first randomized controlled trial to determine the efficacy of breast cancer screening, initiated in December 1963 among female HIP enrollees aged 40 to 64. He also conducted influential epidemiological studies on the incidence of cardiovascular disease and myocardial infarction, including the influence of comorbidities, with funding from the National Heart and Lung Institute. "At that time," Shapiro recalled, NIH research "was primarily disease-oriented rather than service-oriented. Their approach would be epidemiologic whereas health services research approached the problem from a service standpoint."[25]

White was among the loudest voices in the 1960s and 1970s calling for fewer specialists and more general practitioners, with corresponding reforms in medical education to instill physicians with broad interdisciplinary knowledge and an ethos of nurturing trust and communication with patients. White recommended Jack Wennberg for a position as director of the state Regional Medical Program at the University of Vermont, where White had done his earlier work on the Physician's Activity Study, a database of discharge reports from most Vermont hospitals. Wennberg greatly expanded the volume and complexity of the database to track local and regional variations in cost and utilization of medical care. Some of his most striking findings were the direct correlations between the number of surgical specialists and rates of surgical procedures in a defined area, which indicated that the demand was supplier induced rather than proof of more widespread disease in a population. With JHSPH biostatistician Alan Gittelsohn, Wennberg developed small area analysis as a method to measure the utilization and distribution of health services per unit of population. Their 1973 article in *Science* established the existence of large geographical variations in health care usage.[26]

As innovators in population-level studies of medical care and outcomes research, White, Wennberg, and Gittelsohn would later influence the development of clinical practice guidelines in the 1980s. After joining the Dartmouth Medical School faculty in 1980, Wennberg also developed the Dartmouth Atlas of Health Care to accurately describe the use and distribution of medical resources in the United States and to analyze national, regional, and local health care markets, including individual hospitals and affiliated physicians. As an advocate for greater federal funding for outcomes research, Wennberg was involved in establishing the Agency for Health Care Policy and Research (AHCPR) in 1990. As he recalled in an interview, "Our goal was to introduce clinical research into the health services research agenda, which had been dominated pretty much by policy wonks and economists."

At Hopkins, however, health services research had been firmly grounded from the beginning in clinical practice in the Baltimore City Medical Care Program, the Johns Hopkins Hospital, and the East Baltimore and Columbia health plans. Just as Tayback's 1953 study based on Baltimore City Medical Care Program records had shown that Baltimore physicians frequently prescribed costly drugs with no established therapeutic value, Wennberg remarked a half-century later, "What is done with a new technology once it's in the market depends on the inventiveness of physicians, and they're terribly inventive. Untested theories and practices are huge, expensive, and dangerous problems." Tayback's work and Wennberg's comments anticipated the future development of JHSPH research specialties in both patient and drug safety.[27]

The School of Health Services and the Graduate Program in Nurse–Midwifery

In the 1960s, as head of the Division of Maternal and Child Health in the Department of Population and Family Health, Don Cornely had pursued his goal of meeting the intense need for improved pediatric and maternal health care in Baltimore by contributing his expertise to the Johns Hopkins Comprehensive Child Care Center. In the 1970s, he continued this commitment by overseeing the development of two important new JHSPH programs: graduate training in nurse–midwifery and a nutrition program for mothers and their young children.

When Harper retired in 1970, his department's divisions of Population Dynamics and of Maternal and Child Health were split into separate departments, despite his opposition. The decision to split Population and Family Health may have been influenced by the fact that Cornely, although he supported family planning research and policy initiatives, was the father of 13 children. Of 22 JHSPH doctoral dissertations on Baltimore completed between 1960 and 1980, eight were by students in Maternal and Child Health or Population Dynamics, most dealing with infant mortality or teen pregnancy. The two departments came to be nicknamed "Mom" and "Pop."[28]

The Johns Hopkins Hospital nurse–midwifery program had originated in the late 1940s and continued in the 1960s under Alan C. Barnes, chair of Gynecology and Obstetrics, and John Whitridge Jr., director of the Maryland Department of Health Bureau of Preventive Medicine. Although the original 1939 federal guidelines for Children's Bureau training grants had specified that nurse–midwives and social workers could receive specialized instruction along with physicians and health officers, in 1961, Arthur Lesser of the Children's Bureau told Whitridge that nurse–midwives were no longer needed in America. The Children's Bureau also criticized the program as a hospital certificate rather than a university degree and abruptly cut off funding in 1962.[29]

Lesser, however, had lost touch with the direction of American nursing in the 1960s. The development of formal degree programs for nurse practitioners,

including graduate nurse–midwifery programs, grew from the desire to legitimize public health nurses' existing practical responsibilities for making critical
patient care decisions and preventing disease and promoting health in families. As nursing historian Julie Fairman observes, "Public health nurses providing services in the community typically practiced beyond the traditional
boundaries of practice in hospitals or private practices. They were quite independent and less bound by institutional rules." Rural public health required
nurses to cover large geographic areas and provide a wide variety of generalized
services, and this held true to an even greater degree in developing countries.
Whitridge and Maryland health commissioner Edward Davens held appointments as lecturers in Maternal and Child Health, and they committed state
support to continue the training program for a few more years with the goal of
establishing a graduate nurse–midwifery degree.[30]

In 1968, Cornely initiated the transfer of the nurse–midwifery training program from the medical school Department of Gynecology and Obstetrics to
the JHSPH Division of Maternal and Child Health. The program was a good
fit for the division, where Cornely led initiatives to promote healthy pregnancies and optimum pediatric care. He and Ruth Freeman, head of the PHA
Division of Public Health Nursing, cooperated to expand the eight-month
nurse–midwifery program into an accredited two-year MPH specialty track,
which became a major source of growth and innovation for the Department of
Maternal and Child Health and for nursing more broadly in the School of
Hygiene. After Freeman retired in 1970, the nurse–midwifery program became the main focus of public health nursing at JHSPH. Through 1981, an
HEW training grant supported faculty salaries and 12 fellowships. Graduates
were eligible for certification by the American College of Nurse-Midwives, and
many went on to administer or teach in nurse–midwifery programs.[31]

Of the six nurse–midwifery master's programs in the United States, only
the one at Johns Hopkins was not based in a school of nursing and also offered
a combined public health/nurse–midwife program with the option to continue in doctoral studies (the first two nurse–midwives earned DrPHs in 1976).
Bernie Guyer, Cornely's successor noted that Helen Wallace at the University
of California–Berkeley "concentrated on training master's level people who
would go out and run state health departments, and [Cornely] concentrated on
training doctoral level people who had good research skills and who would be
academics. So almost all the academic leadership at that time was Hopkins-
trained." Examples include Patricia Burkhardt (DrPH 1981) at New York
University and ACNM president Judith Rooks (MPH 1974).[32]

Fulltime nurse–midwifery faculty included director Carroll Celentano
and Mary Shean, Jean Cassity, and Jean Huang. The program needed more
faculty but could not fill budgeted positions, so the department enlisted

nurse–midwives from the Baltimore City Health Department, local county health departments, and the Johns Hopkins and Baltimore City hospitals. Johns Hopkins Hospital was the primary hospital base, under the supervision of Ted King, Whitridge's successor as chair of Gynecology and Obstetrics. Other teaching facilities included Baltimore City hospitals, local city and county health departments, Planned Parenthood, and the JHU University Health Service at Homewood, as well as the Indian Health Service Hospital at Fort Defiance, Arizona, and the Navajo Reservation at Chinle.[33]

In October 1969, as the nurse–midwifery program was just getting under way, JHU President Lincoln Gordon appointed Freeman to a committee charged with planning and establishing "programs in the allied health fields [that would] be closely inter-linked with the revised M.D. curriculum, with masters and doctoral programs in the School of Hygiene and Public Health and postdoctoral programs in the School of Medicine, and with pertinent undergraduate, postgraduate and postdoctoral programs in the Faculty of Arts and Sciences." Russell H. Morgan, chair of Radiology in the medical school and Radiological Science at JHSPH, had chaired the Ad Hoc Committee for a School of Allied Health Sciences since 1966. The school was proposed to meet the critical shortage of broadly educated teachers, researchers, and administrators in allied health sciences, with two initial departments, Nursing (to replace the JHH diplomate nursing school) and Clinical Laboratory Sciences, whose faculty would have joint appointments in either Medicine or Hygiene.[34]

The ad hoc committee's report named the "relative lack of health manpower" as the most critical factor in barriers to health care access. Like the postwar public health reformers, the report's authors emphasized the team approach to health care as essential for providing comprehensive care and improving the delivery of services. The Association of Schools of Allied Health Professions was established in 1967, representing baccalaureate programs in medical technology, physical and occupational therapy, medical records, nursing, health care administration, dental hygiene, and medical illustration. That year, Surgeon General William H. Stewart charged the Education Subcommittee of the National Advisory Health Council with studying education for allied health professions and encouraged "creative thinking and experimentation" to address the lack of a coherent structure for education in the allied health professions. Congress passed the Allied Health Professions Personnel Training Act in 1966 and extended the act in 1968, when at least 30 allied health sciences schools or programs existed and the number was expected to double.[35]

Correspondence among the president, provost, and deans revealed numerous weaknesses and concerns about the proposed School of Allied Health Sciences. The proposal relied heavily on the existing faculty and departments for funding and teaching, yet created a new administrative unit under a separate dean, which threatened necessary cooperation from the East Baltimore schools. The Hygiene, Homewood, and medical school preclinical departments all objected to establishing Allied Health Sciences as a division of the medical school. Faculty in the new school were to be oriented toward teaching, which went against Hopkins' strong research tradition and threatened to place the school's faculty on unequal footing with the rest of the university. The university's finances were already under serious stress, and the political situation was extremely unstable, with Congress failing to appropriate money for many health programs that it had passed. The most divisive issue was the proposal to maintain separation between the chair of the nursing department, responsible for nursing education, and the JHH head of nursing services. JHH did not trust the current or proposed nurse training programs to provide adequate supervision of the hospital's nursing services. Finally, standard Hopkins tuition would be prohibitively expensive compared to most nursing schools or other allied health programs and would probably discourage otherwise-qualified applicants.[36]

Dean of Arts and Sciences Allyn Kimball and the Homewood faculty were strongly opposed to establishing either a new undergraduate program or a new division of the university in East Baltimore. Kimball did not believe that the program could attract Hopkins-quality students and faculty, and the program was much too expensive and would negatively affect the already overburdened existing divisions. Kimball pointed to the failed undergraduate business program as a basis for starting new programs within existing divisions, since independent schools were much harder to get rid of if they failed. John Hume shared Kimball's views and thought that any allied health science program should be a small, advanced, specialized graduate program under the medical school.[37]

Despite these objections, in September 1971, the university board of trustees approved the School of Health Services ("allied health sciences" was dropped from the original title). JHSPH assistant professors Kay B. Partridge and Anna Scholl served on the nursing subcommittee of the new school's advisory board. Under Malcolm L. Peterson as dean, the School of Health Services applied principles that had been pioneered at the School of Hygiene. It offered a common curriculum based in the biomedical and behavioral sciences to undergraduate students in nursing, health associates, and clinical laboratory sciences. Health professionals from a variety of disciplines and occupations—physicians, nurses, physician assistants, and laboratory technicians—would work together and learn to collaborate. The new school's objective was to "develop and demonstrate models for educating, training, and staffing health services." Peterson stated to the university board of trustees in

April 1972, "The School of Health Services will educate young men and women to deliver direct patient care in both office and institutional settings. They will fulfill many of the functions which usually have been carried out by nurses and primary care physicians." The school would also prepare managers and administrators of health care services with instruction in health services organization.[38]

Yet after the School of Health Services opened in fall 1973, Peterson publicly deemphasized the nursing curriculum and touted the new roles of health associate and health assistant. The hospital and JHSPH had founded a Nurse Practitioner program, which transferred to the School of Health Services, and faculty from the nurse practitioner program developed a curriculum for a bachelor's nursing education program. Partridge, now director of OB-GYN nursing at JHH, was appointed director of the Nursing Education program in September 1974. According to Susan Carroll Immelt, a graduate of the nursing education program, Partridge was "a strong public-health nurse presence. Public health and research were part of the school's identity [but] those who were expecting a more traditional nursing experience didn't really understand [the community focused curriculum]."[39]

From the beginning, the School of Health Services was plagued by low enrollment and deficiencies in the curriculum that interfered with accreditation by the National League of Nursing. The more traditional curriculum prepared to meet accreditation standards contrasted with the innovative, experimental program envisioned by the program's founders. But the school's worst problems were financial, especially in the context of budgetary demands from other competing socially minded programs within JHMI. By 1972, new operational budgets for the Columbia and East Baltimore health plans exceeded $5 million. For the Office of Health Care Programs, the Health Services Research and Development Center, and the School of Health Services, JHU estimated that it would need between $1 million and $2.5 million annually for five years "to assure success of the new endeavor and give it the needed stability and visibility to ensure the ultimate aims of these programs to bring about meaningful, lasting and needed change in Medical Education and Practice." In a letter to foundation officers following a visit to Hopkins on April 6, 1972, Heyssel and Peterson wrote,

> While the original goal of the Office of Health Care Programs and the Health Services Research and Development Center are only beginning to be fulfilled, we believe that we are well on the way to developing new and reshaping the older Hopkins Institutions as places for new education and much needed applied and basic research in Health Services Delivery in addition to the more traditional activities in Biomedical Research and specialty practice. We now

have the opportunity to couple those programs to a new school dedicated to the training of individuals who are capable of working with physicians and other health workers in new approaches to health services delivery.

As with each new venture rolled out by JHMI, they stressed that the new School of Health Services would "become a demonstration to others in Universities, Area Health Education Centers and non-academic service oriented settings of the validity of team concepts and task analysis for functional education in health delivery."[40]

When Shapiro took over as director of the Health Services Research and Development Center in 1973, its primary focus "was on the research that we were carrying out at Columbia" to determine the effectiveness of newly hired health associates, "who were especially trained [at the School of Health Services] to help the primary care physician and to provide services that didn't necessarily require a doctor." But as the Johns Hopkins Hospital budgets for the East Baltimore and Columbia health plans swelled from the costs of providing both traditional and new types of medical care, the university began to run serious deficits due to inflation and declining federal support for research. Former JHSPH department chair Russell H. Morgan, now dean of the medical school, wrote in May 1972, "We should be prepared no later than next fall to make an all-out effort to recover funds which now are not being collected." The medical school needed to find new funds to replace the annual $800,000 allocation from the state of Maryland, which would terminate that year. Morgan asked Heyssel to conduct a study of areas of the Johns Hopkins Hospital and clinics where there were problems in receiving payment, such as resident supervision of inpatients under Medicaid, Medicare, and third-party carriers, as well as clinical services provided by full-time faculty to Medicaid inpatients and outpatients. Despite the contemporary concerns about cost containment and the physician shortage in the early 1970s, Shapiro later recalled that under the pressure of budget cuts, "the whole issue [of utilizing physician associates] receded in importance." The Columbia health plan was a prepaid group practice HMO that accepted private health insurance purchased by both individual subscribers and employers, but it was never financially stable enough to subsidize the East Baltimore plan, which operated entirely with public funds. During the 1980s, both plans underwent a series of reorganizations before Johns Hopkins sold the Columbia plan and reorganized the East Baltimore plan under the umbrella of its new Johns Hopkins Health Plan. Heyssel applied the lessons learned from the 1970s and launched the Johns Hopkins Health System in 1986, serving as president until his retirement in 1992.[41]

The School of Health Services had received large grants from foundations but had no significant hard money from the university or federal government.

Nursing faculty recruitment in particular was hampered by the program's lack of autonomy or permanent funding. By June 1977, Peterson asked Partridge to resign, and the school as a whole generated a $700,000 deficit in fiscal year 1977. After the Johns Hopkins Board of Trustees voted to close the School of Health Services, the last class graduated in May 1979. The connection between JHSPH and public health nursing has endured, however. In 1983, Johns Hopkins established a School of Nursing in East Baltimore as a new university division and the fourth component of JHMI. JHSPH alumna Martha N. Hill (PhD 1986) served as dean of the School of Nursing from 2001 to 2014 and holds joint appointments in the JHSPH departments of Health Policy and Management as well as Health, Behavior and Society. Hill, internationally recognized for her research on racial disparities in cardiovascular disease, oversaw the creation of a joint MPH–MSN degree program between the two schools. At JHSPH, the Johns Hopkins Education and Research Center for Occupational Safety and Health features a training program in occupational and environmental health nursing, directed by Sheila T. Fitzgerald (PhD 1988).[42]

By contrast, JHSPH's nurse–midwifery program maintained an institutional base primarily within one division of JHMI rather than attempting an unpopular university-wide collaboration. By 1975–1976, 27 nurses were enrolled as JHSPH doctoral students, four under the PHS nurse–midwife grant and 17 with support from the federal Nurse Training Act. Another 40 nurses were earning an MPH, including 12 nurse–midwives and 10 in the Collaborative Leadership Training Program, a PHS-funded training program for public health nursing supervisors. The nurse–midwife program focused on the public health aspects of maternal and child health, integrating its goals with the funding and ideology of the Great Society. It proved to be the "small, advanced, specialized graduate program" that John Hume had wanted instead of the unwieldy School of Health Services.[43]

The Baltimore Origins of WIC

Together with the nurse–midwifery training program and the school's work in improving the quality and administration of personal health services in urban settings, David Paige's maternal and infant nutrition program was the JHSPH initiative that perhaps best fulfilled the Great Society ideals of equalizing access to services that met basic human needs. The stage for Paige's work had been set by two JHSPH International Health faculty, M. Alfred Haynes and George G. Graham. In 1968, Haynes coauthored *Hunger USA 1968*, a study of hunger in the United States by the Citizens' Board of Inquiry and Malnutrition in the United States. Haynes also testified before Congress on the commission's findings that the United States was home to "a sizable number of hungry poor," based on evidence of stunted physical growth and delayed mental development. American children who fell far below national height and weight standards seemed "to conform more to the pattern of developing countries." Haynes had worked as a PHS physician on the Cheyenne River Indian Reservation in South Dakota as well as in Zaire and India. He noted that the study team had found kwashiorkor, a protein deficiency typically associated with extreme poverty in Africa and Asia, on Indian reservations. Malnutrition increased rates of preschool mortality, and in the United States, the highest rates of postneonatal mortality corresponded with the highest rates of poverty.[44]

"Unfortunately," Haynes testified, "medical education is often obsessed with the acute, the rare, the esoteric. Medical students know far more about rare, inborn errors of metabolism which they may see once in a lifetime than they do about the problems of hunger and malnutrition in their immediate vicinity." The Hunger USA study showed that "there is indeed a problem and it is not confined to Mississippi." In 1968, Haynes became the first African American to be promoted to full professor at Johns Hopkins, but he left to become associate dean and chair of Community Medicine at the Charles R. Drew Postgraduate Medical School, developed in the aftermath of the 1965 Watts riots to remedy the lack of medical services for residents of Southeast Los Angeles County.[45]

As a Johns Hopkins pediatric resident, Paige volunteered to work at Baltimore City Hospital, where he encountered the chief of pediatrics, Harold Harrison, a renowned calcium expert and Hopkins medical faculty member, as well as Laurence Finberg, known for his work on electrolytes. Another pediatrics staff member who influenced Paige was George Graham, who in 1961 had founded the Institute for Nutritional Research in Lima, Peru, where he had discovered copper deficiency in children and demonstrated the mineral's role in human nutrition. Graham joined the JHSPH faculty in International Health in 1968 and founded the Division of Human Nutrition in 1976. In addition to collaborating with these three giants in clinical nutrition research and visiting Peru at Graham's invitation, Paige worked in the Johns Hopkins Hospital Harriet Lane pediatric emergency room in the late 1960s. There, he routinely saw iron-deficient infants with stunted growth—many were so weak that they required hospitalization. At the time, breastfeeding was rapidly declining in favor of evaporated milk formula, which poor families frequently would try to stretch by diluting with water. Some mothers gave infants cow's milk, which often caused gastrointestinal blood loss and malabsorption of nutrients.[46]

While earning an MPH at JHSPH, Paige had learned to prevent disease instead of waiting to treat it. As he encountered more sick babies with the same diagnosis, it triggered a clinical recognition of the futility in treating case after case. He reasoned, "I'm writing prescriptions for everything. Why don't we treat under-nutrition by prescribing appropriate foods?" Paige's instructor in population statistics was Matthew Tayback, who was heading a task force for Mayor D'Alesandro that was exploring ways to increase enrollment in the federal free school lunch program. Tayback asked Paige to be a working member, which gave him the opportunity to marry clinical nutrition issues with a public health perspective. The school lunch program helped to ensure that disadvantaged children received adequate nourishment and improved their educational experience, but malnutrition had already negatively affected cognition before age 5. Paige decided he wanted to direct his efforts at pregnancy and the early years of life.[47]

To pursue that goal, Tayback's school lunch committee led to creating a permanent Maryland Food Committee, later reorganized as the Maryland Food Bank. Along with the committee, Paige and his colleagues developed a prescriptive approach to early infant feeding and pregnancy. They started to provide iron-fortified formula to newborns at the newborn clinic in Cherry Hill, a poor, majority-black neighborhood on the south side of Baltimore. Paige remembered, "It was really a mom-and-pop operation, I was doing almost all the work. We started collecting data on heights, weights, and blood characteristics and noted a very high percentage of undergrown children, below the third percentile. Of course, a high percentage of low birth weights. The early data on the benefits of supplementing maternal and infant diets gave us courage to try to expand to a larger population."[48]

In 1971, with a grant from the federal Community Services Administration, an antipoverty agency, Paige's program grew into a statewide voucher program that enabled Maryland mothers to purchase formula and nutritious food. His research generated scientific proof that providing fortified formula to infants in low-income families reduced their risk of malnutrition-related health problems. Paige wanted to demonstrate that the problems he was seeing at Hopkins were not specific to Baltimore City, that malnutrition existed anywhere poverty existed. He and his partners at the Maryland Food Committee coined "IFIF" as the acronym for Iron-Fortified Infant Formula Program. As he remembered, "Our internal conversation was, '*If* we get the money, *if* we can convince the health officers,' so everything was if-if, and it seemed like an appropriate acronym."[49]

The program encountered considerable resistance from many of Maryland's rural counties, where health officers had been disappointed by previous federal programs that came and went. The food vouchers were unfamiliar and untested, and merchants might not accept them. The IFIF program had the greatest potential to benefit residents of the Eastern Shore, the state's poorest, most rural section, but resistance from health officers was also strongest there. During his pediatric residency, Paige had traveled throughout Maryland and down to the Eastern Shore, when others avoided working there. The health officers finally accepted the IFIF program when Paige agreed to continue to cover their pediatric clinics once a month. Paige recalled, "We were in every county, from Cecil County all the way down to Salisbury, and that was quite a trip for us to cover." The Community Services Administration began to see the public relations value of IFIF for proving the value of federal anti-poverty programs, and federal staffers began to promote the Maryland program on a national level as a model community-level intervention to improve nutrition and health status. According to Paige, "It suddenly became bidirectional: our appeal and our funding unleashed interest on the part of the feds, such as the Food and Nutrition Service in the USDA."[50]

Paige first urged Congress in 1971 to "consider mounting a successful program to combat undernutrition in children in the United States [that was] focused on children at the earliest possible moment, i.e. in infancy." Paige's program was among several from around the country chosen as models by the US Senate Select Committee on Nutrition and Human Needs, chaired by George McGovern of South Dakota. In a bipartisan alliance with McGovern and Republican Senator Robert Dole of Kansas, Hubert Humphrey led the push in the Senate to authorize the Women, Infants and Children (WIC) federal nutrition program on a two-year trial basis in 1972, and the program has been reauthorized every five years since 1974. Humphrey was an ideal champion, and WIC was an ideal program: it was essentially a domestic version of his P.L. 480 food aid program, except that it did not involve foreign currencies. WIC was the rare social welfare program that appealed to both big-government liberals and farm-state conservatives.[51]

WIC emerged as a cornerstone national program for which Paige and his JHSPH colleagues were important architects. He would testify before Congress 16 more times and told Congress in 2009,

> WIC has been very successful in lowering the incidence of low birthweight and pre-term birth, which in turn effectively reduces infant mortality and developmental disabilities. Studies by the Centers for Disease Control found that WIC preschoolers show improved weight gain and overall health, as well as a sharp reduction in anemia. At the same time, WIC has been extraordinarily cost effective. Even reducing one or two nights in the neonatal intensive care unit or an extra day of a woman's hospital stay will more than compensate for the cost of WIC benefits. I would argue that we should enroll all Medicaid recipients and all infants, women and children below 185 percent of the poverty level. This is cost effective, it is smart policy, and we will set the tone and provide the health infrastructure to help this population move out of poverty.[52]

After food stamps and the school lunch program, WIC is the third-largest federal nutritional assistance program. Designed to prevent the serious health

consequences of malnutrition, it provides nutritious foods, nutrition education, and referrals to health care and other social services. By 2002, participation in WIC had grown to include almost half of all infants and one-quarter of
children aged 1 to 4 nationwide.[53]

The Departments of Mental Hygiene and Behavioral Sciences

In addition to fueling the growth of health services research, nurse–midwifery,
and WIC, Great Society programs such as Medicare, Medicaid, and the Office
of Economic Opportunity provided federal grants that enabled JHSPH to attract a critical mass of sociologists, which fostered the formation of disciplinary
clusters within departments. Mental Hygiene was dominated by psychiatrists
and psychologists, and more physicians joined Chronic Diseases, which merged
with Epidemiology in 1970. Bright, Monk, and most of the sociologists changed
their primary appointment to Behavioral Sciences, whose faculty by 1978 included only one physician, David M. Levine. Levine, Pearl S. German, and
nearly all the early doctoral graduates in Behavioral Sciences joined the department's faculty, as did Social Relations graduates Laura Morlock and Carol
Weisman. The first doctoral graduate in Behavioral Sciences, Kay B. Partridge
(PhD 1971), joined the faculty of Public Health Administration in 1971 and
was assistant director of the Public Health Research Training Center in Hagerstown, Maryland. With her doctoral adviser Paul White, Partridge analyzed
the decision-making process among community members and health professionals at the East Baltimore Community Health Center, with special attention to the allocation of health resources.[54]

Yet despite the crystallization of disciplinary groups, JHSPH continued to
foster remarkably free collaborations among the basic, clinical, and social sciences. For example, in the Baltimore Study of Women's Health survey conducted by the Department of Epidemiology in 1973, the 27-page questionnaire
requested data with potential relevance to a range of disciplines from clinical
medicine to behavioral science to genetics (table 9.1).

NIH grants substantially expanded clinical and basic science activities
throughout JHSPH, even in departments not traditionally oriented toward
laboratory investigation such as Mental Hygiene. The department was an early
pace-setter in alcohol and drug abuse epidemiology, and its faculty served as
key consultants to develop the substance abuse research programs of NIMH
and two new NIH institutes: the National Institute on Alcoholism and Alcohol Abuse (NIAAA) and the National Institute on Drug Abuse (NIDA). During the 1970s, federal grants for substance abuse prevention and treatment
were the primary source of growth for the department.

Substance abuse research drew insights from social science, clinical medicine, and basic science. After the Department of Mental Hygiene recruited

TABLE 9.1
1973 Baltimore Study of Women's Health Survey Questions

Category	Question Description
Social/economic factors	Age, race, marital status, education level, religion, respondent's occupation, and family income
Medication use	Vitamins, antipsychotics, birth control pills and female hormone pills/injections, and medicines given to prevent miscarriage
Radiation exposure	Number and type of X-rays, medical treatment with or occupational exposure to radioactive materials
Sexual and reproductive history	Age at first menstrual period, irregular or uncomfortable periods and whether respondent saw doctor and/or took medication, number/length/outcome of all pregnancies, whether children were breastfed and how long, had respondent entered menopause, was there trouble and was it treated with pills, injections, or hysterectomy, "Have you ever had an operation on any of your female parts?", were ovaries removed, were you sterilized, age at first sexual relations, frequency of sex, use of contraceptives, number of times married, date and age at marriage, did husband have vasectomy, was it difficult to get pregnant
Breast health	"How would you classify yourself as to bosom size—small, medium, large, and cup size?", "Have you felt your breasts for lumps?", effects of periods on breast swelling, tenderness
Genetics	Questions about birth family and offspring: causes of death and history of heart disease, stroke, breast disease, or cancer

Mandell in 1968, he formalized the alcoholism counselors training program in 1971 as an MPH track. A few years later, with an NIAAA training grant, the program prepared epidemiologists and administrators for substance abuse treatment programs—the first of its kind in the country. By the 1980s, many directors of state programs were Hopkins graduates. Yet the NIH began to tighten requirements for training grants, and applicants had to prove that their program was filling a shortage in a high-priority professional field. The counselor training program was ultimately a casualty of the debate over whether the state directors should have an MPH and background in public health administration. As state public health agencies became more politicized and turnover increased, the demand for administrators with public health training waned. As Mandell admitted, "We lost that battle."[55]

Lemkau had tapped Mandell to lead new research initiatives that focused on preventing and treating drug and alcohol abuse, and these initiatives drew from a wellspring of federal mental health grant programs. Mandell, a clinical and social psychologist, had been on the front lines of New York City's heroin epidemic while working with disadvantaged urban youth at the Staten Island Mental Health Society's Wakoff Research Center. As a member of New York

Governor Nelson Rockefeller's commission on drug abuse, he had assisted in establishing therapeutic communities to fill the gap in the mental health system, which excluded drug addicts and alcoholics from treatment.[56]

Unlike alcohol or tobacco, narcotics were illegal and popular culture invariably demonized drug users. When the PHS Narcotic Hospital at Lexington, Kentucky, opened in 1935, Surgeon General Hugh Cumming had called narcotics addiction an endemic but treatable disease whose victims could be rehabilitated and returned to society. The majority of work in psychopharmacology had been done at the hospital's Addiction Research Center, led by Abraham Wikler, who published *The Relation of Psychiatry to Pharmacology* in 1957. Yet until the late 1960s, psychiatry was dominated by psychodynamics, and most psychiatrists considered addiction research a professional backwater. Public opinion and federal funding coalesced around finding a solution to America's drug problem, portrayed in a series of often sensationalistic exposés of the heroin epidemic that struck inner cities and returning Vietnam veterans.[57]

Mandell was among a new breed of policy-oriented mental health researchers who fixed their sights on drug abuse and brought a previously obscure field to the forefront of psychiatry. Others included Danny Freedman, chair of psychiatry at the University of Chicago and among the top experts on LSD and hallucinogens, and Jerome H. Jaffe, a leading advocate of methadone maintenance treatment for heroin addiction who became the first drug czar in 1971 under President Nixon. As Jaffe recalled, "We probably broke all the rules for psychiatry as we had been taught it—that you maintain your distance, you don't form personal relationships. The passivity of [psycho]analysis was not appropriate in the arena in which I found myself."[58]

The urban drug crisis gave addiction researchers new prominence and funding but also exposed them to policymakers' unrealistic expectations and the risk of very public failure. After NIMH founding director Robert Felix retired, another JHSPH alumnus, Stanley F. Yolles (MPH 1957), served as director from 1964 to 1970. Although Yolles had earned a master's in parasitology from the Harvard School of Public Health and fought insect-borne diseases in the Caribbean during the war, he decided to pursue psychiatry because he "could no longer be satisfied with a one-to-one relationship with a microscope." Like Felix and many other Mental Hygiene alumni, Yolles had worked with drug addicts at the PHS Hospital in Lexington, Kentucky, where he abolished the use of bars and handcuffs to restrain patients. The experience galvanized his commitment to finding more humane and effective methods for preventing and treating drug abuse.[59]

As NIMH director in the turbulent 1960s, Yolles denounced what he saw as "stupid, punitive laws" that criminalized drug use. He testified before Congress that strict penalties failed as a deterrent, since addiction was a medical and social problem. Yolles made headlines by calling for abolishing mandatory sentences and giving judges greater discretion to deal with drug users, especially first-time offenders. Regarding marijuana possession, he knew "of no clearer instance in which the punishment for an infraction of the law is more harmful than the crime." This view would later be famously advocated by President Jimmy Carter early in his term, until Peter Bourne, special assistant for health issues, forced Carter to backtrack after a scandal erupted over Bourne's own use of illegal drugs and connections with the National Organization for the Reform of Marijuana Laws. Although Yolles persuaded the Justice Department to reduce federal penalties for marijuana, he also angered the Nixon administration, which worsened conflicts over the budget and direction of NIMH. When the administration announced that Yolles had been dismissed, he penned a resignation letter the same day in which he accused Nixon of "abandonment of the mentally ill."[60]

In the 1970s, federal mental health policy was redirected toward alcohol and drug abuse treatment services and program evaluation. NIMH was reorganized in 1973 as a unit of the new Alcohol, Drug Abuse and Mental Health Administration (ADAMHA), which also included NIAAA and NIDA. These entities provided strong financial support for research on substance abuse and also lay the foundation for the major expansion of the treatment system. As Mandell recalled, when Nixon charged him and Richard A. Lindblad, associate director of NIDA, with creating a network of drug addiction treatment services, there was no precedent, so they based their proposals for drug abuse clinics on the alcoholism model. By 1973, the treatment programs had been up and running for several years, and Nixon selected Mandell to evaluate the NIMH grant program in drug abuse research. On September 11, 1973, the president announced to a White House conference on the heroin problem that "we have turned the corner on drug addiction in the United States." Yet Mandell could not find strong evidence that NIMH grant-supported programs were achieving better results than those without federal support. Nixon was furious and sent Mandell packing back to Baltimore. When Dean Hume heard what had happened, he said philosophically, "Presidents come and go but the university remains." Still shaken from his encounter with Nixon, Mandell was so relieved to hear Hume's encouraging response that "I could have kissed him."[61]

Alcoholism proved somewhat less politically hazardous than drug abuse. To house a residential alcoholism treatment facility, Mandell and Schneidmuhl converted Baltimore's Old Bohemian brewery, where workers had previously lived onsite. Instead of simply releasing patients with no follow-up, as existing hospital programs did, the residential program used the period immediately after detoxification to educate recovering alcoholics and connect them with outpatient resources. This evolved to become the Johns Hopkins Hospital comprehensive alcoholism treatment program, which Mandell launched with a grant from NIAAA.[62]

In 1972, Mandell also established the JHU occupational alcoholism treatment program, which offered outpatient counseling and medical services as well as inpatient detoxification to 130,000 employees of 12 Baltimore companies. The program received funding from the US Department of Labor to prevent job loss among problem drinkers as well as to counter the negative effects of workplace alcoholism on productivity, and it became a model for other employee treatment programs. But when Department of Labor policy precluded Mandell from maintaining control of the data generated by the program, Dean Hume made him return the $300,000 grant. Perhaps Mandell's most far-reaching research on the epidemiology of substance abuse was an NIAAA study begun in 1979 of relationships among alcohol control policies, characteristics of counties, and sex- and race-specific liver cirrhosis mortality in over 3,000 US counties and 100 cities.[63]

Mandell's alcohol research also included a robust NIH-funded laboratory program, based on the premise that "since the proper control over genetic, environmental and nutritional variables is difficult in a population of alcoholic patients, investigations using animal models are desirable." When David E. Davis left Pathobiology in 1960, his Division of Vertebrate Ecology (described in chapter 10) was transferred to Mental Hygiene and renamed the Laboratory of Comparative Behavior. Mental Hygiene maintained its earlier ties to the Pathobiology studies of population ecology, and the laboratory trained students to observe and analyze the social behavior of animals in the field to understand how different species maintained their survival through mechanisms such as mating and aggression and how these behaviors were governed by hormones, heredity, learned experience, and environment. In the Department of Biochemistry, Bacon Chow's research team studied pregnant rats to analyze the effects of low-protein diets on the physical and behavioral development of offspring. The researchers also tested methods of reversing these adverse effects following birth and found that feeding the offspring crude pituitary extract could prevent both physical and behavioral abnormalities from developing.[64]

With this promising foundation, Mental Hygiene began offering a PhD in comparative animal behavior in 1965, directed by Edwin Gould, whose research on bats and shrews involved observation of mother–infant interactions (otegeny) and communication during echolocation. Gould also studied homing behavior in turtles by fitting them with tiny radio sets to track them as they crawled down the halls of the School of Hygiene. During the 1970s, Gould's research was well funded by the National Science Foundation and the National Institute of Child Health and Human Development. Mandell also used animal models to study infant development and behavior by observing the effects of maternal alcohol use on rats and their young. With their similar research interests, Mandell and Gould taught a course on comparative mammalian behavior and infant development.[65]

By the early 1970s, researchers from several countries had identified maternal alcoholism as a factor in birth defects and premature birth, and they had also observed withdrawal symptoms in infants born to alcoholic mothers. But studies of human alcoholic mothers were complicated by additional variables such as race and socioeconomic status, as well as levels of nutrition, prenatal care, stress, and anxiety, which made it difficult for researchers "to divide the factors and isolate the problems caused by the ethanol component, particularly in prospective studies." In his NIAAA grant project, Mandell used rats to study the effects of gestational ethanol use on prenatal development and the offspring's subsequent behaviors. Experimental and control groups of mothers were compared for performance on development and behavioral tests. To test their offspring's proclivity to consume alcohol and to build a metabolic tolerance for it, the young rats were equipped to self-administer ethanol intragastrically by pressing a lever. The results showed that some rat lines preferred consuming alcohol and others did not, indicating a genetic susceptibility to alcoholism. To isolate the effects of ethanol from those of nutritional stress, Mandell replaced the calories from ethanol intake with an equivalent amount of carbohydrate and also fed the control and experimental animals in pairs.[66]

In fall 1970, the Center for Urban Affairs became the Center for Metropolitan Planning and Research, superseding the center's initial focus on inner-city Baltimore. After the director, Sol Levine, left Hopkins for Boston University in 1972, JHSPH's involvement with the center ended. Gordon's successor as JHU president, Steven Muller, moved the center to the Homewood campus and shifted its scope even farther afield to emphasize international issues. Although the fate of the Center for Urban Affairs may have reflected the rapid cooling of social justice activism in establishment circles under the Nixon administration, university officials also likely did not see a continued need for two different urban institutes and chose to devote their resources and attention to the Office of Health Care Programs, with its narrower commitment to health care, rather than the more diffuse Center for Urban Affairs.[67]

Levine's departure was a major setback for Behavioral Sciences, since he took several other faculty with him. This left two factions struggling for control, with faculty morale low and the department's future uncertain. Faculty member Arthur H. Richardson urged Dean Hume to consider a merger of the departments of Behavioral Sciences and Mental Hygiene, which would follow the pattern of other schools of public health. Kerr White emphasized to the search committee that basic sciences and social sciences should be prerequisites for admission to schools of public health rather than part of the core curriculum, an attitude that was upheld in the Milbank Memorial Fund's 1976 report, *Higher Education for Public Health.*[68]

In 1973, the search committee awarded the chairmanship to Paul White, whose research interests included health care organization, drug abuse treatment evaluation, and decision-making processes in regional medical care programs. "In the '60s," he remembered, "there was a lot of hope, and they thought things could get done. And then I had participated in some of that, trying to realize that hope." He taught courses on organizational functioning and planned change, highly relevant topics for the tumultuous 1970s. White used examples to make his students "properly cynical rather than hopeful. I mean a helpful cynicism. I would tell them instead of a cautious optimism, we will study some confident despair. And try to focus on why organizations fail, rather than why they work. Because looking at the failures, you can learn more."[69]

The highly interdisciplinary nature of Behavioral Sciences prepared students well to go out and solve real-world public health problems, but the low number of dedicated full-time teaching faculty weakened the department's cohesion and funding. White, for example, held joint appointments in International Health, Mental Hygiene, and Social Relations. He remembered, "The collaborative model had everything against it. We couldn't become a programmatic department. With that organization, with no one paying attention, we got almost no funding. Often we had major money, but we [weren't] the titular P.I." Behavioral Sciences excelled in teaching and offered two popular MPH courses, Social Behavior in Public Health as well as Health Professions and Health Organizations.[70]

When Paul Lemkau announced that he would retire in mid-1974, Dean Hume appointed a search committee to find a new chair of Mental Hygiene. Abe Lilienfeld, a key collaborator in the department's early studies of prematurity and developmental disabilities, had just retired as chair of Epidemiology and was appointed interim chair of Mental Hygiene. The search committee surveyed the current state of the fields of mental health and psychiatry, which were "in confusion and disarray" because "the amateur counsellors and encounter groups are taking over." According to the committee, half of all medical school psychiatry departments were led by acting chairmen. Moreover, only four schools of public health housed departments of mental hygiene or the equivalent (and all but the department at Johns Hopkins would fold by the decade's end). The committee concluded, "The need for new initiatives in the field of Mental Health is apparent."[71]

Hoping for bold young leadership, preferably embodied in a woman or an ethnic minority, the search committee would meet 52 times over a period of a year and a half. As had been the case during the Behavioral Science chair search the year before, the Mental Hygiene search committee faced fiscal pressures from the university for some form of merger involving Mental Hygiene, Behavioral Sciences, and Psychiatry, but all three remained independent departments. The selection process was slowed by both a paucity of applicants and new federal affirmative action hiring guidelines. The committee approached New York psychiatrist June Jackson Christmas, the founder and director of the Harlem Rehabilitation Center who had served as New York City's Commissioner of Mental Health, Mental Retardation, and Alcoholism Services and who would become the first black woman president of the APHA in 1980. After Christmas declined to apply, search committee chair Phil Bonnet reported, "Returns from ads were disappointing—no women—no blacks—no other minorities." Only seven applications were received, all from men, "none with special qualifications."[72]

JHSPH alumnus Alan Miller was also invited to apply for the position but declined to become dean of students at Albany Medical College. Miller suggested his longtime New York colleague Ernest M. Gruenberg, who had headed the state's Mental Health Research Center and was now chair of psychiatry at Columbia University, and Gruenberg accepted the chairmanship in May 1975. In addition to his considerable administrative experience in mental health agencies, Gruenberg had published extensively on mental health epidemiology and the distribution of mental disorders in populations, specializing in evaluating the effectiveness of integrated services to treat schizophrenia.[73]

Gruenberg and Mandell's success in attracting federal grants from a range of agencies enabled Mental Hygiene research activities and fellowship support to grow. In 1970–1971, the Department of Behavioral Sciences had been significantly larger than the Department of Mental Hygiene as measured by budget, faculty, and student enrollment, and both departments received roughly three-quarters of their funding from federal grants. But by the end of the decade, federal grants enabled Mental Hygiene's budget to more than triple, while Behavioral Sciences' budget shrank and became dependent on general funds for nearly two-thirds of its support. In 1987, Behavioral Sciences was merged to become a division of the Department of Health Policy and Management.[74]

Conclusion

The Johns Hopkins Medical Institutions' relationship with East Baltimore has spanned nearly 130 years since Johns Hopkins Hospital opened in 1889. This relationship has enabled the university to attract high levels of public and private funding that has been essential for JHMI's operations and growth. In turn, both federal guidelines and neighborhood activism—as well as advocacy from within by faculty, staff, and students—have held Johns Hopkins accountable to fulfill its commitment to serving the community and increasing race and gender diversity in hiring and admissions.

JHMI was less successful in remaining dedicated to providing affordable primary health care to the community in the face of major financial and administrative obstacles, as well as ongoing distrust from East Baltimore leaders and residents. JHMI also struggled to integrate the goal of community outreach with its core mission of training elite medical and public health researchers. As had been the case with JHSPH and the EHD in the early 1950s, the East Baltimore clinical care programs could not fully meet the university's need for workable clinical and field training sites for students in its flagship medical and public health degree programs (the MD and MPH). As early as 1966, the university's long-range plan protested that "the population of East Baltimore is less and less representative of the national needs for medical care, and the medical institutions must look elsewhere for the populations to be used for innovation in methodology and for realistic education of students." Finding sites with sufficient patient diversity in health conditions and socioeconomic status was, according to the medical school's dean, Thomas Turner, "the greatest single problem faced by the clinical departments in the Medical School." Put another way, the health problems of affluence—heart disease, cancer, and stroke—and the challenges of rare but scientifically interesting conditions were given priority over the health problems of poverty. From the beginning, the Columbia plan represented competition for the East Baltimore programs, which struggled to maintain their public financing under a patchwork of grant programs. At the same time, the university's finances were suffering under inflation and Nixon's austerity budget.[75]

The role of Johns Hopkins in Baltimore drives home the truth of policy historian Guian A. McKee's observation that "in the United States, healthcare policy has operated as a critical but largely unrecognized form of urban policy." Since World War II, both the university and the School of Hygiene and Public Health have had an uncanny ability to leverage federal funding for national defense, medical research, health services, higher education, and even urban renewal, which transformed Johns Hopkins into a federally funded private university and the largest employer in Baltimore. The schools of Medicine and Hygiene became the top-ranking federal research grant recipients among their peer institutions. By contrast, Baltimore during the mid-twentieth-century seemed to be perennially on the losing end of government programs that promised but failed to deliver improvements in housing, transportation, education, civil rights, and economic development.[76]

JHSPH was both part of JHMI and distinct from the medical school and hospital. The local context of education and research activities has always profoundly shaped the development of universities, but this was particularly true for schools of public health, which were by definition obligated to public service in ways that medical schools and even hospitals were not. The School of Hygiene played a critical liaison role between the university and the city government as well as civic and professional groups involved in health, such as Planned Parenthood and private physicians. These connections were fundamental to establishing and building successful research, education, and patient service programs that were rooted in the school's forte in social and behavioral sciences, such as those in sexually transmitted diseases, family planning, maternal and child health, and substance abuse.

Local geography was just as important as national politics in shaping the development of JHSPH, particularly during times of social upheaval. The school's setting in East Baltimore, which had played a starring role in the US State Department's globally promoted 1947 documentary, over the next two decades became a recruiting liability. This was true not because of the riots per se but because their root causes—the surrounding neighborhood's poverty and the university and hospital's lingering discriminatory treatment of local blacks—remained so plainly visible. Ann Skinner, who began working in the Health Services Research and Development Center in 1972, remembered that buildings constructed immediately after the riots, such as the post office and one of the University of Maryland School of Medicine buildings, "essentially had no windows. And you can't get into it except up this one really narrow single-person-width stairway. It was terrifying—because I used to go over there for meetings a lot. . . . It just looks like it's been built to withstand any attempt to invade." Local politics and geography likewise shaped the school's work overseas. Based on the strongly stated foreign policy priorities of the Kennedy and Johnson administrations, as well as the personal backgrounds and research interests of JHSPH faculty, the school had decided to base all three of its primary international health research projects in South Asia. This geographical logic had seemed undeniable in 1960 but became a serious disadvantage in the 1970s, when the governments of India and Pakistan erupted in civil unrest and Bangladesh declared its independence from Pakistan. Although JHSPH would continue to expand and develop new partners over the decades, the school remained committed to improving the health of populations in both East Baltimore and South Asia, which are still pillars of its work in the twenty-first century.[77]

CHAPTER TEN

The Environmental Revolution in Public Health

In 1970, the radio waves hummed with environmental health messages. Joni Mitchell asked farmers to put away their DDT and the Kinks complained that the air pollution was a-foggin' up their eyes. The next year, Marvin Gaye released "Mercy, Mercy Me (The Ecology)," which worried about the blue skies disappearing, mercury-filled fish, and radiation above and below ground. One higher education journalist noted that "pollution, ecology and the preservation of resources seem to be glamour offerings of the current academic year." Universities rushed to found environmental studies courses, conferences, and interdisciplinary programs. But the main impetus for environmental science programs came from schools of agriculture, forestry, and engineering, with some schools and departments appending "environmental science" to their names.[1]

Most schools of public health did not leap at the chance for federal sponsorship of environmental health research: of six NIH Environmental Health Institutes established by 1974, only one was based at a school of public health. The traditionally apolitical stance of schools of public health was also a factor in their reluctance to engage in debates over environmental issues that were often highly charged and that challenged universities, in the words of one school of public health representative, to "make some fundamental choices between academic study and social activism." Environmental health in the

1960s and 1970s represented both a renewal of traditional public health activities in sanitation and medical ecology, as well as a new source of federal funding for schools of public health. At JHSPH, the departments of Sanitary Engineering (renamed Environmental Health in 1961) and Parasitology (renamed Pathobiology in 1955) had both been among the school's founding departments, leading the charge against parasitic and water-borne diseases. The newer departments of Environmental Medicine (founded in 1950) and Radiological Science (established as a division of Environmental Medicine in 1958) evolved beyond their original Cold War mandates to embrace a broader and more powerful exploration of the molecular mechanisms underlying the relationships among environment, agent, and host. Yet the events that culminated in the creation of a new Department of Environmental Health Sciences (EHS) in 1976 demonstrated the conflicts among faculty over what constituted "true" public health research—and what kinds of faculty interests deserved to be recognized with promotion and tenure as well as dedicated space in an overcrowded building.[2]

The X-Ray Vision of Russell Morgan

The mushroom clouds that ended World War II and the devastation they wrought were etched in the minds of a whole generation who grew up fearing the possibility of nuclear war. The US Atomic Bomb Casualty Commission initiated extensive health studies on survivors of Hiroshima and Nagasaki in cooperation with the Japanese National Institute of Hygienic Health Sciences. Such research on the long-term health and developmental effects of a single high-level radiation exposure also raised new questions about the risks of compounded exposures over time to common sources of low-level radiation, such as X-rays in hospitals or even in shoe stores to measure customers' shoe size. With the advent of cheap, lightweight, mass-produced Geiger counters in the late 1940s, sales skyrocketed as advertisements urged consumers to protect themselves against the hidden danger of radiation or, alternatively, strike it rich by finding a uranium deposit. The transfiguring power of gamma rays became a stock of popular culture, such as the Stan Lee comic heroes Spider-Man, Hulk, and the Fantastic Four.[3]

At JHSPH, the 1956–1957 De Lamar Lectures were devoted entirely to talks by seven members of the Health Division of the Los Alamos Scientific Laboratory. Interest in radiation health courses was also growing among MPH students, particularly military officers. To develop the field of radiobiology, Stebbins solicited the advice of several prominent scientists, including microbiologist Victor P. Bond of the Brookhaven National Laboratory. Bond wrote to Stebbins, "Our greatest hope of getting the necessary answers to the problems of low-dose effects in man lies in the application of Public Health epidemiological approaches, which have not been utilized adequately as yet in this respect."[4]

In 1958, without the medical school's prior approval, Stebbins boldly requested startup funding from the Rockefeller Foundation, which had awarded grants to the schools of public health at the University of Pittsburgh and Harvard to establish programs in environmental and occupational radiation exposure. He further crossed Thomas Turner and the medical school administration by luring away Russell H. Morgan, who had chaired the Department of Radiology since 1946. Morgan had a strong public health background, since he had come to Hopkins from the PHS Division of Tuberculosis and, more recently, had chaired the Surgeon General's National Advisory Committee on Radiation, which issued its first report in 1959. The report had urged the PHS "to assume a major role both in the formulation of national policy and the initiation of comprehensive programs in the control of ionizing radiation in the United States." Radiation's "great and substantial benefits to mankind" for diagnosis and therapy had to be carefully balanced against preventing the many health risks associated with human exposure to radiation from environmental and medical sources.[5]

In 1962, as the PHS prepared to launch a major extramural research program in radiation control, Morgan accepted the full-time chairmanship of the JHSPH Department of Radiological Sciences, purposed with "determining the effect of all forms of radiation on biological processes, thus enabling scientists to establish and promote adequate health standards." Morgan drew upon the existing joint Department of Biophysics for expertise in the chemistry and physics of radiation, as well as assembled representatives from the fields of molecular biology, biochemistry, genetics, pathology, radiology, and nuclear medicine, allowing the faculty to become effective contributors to solving "the research problems of their biomedical colleagues in other parts of the University." No other academic radiological research programs were based in schools of public health, and none approached the disciplinary breadth of the one at JHSPH, composed of three divisions: Radiobiology, Radiochemistry, and Morgan's own Division of Radiophysics. After the mass exodus to the medical school in 1957, Morgan took on Turner's mantle in the School of Hygiene by redeveloping the basic sciences and establishing stronger links with the science departments in Medicine and at Homewood.[6]

Morgan chose to base his department in JHSPH because Stebbins promised him modern, ample research space and administrative support for the master's and PhD programs in nuclear medicine, neither of which the medical school could provide. Between 1961 and 1986, 180 MDs and 47 non-MDs graduated from Radiological Science, as well as over 200 postdoctoral students. Many Radiological Science PhDs joined the faculty, and several alumni applied radioisotope tracer techniques to develop new tests for infectious disease and nutritional deficiencies. Yasuhiro Sasaki, the third of 35 Japanese researchers to study nuclear medicine at JHSPH, used carbon-14 lactose from patients' breath samples to detect the absorption of lactose and screen for lactose intolerance. Sasaki later directed the Japanese Department of Radiological Sciences. Morgan noted that his department's organization and research were "based on the belief that a productive working relationship between the clinician and the basic scientist is possible," and he established a university-wide PhD program in cancer research with the medical school and Homewood science departments. Another Japanese student who studied the health effects of radiation was pediatrician Kanji Iio (MPH 1964), who helped to conduct the landmark Child Health Survey from 1957 to 1961 at the Nagasaki Laboratory of the Atomic Bomb Casualty Commission. The US government awarded Iio an NIH fellowship to earn an MPH at Johns Hopkins, and he returned to join the faculty of the Department of Child Health at Osaka City University and later at Kyoto University.[7]

Radiological Science received nearly $1 million in startup funds from the PHS Division of Radiological Health, the NIH, and the Avalon Foundation. A $1.5 million private gift established Radiological Science as the second endowed department in the school's history (the first had been Raymond Pearl's short-lived Department of Biology). The department's grants underwrote construction of modern new research facilities that were crucial for attracting ongoing external funding, since granting agencies required proof that existing facilities and equipment were adequate to support proposed projects. The department grew so quickly that it was assigned its own wing in the new addition to the Hygiene Building, which provided a total of 30,000 square feet on five floors, nearly the size of the entire original building.[8]

The Radiological Science Wing was quickly filled with expensive new space-age equipment funded by NIH grants. One of the most important legacies of Radiological Science would be to promote the adoption of modern computing throughout the School of Hygiene, whose catalogs featured the mainframe computer as an icon of 1960s Big Science. During the planning for the new Basic Sciences Building in the late 1950s, Kenneth Zierler in Environmental Medicine had urged the medical school to include a biostatistics computer center that would enable researchers to analyze "complex data obtained from biological experiments." Zierler specified that "the center should include both an analog and a digital computer" and estimated their combined cost at $40,000 (about $320,000 in 2015). At the same time, NIH director James Shannon began urging the agency's researchers to adopt computing for biomedical research and purchased an IBM 650, housed in the basement of Building 12 on the Bethesda, Maryland, campus. The computer weighed three tons and required a 200-square-foot air-conditioned room with reinforced floors and high-voltage outlets. But NIH researchers were suspicious of the new machine and viewed their work as experimental and qualitative, and therefore ill-matched to an oversized calculator. Admittedly, the complexity of biomedical research did not produce quantitative data or simple equations that computers could manipulate. The 650 was a first-generation computer that could only process specially prepared data after a series of complex steps, using routines written in the opaque computing language FORTRAN. Therefore, unlike their colleagues in areas such as physics, who readily adapted to using computers in the 1950s, most biologists and physicians considered computers useless circa 1960.[9]

Morgan made JHSPH an early adopter of biomedical computing and also secured NIH funding during the 1960s to develop prototype computing systems for clinical use at Johns Hopkins Hospital. He selected the IBM 1401, far superior to the NIH's IBM 650 but smaller and cheaper than the massive IBM 7090 scientific mainframe and the even larger STRETCH supercomputer, introduced in 1961. The 1401 was designed for accounting tasks and monthly reports, and IBM marketed it to business managers to replace the then-standard large, unwieldy, single-purpose electromechanical machines that programmed operations via levers, knobs, and plugboards. It was a stored program computer that allowed programmers to write and share applications loaded from punched cards or magnetic tape, eliminating the need to physically reconfigure the machine for each task. Morgan began renting the IBM 1401 in 1962 for the colossal rate of $50,000 per year. The department recovered most of this cost by charging other grant-funded projects in the school for computer time at the NIH-approved rate of $70 per hour.[10]

The largest computerized project at JHSPH was Morgan's comprehensive analysis of dosimetric data from diagnostic X-rays. The project's special X-ray exposure facilities and the computer and electronics laboratory occupied about half of the first floor and employed three full-time personnel: an electronic engineer and computer programmer, a computer operator, and an electronic technician, as well as a half-time machinist. The project consumed an estimated $5,000 annually in computer supplies, including punch cards, computer paper, vacuum tubes, transistors, diodes, capacitors, and resistors. For 600 computer hours, Morgan requested $42,000 from the NIH—nearly twice the total cost of personnel. In his budget justification, Morgan told the PHS grant reviewers that this was still reportedly 60 percent below the market rate and so "computer charges for this project therefore are relatively low."[11]

His research on the minimum necessary dose of radiation for accurate diagnostic X-rays cemented his reputation as one of the foremost authorities on radiation exposure in medical environments for patients and health professionals.[12] Over a seven-year period, Morgan's team took over 10 million dosimetric measurements on 1,500 individuals "of widely ranging [physical] characteristics" to conduct a quantitative evaluation of how these factors influenced the radiation doses received by human tissues during diagnostic X-ray exams. Exposure was varied through the ranges of field size, field position, half-value layer (the measure of thickness of a material at which the incident energy is weakened by 50 percent), and beam projection angle. Morgan described the procedure for the 20 full-body scans on each study participant: "An x-ray beam, 2 cm in cross-section, systematically scanned each individual from side to side and from head to toe in a manner similar to that in which the electron beam of a television viewing tube scans the tube's face plate. During the scanning process, the instantaneous doses received at seven preselected regions of the body were measured in digital form by a series of highly sensitive, tissue-equivalent dosimeters and the resultant data recorded on magnetic tape."[13]

The result was over 5,000 tables to predict the radiation doses received by various population groups from diagnostic X-rays, based on "height, weight, age, race and sex." Dosage values were calculated according to the type of examination, such as chest or lumbar spine, as well as the exposure to "the male and female reproductive organs, the hematopoietic system, the thyroid gland and the lens of the eye." Computer data analysis revealed patterns that would prove crucial in minimizing patients' exposure to radiation during diagnostic procedures. Morgan's tables provided the first reliable estimates of the extent of radiation exposure from medical X-rays, based on the numbers of persons exposed in the population and on the types of examination they received. The study also produced graphic data that enabled radiologists to use patients' height and weight measurements to predict the landmark position and body width and thickness to ensure optimum image quality and correct exposure level.[14]

In the 1950s, Roger Herriott, chair of Biochemistry, had conducted the first JHSPH research on DNA, which dealt with photoreactivation repair of DNA damaged with ultraviolet light, mutagenesis, and genetic transformation of cells by exogenous DNA. Biochemistry faculty and students worked closely with members of the Radiological Science divisions of Radiobiology and Radiochemistry to further expand molecular-level research on genetics and the mechanisms of cell mutation, damage, and repair occurring in healthy, diseased, and injured organisms. Another important collaborator was Allyn W. Kimball, chair of Biostatistics from 1960 to 1966, who had spent a decade as chief of biological statistics at the Oak Ridge National Laboratory and published widely on statistics in radiation biology and genetics.

The Division of Radiobiology, directed by Roland F. Beers, studied the adverse effects of radiation on the enzymatic synthesis of nucleic acids, which caused mutations through either structural damage to genetic material, interference with gene replication, or both. His lab observed the relative radiation sensitivity of normal and cancerous tissues, findings that were essential for developing effective radiation therapy for cancer. To create cells that were resistant to antibiotics, viruses, or radiation, Beers also studied the differential sensitivity of human and mammalian chromosomes to conditions such as anoxia, which could act as a protective environment against radiation. These experiments yielded valuable knowledge about the genetic control of resistance and its acquisition through cell transformation.[15]

Although much of the Radiobiology division's work involved basic research on fundamental biomolecular processes, its studies of radiation damage provided insights into many other causes of disease and injury. To better understand the role of hydrolytic enzymes in injury, inflammation, and repair, Arthur Dannenberg compared lesions caused by an infectious agent, tuberculosis, with those from a noninfectious agent, radiation. Dannenburg's team also tested whether stimulating or inhibiting specific enzymes could alter the course of disease by administering hormones and antibiotics to tuberculous or irradiated animals. Shih Yi Wang exposed nucleic acids to ultraviolet radiation to determine its effects on molecular structure and resulting changes in cellular functions, which he developed into patented methods for inactivating viruses and bacteria and reversing cellular damage. Wang became one of the foremost experts on the photochemistry and photobiology of nucleic acids, a field that has produced revolutionary insights into the effects of ultraviolet rays on not only carcinogenesis but also cell death, growth delays, and mutations. Wang and the department's research associates from China, Thailand, Czechoslovakia, Japan, India, and Australia were among the many highly trained foreign researchers who began studying and working in US universities during the rapid advance of biochemistry and molecular biology in the 1960s and 1970s.[16]

The Radiobiology division's square footage increased from 2,000 in the old building to 8,500 on two floors in the new wing. This extremely high-tech specialty employed techniques such as photochemical analysis and proton magnetic resonance, which required the purchase of a Geiger counter, electrophoretic equipment, a rotary dispersion polarimeter ($21,000), an analytical ultra-centrifuge ($26,500), time-lapse cinematography apparatus ($13,000), and an electron microscope ($33,000). Success begat success. In 1963, the NIH awarded the department two five-year grants totaling nearly half a million dollars for research on radiation damage to cells and to develop better diagnostic methods using radioactive tools. All of the senior investigators on NIH grants were MDs–PhDs in fields such as immunology and biochemistry.[17]

The JHSPH Division of Radiochemistry was also home to Henry N. Wagner Jr., one of the founders of nuclear medicine, which uses molecules labeled with radioisotopes to study the structure and function of organs in living patients. The resulting images give physicians the unique ability to examine these processes visually over time to reveal abnormal regions and to differentiate healthy from diseased physiological states. John G. McAfee and Wagner cofounded the Johns Hopkins Hospital Division of Nuclear Medicine in 1959, which received $90,000 from the hospital and university to purchase nuclear counting and lab equipment. The following year, Morgan brought the nuclear medicine group into the Department of Radiological Sciences to form the Division of Radiochemistry, which was originally housed in the Biophysics Building of the medical school, and retained close ties with that department.[18]

McAfee, a radiologist, and J. M. Mozley, a physicist and chemical engineer, had built the first nuclear imaging rectilinear scanner at Hopkins in 1957, which produced two-dimensional images by moving down the length of the patient's body. By 1962, nearly 80 percent of US hospitals with more than 100 beds had a unit that received radioisotopes for clinical and research use from the Atomic Energy Commission. Yet according to a national survey of existing total body radiation counters that Mozley conducted for the PHS Division of Radiological Health, current machines for patient diagnosis had many flaws. McAfee wrote an NIH grant to "design and construct a total body counter for humans, for optimum performance as a system for diagnostic studies rather than for the measurement of body burdens of natural and fallout radioactivity."[19]

A key concept in McAfee's proposal for the division was to foster the interchange of ideas between nuclear engineers and physicians by establishing an instrument development laboratory in the allied fields of nuclear instrumentation and radiochemistry. Up to that time, nuclear medicine had developed in hospital laboratories and drug companies, largely isolated from the physical sciences even though its diagnostic techniques were dependent on advances in areas such as nuclear physics, chemistry, instrumentation, and data processing. McAfee convinced NIH grant reviewers that by combining the power of all these disciplines within one institution at Johns Hopkins, the Division of Radiochemistry would solve "major problems in radiochemical syntheses not even attempted by the radiopharmaceutical industry."[20]

The proposed machine used a ring made of three-inch sodium iodide crystals, through which "the patient's body, supported on a light frame, will be mechanically moved [lengthwise] from head to foot, so that radioactivity from all areas of the body will be detected with equal sensitivity. The overall increase in detection efficiency will be approximately 30 times that of existing counters [that used] a single 8" × 4" sodium iodide crystal." This machine, called a scintillation scanner, was the first in a series of scanners developed as a joint project of Hygiene, Medicine, and Johns Hopkins Hospital with NIH funding that would be renewed every five years for over 40 years. The scanner achieved greater accuracy by moving the patient's body through the stationary ring of sodium iodide crystals, which reversed the design of previous scanners and became the standard through the late 1970s. By the early 1980s, JHSPH Radiochemistry faculty had produced one of the first prototypes for the positron emission tomography (PET) scanner. Wagner himself was the first person to have a lung scan (in 1961) and to undergo PET imaging of dopamine and opiate receptors in the brain (in 1983).[21]

Radiological Science used large numbers of expensive, highly complex, and sensitive electronic instruments. The NIH grant budgets for personnel and expenses were "increased approximately 5% per year to provide for the anticipated annual increase in cost of these items." In addition to designing and constructing new nuclear instruments for medical research and diagnosis, the research program involved radiochemical synthesis carried out by an organic chemist and a pharmacist using electrophoresis, chromatography, a spectrophotometer, and beta-gamma monitors. Neutron activation analysis, a sensitive in vitro technique developed in the 1960s, facilitated multielement analysis of trace elements in biological samples.[22]

The significance of the Division of Radiochemistry's activities for medical research and clinical application was clear and had resulted, for example, in revolutionary diagnostic imaging technologies that fused anatomical X-ray images with radioisotope studies to visualize previously hidden organs and physiological processes. The public health significance of these activities was less evident, and in one single-spaced grant proposal, McAfee did not state the project's implications for population and environmental health until page 23, and then only in rather vague terms: "There is increasing evidence that certain trace elements, environmental contaminants of our urban-industrialized society, may be associated with human disease."[23]

The Dilemma of Sanitary Engineering

Along with the hazards of radiation from industry, nuclear testing, and medical procedures, JHSPH was an early national leader in two other areas of environmental health research: methods of preventing airborne infections and the impact of housing on child health. During the 1950s, the school's complementary research projects on toxicology, air hygiene, and the health effects of housing reflected the growing public health importance of identifying risk factors. In the epidemiological triangle of agent–host–environment, Anna Baetjer and Richard Riley in Environmental Medicine employed classic basic science methods rooted in physiology and biochemistry to examine pathogenic agents (lead, tuberculosis bacilli), while in Public Health Administration, Daniel Wilner's broader social approach labeled the environment of slum housing as a risk factor correlated to urban poverty but failed to identify the specific harmful agent(s). Baetjer began with clinical evidence of lead poisoning in a group of Baltimore children, then conducted trial-and-error animal testing to quantify lead's hazardous effects. Likewise, Riley used guinea pigs to prove the hypothesis that irradiating air would prevent tuberculosis by halting the spread of airborne droplet nuclei. Baetjer and Riley's work fit within the emerging paradigm of epidemiology that linked smoking and lung cancer. Wilner, however, began with the environment. Instead of lab tests, Wilner relied on long-term observation of two groups of children living in slums versus public housing to document disparate outcomes for their behavior and education as well as health.[24]

Ironically, however, after Wilner left Hopkins in 1960 to join UCLA's new school of public health, interest in the health effects of housing quickly faded, both in Baltimore and nationally. As medical historian Samuel Kelton Roberts has observed, "The last decades of incurable tuberculosis coincided with the first decades of federal housing policy. This relationship has been forgotten: after the urgency of tuberculosis in housing politics receded after 1960, the claims of liberal public health in many ways seemed to lack an organizing epidemiological principle to anchor a critique of urban policy." Ultimately, the most important lasting effect of Wilner's work may have been the ways in which his interdisciplinary social science and statistical methods anticipated the future shift in public health research away from single causes toward understanding the interactions among multiple factors. Morgan, Baetjer, Riley, and Wilner's research positioned the school to seize opportunities offered during the 1960s by the surge of federal environmental health initiatives under the PHS and NIH and further expanded in the 1970s by the Environmental Protection Agency (EPA), Occupational Health and Safety Administration (OSHA), and Food and Drug Administration (FDA).[25]

In a 1957 proposal to restructure the Department of Sanitary Engineering, Abel Wolman and his colleague Cornelius Krusé fired an early salvo at environmentalists who dared to trash the virtues of technology. As engineers, they championed "the classical concept of building public health on . . . permanent environmental alteration," and they ridiculed "the fast growing concept in this country that water supply, waste, food and vector control are no longer 'important enough' to command much attention." To remain relevant yet true to core sanitary engineering principles, Wolman and Krusé argued that the department must engage in new areas of research, including evaluating the impact of chemicals in the water supply on chronic diseases, dental health, and pregnant mothers; applying advances in virology to develop new filtration techniques; and defending "the water resource against increasing pollution and consumption load imposed by the growth of our cities and industry." They predicted that water pollution would outstrip domestic waste disposal in importance as a future public health problem, due to "the increasing industrial load of complex materials from physiologically toxic to radioactive agents." Such hazardous in-dustrial waste in the water supply would overwhelm current concerns about the cost of water treatment for domestic use, including its impact on wildlife, recreation, farming, and fishing. The sheer scale of industrial water pollution, Wolman and Krusé claimed, required that "a whole new set of disciplines must be marshaled."[26]

Public concern was building over the dangers of what Wolman termed "the byproducts of civilization," such as the ubiquitous building material asbestos and the insecticide DDT. Through the 1950s, federal environmental quality efforts had focused primarily on water but now broadened to include air, radia-tion, and the impact of manmade chemicals on plants and wildlife as well as people.[27]

The publication of *Silent Spring* (1962), the environmental movement mani-festo by Rachel Carson, vaulted the previously apolitical discipline of ecology into the forefront of policy debates. Carson, who had earned a master's degree in marine biology at the Johns Hopkins Homewood campus, drew upon the population biology theories of her one-time professor, Raymond Pearl, who headed the JHSPH Department of Biology during the 1930s. While *Silent Spring* specifically warned of the dangers of agricultural use of DDT and other pesticides, Carson's advocacy was a critical factor in enlarging the parameters of the pollution issue beyond human health to consider the overall effects on ecosystems and biodiversity.[28]

In the early 1960s, a rapid changing of the guard invigorated both the en-vironmental movement and the four Hygiene departments that focused on environmental health. In 1961, Riley was appointed chair of Environmental Medicine, and Russell H. Morgan was appointed chair of the new Department of Radiological Science, which evaluated the hazards of radiation from indus-try, nuclear testing, and medical procedures. Wolman's successor as chair, Cor-nelius Krusé, struggled to defend Sanitary Engineering's relevance to current practice under pressure from both JHSPH administrators and PHS officials. Sanitary engineering, once a core public health discipline, was often pushed aside rather than included in the "new" environmental health.[29]

Krusé had observed in 1957 that "the 'golden age' of communicable disease control through environmental sanitation is all but over. . . . Our traditional areas of water, liquid and solid waste, food and housing are becoming more complex and require for solution most highly developed integrations of biology [and] biochemistry with physical science and engineering." The mounting challenges posed by new and existing environmental health problems required "the kind of bacteriology and chemistry in which our basic science depart-ments have professed no interest at all." Krusé admitted that the School of

Hygiene's existing sanitary engineering program "could not attract high level research interest" and turned his sights to air pollution, which he identified as a "goldmine" for attracting research funding. With Richard L. Riley, one of the few remaining Environmental Medicine faculty, Krusé proposed to develop a concentration on industrial ventilation, including control of infectious biological agents within factories and limiting the atmospheric diffusion of radiation wastes and general stack emissions. Yet the central dilemma of modern environmental health was that advances in conventional water purification and waste disposal could "no longer be measured in terms of reduced death rates from communicable disease," and it was equally difficult to prove that long-term exposure to air pollution was a direct cause of chronic disease morbidity and mortality.[30]

Krusé was being groomed to succeed Abel Wolman as chair, so he took a sabbatical to earn a DrPH in environmental health at the University of Pittsburgh. Krusé returned to JHSPH in 1961 as professor and chair of sanitary engineering, but he would find interdisciplinary collaboration an elusive goal at Hopkins. From 1937 to 1961, Abel Wolman had chaired both departments of sanitary engineering in the schools of Engineering and Hygiene, which he described as "riding two circus horses." With Wolman's retirement, the horses went their separate ways, and John C. Geyer was named chair of Sanitary Engineering at Homewood. Although all faculty in both departments received joint appointments and Krusé suggested merging the graduate programs, the two groups remained more loyal to their home disciplines than to bridging the Hygiene–Engineering divide. These tensions influenced Krusé when he renamed the department. He at first replaced "sanitary" with "environmental," listing the department variously as Environmental Hygiene, Environmental Health Engineering, and Environmental Engineering Science, and then dropped "engineering" altogether in 1966 for the shorter Environmental Health. The similarity to the Department of Environmental Medicine, however, at times caused confusion.[31]

But despite the changes in departmental letterhead, the Municipal Sanitation course preserved the basic content of the longstanding sanitary engineering course: "activities of regulatory agencies in discharging legal responsibilities in municipal sanitation matters including the broad areas of public water supplies, public sewage treatment, milk and food sanitation, solid waste collection and disposal, and industrial environmental problems," including air pollution. Students made field visits to water and sewage treatment plants, a dairy farm, a food processing plant, and a refuse collection and disposal facility. Likewise, the Department of Environmental Health's research in the 1970s remained focused on sanitary engineering and explored the action of halogen and other disinfectants on disease-causing microorganisms in water and sewage, as well as improved methods of disinfecting and evaluating levels of pathogens in water and wastewater.[32]

During his tenure as chair, Krusé kept his department out of the limelight and largely independent of federal funding. In contrast to the flashy, sometimes confrontational brand of environmentalism being promulgated by the PHS and many eco-activists, Krusé attacked the problems of environmental health with time-tested orthodox methods, which he skillfully passed on to his students. In the 1960s, when students became more critical of teaching and course content, some objected that engineering was irrelevant. Krusé, like Wolman before him, strongly believed that an appreciation of engineering was precisely what public health practitioners needed most.[33]

The Pathobiology Menagerie

If Environmental Health hewed a traditional course, Pathobiology was the school's iconoclast. In the twentieth-century search for new advances against agents of mass disability and death, animal models were the scientific bridge from guesses to guarantees. The term *pathobiology* had been in use since the 1880s, sometimes as a synonym for *pathology*, but also denoting the biological processes associated with disease. Rudolf Virchow and William Osler, giants in the fields of pathology and medicine, respectively, were outspoken advocates of the medical value of studying veterinary pathology and using knowledge obtained from animals to understand physiology, immunology, and pathology in humans. Early public health leaders, including William Welch, Daniel Salmon, and Theobald Smith, all promoted the importance of comparative pathology for public health, not only in controlling zoonotic diseases and ensuring the safety of animal products, such as milk and meat, but also for insights into the fundamental mechanisms of disease.[34]

Schools of medicine established programs in comparative pathology, and veterinary schools established departments of pathobiology. By midcentury, Johns Hopkins faculty in both Medicine and Hygiene had begun to think more holistically about the biological and pathological relationships among pathogens, parasites, animals, human beings, and their environment. In 1946, Arnold Rice Rich, chair of the medical school's Department of Pathology, proposed to establish a new program in comparative pathology, which he defined as "a systematic approach to the understanding of the reactive and adaptive processes that constitute disease and recovery, by means of studying the development and significance of those processes up (or down) the evolutionary phylogenetic scale of animals." Although Medicine awarded Rich initial funding to get the program started, it was Hygiene that fully realized a program in comparative pathology and medical ecology.[35]

Since the school's founding, JHSPH researchers had developed mutually reinforcing strengths in medical ecology and animal models of disease. The laboratory yielded knowledge of how pathogenic agents behaved in simplified, controlled conditions, which was necessary for creating new vaccines and diagnostic tests. Field observation of the complex, unpredictable natural environment produced insights into precisely how disease spread from vector to host and outward into animal and human populations. If animal models helped fashion the "magic bullets" against disease, medical ecology was the rifle scope that enabled epidemiologists to identify and zero in on the most effective targets for intervention.

As noted in the first three chapters, the school's research on bird malaria and the use of primates to study the virology of polio yielded two of the faculty's most lasting contributions to the science of public health. Rats were the most commonly used experimental animal, first brought to the school in 1918 by E. V. McCollum for his experiments on vitamin deficiency. JHSPH laboratories also housed smaller numbers of other mammals whose anatomical and physiological characteristics were matched with various diseases. For example, guinea pigs were used to study tuberculosis, and rabbits and sheep to study syphilis (the sheep, who only had to supply blood samples for use in Wasserman tests, grazed on the school's front lawn along Monument Street).

Dogs were essential for developing the Department of Parasitology's quantitative experimental approach, which its faculty and alumni extended to parasitology laboratories throughout the world. In the 1920s, the department's studies of host–parasite relations in dog hookworm had revealed that well-fed dogs developed immunity, while a poor diet led to heavy hookworm infestation, even in dogs that had been previously resistant. The dog studies guided Gilbert F. Otto in his investigations of hookworm infection in southern children, which established that dietary deficiencies adversely affected immunity to hookworm infection—one of the earliest of the school's many discoveries on the links between malnutrition and susceptibility to infectious disease.[36]

The first article published in *Science* by a JHSPH faculty member did not outline a grand theory on disease control but rather a simple method for devocalizing dogs. Justin Andrews began his 1926 article with the observation, "In a laboratory situated within a residential district, it is frequently somewhat of a problem to keep a number of experimental dogs because of their persistent barking during their cage confinement." Apparently, however, Andrews's method was not always employed. Until the 1980s, JHSPH students who took classes in the East Wing Auditorium (now Sheldon Hall) regularly heard barking from the laboratory kennels in the basement below.[37]

Dogs were so important to the school that they were the focus of the first—and perhaps only—instance of formally sanctioned political activism in JHSPH history. In 1950, Baltimore City voters considered a proposed referendum to prohibit health department officials from turning over impounded stray animals to medical institutions for education and research. As the "quiet decade" of the 1950s began, Johns Hopkins Hygiene and Medicine faculty, staff, and students took to the streets and went door to door with their University of Maryland counterparts and members of the Maryland Society for Medical Research. Their efforts overwhelmingly defeated the referendum by a ratio of four to one, and the victory was trumpeted in the pages of the *American Journal of Public Health*.[38]

The war had drawn attention to the problem of controlling rodents, which spread typhus fever, plague, and leptospirosis. David E. Davis joined the Department of Parasitology in 1945 to direct the Baltimore rat control study begun under NRC auspices by behavioral psychologist Curt P. Richter in Psychiatry, assisted by JHSPH parasitologist John T. Emlen (Richter, who established the psychobiological laboratory in the Phipps Psychiatric Clinic in 1922, was an expert in animal behavior, famous for his work on biological clocks in humans and animals). Davis became known as "the rat man" and conducted elaborate studies of rat populations, stress, and behavior by trapping them in urban residential blocks and designing artificial habitats for them inside the school and in nearby vacant lots. In 1950, Davis received a PHS grant to establish the Division of Vertebrate Ecology, broadening his initial rat research to encompass a multispecies approach to comparative pathology with a focus on the implications of animal behavior for understanding human populations.[39]

Paul Lemkau, head of the PHA Division of Mental Hygiene and a contributor to Davis's courses, told Turner that "the teaching of vertebrate ecology has, in my estimation, shown more originality of thinking about relating human behavior as observed to the science dealt with in courses. . . . Pathobiology certainly must concern itself in an unembarrassed way with psychologically induced behavior as well as physiologically induced behavior, and when it does this it will more nearly prepare the student for the real world and not one artificially restricted to what can be exquisitely measured, weighed and analysed." Lemkau's comment indicated the broader shift during the 1950s toward investigations of the disease-causing roles of social and environmental factors and individual behavior patterns.[40]

The concept of pathobiology in public health elevated comparative pathology to the population level, just as three major funding streams were coming online or greatly increasing in the late 1950s: NIH categorical disease research, environmental health and toxicology, and social and behavioral psychology related to urban problems and global population growth. With assistance from Davis, Frederik Bang would transform Parasitology into a wide-ranging research program in medical ecology, comparative behavior, and population biology, including the parasitology and epidemiology of polar animals in collaboration with the PHS Arctic Health Research Center.[41]

In 1964, just two years after the publication of Carson's *Silent Spring*, the PHS prepared to "revolutionize the entire approach to environmental health hazards" by inviting universities to develop interdisciplinary Institutes for Environmental Health Studies. In its application guidelines, the PHS declared, "Environmental health problems *cannot be approached solely within the traditional teaching-learning framework*. They require ingenuity, new methodology, new instrumentation, field study, and *unorthodox attack*." The new program placed a premium on interdisciplinary approaches that reflected the "interrelationship among environmental health problem areas. The hazards we seek to prevent or control do not necessarily assert themselves as a 'single agent insult,' and there is need to consider the total cause-and-effect relationship of man to his environment." To study this relationship, the new environmental health institutes would apply multidisciplinary scientific resources, with special attention to the "interrelated aspects of the biological, physiological, and social components of our rapidly changing environment."[42]

In the formulation of the PHS, the brave new discipline of environmental health science would concern itself with measuring and evaluating the health effects of exposure to environmental agents, whether long or short term. The brochure noted, "While ultimate concern is in the direction of human illness, there is also interest in proposals involving animals and other biological systems which may provide information related to the human problems." This had been the founding principle of Fred Bang's Department of Pathobiology, and indeed, the School of Hygiene was teeming with different animal species used for research in nearly every department. Turtles wandered down the hallways for the Mental Hygiene Division of Comparative Behavior's studies of orientation behavior, and bats were used for observing mother–infant bonding. The basement housed a 5,000-gallon seal tank.[43]

For William and Brenda Sladen's studies of Antarctic birds, Pathobiology secretary Ethel Poplovski helped care for the penguins who lived at the Eastpoint Shopping Center, where they occupied a corner window in the Hochschild–Kohn department store and became perennial favorites of local children. The penguins, named Ernie, Donna, Debbie, and Peter, arrived from the Cape Peninsula of South Africa in July 1963. The rest of the School of Hygiene menagerie was generously funded by an influx of PHS and NIH grants to Environmental Medicine, Radiological Science, and especially Pathobiology, but never more than a pittance for Sanitary Engineering. Environmental research represented the single largest source of external funding for the school during the first half of the 1960s, when total PHS research grants to all departments averaged between $1.5 and $2 million annually. Beginning in 1965, the Johnson administration accelerated support for ecological research from a variety of federal agencies, from the National Science Foundation to the Smithsonian, and the school's environmental health programs benefited accordingly.[44]

In 1966, William Sladen and Fred Bang met with JHU President Milton Eisenhower to discuss the Hopkins Field Station, a part of the Smithsonian Institution's Chesapeake Bay Center for Field Biology, located seven miles south of Annapolis. Sladen described his vision for the field station's investigations of "major problems of man's adaptations to his own environments," which would train graduate students in terrestrial and estuarine field ecology, comparative animal behavior, wildlife diseases, and health-related problems of pollution and conservation. The unique program in the field biology of populations would train master's, doctoral, and postdoctoral students to conduct research in both real and simulated natural environments.

Sladen's justification for increasing the field station's funding could have been ghost-written by Rachel Carson. He warned of the environmental dangers of increasing human population and urban and industrial development, concluding that "human activities are threatening to contaminate the entire world. Even Antarctic penguins and seals are now carrying pesticides in their bodies." Sladen emphasized the unpredictable consequences of ecological changes that had "in large measure preceded our knowledge of their effects, both acute and chronic, on man and animals." As whole species of animals and plants disappeared or diminished in number, the resulting disruptions to the food supply and the environment's capacity for self-renewal could, he warned, be disastrous for humans. Sladen succeeded in expanding the field station, and in 1969, the Department of Pathobiology created the Division of Ecology and Comparative Behavior, which Sladen headed until 1983. Sladen, an international authority on swans, would be the basis for the character Dr. Killian in the 1996 movie *Fly Away Home*.[45]

In cooperation with the Department of Environmental Medicine, the Division of Ecology and Comparative Behavior conducted a study of trace metals in the Chesapeake Bay ecosystem, focusing on the ways that sentinel organisms such as bottom-feeding migratory birds could serve as monitors of pollution levels. Charles Rohde, who joined the Biostatistics faculty in 1965, was an expert on statistical ecology who worked with many of the environmental scientists on the JHSPH faculty. He remembers "mucking around in an island in the Chesapeake Bay with Bill Sladen looking for turtles that he had marked." The island was a few miles downwind of Aberdeen Proving Grounds and had been bombarded for decades by all kinds of shells and explosive devices. To determine whether these activities had any lasting effects on the natural inhabitants of the island, the researchers selected turtles, since their home range was so small, rarely more than 100 yards from their birthplace. Rohde advised Sladen on how to compile and analyze the voluminous data from tracking the baby turtles.[46]

Another environmental application of statistics was Rohde's use of composite sampling to measure biodiversity and to determine the oxygen content of the Chesapeake Bay. Instead of measuring the content of 1,000 samples individually, composite sampling could divide the lot into 10 groups composed of 100 combined samples and take one sample from each batch. The technique had first been used during World War II to test soldiers for sexually transmitted diseases, since individual testing would have been too expensive. By combining the blood samples from each platoon and taking a single sample for the group, a negative result could clear them all at once or, if it was positive, the group would be retested individually. Composite sampling has also been used to detect spoilage in food processing plants, was "rediscovered" for AIDS testing, and has been used in mass data applications such as evaluating Superfund sites.[47]

Under both Alan Ross (chair from 1966 to 1981) and Chuck Rohde (chair from 1981 to 1996), one of the main goals of Biostatistics was to "infect" the rest of the school and the university with a passion for good data and healthy skepticism. Rohde advised a senior biologist at Homewood who was writing a grant proposal to study the potential effect of nuclear power plants, which would raise the temperature in the Chesapeake Bay, on the spawning patterns of the striped bass. The biologist proposed to incubate samples of 10,000 eggs at the current temperature of the bay and then increase the temperature in 5-degree increments with each sample and then count the proportion of fertile eggs after several days. Rohde asked the biologist, "Where did you get the eggs?" and he replied, "Well, we caught this female fish, and that's where all our eggs came from." Then Rohde asked, "Do all striped bass spawn at the same temperature?" At that, the flustered biologist asked Rohde to leave. "So there was an example of a totally useless experiment. The sample size was one, but there were thousands of dollars put into this study of one fish."[48]

G. Carleton Ray was an expert on polar marine mammals, and his research was part of the school's work on population ecology—studying disease and population changes in animal models to better understand implications for human populations, as well as human health from an ecosystem perspective. While at Johns Hopkins, he was the primary person responsible for passing the federal Marine Mammal Protection Act of 1972—the original "save the whales" law.

The National Institute of Environmental Health Sciences

By 1970, more than 30 environmental scientists were spread among the Pathobiology Division of Comparative Ecology and the departments of Environmental Health and Environmental Medicine. The 40 faculty in Radiological Science primarily focused on basic science research with little direct environmental application. The Department of Pathobiology needed no prompting to pursue environmental research, but Stebbins forwarded the PHS environmental health institute brochure to Anna Baetjer and Richard Riley in Environmental Medicine, Cornelius Krusé in Sanitary Engineering, and Russell Morgan in Radiological Science. In a handwritten memo, Stebbins instructed the four faculty to "decide whether this would be wise." Morgan opposed an environmental health institute at Hopkins, both as an administrative strategy and specifically as it was proposed by the PHS. He particularly questioned the guide's introductory statements about the need for an unorthodox ecosystems approach, which seemed to bypass implications for human health: "even members of Congress have found [these statements] hard to believe when they have appeared in background material supporting the Environmental Health Program of the Public Health Service."[49]

Although neither Baetjer nor Krusé registered an opinion in favor of founding an Environmental Health Institute at Hopkins, Krusé went on to serve on the advisory committee formed in 1965 to establish a new National Institute of Environmental Health Sciences (NIEHS). Through the 1950s, the NIH had focused almost exclusively on the cellular, molecular, and later the genetic aspects of medical research, with little attention to either an environmental or population health approach. In 1965, responsibility for air pollution research shifted from the NIH to the new PHS Division of Air Pollution, but it returned to the NIH in 1969, when Congress authorized the creation of NIEHS in response to growing national concern about the health risks of chemicals and other environmental agents. It was the first institute to depart from the NIH's traditional emphasis on the medical sciences with a name that did not contain an organ system, disease, or medical subfield.[50]

Although all schools of public health continued to teach environmental health courses and most retained public health–minded engineers on their faculties, only Johns Hopkins, North Carolina, Harvard, Michigan, and Pittsburgh committed major institutional resources and faculty lines to maintain and expand their programs in environmental health and related fields. Harvard had established a Division of Environmental Hygiene in 1960, which joined the public health departments of Industrial Hygiene and Physiology as well as the arts and sciences Department of Sanitary Engineering. To promote interdisciplinary collaboration in environmental health, Harvard combined these three departments and moved them into an elaborate new research facility, citing Carson's *Silent Spring* as an intellectual catalyst. During the 1960s and 1970s, environmental health research was a major driver of the overall growth of the five schools of public health with strong environmental emphases.[51]

The development of the Department of Environmental Sciences and Engineering at the University of North Carolina (UNC) School of Public Health provides another instructive comparison to Johns Hopkins. UNC's Department of Environmental Sciences and Engineering faculty had already grown from seven in 1960 to 33 in 1968. These faculty were subdivided among programs in sanitary engineering and water resources, environmental and food sanitation, environmental chemistry and biology, air and industrial hygiene, and radiological hygiene, with 19 doctoral students. NIEHS was the first institute to be located remotely, in North Carolina's Research Triangle Park. UNC leveraged its location in Chapel Hill, a short distance from NIEHS, just as JHSPH had benefited as the school of public health closest to the main NIH campus in Bethesda, Maryland. By founding an Environmental Health Institute in collaboration with NIEHS, UNC further accelerated the expansion of the department and the school.[52]

Unlike UNC, most schools of public health did not take active roles as either centers for NIEHS research or as leaders on environmental justice issues. At a meeting of the Association of Schools of Public Health in the late 1960s, Abel Wolman told the deans that they were too indifferent to environmental health problems. He begged them "to extend themselves beyond the infectious disease problem" and advance the epidemiology of environmental diseases. "You have defaulted," he charged. "Your voices are rarely heard nationally in this country" on either environmental health specifically or public health more broadly. One of the most controversial issues at the time was asbestos, which Irving J. Selikoff had identified as the primary cause of mesothelioma in 1963. Scientists also debated whether asbestos was harmful when ingested in drinking water. WHO had only recently issued its first guidelines on safe drinking water in 1958, and the EPA did not yet exist. Wolman chided the public health deans, "I don't hear a single voice out of any school of public health in the United States or Canada."[53]

Wolman singled out Andrew J. Rhodes, dean of the University of Toronto School of Hygiene, for downplaying the significance of environmental issues for public health. Rhodes, a microbiologist famous for his use of electron microscopy to identify viruses, represented the medical and public health establishment's conventional focus on the direct transmission of pathogenic organisms at the expense of broader environmental factors. But public health departments had likewise deemphasized environmental health. By fiscal year

1978, US state and territorial public health agencies spent three-quarters of their total budgets on personal health services and only 7 percent on all areas of environmental health, including consumer protection, sanitation, and air and water quality. In only one-third of states and territories was the health department designated as the lead agency under the Environmental Protection Act.[54]

Part of Wolman's ire may have stemmed from the fact that JHSPH, like most other schools of public health, was drifting away from its once-strong ties to the engineering school. A 1973 Josiah H. Macy Jr. Foundation report concluded that "present mechanisms do not appear capable of ensuring a stable base for such cooperation [between schools of engineering and public health]." In 1972, a joint APHA–ASPH committee would issue new accreditation standards that included "environmental monitoring, analysis, and manipulation" as one of the fundamental skills that master's degree students should learn. By 1978, the American Board of Preventive Medicine would designate environmental health as "one of the major content areas of preventive medicine." The board refused to recognize MPH degrees from schools of public health that did not require a course in environmental health.[55]

Despite Wolman's criticisms of academic public health as too uninvolved in environmental health, he and Kruse dragged their feet when Stebbins urged them to take advantage of new PHS federal training grants to develop programs in community air pollution and environmental health. The department's only such grant was from the PHS Division of Community Health Services for training in sanitary microbiology. Another funding opportunity came from the PHS Division of Environmental Engineering and Food Protection to develop short-term training in urban planning for environmental health. One goal of the program was "the rapprochement of health agencies and planning agencies at local and state levels." M.I.T. and Georgia Tech offered two-week summer courses in city planning for environmental health officials, but Hopkins declined to participate. Baetjer served on the board for the Atomic Energy Commission's Industrial Hygiene Fellowships, and she asked Kruse to offer the necessary industrial hygiene engineering and chemistry courses in order for the School of Hygiene to qualify. But Environmental Health remained resolutely focused on traditional sanitary engineering problems of water supply and sewage treatment, along with Kruse's ongoing work in malaria control. Despite Kruse's early plans, new research in air pollution was concentrated in the Department of Environmental Medicine.[56]

Wolman, who had served as a consultant to a host of federal agencies since the New Deal, became more critical in the 1970s of the federal approach to environmental standards. The 1972 Clean Water Act introduced the stringent new goal of "zero discharge," or reusing all industrial wastewater for processes inside the plant so that no toxic pollutants would be released into waterways. In a 1981 oral history interview, Wolman scoffed at what he viewed as the naïve goals of "zero population growth and zero risk" that dominated the public health and environmental movements of the 1970s. He denied that "the control of the environment to the nth degree is the most important social problem in the United States. . . . Since Congressional directives are highly general, Federal agencies interpret them very broadly and too zealously."[57]

Environmental Medicine and the Growth of Toxicology

Aside from the more independent-minded Department of Environmental Health, NIEHS provided essential support for the JHSPH departments of Pathobiology, Radiological Science, and Environmental Medicine, all of which maintained close ties to the medical school. Environmental Medicine proved most loyal to the NIEHS mission of quantifying and reducing the effects of environmental pathogens on human health. During the 1950s, Environmental Medicine had shared its faculty and cooperated closely with the Department of Medicine's Division of Physiology. Accordingly, Environmental Medicine's research was clinically oriented and focused on four main areas: pulmonary and cardiovascular physiology, applied environmental and occupational physiology, environmental toxicology, and audiology and speech. In their 1957 forecast of future trends, Krusé and Wolman had declared that "a department of Environmental Hygiene in a School of Public Health should strive to shorten the lag between theory and practice in the emerging areas of noise, radiation, accident, toxic materials, etc. It should go further than merely enumerating environmental hazards and explaining their causation." The Department of Environmental Medicine fulfilled this charge by excelling in two related fields of highly applied research, air hygiene and toxicology.[58]

Just as measures to purify public water systems had radically reduced rates of intestinal diseases, air hygiene researchers posited that removing infectious organisms and toxins from the air could reduce the incidence of respiratory diseases such as asthma, emphysema, influenza, and tuberculosis. After becoming chair of Environmental Medicine in 1961, Richard L. Riley had expanded the department's research on indoor air pollution, which he argued was more dangerous than atmospheric pollution, since the concentration of pollutants could increase dramatically within built environments, particularly in industrial plants. Riley warned that the danger of infection from airborne diseases was increasing as people spent more time indoors and air conditioning became more widespread. He consulted with the National Aeronautics and Space Administration on methods of protecting astronauts from airborne infections by irradiating the air in space capsules. In the seventh-floor corridors of the Hygiene Building, he used ultraviolet lights to disinfect circulating air as part of experiments to measure and reduce the concentration of germs. Riley advocated the installation of ultraviolet lighting in the ceilings of public buildings to prevent airborne diseases, including chickenpox, influenza, measles, mumps, and smallpox, as well as tuberculosis. As a member of both the National Heart Institute Cardiovascular Study Section during the 1960s and the Environmental Health Sciences Study Section in the early 1970s, Riley helped to elevate the scientific profile of environmental research to the level accorded to the traditional categorical disease institutes within the NIH. He also served as president of the American Thoracic Society in 1977 and won the Edward Livingston Trudeau Medal from the National Tuberculosis and Respiratory Disease Association.[59]

Environmental Medicine is a clear example of JHSPH's marked shift from dependence on defense-related funding in the 1950s to embracing R01 grants, the NIH's original research project grant that was the mainstay of the agency's extramural program. In 1964, the department had discontinued its contract work for the US Air Force and consolidated its research support under the NIH for projects on the mechanics of lung physiology, including airway obstruction, systemic circulation, and pulmonary gas exchange. The Department of Pediatrics collaborated with Environmental Medicine on problems of pollen allergy in children and on the epidemiology of respiratory disease, particularly asthma, among low-income children. More effective methods of air sanitation could potentially solve both these problems. The role of surfactant in pulmonary mechanics was a particularly fruitful area of cooperation between Pediatrics and Environmental Medicine. In 1959, Mary Ellen Avery in Pediatrics discovered that neonatal respiratory distress was caused in premature infants by their lack of alveolar surfactant coating, which helped the lungs expand by reducing surface tension and the pressure differential necessary for lung inflation. Environmental Medicine faculty contributed to these studies by elucidating the physiological mechanical principles and pathophysiology in a variety of clinical problems. Their work also led to improved diagnostic tests for determining the reversibility of airway obstruction.[60]

Between 1965 and 1970, the central focus of the Department of Environmental Medicine was its air hygiene research project, one of the first projects to be funded by the PHS Division of Air Pollution. The lead investigator, Donald F. Proctor, had joined the Hopkins medical faculty in 1945, initially as a professor of laryngology and otology and later of anesthesiology. Through the 1950s, Proctor's research had dealt with tuberculosis, respiratory air flow, and bronchial obstruction. He was also an early advocate of using irradiation of lymphoid tissue to reduce swelling and prevent disease and deafness, and he was involved in the Division of Audiology and Speech's PHS study of nasopharyngeal irradiation to prevent deafness. In the early 1960s, Proctor began working with Riley and Sol Permutt on lung inflation and pulmonary pressure.[61]

In 1967, Proctor achieved local renown by calling for a ban on cars in Baltimore City and the establishment of a state agency to regulate air, land, and water pollution. His research indicated that air pollution caused irritation and watering of the eyes, coughing, nasal irritation, and increased symptoms of asthma, bronchitis, and emphysema, as well as could cause death in patients with heart and respiratory disease. He told the Metropolitan Conference on Air Pollution, "If we allow ourselves to be persuaded that evidence is not strong enough at this time to clean the air then we are dooming thousands to death in the 20 years it will take to clean the air." Proctor voiced the lament of air pollution researchers that "we can't prove in a court of law which specific pollutant, or combination of pollutants, in the air we breathe causes which specific adverse health effects. But we have to say that at the present time the evidence shows there are plenty of things in the air that are harmful to human health." Proctor, however, echoed Riley by stressing that cigarette smoking and poor indoor air quality posed greater threats than most atmospheric pollutants. In 1982, Proctor testified at a hearing convened by the Texas Air Control Board on raising the Asarco smelting plant's allowable sulfur dioxide emissions levels. Proctor's laboratory studies had found no ill effects from human subjects breathing much higher concentrations for up to six hours, so that the higher proposed levels "were not a health hazard."[62]

In a 1969 journal article, Proctor and his coinvestigators asked, "How does one explain the slow progress made toward the control of airborne disease in comparison with the dramatic progress in the area of waterborne disease?" Control efforts against waterborne disease had emphasized preventing the etiological factor from reaching the host, while those against airborne disease had focused on developing artificial immunity, "an approach which offers no help in the noninfectious diseases associated with industrial exposures or air pollution." Based on his observation that "the role of the nose in both infectious and noninfectious airborne disease has only recently come under investigation," Proctor and biochemist George W. Jourdian conducted in-depth research on nasal airflow and the role of the nasal passages as the primary "defense against inhaled particles" and therefore a key factor in industrial exposure to airborne contaminants. Proctor's group attempted to establish baselines to determine normal nasal airflow resistance and mucociliary clearance, as well as the type and location of airborne particles deposited in the nose, with attention to the effects of environmental variations. Breathing aerosols, for example, deposited particles in the anterior nares.[63]

In 1972, Riley established a three-year training program in industrial environmental health, comprising the MPH and two additional years of industrial health field experience. The Department of Environmental Medicine also began new research on the underlying causes of alcoholism, and the department's Lung Center conducted studies of chronic bronchitis and emphysema with the Department of Epidemiology and the medical school's human genetics program.[64]

Cause-and-effect relationships are much more difficult to detect in observational studies than in clinical trials, and this difficulty is multiplied when attempting to detect links between specific health problems and long-term, low-level exposures to chemicals rather than acute exposure to infectious agents. Anna Baetjer had joined the Department of Physiological Hygiene in 1924 and remained its only faculty member for much of the 1930s and 1940s while teaching a full range of courses, conducting original research, and serving as a consultant for a wide range of industrial, government, and military organizations. During the 1960s, one of Baetjer's primary research projects dealt with communicable disease—the effects of temperature and humidity on respiratory virus infections. Most previous research on environmental factors in viral lung infectious had been conducted on tissues in vitro (i.e., using test tubes and tissue cultures), but Baetjer exposed chicks and other live lab animals in vivo to varying temperatures and levels of humidity to measure the effects on the cilia-mucous mechanism of the respiratory tract, which functioned to remove foreign droplets and particulates, including infectious agents.[65]

Along with her work on chromate dust as a carcinogen, Baetjer's other major PHS grant project gauged the effects of toxic organic chemicals on laboratory animals in combination with the effects of dehydration and electrolyte changes associated with high temperature and humidity as well as extreme cold, which provided relevant comparisons for industrial workers and military personnel in similar conditions. Her prior research had demonstrated that dehydration increased susceptibility to lead poisoning, but the effects of lead were difficult to measure in small animal tissues, especially while maintaining a state of dehydration for prolonged periods. Baetjer now used three common environmental chemicals with different toxic properties: parathion, an insecticide; aniline, an organic compound used in industrial chemical production; and trichloroethylene, an industrial solvent also commonly used as a powerful anesthetic. She applied insights from both the virus and chemical toxicity projects to conduct a study of the influence of temperature and humidity on the toxicity of chromium compounds and their rates of clearance from the respiratory tract. She also emphasized the importance of her research for understanding the health effects of air pollution, bronchitis, and asthma, all of which she hypothesized were compounded by high humidity.[66]

Radiological Science faculty provided key assistance to Baetjer, Permutt, and Proctor in their research on environmental factors in respiratory viruses and airway obstruction. Baetjer and Proctor worked with nuclear medicine expert Henry Wagner to study the mucociliary clearance of particles from the upper respiratory tract, including the effects of cigarette smoke and viscose rayon fibers (commonly inhaled by textile mill workers) on particle transport. Their research emphasized the mechanism by which insoluble particles, tagged with radioactive iodine, were cleared after being deposited in the lungs. This knowledge was important for understanding the body's defenses against inhaled toxins. Radioactive tracers could also be used in testing the absorption and excretion of diagnostic or therapeutic compounds to determine drug action and correct dosages. To track the distribution of radioactive materials in different types of animal tissues following administration by various routes, researchers in the Division of Radiochemistry also developed and evaluated new compounds with localizing properties for specific organs or tumors.[67]

The use of radioactive tracers in animal distribution studies would be a critical tool for the environmental toxicology program that Baetjer established in 1963. After pharmacologist Robert J. Rubin joined the Environmental Medicine faculty in 1964, he and Baetjer codirected the PHS training grant in biochemical toxicology. Rubin went on to direct the Division of Toxicology in the Department of Environmental Health Sciences from 1977 to 1979 and the program in biochemical toxicology from 1983 to 1987, when he was appointed deputy director of the NIH Center in Environmental Health at JHU. Rubin and his advisee Rudolph J. Jaeger (PhD 1971) were among the earliest researchers to raise questions about the potential hazards of DEHP, commonly used as a plasticizer for polyvinyl chloride (PVC) medical devices, including blood storage bags. In the early 1970s, one billion pounds of DEHP were manufactured in the United States annually for plastic wrappings and to plasticize clothing, floor accessories, medical products, and other items.[68]

In 1971, Jaeger and Rubin discovered that DEHP from blood storage bags traveled into the bloodstreams of patients who had received transfusions, and they published their first findings that large doses of DEHP could cause blood clotting in the lungs and kill heart cells in tissue culture. They also speculated that it could be a possible factor in "lung shock," a potentially fatal condition reported among wounded Vietnam soldiers who received battlefield transfusions, in which capillary vessels are blocked from transporting oxygen into the bloodstream. In 1975, Rubin concluded on the basis of a two-year study that DEHP may cause severe lung damage or death. Rubin called for manufacturers of the bags to remove them from the market and to substitute a nonleaching plasticizer. He also studied autopsies of patients who had died after receiving transfusions to determine whether DEHP was implicated. Rubin said of DEHP, "We know it won't kill you at levels to which man is exposed, but the effects of low and chronic exposure, as we encounter every day, are not known."[69]

The politics of environmental health have continued to divide both governmental agencies and academic experts. Based in part on Rubin and Jaeger's research, the EPA classified DEHP as a probable human carcinogen since "orally administered DEHP produced significant dose-related increases in liver tumor responses in rats and mice of both sexes." EPA deemed the available human carcinogenicity data on DEHP inadequate, but the FDA concluded in 2009 that DEHP was not hazardous to humans, noting that "although the toxic and carcinogenic effects of DEHP have been well established in experimental animals, the ability of this compound to produce adverse effects in humans is controversial," since no human studies to date had shown adverse effects.[70]

Rubin was soon joined on the Environmental Medicine faculty by a second public health–minded pharmacologist, Alan M. Goldberg, an expert on cholinergic biology, neurotoxicology, and in vitro methodology. Goldberg's research initially focused on pesticides, in collaboration with the medical school Department of Neurology, and he also started teaching toxicology courses. Up to that point, other than Baetjer's work described above, the only department doing work on pesticides was Pathobiology, which included studies of both pesticide resistance in mosquitoes and the extent of DDT's encroachment into marine birds and mammals. Goldberg recalled that working on pesticides "was a way to get into the environment at the mechanistic level," that is, to advance environmental health through laboratory investigation designed to understand the fundamental basis of toxicity. He recalled proudly that he "became Anna's last student" when she helped him prepare to serve as an expert witness. Baetjer taught him everything she knew about chromium, and they spent many hours in discussion and readings. Goldberg never did testify but relished the chance to learn from Baetjer. He also learned glassblowing to make his own micropipettes, since standard lab glassware was not small enough for toxicology work.[71]

One of Goldberg's first postdoctoral trainees was Ellen K. Silbergeld, who switched her career plans to environmental health after attending the first Earth Day in 1970. She remembered the initial rush of being "captivated and swept up into the environmental movement." After meeting Abel Wolman's son M. Gordon "Reds" Wolman, who chaired the Department of Geography and Environmental Engineering at Johns Hopkins, Silbergeld earned a PhD in environmental engineering and then came to JHSPH to work with Goldberg. Her excitement had spread to toxicology, which she described as "the science that answers the question, Why is this thing hazardous? What is it about lead that makes it dangerous? And then it's like Alice going down the rabbit hole, because you start getting deeper and deeper, particularly if you have a great mentor, into the actual mechanisms and biological and cellular events."[72]

Silbergeld observed that NIEHS, EPA, and OSHA became places that would "support and really dignify the field of toxicology as something that was not a handmaiden to other things that toxicology had been captive to," since it had primarily been a subfield of pharmacology. Goldberg encouraged her "to get away from just asking what's killing things, and into understanding more subtle forms of damage and disabilities," which paralleled the larger shift in public health away from a primary focus on mortality and toward greater attention to reducing morbidity and preventing injury. One of the pair's early forays into neurochemistry research was made possible by the repository of World War II–era chemical compounds that had been seized from Nazi Germany and stored at Edgewood Arsenal, a US Army facility outside Baltimore that housed the Chemical Warfare Service research and development division. Two Department of Environmental Medicine faculty were Army veterans who had been stationed at Edgewood, and they arranged to make the chemicals available to Johns Hopkins researchers. By the 1970s, such an exchange had no connection with defense research; the chemical agents had highly specific actions and so were very interesting probes for neurochemistry research and identifying specific nerve chemical pathways. To indicate how much faculty attitudes had changed since the heyday of defense-related research in the 1950s, Silbergeld asserted that "if anybody had said to us, 'Would you like some money from the Defense Department so you could do some more work?' I think we would have run out of the room."

For example, QNB (3-quinuclidinyl benzilate) was a highly specific ligand that would bind to cholinergic receptors, and with a radioactive tag, it could be used to visualize the location of cholinergic neurons in the brain. Using such techniques to illuminate the cholinergic nervous system (which uses acetylcholine as its neurotransmitter), Goldberg and Silbergeld could examine animal brain slices or cell cultures to learn whether exposure to hazardous substances such as lead would change the system's neurochemistry. They determined whether changes had occurred by comparing the densities of receptors or pathways in the exposed versus unexposed samples.[73]

Goldberg collaborated with Silbergeld and Environmental Medicine colleague John Fales to study the effects of low-level exposure to lead, which caused hyperactivity in mice and reversed normal responses to drugs (e.g., sedatives caused excitement and stimulants had a calming effect). They connected these findings with the potential role of lead poisoning in hyperactivity and other childhood behavioral and neuromuscular disorders. Such research helped to establish lead poisoning, which previously had been studied primarily as an adult occupational hazard, as an environmental problem uniquely suited to NIEHS as distinct from other NIH institutes. Although the EPA and CDC also pursued interventions that resulted in significantly decreasing blood lead levels, NIEHS stood out for continuing to fund basic science investigations of the health effects of lead after the initial regulations had been issued.[74]

By reopening questions about the toxicity of low-level lead exposure, NIEHS research lay the groundwork for more stringent regulations, including the removal of leaded gasoline from the market. After Silbergeld completed her fellowship at JHSPH in 1975, she was appointed to head the Behavioral Neuropharmacology Unit at the National Institute of Neurological and Communicative Disorders and Stroke, where her research showed that in adults, lead poisoning resulting in muscle weakness was not caused by a direct effect on the muscle but by an interruption in neurotransmission. She also served as director of the Toxic Chemicals Program at the Environmental Defense Fund, and her 15 years of research and advocacy helped to convince federal policymakers to ban lead from gasoline after 1995. She would return to the EHS faculty in 2002.[75]

Conclusion

In the 1950s and early 1960s, federal funding for defense-related research had fostered the school's programs in lung physiology, air hygiene, radiation hazards, and environmental toxicology. Subsequently, these programs benefited from the wave of environmentalism launched by Rachel Carson and institutionalized by the Nixon administration's establishment of the EPA, OSHA, and NIEHS. National defense and environmentalism were distinct but complementary channels of influence, broadening and deepening the resources available for open-ended investigations of environmental health questions from the cellular to the population levels. Without the fears of atomic radiation that prompted the PHS to fund the Department of Radiological Science, JHSPH toxicologists would not have had the early, direct access to radioactive tracers so critical to revealing the molecular mechanisms of poisoning from lead and other heavy metals. But interest in radiation as a health hazard had waned by 1971, when Russell Morgan was appointed dean of the School of Medicine and vice-president of health services for the university. Henry Wagner took over as interim chair of Radiological Science.

The "new" environmental health was a response to two extremely daunting challenges faced by mid-twentieth-century public health: that its methods were either too weak or too powerful. Some of the most spectacular public health "miracles" had proved to be illusory, since pathogens could develop resistance over time to control agents that were initially effective. For example, widespread use of DDT had resulted in insecticide-resistant mosquitoes, overuse of chloroquine had created drug-resistant malaria strains, and heavy prescription of antibiotics led to multidrug-resistant tuberculosis and methicillin-resistant

Staphylococcus aureus (MRSA). Environmental health approaches that drew from epidemiology, population biology, and toxicology offered an alternate strategy for interrupting disease transmission, with the promise of reversing and preventing damage to both human health and the natural environment.

Even more problematic than these setbacks, however, was the degree to which the public health profession was haunted by its pre-1960 successes in controlling infectious disease with antibiotics and vaccines. After rates of formerly terrifying epidemic diseases declined to near zero and this became the new norm, American health agencies faced increasing difficulty in mobilizing public and political support for simply continuing to do the same thing. In the international context, observers ranging from Albert Sabin to Lyndon Johnson had expressed the belief that public health campaigns against disease had been "too effective," causing population growth to outpace available resources (at this juncture, few acknowledged that the less-fecund industrialized West exacted a much higher per-capita toll on natural resources). Poor countries then faced the paradox that lack of resources led to famine and civil war, which replaced infectious diseases as causes of excess mortality. Population-level family planning, as discussed in chapter 7, dovetailed with efforts to limit human environmental impact by both curtailing pollution and conserving natural resources. Environmental health research at JHSPH expanded knowledge of the health effects of pollution and environmental degradation on both humans and animals, which represented an important contribution to the broader arguments for environmentalism.

While critics of developing-world health campaigns averred that they had slashed death rates too rapidly, Ernest M. Gruenberg, chair of Mental Hygiene, opined in the *Lancet* that chronic diseases in the industrialized countries were "the new diseases of medical progress." Most forms of communicable disease, although they could spread rapidly and kill many, were still more preventable and curable than noncommunicable disease. Speaking as an epidemiologist who strove to prevent disease from ever developing, Gruenberg claimed that new treatments that arrested but did not eliminate disease, such as chemotherapy for cancer and angioplasty for heart disease, had resulted in "a new rising tide of disease and disability produced [by] well-intentioned health services." While health services researchers sought ways to expand access to medical care and to improve the functional and financial economy of health service delivery systems, Gruenberg contended that "more systematic application of [life-extending] techniques will still further raise the prevalence of disease and disability and thus heighten the need for even more medical care and social services," which he called "the failures of success." Gruenberg urged his fellow epidemiologists to redouble their efforts to find more effective preventive methods.[76]

During the 1960s, as sanitary engineering had made the transition to environmental engineering, the field had lost its traditional public health focus. At the same time, schools of public health and other research centers had deemphasized environmental engineering, particularly its subdisciplines of chemistry and physics, which in turn undermined investment in the research infrastructure needed to address "new" environmental problems posed by chemical impacts. When public concerns over environmental health reemerged in the 1980s and 1990s, these policy debates were largely divorced from their historical roots in public health, a separation that was reflected in the national, state, and local regulatory agencies responsible for enforcing environmental protection policies.[77]

Meanwhile, at JHSPH, Dean Hume had formed a schoolwide Committee on the Environment in 1972 to guide the development of new research and training programs. The committee's deliberations, together with the departure of Russell Morgan and pending retirements of Richard Riley and Cornelius Krusé, resulted in a 1976 merger of the departments of Radiological Science, Environmental Medicine, and Environmental Health to form a single Department of Environmental Health Sciences. The new department was chaired by Gareth Green. In 1978, the department's future was by no means clear. In a letter to JHSPH faculty inviting them to serve on a committee to review the field of environmental health engineering, Green wrote, "The School of Public Health and the Division of Environmental Health Engineering in particular are at a major turning point in the history of public health practice. At the moment the School is ill prepared to respond to the demands in air pollution control, industrial hygiene and safety, occupational health, toxic substances control, accident prevention and safety management, solid waste disposal and waste water management, and related areas where control technology might conceivably reduce the burden of accident and illness, morbidity and mortality in industrialized civilizations." As the next chapter will show, Gruenberg's concerns about strengthening prevention and Green's desire to reconfigure and expand his department would be substantially addressed through a close alliance between Environmental Health Sciences and Epidemiology. Through this alliance, the school's faculty made major strides toward preventing chronic disease by applying risk analysis to study and quantify the health effects of everything that human beings consumed, touched, and breathed.[78]

CHAPTER ELEVEN

Chronic Disease Epidemiology

Chronic disease epidemiology at Johns Hopkins is synonymous with two names: Abraham M. Lilienfeld and George W. Comstock, who both helped establish and propagate the field in America and globally. Lilienfeld headed the Department of Chronic Diseases from 1958 to 1970, when it was merged with the Department of Epidemiology; he then chaired Epidemiology from 1970 to 1974. Comstock had been appointed lecturer in Epidemiology in 1956 immediately after earning a DrPH under department chair Philip E. Sartwell. Comstock joined the full-time Epidemiology faculty in 1962 at the rank of professor, when he was appointed director of the PHS Training Center for Public Health Research in Hagerstown, Maryland. When Lilienfeld died in 1984, he had worked at JHSPH a total of 30 years (including his earlier stint on the Public Health Administration faculty), and Comstock taught for nearly 50 years, until shortly before his death in 2007.[1]

Lilienfeld and Comstock arrived at JHSPH at a critical moment in the late 1950s, as public health began to experience a financial and ideological crisis. The new NIH paradigm increasingly excluded public health researchers, educators, and professionals and instead privileged the life sciences, particularly molecular and cell biology. Many seasoned observers were doubtful about the overall future of public health research. In 1957, Jack Haldeman, medical director and chief of the Division of General Health Services of the Public Health Service Bureau of State Services, wrote an internally circulated paper, "Research in Public Health." His first sentence admitted that "there is general agreement that research in the science of public health has not kept pace with laboratory research in the basic sciences or with research in clinical medicine." Haldeman also attempted to answer the nagging and elusive question, "What is public health research?" proposing to define its scope and most important priorities. He identified the distinguishing feature of public health research as being oriented toward the community, "rather than to the study of an individual, an organ, a cell, or a specific disease." He also placed an emphasis on prevention and protection, with the goal of "effectively translat[ing] results from laboratory, clinical, or other forms of basic research into practical application to health problems of the community."[2]

Lilienfeld and Comstock helped drive the growth of chronic disease research at JHSPH, particularly on cancer, that would fulfill Haldeman's ideal and bridge the widening medicine–public health gap in scientific research between the NIH and the PHS. JHSPH graduates had already begun to inculcate the agencies that employed them with high-quality public health methods. The work of Robert Felix and Morton Kramer in introducing top-notch biostatistics into the NIMH was noted in chapter 2. James Watt (DrPH 1936), director of the National Heart Institute from 1952 to 1961, established epidemiology as an equal discipline administratively and conceptually within the NIH. According to cardiovascular epidemiologist Henry Blackburn, "All cardiovascular epidemiology, and much of population approaches in the other NIH institutes, comes from his having established this equality. Don't think that the heads of NIH, the elites from the laboratories and from the clinics, would give epidemiology a crumb if he hadn't fixed that into administrative policy!"[3]

This chapter continues the story in chapters 3 and 10 of the school's early work on cancer. It also traces the development of large-scale epidemiological cohort studies beginning in the 1960s, as well as the reasons for the faculty's increased attention during the 1970s to environmental epidemiology as a critical aspect of understanding cancer risk.

Chronic Disease under Lilienfeld

During the first postwar decade, the fight against chronic disease had been waged primarily by medical researchers intent on finding treatments, not public health workers focused on prevention. When JHSPH began to enter the field of chronic disease in the 1950s, it had borrowed two of the primary tools developed for fighting infectious disease. One was statistical and epidemiological surveys to establish accurate baseline rates of incidence and prevalence, such as the EHD and Commission on Chronic Illness studies. The second was diagnostic tests for mass screening programs. By 1960, the number of effective diagnostic methods was increasing. For cancer, they included the Pap smear, breast self-examination, blood tests, and X-rays. Stebbins declared in 1965 that improvements in secondary methods of prevention—early diagnosis and treatment after onset—were "undoubtedly of greater importance [than primary prevention], in terms of possible action." The mass application of modern methods of detecting and arresting chronic diseases was, "in light of our present knowledge, the most effective means at hand for the mitigation of the human, social, and economic losses resulting therefrom."[4]

Beginning in the late 1940s, Johns Hopkins radiologist Russell H. Morgan had endeavored "to simplify the x-ray procedure and to encourage mass examinations throughout the population." To detect cancer of the stomach and other abdominal organs, Morgan and his coinvestigators adapted the small-film photofluorographic methods used for mass chest X-ray exams for early detection of tuberculosis. In 1957, Stebbins initiated three major types of studies in PHA: (1) to develop and evaluate health agency programs for the early detection and treatment of chronic illness, (2) to analyze and solve problems in medical care programs, and (3) to improve rehabilitation for stroke patients. The studies were conducted in hospitals and health departments across Maryland and Virginia. One recommendation that emerged was to X-ray all patients admitted to the hospital, regardless of the precipitating cause, since "asymptomatic chronic illness may remain undetected in even the best hospitals." X-rays were among the tools used in multiphasic screening, which administered a comprehensive battery of tests to detect disease. Multiphasic screening was developed in the 1950s by the Commission on Chronic Illness (discussed in chapter 3) and further refined in the 1960s by Morris Collen at Kaiser Permanente, who used automated computing to simplify procedures and maximize efficiency. Kaiser Permanente conducted multiphasic screenings, including blood samples, on approximately 113,000 individuals in Northern California between 1964 and 1971. The blood samples were collected to create the earliest serum bank used for epidemiologic research. The serum of participants who were later diagnosed with cancer and other chronic diseases could be studied and matched with demographic and clinical data in studies designed to identify the precursors of these diseases. Other similar serum banks would be established in the early 1970s at the Johns Hopkins Training Center for Public Health Research in Hagerstown, Maryland, as well as in other locations in the United States, Norway, and Sweden.[5]

Stebbins wanted to expand the school's work in chronic disease research, which was not yet a major focus in Epidemiology under Sartwell. After renowned syphilis expert J. Earle Moore died in late 1957, Stebbins took the opportunity to offer the directorship of the Division of Chronic Diseases and a full professorship to Abe Lilienfeld, then only 37 but eminently qualified. Under Lilienfeld, Chronic Diseases both met the NIH's requirements for rigorous scientific research and retained the interdisciplinary nature and community health practice aspects of the school's earlier work in the EHD. Chronic Disease students learned the medical social work and public health nursing aspects of chronic disease along the full spectrum of prevention, treatment, and rehabilitation, which reflected Lilienfeld's goal of integrating "the clinical, epidemiological, genetic, and public health administrative aspects of chronic diseases." Courses taught methods of conducting multiphasic screening and community surveys of chronic illness, as well as administrative aspects of rehabilitative services and long-term home and hospital care.[6]

Lilienfeld's approach to chronic disease was guided by two disciplines that rose to broad influence in the 1950s: social sciences (discussed in chapter 8) and medical genetics. In 1953–1954, Lilienfeld had introduced the first JHSPH course to deal substantially with chronic disease, Human Genetics, which he taught with three eminent Hopkins geneticists, Bentley H. Glass in the Homewood Department of Biology, Barton Childs in the Department of Pediatrics, and Victor A. McKusick, head of the Division of Medical Genetics in the Department of Medicine. In 1958, with generous NIH support from the cancer, heart, and arthritis institutes, Lilienfeld and McKusick established the joint Epidemiologic and Biometrical Research Unit at the Moore Chronic Disease Clinic at Johns Hopkins Hospital. This collaboration offered specialty training to medical and public health students in clinics treating venereal disease, hypertension, collagen diseases, genetic conditions, disabilities requiring rehabilitation, sarcoidosis, and cancer.

Lilienfeld and Bernice H. Cohen (MPH 1959) played leading roles in establishing genetic epidemiology as a scientific discipline and defining its importance for public health. Cohen earned a PhD in 1958 at the School of Medicine under one of the twentieth century's most influential geneticists, H. Bentley Glass. At Lilienfeld and McKusick's urging, she enrolled for an MPH at JHSPH. With appointments in three university divisions in the departments of Epidemiology, Biology, and Medicine, Cohen served on the University Committee on Human Genetics and would later found the nation's first formal training program in genetic epidemiology at Johns Hopkins in 1979. Described by her colleagues as serious, determined, and exceptionally hardworking, Cohen was "a forceful teacher" who held her many graduate students and postdoctoral trainees to high standards.[7]

Together with Roger Herriott's research on viral DNA in the Department of Biochemistry, the Department of Chronic Disease was the birthplace of genetic research and teaching at JHSPH. Biostatisticians George M. Tallis and

Helen Abbey introduced courses in statistical genetics in the mid-1960s. With P. C. Huang in Biochemistry, Cohen and Lilienfeld edited the 1978 volume *Genetic Issues in Public Health and Medicine*, which provided medical and government decisionmakers with the first overview of the most salient genetic issues and assessed their "social, political, legal, economic, and moral-ethical impact."[8]

Lilienfeld's expertise in genetics complemented his efforts to expand cancer research across the Johns Hopkins Medical Institutions. He had left Hopkins in 1954 to become chief of statistics and epidemiology at the Roswell Park Memorial Institute of the New York State Health Department, where he continued to work closely with Morton Levin, the department's assistant commissioner for medical services. Lilienfeld's first article on cancer, published in 1955, was on the age distribution of female breast and genital cancers. The following year, he and Levin reported findings from the first retrospective controlled study of the relationship between cigarette smoking and bladder cancer, which found a significant association among males but not females. In one of the earliest surveys of socioeconomic and personality characteristics of smokers versus nonsmokers, Lilienfeld found that smokers changed jobs significantly more often than nonsmokers. He attributed the difference to neurotic traits or to psychological pressures from other causes that triggered both smoking and job changes in response. The school's faculty in Epidemiology, Behavioral Sciences, and Mental Hygiene would go on to conduct major studies of the connections among depression, smoking, and cancer in the 1970s.[9]

With Lilienfeld's return to JHSPH in 1958 to direct the Division of Chronic Diseases, the number of faculty publications on cancer research accelerated. That year, he published a *Journal of Chronic Diseases* article, "The Epidemiologic Method in Cancer Research," that would set him on the path to becoming the father of chronic disease epidemiology, particularly that of cancer. With Jerome Cornfield, chair of Biostatistics from 1958 to 1960, and others, Lilienfeld coauthored the influential 1959 review of recent evidence linking smoking and lung cancer. Lilienfeld and Cornfield called the rising lung cancer death rate in all countries "the most striking neoplastic phenomenon of this century." They determined that in diseases with a suspected link to smoking, once the incidence rate in the population is established, case-control studies can be used to estimate the relative risk of disease as a function of smoking status. In the historic 1959 review, using Bayes' rule and NIH data, Cornfield was the first to use logistic regression, which provides the odds ratio, the standard measure of excess risk of mortality. He calculated the relative risk for lung cancer among smokers, which equaled the lung cancer death rate in smokers divided by that in lifelong nonsmokers. Cornfield left Hopkins in 1960 to become chief statistician at the National Cancer Institute.[10]

JHSPH research on smoking and cancer during the 1950s culminated when Levin, Lilienfeld, Lewis C. Robbins (MPH 1938), and Surgeon General Leroy Burney, all JHSPH alumni, drafted the initial 1959 surgeon general's report on smoking and lung cancer. Levin, Lilienfeld, and Hopkins epidemiologists Raymond Seltser and Alexander Gilliam were consultants on the second, more widely publicized 1964 surgeon general's report, *Smoking and Health*. William Cochran, who was now at Harvard, was a member of the Advisory Committee to the Surgeon General. Unlike Levin, Cochran continued to smoke after he authored the 1964 report's most important chapter, "Criteria for Judgment," which laid out the rationale of "the multiple etiology of biological processes." Since not all smokers developed lung cancer, cigarette smoking was not an absolute cause in the same way that the tubercle bacillus was the invariable cause of tuberculosis infection. After two decades of collaboration with Lilienfeld, Levin would join the JHSPH Epidemiology faculty in 1967, and his testimony on the health hazards of smoking was crucial to legal victories in cases against American Tobacco in 1964 and Liggett and Myers in 1969. Stebbins and John Hume were among the many frequent visitors to the basement cigarette vending machine until 1969, when the Hygiene Advisory Board voted to discontinue cigarette sales in the building at the urging of the Johns Hopkins Medical Student Society. Yet through the 1970s, clouds of cigarette smoke were a common sight and smell in JHSPH offices, conference rooms, and classrooms, which provided ashtrays for the convenience of the school's many smokers. Even the Johns Hopkins Hospital did not become a completely smoke-free campus until July 1, 1988.[11]

Throughout his career, Lilienfeld worked closely with medical colleagues, but he ensured that Chronic Diseases also welcomed an interdisciplinary group of students and faculty from statistics, sociology, genetics, and nursing. Tieless, crewcut, and often disheveled, Lilienfeld was, in Margaret Bright's words, "an innocent, unsophisticated in a way. He was just so friendly to everybody, he did things that nobody else would do, silly things to make us relax." As chair, he settled disagreements among the faculty by loading them all into his Volkswagen bus and driving to a hotel, where he would pull out the wine and get them talking and drinking until they resolved the problem.[12]

Lilienfeld was an early opponent of discrimination on the basis of race, sex, or religion. In 1960, when there were no other African Americans on the faculty or administrative staff and very few black students, Earl Diamond in Chronic Disease hired a black research assistant. After hearing that other women on the staff had refused to eat with the new assistant in the basement cafeteria, Lilienfeld convened all the faculty and staff that afternoon and announced that the school was going to hire whoever was qualified, irrespective of race, and anyone who disagreed should submit their resignation. In 1961, Lilienfeld hired the first African-American instructor at JHSPH, Ralph J. Young (profiled in chapter 1), and also recruited George D. Miller, another early black faculty member from 1972 to 1977, recognized for his work on the Baltimore stroke mortality study.[13]

The Johns Hopkins Training Center for Public Health Research

When Lilienfeld had arrived in 1958 to direct the Division of Chronic Diseases, the Department of Epidemiology had only three full-time faculty: Sartwell, Raymond Seltser, and Howard Howe, who was about to retire. Sartwell was an expert on tuberculosis, and his department's TB program drew on Comstock and several other part-time faculty, including Russell Morgan, Miriam Brailey, Charlotte Silverman (head of epidemiology for the state health department), and Robert E. Farber (head of epidemiology for the city health department). Yet tuberculosis was held in such low regard among students that only one registered for the Epidemiology of Tuberculosis course in 1957–1958. That year, the medical school stopped requiring epidemiology.[14]

Comstock took over the Epidemiology of Tuberculosis course in 1963, and he transformed it into one of the most popular courses in the school's history. In addition to Sartwell, his DrPH adviser, Comstock traced his epidemiological lineage to Carroll Palmer, founding director of the PHS Division of Tuberculosis; Palmer, in turn, had been influenced by Frost and Reed. Comstock's studies of vaccination against tuberculosis with the bacillus Calmette-Guérin (BCG) vaccine in Muscogee County, Georgia, definitively showed that the vaccine had limited effectiveness, which helped to convince Palmer and the PHS to reject BCG vaccination in the United States. Comstock and JHSPH colleagues later conducted a 60-year follow-up of BCG's long-term efficacy, which confirmed the earlier findings.[15]

Comstock was a consummate teacher and mentor. He delighted in using an array of methods for randomizing the selection of students for class presentations, which both added a playful note and demonstrated randomization as a key principle of epidemiological research. Among the randomization props he used were a set of toy soldiers (one had the message "please discuss problem" taped under the base); fortune cookies, one with a special message placed carefully inside with tweezers before class; and walnuts with a silver nut indicating the winning student. He would reward good answers from students by tossing them a Hershey's kiss. In lab discussions of case studies and problem sets, Comstock purposefully grouped students at tables to include a variety of levels of medical training, ages, and nationalities, so that each participant could bring their own perspective to the discussion.[16]

As director of the Training Center for Public Health Research in Hagerstown, about a two-hour drive from Baltimore in Washington County, Comstock played a critical role in expanding the school's work in three main areas: the epidemiology of cancer, heart disease, and stroke; large-scale cohort studies; and community survey research and preventive health methods. Prior to 1965, relatively few JHSPH faculty were conducting cancer research. In addition to Lilienfeld's group in the Epidemiologic and Biometrical Research Unit, Radiological Science faculty used radioactive tracers to compare normal and tumor tissues and to study the mechanism of action of the antitumor drug mithramycin. Pathobiology faculty conducted studies of Rous tumor virus using blood samples and tissue cultures to examine the conversion of cells from normal to tumorous and vice versa. They also made ecological surveys in wild bird populations to study the epizoology and antigenic relationships of Rous and pox viruses in birds. In Epidemiology, Sartwell and Comstock surveyed residents of Washington County, Maryland, to determine the role of obstetric history, attitude toward the medical profession, physical condition, history of major illness and irradiation, knowledge about cancer, and knowledge of exfoliative cytology in determining participation in Pap smear screening for cervical cancer.[17]

It was not until after Lilienfeld had served as staff director of the President's Commission on Heart Disease, Cancer and Stroke that the departments of Biostatistics, Epidemiology, and Chronic Diseases began large-scale epidemiological studies of the top causes of US mortality. On October 6, 1965, Johnson signed into law the Heart Disease, Cancer, and Stroke Amendments of 1965, which authorized grants to establish cooperative regional research and training programs among schools of medicine and public health, research institutions, and hospitals, as well as for demonstration projects in patient care in the fields of heart disease, cancer, stroke, and related diseases.

Comstock was highly attuned to social and cultural factors as codeterminants of risk for chronic disease. A *Time* magazine article titled "Nice Guys Finish Last" reported on Comstock's findings from his studies of the relation of socioeconomic factors to disease in the population of Washington County. "Regular churchgoing, and the clean living that often goes with it, appear to help people avoid a whole bagful of dire ailments and disasters," including heart disease, cirrhosis of the liver, tuberculosis, cervical cancer, chronic bronchitis, fatal one-car accidents, and suicides. The health benefit that correlated most strongly with weekly church attendance was reduced rates of arteriosclerotic heart disease, which Comstock found was nearly 90 percent higher among non-churchgoers. Comstock also authored a series of articles with Epidemiology colleagues Moyses Szklo and Knud J. Helsing on the impact of bereavement and widowhood on mortality. They found that mortality rates based on person-years at risk were similar for widowed and married women but significantly higher for widowed versus married men, even after adjusting for demographic, socioeconomic, and behavioral variables. Widowed men who remarried had far lower mortality than those who did not remarry, but this difference was not observed among widowed women. Multiple regression analysis also showed that, for both sexes and independently of other factors, moving into a nursing home or other long-term care facility was associated with higher mortality than any other residential status, and living alone also increased mortality risk.[18]

In the fall of 1974, Comstock and the Johns Hopkins Training Center for Public Health Research initiated a major NCI-funded study of serologic precursors of cancer by collecting blood samples from 25,620 Washington County residents. One set of samples was stored at the Hagerstown Hospital and the other at JHSPH in Baltimore. A cancer registry was established in Washington County to determine which of the blood sample donors developed cancer. Comstock's work began just after the Third National Cancer Survey, conducted from 1969 to 1971 to provide comparison data for the two previous surveys conducted in 1937 and 1947.[19]

One purpose of the Campaign Against Cancer and Stroke study, known as Operation CLUE, was to determine whether the abnormal levels of hormones, viral antibodies, and other factors seen in victims of certain cancer antedate or follow development of the disease. The presence of serologic changes before the development of cancer would indicate an etiological relationship, and the changes might also be useful in predicting subsequent cancer in individuals, thus identifying the need for intensive follow-up. In the early 1980s, Comstock was among the first to develop a new methodology for epidemiological research, the nested case-control study. These studies are extremely time-saving and cost-effective, since they use data and samples (blood or other substances) already collected from previous prospective studies to answer new questions. Prospective studies measure possible risk factors in large numbers of persons without disease and follow them forward in time to ascertain who develops the disease or other outcomes being studied. Nested case-control studies select cases that were subsequently detected through follow-up and match them with controls who did not develop the outcome of interest. Baseline factors and analysis of stored samples are then compared between the two groups to detect associations with the outcome of interest. This clever approach mitigates the limitations of both classic prospective studies (which involve years of follow-up and are limited to the initial factors measured at baseline) and case-control studies (which entail difficulties in selecting controls and measuring risk factors after the disease or other outcome has already occurred). One of Comstock's first nested case-control studies used the CLUE samples to determine whether patients with Hodgkin lymphoma had elevated levels of antibodies to Epstein-Barr virus before they were diagnosed. He also collaborated with

Nancy Gutenson of Harvard to pool his samples with those from other prospective studies. B. Frank Polk in Epidemiology directed another very early nested case-control study. With funding from NHLBI, Polk's team used samples from the Multiple Risk Factor Intervention Trial (MRFIT) to analyze the connection between the presence of vitamins in the blood and cancer risk.[20]

In addition to social, behavioral, occupational, and environmental risk factors for chronic disease, JHSPH epidemiologists also began to evaluate the risks and effectiveness of new drugs and medical technology. Sartwell chaired the initial reports of the FDA Advisory Committee on Obstetrics and Gynecology on both oral contraceptives (1966) and intrauterine contraceptive devices (1968). Sartwell and his coauthors determined that birth control pills, which contained much higher levels of estrogen when they were first introduced in 1961 than do current oral contraceptives, were associated with an increased risk of blood clots. His work received national media coverage when the committee's findings were announced in 1970. Sartwell expressed shock at one of the study's revelations: the large amount of medication American women were taking. According to detailed lists from study participants, "it was common for a patient to have been taking several analgesics, a tranquilizer and a variety of other kinds of pills," both prescribed and over-the-counter. He doubted that the women's physicians were fully aware of the variety and speculated that unrecognized drug interactions were likely. Sartwell observed, "Drugs are used to excess in our culture. The amount of benefit and harm to a given patient from a given therapy cannot be accurately predicted; the risk-benefit ratio is a stochastic quantity. The most capable physician might be said to be the one who can most accurately estimate this ratio."[21]

After Sartwell retired in 1970, Chronic Diseases was merged with Epidemiology and Lilienfeld served as chair from 1970 to 1974. His successor was his protégé Leon Gordis (MPH 1965, DrPH 1968), an expert on the epidemiology of pediatric chronic lung diseases, prevention of adolescent pregnancy, and evaluation of health services. From 1961 to 1965, Gordis served as the PHS field officer for the Maryland state heart disease control program, and after joining the Epidemiology faculty in 1971, he directed the Epidemiology and Statistics Center of the Maryland Regional Medical Program for two years. His study concluded that use of anticoagulants after hospitalization for a heart attack reduced death rates threefold. Gordis served as chair from 1975 to 1993, with joint appointments in Pediatrics and Health Policy and Management. He named occupational health and evaluation of health services as two areas of expansion for the department, as well as greater involvement with other Hygiene departments and with Johns Hopkins Hospital clinical programs, including a training program in pediatric epidemiology.[22]

Like Lilienfeld and Comstock, Gordis was extremely dedicated to teaching and restored the epidemiology requirement in the medical undergraduate curriculum. In 1980, he secured a three-year, $675,000 grant from the Andrew W. Mellon Foundation to expand courses on clinical epidemiology for medical and public health students and residents, taught by JHSPH faculty in the Johns Hopkins Hospital's clinical setting. Gordis directed the program with Moyses Szklo (MPH 1972, DrPH 1974), an associate professor of epidemiology who headed the department's Clinical and Chronic Disease Epidemiology program. Gordis emphasized that "physicians need to become intelligent consumers of research data so that they will be able rationally to apply the findings of research to the clinical care of patients. The basic process of decision-making in clinical medicine rests on an understanding of quantitative and statistical concepts and their application to population-based data, and that's what epidemiology is all about." The grant also established a two-year clinical epidemiology fellowship program, directed by Paul Whelton and supported a research component for studies on environmental risk factors for specific diseases, the effectiveness of new therapeutic approaches, and "shoe leather" epidemiology. By 2000, Gordis had taught the Epi 1 Introductory Epidemiology course to approximately 10,000 public health and medical students.[23]

Microwaves in Moscow

Over the school's history, defense-related problems often had served as the catalyst for developing new public health tools and methods. But sometimes the process could also work in reverse: existing public health techniques could be adapted to answer a national security question. In the late 1970s, JHSPH was featured on the *CBS Evening News* and in *The New Yorker* for its role in settling a conundrum from the annals of Cold War diplomacy by marshaling its expertise in biocomputing and risk analysis.

As mentioned previously, the Department of Radiological Science had promoted the adoption of modern computing throughout the school, and the Department of Biostatistics had made fundamental contributions to the development of record linkage as a major information management tool for analyzing medical and public health records. By the early 1960s, Sartwell, Comstock, Lilienfeld, and their colleagues were using computerized record linkage to analyze large groups of hospital, clinical, and survey records for epidemiological research, such as to determine the familial occurrence of a particular disease. Along with Morgan in Radiological Science, biostatistician Alan M. Gittelsohn was a pioneer in employing sophisticated computer analysis to mine health data for information that could guide health departments toward preventing sickness and death across populations. Gittelsohn had worked for 15 years as a biostatistician for the state health departments of New York and California before he joined the Biostatistics faculty in 1964. At the federal and state levels of government, Gittelsohn had identified "significant deficiencies in the areas of information quality, trained personnel, and capabilities for mass data processing, data reduction and data analysis."[24]

The backlog of unprocessed data posed serious dangers. Gittelsohn's concerns were in line with those of Senator Hubert Humphrey, who warned that American researchers were squandering scientific capital because they lacked coordination and organization of their information. As he had with public health training grants and international health research, Humphrey advocated congressional support for the computerization of health research, and of science and engineering generally, as a strategy for maintaining intellectual and technological superiority over the Soviet Union and enabling the United States to extend humanitarian aid to its allies. He also saw the practical importance of more efficiently indexing scientific information emanating from the rapid expansion of research by government, universities, and corporations.[25]

Gittelsohn's first NIH grant application in 1964 proposed to "investigate and develop automated processes for maximizing the information derived from the state-wide registration system for births, deaths, and marriages," which would form the basis for detailed analyses of births and deaths in New York State. As an example of how Humphrey's ideas could be applied, Gittelsohn used California, where a fivefold increase in chronic pulmonary emphysema mortality during the 1950s went undetected because there was no routine analysis of trend data. The change had only become apparent through reports of increased cases by private physicians. Neither did most states undertake ongoing analyses of fetal, perinatal, infant, and early childhood mortality patterns, even though this would effectively highlight problems and suggest ways to concentrate maternal and child health program efforts. As "the most striking case in point," Gittelsohn cited the recent high-profile tragedy of an estimated 20,000 babies born with phocomelia (absence of the proximal portion of one or more limbs) to primarily European mothers who had taken the drug thalidomide to counteract morning sickness. Gittelsohn asserted that "examination of the incidence data could have led to a significant reduction in the lag between introduction of the drug and discovery of its effects." His research at JHSPH linked information on live births with childhood death records to examine the trends in the incidence of congenital malformations. He then tested the associations between these trends and concurrent environmental changes. Gittelsohn's research continued and expanded the school's significant body of research on teratology and the epidemiology of premature birth and developmental disabilities. "The surface of the prematurity problem has only been scratched," Gittelsohn declared. "Insufficient exploration has been made into the possibility of developing family data and fertility data through linking marriage and successive birth record data."[26]

With the NIH award, Gittesohn employed multidimensional frequency tabulation of the large data files to detect variations in events such as congenital malformations and fetal/neonatal mortality. By cross-referencing different types of vital records (e.g., birth records with infant mortality data, maternity records with birth records for multiple siblings) and analyzing the data with an IBM 7094 computer programmed with algorithmic languages, Gittelsohn could produce frequency tables that demonstrated linkages among the records. His research was designed to address "the inability of state health departments to efficiently and thoroughly utilize data obtained through the vital registration mechanism."[27]

Gittelsohn went on to become one of the leading experts in applying surveillance techniques to large health data sets, which provided the foundation for the National Death Index database maintained by the CDC National Center for Health Statistics (NCHS). The NCHS would evolve to allow researchers to access multiple population health data sets that link factors that influence disability, chronic disease, health care utilization, and all forms of morbidity and mortality. NCHS would link its data with other sets from the Environmental Protection Agency, Centers for Medicare and Medicaid Services, and Social Security Administration. As a measure of the exponential magnitude of change in both computing and electronic health records management, in 1982, Gittelsohn expressed gratitude for the many hours that Hygiene faculty and graduate students had devoted to assisting him with the "impossible" task of processing "three billion bytes" (3 gigabytes) of data from the original national mortality database of 21 million death records from 1968 to 1978. Nearly 40 years later, today's individual desktop computers commonly have hard drives with 1 or more terabytes of storage, about 200,000 times the storage capacity of the first hard drive introduced in 1980.[28]

Gittelsohn and Jim Tonascia led in developing the early computing software for data management in epidemiological studies and large data sets. Tonascia, with a joint appointment in Biostatistics and Epidemiology, contributed to wide-ranging research on cancer, heart and vascular disease, and the reliability of drug histories from patients versus physicians. In the late 1970s, Tonascia introduced the course Problems in Data Analysis, and he and the students served as a test site for updating SPSS statistical software (the abbreviation stood for Statistical Package for the Social Sciences, first introduced in 1968, which was the premier mainframe computer program for batch processing data on punch cards). Students and faculty wrote their own software routines and exchanged them with each other.[29]

Tonascia and Gittelsohn's students were the first generation at JHSPH to use computers to process data for their dissertations. At the end of the day, students would bring their boxes of punch cards to the card-reading machines on the second and third floors and get in line to read in their jobs. The next morning, they went to pick up their printout from the mainframe in the basement of the medical school's Turner Building. One of Tonascia's early students, David Celentano, remembered how unforgiving the early computer programs were. "You knew there was a problem when your printout was only three pieces of paper. Because obviously the job had failed, because you left out a semicolon or a comma or something. I would often go for two weeks without getting anything done, because I kept having little tiny errors."[30]

The Department of Biostatistics had a long track record of consulting for an array of public and private organizations as well as for Hopkins faculty across the university. As Biostatistics chair Alan Ross observed, "Statisticians need regular contact with the substance of scientific inquiry if they are to maintain their technical skills." Frequently, consulting problems contained "statistical aspects that deserve[d] attention on their own merits, either within the context of the client's problem, or, occasionally, as statistical problems to be abstracted and analyzed with more generality." Many of the department's faculty publications and student theses traced their origins to consultation problems, often those primarily of interest to national security agencies. Hopkins biostatisticians channeled their passion for good data by developing and applying techniques that extracted maximum information from the data. The department's strengths dealt with strategies and tactics for assessing and clarifying relationships among variables that expressed observable environmental, population, and biomedical characteristics.[31]

Gittelsohn and Tonascia found a golden opportunity to put their software to work when the US State Department requested JHSPH to conduct a massive evaluation of the health risks associated with microwave exposure. In 1953, the Soviet Union had begun beaming low-intensity, nonionizing microwave radiation at the US embassy in Moscow. The State Department was aware of and monitoring the levels of radiation, but in mid-1975, the levels and duration began to increase, reaching 18 microwatts per square centimeter for up to 20 hours per day (still much lower, however, than the 100,000 microwatts per square centimeter that had been associated with the risk of developing cataracts). The embassy installed screens on the exterior windows that blocked most of the radiation, but when the embassy's employees were informed of the problem, many became alarmed and wanted to leave Moscow. The US Senate Foreign Relations Committee created a subcommittee to investigate concerns over whether microwave exposure had caused health problems for Moscow embassy personnel and their families, including offspring born after the exposure occurred. To answer this question, the State Department contracted with JHSPH to conduct a comprehensive study led by Lilienfeld. The project warranted an enormous two-issue story in December 1976 in *The New Yorker* by Paul Brodeur, the first journalist to write extensively on the health hazards of microwaves.[32]

Lilienfeld and coinvestigators Charlotte Libauer and Susan Tonascia, both research associates in Epidemiology, examined 13,000 US State Department employees and their families. Some had been exposed to microwave radiation at the US embassy in Moscow between 1953 and 1976, and the rest were controls who had worked or lived near eight other Eastern European embassies. Tonascia directed the data analysis of records such as death certificates, medical records, and health questionnaires. In only eight months, he wrote 100 computer programs to manage the study and another 50 for data analysis. The final computer printout produced a 12-foot stack of 8,000 pages. On June 27, 1977, and again on November 20, 1978, Walter Cronkite reported on the *CBS Evening News* that the Johns Hopkins study had definitively shown that there had been no statistically significant differences in the cancer rates or other health outcomes for exposed versus nonexposed State Department employees, but some former Moscow embassy employees remained unconvinced.[33]

Although Lilienfeld's team had concluded that low-level microwaves were not hazardous, others from JHSPH would, more than three decades later, warn of risks associated with another ubiquitous source of low-frequency nonionizing radiation: cell phones. Lilienfeld's postdoctoral fellow, Devra Lee Davis (MPH 1982), published *Disconnected* (2014) on the hazards of cell phone radiation. Davis, a leading environmental health advocate, author, and policy adviser, also wrote *When Smoke Ran Like Water: Tales of Environmental Deception and the Battle against Pollution* (2002), a National Book Award–nominated memoir about the 1948 toxic fog that descended on her hometown outside Pittsburgh. Jonathan Samet, chair of Epidemiology from 1994 to 2008, chaired a committee of physicians and scientists established in 2011 by the International Agency for Research on Cancer that concluded that long-term cell phone use that involves close contact with radiofrequency electromagnetic fields may increase the risk of glioma, a malignant type of brain cancer, and tumors of the inner ear. To date, most major health agencies, including the NCI, have ruled that existing evidence is inconclusive and further study of the question is warranted.[34]

Johns Hopkins epidemiologists conducted many other studies on the potential risks of various types of higher frequency ionizing radiation, which contain enough energy to charge an atomic particle. In a novel connection of the school's research interests on smoking, lead poisoning, radiation, and environmental health, Edward P. Radford in Environmental Medicine had conducted studies in the 1960s that detected the presence of radioactive polonium 210 in tobacco that made its way into the lungs of smokers. He built on this research to propose a new theory on how smoking caused lung cancer, featured on the *NBC Evening News* in 1974. He blamed radioactive lead dust that settled from the environment onto tobacco leaves and was then inhaled by smokers. Radford was an expert on radiation and environmental hazards who headed the Maryland state siting committee on nuclear power plants. Shortly after the Three Mile Island nuclear plant near Middletown, Pennsylvania, partially melted down in March 1979, Radford chaired a committee of the National Academy of Sciences that released initial findings that 0.5 percent of Americans would develop cancer during their lifetimes from manufactured sources of radiation such as power plants and X-rays. The nuclear power industry contested the report, which was used by the EPA to update its radiation protection standards after Three Mile Island, the most serious commercial nuclear plant accident to date. Moreover, the 21-member committee was deeply divided, which caused such bitter public acrimony that the Academy withdrew the report and issued a revised paper the next year. It replaced Radford's model, showing risk existed, albeit small, even at the lowest levels of exposure, with another model that established a threshold below which there was no harm.[35]

Other JHSPH faculty and alumni, as well as later studies by other scientific bodies, upheld Radford's ideas on radiation risk. Beginning in 1958, Sartwell and Raymond Seltser were among the first researchers to raise awareness of risks associated with overexposure to X-rays for patients and health professionals. They subsequently teamed with JHSPH epidemiologist Genevieve Matanoski to publish their updated findings in 1975. Lilienfeld had worked in the mid-1950s with Irvin D. J. Bross, director of biostatistics at the Roswell Park Memorial Institute in New York. Bross, like Radford, ran afoul of the nuclear industry and warned stridently against the health hazards of even low-level X-rays. In a congressional hearing regarding the Department of Energy's decision to cut funding for his study of the hazards of low-level radiation, Bross charged that "Big Science was committed to the Big Lie that 'Low level radiation is harmless,' in order to protect the weapons testing program from the furor over fallout."[36]

Even Russell Morgan later admitted that there were better ways to prevent cancer than X-raying everyone admitted to a hospital. Ironically, although he had promoted X-rays as a key aspect of multiphasic screening in the 1940s and 1950s, he shifted during the 1960s to *reducing* unnecessary exposure to X-rays and other radiation as a potential health hazard. X-ray screening pointed to a larger crisis of confidence in mass diagnostic tests, including the decline of multiphasic screening programs due to objections from physicians and the public. Computerized multiphasic screening had been held up as an effective method of both preventing disease and reducing treatment costs, but by the end of the 1970s, multiphasic screening was criticized for its large initial and continuing operating expenses, as well as its impersonal nature and patients' fears of computer errors. Even the less dangerous mass screening tests, such as the blood test for syphilis that became a standard requirement for marriage licenses, were later proven to be wasteful in light of the comparatively tiny number of infections they detected. Lilienfeld noted in 1980 that cytological screening programs (i.e., routine Pap smears) had possibly contributed to the decline in uterine cancer mortality, but he also acknowledged that "the evidence for the efficacy of these programs is by no means clear," since the decline could also have been explained by the simultaneous increase in the frequency of hysterectomies.[37]

In 1976, Bross harshly criticized the American Cancer Society's mass mammography screening program for women under 50, citing a 1972 article coauthored by Lilienfeld on diagnostic radiation as a factor in the epidemiology of adult leukemia. Gordis would chair a 1997 NCI panel that concluded, after an exhaustive study, that the evidence did not support routine screening mammography for women in their 40s. Although the panel's advice was not heeded at the time, in October 2015, the American Cancer Society upheld the 1997 recommendations when it revised its guidelines to balance the benefits of screening the groups at greatest risk with the potential harms of unnecessary radiation and false-positive results.[38]

Conclusion

In the last years of his career before his death in 1984, Lilienfeld focused on understanding the causality of so-called weak associations where the risk was relatively small, less than twofold, but the exposure or risk factor was present in a large proportion of the population. He studied the effects of confounding factors and interviewee/interviewer bias, as well as ways of strengthening the sensitivity of measurement and risk assessment, particularly in determining carcinogenicity. In 1980, he summarized his thinking in an overview chapter for a textbook on cancer epidemiology. Past epidemiological studies had focused on determining the relationships between cancer and broad population characteristics such as socioeconomic status and individual behaviors and lifestyle. Within these broadly identified groups, researchers had targeted specific categories of etiological factors to develop specific hypotheses about their role in the epidemiological distribution of different types of cancer. But even weak associations could have a major impact if they were distributed across a large enough population group. Lilienfeld emphasized that the epidemiological data from these studies "strongly suggest that *a vast majority of cancers, approximately 75% to 80%, result from etiological factors in the environment.*"[39]

A primary example of the importance of environmental risk was mortality from lung cancer, which had increased during the twentieth century to become the most common fatal cancer in men. "When such a marked increase occurs during such a short period of time," Lilienfeld wrote, "it strongly indicates that an agent introduced into the environment of the exposed population has been the major factor responsible for the increase. Genetic factors cannot be responsible for a marked increase within a short period of time." He surmised that the marked decline in gastric cancer mortality was also probably primarily environmental. Since lifestyle and environmental factors varied among countries, Lilienfeld called for additional international comparative studies to better understand the underlying causes of differences in incidence and mortality for cancer. He cautioned that epidemiologists must be careful to rule out artificial differences resulting from data-collecting errors in causes of death and census surveys of populations. Solving such problems had long been the focus of efforts by the JHSPH Department of Biostatistics to improve the quality of data collection and analysis in contexts ranging from the Eastern Health District to the International Classification of Diseases to the Commission on Chronic Illness. Lilienfeld also noted that studies of international migrants could be useful in determining the relative importance of environmental versus genetic factors in various types of cancer by comparing mortality data in the migrants' country of origin versus their new country. Lilienfeld and his departmental colleagues Morton Levin and Irving I. Kessler compared cancer mortality in foreign-born US residents versus rates in their countries of origin for 1959–1961 and found that migrants' death rates approximated those of the United States, "suggesting that changes in the environment and/or living habits are of etiologic importance." Within the United States, mortality from gastric cancer and leukemia showed marked regional differences.[40]

By the late 1970s, Comstock had shown a similar shift in emphasis toward environmental hazards. He examined drinking water as a logical source of both risks and remedies for chronic disease. With his doctoral student John R. Wilkins (DrPH 1978) in Environmental Health Sciences, Comstock analyzed 31,000 residents of Washington County, Maryland, to determine sex- and site-specific cancer incidence rates with reference to age, socioeconomic status, smoking history, and source of home drinking water. The study identified three historical cohorts that had each experienced a different degree of exposure to chloroform and other chlorination by-products. Adjusting for the influence of the other factors, the cohort that grew up drinking chlorinated surface water had higher rates of cancer of the bladder in men and the liver in women than the cohort that had drunk unchlorinated ground water.[41]

Comstock also examined the relationship between heart disease and mineral content in drinking water. If cardiovascular disease mortality was even slightly elevated by a component of drinking water, he reasoned, altering its composition could prolong many lives. Comstock emphasized that water treatment, since it was applied at the community level, had proven to be more effective and less expensive than preventive health measures that had to be administered to individuals. In a review of two decades of the literature positing water composition as an explanation for geographic variance in death rates from heart disease, he concluded in 1978 that "the association between water hardness and cardiovascular disease seems unlikely to be directly causal. Indirect causality, or direct causality only under certain conditions, are better possibilities." Comstock had discussed his work with Abel Wolman, who praised its relevance to David A. Hamburg, president of the Institute of Medicine. Comstock's report for the National Research Council US National Committee for Geochemistry, Wolman wrote, could help guide the Environmental Protection Agency's efforts to determine collateral issues and standards for drinking water. It was also "highly important to the thousands of water purveyors in the U.S. and throughout the rest of the world."[42]

During the 1970s, innovations in computing and toxicology had driven the rapid expansion of research on the epidemiological links between cancer and environmental health at JHSPH and nationally. But as JHSPH toxicologists were beginning to make bold claims about the hazards of a growing list of chemicals and manmade substances, some of their colleagues were working to refute such claims. According to Wolman, the EPA had "jumped the gun epidemiologically" regarding the potential link between chloroform-like halogens or trihalomethanes and cancer. With little epidemiological evidence, on the basis of animal testing alone, the EPA had issued a directive that by 1981, drinking water levels of these substances must be fewer than 100 parts per billion. Wolman criticized the EPA directive's universal application despite the great variations in conditions across the United States and also charged that "verification of its public health significance is still non-existent, or certainly belated."[43]

Ironically, this was the same era when the NCI was facing mounting public criticism that it had allowed the American Cancer Society too much influence over research grant policy, and therefore, the NCI was neglecting the environmental aspects of cancer research except for cigarette smoking. But Wolman emphasized that "regulatory agencies may do more damage by insistence on speed, and on what they consider to be the Delaney Amendment intent [which required the U.S. Food and Drug Administration to ban any food additives that were known to cause cancer in humans or animals], than actual standards warrant." As proof, Wolman cited the work of JHSPH epidemiologist Irving Kessler, who in 1978 was among the first to refute the alleged connection between bladder cancer and the artificial sweeteners saccharine and cyclamate.[44]

More recent assessments of the evolution of federal environmental health policy and operational strategy reflect Wolman's concerns. Bernard D. Goldstein, chair of Environmental Health Sciences at the University of Pittsburgh, has criticized "the command-and-control approach" using regulatory dictates to decrease major sources of end-of-pipe air and water emissions. This "relatively inflexible, legalistic approach" was highly successful in cleaning up visible air and water pollution, but it did not answer the need for more sophisticated approaches to manage pollution from indoor sources (which, as JHSPH researchers successfully demonstrated in the 1990s, cause worse health effects than ambient sources) or other forms of pollution that are difficult or impossible to centrally control. "Meeting these new challenges," Goldstein wrote, "requires a public health approach, including an enhanced scientific capability to measure exposure in the target human or ecosystem rather than at the end of the pipe, a better understanding of the relation between external dose and target organ toxicity, and translation of advances in analytical chemistry and molecular biology to develop better biological indicators of exposure, effect, and susceptibility."[45]

One of the main solutions to these problems was the development of molecular biomarkers in the 1980s by JHSPH scientists. Since toxicogenomics was a subfield of molecular biology with strong public health elements, many programs were based in schools of public health. At JHSPH, the Department of Radiological Science's strengths in radiobiology and radiochemistry fundamentally shaped the school's work on the genomics of environmental health. Beginning in the 1970s, the new genomics were applied to discovering the underlying causes of small risks in large populations. More recently, coupling genomics (the study of genetic material such as DNA) with proteomics (the study of proteins) and metabolomics (the study of metabolites, or the chemical traces left behind by specific cellular processes) has enabled public health scientists to decipher cause-and-effect relationships in new ways.[46]

The departments of Epidemiology, Radiological Science, Environmental Medicine, and Pathobiology had all made early contributions to the technology-driven science of epigenetics. One of the field's groundbreaking discoveries was on the role of aflatoxin B1 in the development of liver cancer. John D. Groopman, who joined the EHS faculty in 1989 and chaired the department from 1993 to 2011, conducted in-depth human and animal studies on the intake, excretion, and metabolism of aflatoxin, a by-product of the fungi *Aspergillus flavus* and *Aspergillus parasiticus* in corn and nuts. Groopman was later

joined by EHS faculty member Thomas Kensler, and their work was fundamental to developing biomarker technology to assess exposure to environmental health risks. Applying these biomarkers to human populations demonstrated
a strong relationship between hepatitis B virus exposure and aflatoxin in the
development of liver cancer, where individuals who are both positive for the
virus and exposed to aflatoxin are 60 times more likely to develop liver cancer
than those who are positive for the virus but unexposed to aflatoxin. Groopman and Kensler's work paralleled that of their colleague Keerti Shah in the
Department of Immunology and Infectious Diseases, who linked another virus, human papillomavirus (HPV), with cervical cancer, also using the combination of intensive epidemiological fieldwork, clinical trials, and powerful
laboratory methods of analysis. Cervical cancer is the only major human cancer with a single infectious cause, the discovery of which led to the development of a vaccine recommended for adolescents since 2006. Toxicologists and
virologists have traditionally focused on the effects of chemicals and microorganisms on human health, but epigenomics is now capable of tracing the roots
of those adverse effects in human populations to discover the causal agents.
Groopman, Kensler, and Shah's work revisits the blurred boundaries between
infectious, chronic, and environmental categories of disease that were so characteristic of Lilienfeld and Comstock's careers as well as those of the school's
early faculty, such as Wade Frost, Kenneth Maxcy, Anna Baetjer, Fred Bang,
and J. Earle Moore.[47]

CHAPTER TWELVE

Federal Funding and Its Discontents

JHU president Milton Eisenhower had declared in 1957, "Federal funds do not and should not finance the broad program of the University." Despite this conviction, within seven years government agencies supplied 47 percent of all revenues at Johns Hopkins University, not including indirect costs or the federally sponsored Applied Physics Lab. In the School of Hygiene, government grants and contracts dwarfed all other income sources. By contrast, government grants provided only 58 percent of the medical school's $22.2 million in 1965–1966 nonclinical revenues, with another 24 percent from private gifts and the remainder from endowment income and tuition. Eisenhower observed that federal project grants to investigators at Hopkins had resulted in "a tendency toward haphazard, unplanned growth," which removed control of the school's future development from the faculty and made it subject to the federal grant-making process. Between 1962 and 1970, JHSPH created eight new departments, largely with federal grants; during the following seven years, 10 of the school's departments underwent mergers to form four departments, resulting in a net gain of only two departments (tables 12.1 and 12.2).[1]

TABLE 12.1
JHSPH Departments with Largest Budgets

1960	1970	1980
Pathobiology	Pathobiology	Environmental Health Sciences
Chronic Disease	Medical Care and Hospitals	Epidemiology
Environmental Medicine	Radiological Science	Health Services Administration

TABLE 12.2
Changes in JHSPH Departmental Structure

Funding Source	Department	Year Created	Type of Change	Year	Resulting Department
NIH	Biochemistry	1917	None		Biochemistry
NIH	Biostatistics	1917	None		Biostatistics
NIH, USAID	Pathobiology	1955	None		Pathobiology
Children's Bureau, NIH	Maternal and Child Health	1961	Renamed Population and Family Health in 1967, then split	1970	Population Dynamics / Maternal and Child Health
NIH	Mental Hygiene	1961	None		Mental Hygiene
NIH	Chronic Diseases	1961	Merged with Epidemiology	1970	Epidemiology
PHS, NIH	Radiological Science	1961	Merged with Environmental Health and Environmental Medicine	1976	Environmental Health Sciences
USAID	International Health	1967	None		International Health
	Behavioral Sciences	1967	None		Behavioral Sciences
PHS	Medical Care and Hospitals	1969	Merged with Public Health Administration	1976	Health Services Administration

Federally Fueled Growth in Funding and Enrollment

Throughout the 1960s, the Association of Schools of Public Health convinced Congress to steadily increase Hill–Rhodes formula and project grants for teaching, which enabled almost 60 percent of public health graduates to receive traineeships during the 1960s and 1970s. Schools of public health thus enjoyed an early lobbying success well in advance of most other fields of higher education, including medicine. The Association of American Medical Colleges did not establish a strong legislative program until 1969, when it moved its national headquarters from Evanston, Illinois, to Washington, DC. Using Hill–Rhodes as a template, Congress authorized a broad spectrum of medical education and training programs for all categories of health professionals, including facilities construction and student scholarship and loan programs under the 1963 Health Professions Educational Assistance Act, 1964 Nurse Training Act, 1965 Regional Medical Programs Act, 1966 Allied Health Professions Personnel Training Act, 1968 Health Manpower Act, and 1971 Comprehensive Health Manpower Act. Yet when Columbia's dean of public health, Ray E. Trussell, met with federal representatives of the Bureau of the Budget in 1967, he complained that they "knew very little about the schools of public health and got very little information from the Public Health Service." Neither did the staff of the new Division of Allied Health Manpower in the Bureau of Health Manpower understand what the schools were doing. Stebbins remarked in the JHSPH annual report that 1967–1968 had been "a year marked by an abrupt shift of priorities in the Federal Government and the rude awakening of the Health professions to the fact that the 'honeymoon is over.' "[2]

During the 1960s, the health sector of the US economy increased from $25 to $60 billion, a 30 percent increase in the share of gross national product. The year 1968 marked a major political and administrative turning point for all health-related federal agencies, particularly the PHS. Senator Lister Hill retired after 14 years as chair of the Labor and Public Welfare Committee and the Health Appropriations Subcommittee. Another important patron of federal medical research, Rhode Island Congressman John E. Fogarty, died. In addition, the 1968 reorganization of the Department of Health, Education, and Welfare separated the NIH from the PHS as an independent agency. The PHS also transferred to the Food and Drug Administration its traditional duties of protecting milk, shellfish, food, and water, as well as promoting sanitary practices in interstate transportation and food establishments. Although the 1968 Radiation Health and Safety Act created a new PHS Bureau of Radiation Health, it was also transferred to the FDA only three years later. After passage of the 1970 Clean Air Act and President Nixon's executive order establishing the Environmental Protection Agency, the remaining environmental health functions of the PHS were shifted to EPA. During the 1970s, HEW's leadership underwent constant turnover with six secretaries and five assistant secretaries for Health and Scientific Affairs.[3]

These changes hit with particular force at Johns Hopkins, the top federal grant recipient among schools of public health. By 1970, the Hill–Rhodes federal traineeships had increased to nearly $500,000 annually, which had expanded JHSPH enrollment by 160 percent since 1960. Yet the school's endowment had increased only 20 percent, versus 58 percent for the university.

During this decade, JHSPH annual expenditures had ballooned by 460 percent, compared to 330 percent across the university. The school's own 10-year plan acknowledged that lack of hard support for faculty was "a major weakness," since JHSPH had been unable to muster sufficient long-term nongovernmental general support "to guarantee a continued high quality of instruction to all our students." With 86 percent of JHSPH revenue from federal sources versus 53 percent for the university, the school's leadership declared, "It is obvious that such dependence on Federal funds, a large portion of which are derived from restricted grants, jeopardizes the ability of the School to maintain its independence in the establishment of its own academic priorities. If it is to remain an independent, private institution, a more favorable ratio of unrestricted, private support to public funding must be secured." Dean Hume set the goal of increasing the endowment and private gifts by $1 million annually to provide at least 25 percent of revenues, a target that has never been reached even after nearly half a century of expanding the school's development efforts.[4]

In early 1969, JHSPH's long-range plan predicted drastic changes in curriculum during the next 10 years. Instead of the majority of graduates receiving the MPH degree, "the generalist degree is losing its value and appeal for the U.S. student. On the other hand, the increasing desire of the new generation of medical students to become involved with the community will make the School of Hygiene and Public Health an increasingly popular base for postgraduate and residency training." As predicted, the demand for graduate and postgraduate training increased, but the MPH would remain the flagship degree for US students, despite periodic announcements of its imminent demise. The school proposed to develop "a true core curriculum which will become the responsibility of a single faculty group which will include representatives of each of the disciplines now contributing to the teaching program for MPH students." Not until July 1976, however, did Dean Hume appoint a Committee to Reexamine the Organization of Research and Teaching of Administration, charged with developing a core curriculum in administration in collaboration with the departments of Mental Hygiene, International Health, Maternal and Child Health, and Population Dynamics. The MPH curricula remained in flux throughout the 1970s, and this major handicap was not solved until after Dean D. A. Henderson appointed a full-time director and an advisory committee to reorganize the MPH program in 1980.[5]

The half century from 1960 to 2010 was characterized by the dramatic growth of American higher education, measured by total enrollments, degrees granted, and expenditures. The period was notable for the comparatively greater growth of bachelor's and master's versus doctoral programs, as well as public versus private institutions. The health sciences were among the fastest-growing

disciplines, and federal sponsorship fueled the expansion of public health doctoral programs through both individual research fellowships and departmental
training grants. By 1970, US schools of public health awarded one-third of
all doctoral degrees in the health professions. Traditionally, schools of public
health had conferred either the DrPH for physician administrators or the ScD
for scientists. These degrees had grown out of the longstanding connection between schools of medicine and public health, since most schools of public
health established before World War II had begun as departments within
medical schools. By 1968, Yale remained the only public health degree program
housed in a medical school department, and schools of public health were becoming more interdisciplinary. The PhD would eclipse the traditional public
health doctoral degrees by the mid-1970s, when doctoral enrollment reached
18 percent of the total at schools of public health nationwide.[6]

New PhD programs strengthened intramural relationships between schools
of public health and schools of nursing, dentistry, allied health professions,
liberal arts, sciences, and engineering. During the 1960s, JHSPH expanded its
cooperative interdisciplinary programs with the Homewood departments to
include social science and public health, comprehensive health planning, environmental health studies, and population studies. Between 1960 and 1980, the
school's overall enrollment increased sixfold and doctoral enrollment increased
tenfold, with doctoral students comprising a majority by 1970. Johns Hopkins
had always led in producing public health doctoral graduates, and in 1983,
JHSPH still awarded 20 percent of all doctoral degrees granted by the 23 US
schools of public health.[7]

As PHS traineeships became the leading sponsor of graduate public health
students, student bodies at all schools of public health changed accordingly.
Schools of public health became more like graduate schools and less like
professional schools, and enrollments of health professionals from medicine,
dentistry, and nursing steadily declined. An ASPH survey of all new public
health students who enrolled between 1974 and 1978 found that nearly half had
no prior health-related experience of any kind. Only about one-quarter of students had prior academic specialization in the health sciences, including
roughly 10 percent in medicine or dentistry and another 10 percent in nursing.
Between 1950 and 1970, the proportion of physicians in the entering MPH
classes at all schools dropped from 41 percent to 19 percent, and by 1974–1975,
they represented less than 5 percent of public health students at the largest
school, the University of Michigan. Among public health applicants, however,
one in five was a foreign physician. To encourage more US physicians to enroll,
many schools initiated joint MD–MPH programs with medical schools, which
benefited from generous federal stipends supported by the NIH Medical Scientist Training Program launched in 1964.[8]

The feminization of public health graduate programs during the 1960s and 1970s was driven by the growing number of schools established at state universities, which enrolled proportionally and numerically more women than did private schools of public health, and by the rapid expansion of health services administration, which by 1987–1988 produced nearly 60 percent of all graduate public health degrees awarded by all types of schools (nursing and engineering as well as public health). JHSPH's elite graduate program in nurse–midwifery and its degree offerings in health services research and administration attracted more women, who comprised a majority of the school's graduates for the first time in 1981 (yet as late as the mid-1970s, the school's main building had far fewer restrooms for women than for men).[9]

The number of women had begun to rise in public health before most other fields of graduate education. In US higher education generally, the gender ratio for master's and bachelor's degrees tipped to favor women beginning in 1982 and has since only increased. By 2008–2009, one-third more women than men received bachelor's degrees, and 44 percent more women than men received master's degrees. For doctoral degrees, however, the ratio was just the opposite, with 44 percent more men than women recipients. In schools that awarded master's degrees in health fields, the gender ratio of master's degrees had long favored women and had begun to favor female doctoral graduates by 1983–1984. In 1968–1969, one-third of graduate public health degrees were awarded to women, but females did not outnumber males until 1978–1979. By 1987–1988, schools of public health graduated half again as many women as men at both the master's and doctoral levels; in health services administration programs, the ratio was even higher.[10]

Thus, by the 1970s, the student bodies in schools of public health were younger and more heavily female; had less professional experience; were less likely to come from health professional backgrounds, especially medicine; and were more likely to pursue doctoral degrees, especially the PhD.

The NIH and Schools of Public Health

As more new schools of public health opened their doors during the 1960s, their deans and faculty looked optimistically to the NIH, which had fueled the rapid postwar growth of medical schools. The PHS and NIH (which remained a PHS subdivision until 1968) recognized that the medical and public health workforce needed far more chronic disease specialists in fields such as oncology, cardiology, rehabilitation, biostatistics, and epidemiology, and the schools of medicine and public health at Johns Hopkins received a significant share of federal institutional training grants in these fields. In 1954, only five doctoral and two Master of Science students had been enrolled in the Department of Biostatistics at Johns Hopkins, the country's oldest and strongest department. That year, JHSPH received PHS grants to establish a new Division of Chronic Diseases and to increase the number of students and strengthen the faculty in Biostatistics.[11]

Schools of agriculture such as those at North Carolina State, Iowa State, and the University of Wisconsin had established many of the early departments of statistics and also initially dominated the field of genetics. Raymond Pearl and William G. Cochran were both highly trained in experimental agriculture and Lowell Reed in mathematical statistics, but none of the three chairs of Biostatistics during its first 40 years had any formal training or experience in public health before coming to Johns Hopkins. Through the 1960s, Hopkins and other schools of public health still recruited many of their faculty from outside public health with expertise in statistics or other readily applied fields such as industrial management and toxicology. Charles Rohde recalled that when he arrived at JHSPH in 1964 to begin a postdoctoral fellowship, "Biostatistics and statistics in those days were not at all interested in public health. We were statisticians, every one of us. Almost no one [on the faculty] had a degree in biostatistics, except for Helen Abbey," who had studied with Reed, Merrell, and Cochran.[12]

In 1962, the NIH Division of General Medical Sciences began to award general research support grants to schools of medicine, dentistry, osteopathy, and public health, which provided unrestricted funds for research training and faculty support in the sciences basic to health. The NIH also established Research Career awards to provide stable incomes for research personnel and free them from dependence on short-term grants. These new initiatives resulted from criticisms that categorical research funding was undermining the essential teaching missions of health professional schools and also from medical research manpower studies that called for a doubling of scientific personnel between 1962 and 1970. During the 1960s, the Department of Biostatistics received 50 or more unsolicited employment requests every year from academic, industrial, and government sources.[13]

As a member of the NIH Training Committee on Epidemiology and Biometry from 1960–1963 and its chair in 1972–1973, Biostatistics chair Allyn W. Kimball was instrumental in expanding federal support for biostatistics graduate programs in schools of public health. Before Kimball became chair, the biostatistics training grant had provided only $18,000 annually for the first six years, but in 1962, the grant jumped to $132,500 and had reached $171,000 by 1966–1967. The grant supported five master's, 10 doctoral, and two postdoctoral students, as well as portions of the salaries for 12 teaching faculty and three secretaries. These funds enabled Kimball to recruit a strong group of faculty to expand the department, including David Duncan, George M. Tallis, Miles Davis, Alan M. Gittelsohn, Richard Royall, and two faculty who became department chairs, Alan Ross and Charles Rohde. Since biostatistics was not in and of itself a lucrative field for research grants, the NIH training grant ensured a secure base for the department's expansion and enabled faculty to focus on teaching advanced graduate students.[14]

The NIH's decision to terminate its biometry training grants program in 1974 was particularly devastating for the Department of Biostatistics, which had little external research support. Alan Ross warned Dean John Hume, "There is no question that Biostatistics is in for serious financial difficulties and probably some painful adjustments." A 1978 departmental self-study confirmed Ross's prediction. At their height, NIH training grants had supported 18 students and provided $80,000 annually in salary support. As scholarships dried up, the quality of students in Biostatistics noticeably declined, and the number of full-time PhD students dropped from 20 in 1973–1974 to only four in 1977–1978, even as doctoral enrollments at the school were at an all-time high. The gutting of the PhD program would rob faculty of valuable assistance in carrying out research, grading papers, and providing laboratory instruction for service courses. The self-study called the acute shortage of full-time students "the most serious limitation in operation of this department. . . . Without sufficient tuition and stipend funds, we cannot attract and keep superior students. The brisk job market for our graduates shows no signs of diminishing." The report predicted a shift from PhD toward master's students, but the department could only survive the contraction in numbers, and funds "provided that a few high caliber, full-time students can be attracted and retained in the PhD program."[15]

Even as NIH support for academic research and training programs was waning, the pipeline could not keep pace with federal and private-sector needs for graduates in the high-demand areas of biostatistics and epidemiology, who provided crucial expertise for designing chronic disease research protocols and analyzing the complex, voluminous results of population studies. A congressional investigation of the NIH in 1976 even acknowledged that "epidemiology has produced most of the research findings indicating the cause of chronic disease." The investigation focused attention on the shortage of epidemiologists in "almost all the important disease areas" and recommended that NIH administrators take "vigorous action to foster epidemiological resources and epidemiological research." Notwithstanding the success of the most well-known NIH-funded epidemiological study, the Framingham Study of coronary artery disease, the congressional report described NIH funding for epidemiology as "pitifully small." And despite the stated enthusiasm of the various NIH directors, few institutes had viable epidemiology programs, which some blamed on the difficulty of recruiting epidemiologists.[16]

These criticisms harkened back to Wade Hampton Frost's 1923 observation that "our knowledge of infectious disease has become somewhat unbalanced, relatively more complete on the experimental than the epidemiological side; and that there is urgent need at present to build up the more detailed epidemiological knowledge which is necessary to make the experimentally established principles more directly applicable to practical prevention." The NIH—and its favorite grantee, the Johns Hopkins School of Medicine—had piled on a great deal of the experimental weight that had tipped the balance against practically applied epidemiological knowledge. At the same time, Lilienfeld criticized what he saw as some of the downsides of epidemiologists' intense involvement in NIH research and clinical trials. In a 1984 article in *Public Health Reports*, he reflected that epidemiology always had been closely linked with the public health movement and health policy, but in the past 30 years (the period of NIH ascendancy), there had been "a general tendency for epidemiology to ignore its natural and historical relationship with public health, and much health policy has tended to ignore the need for epidemiologic consideration."[17]

In addition to sponsoring federal training grants and fellowships, the NIH powerfully shaped the development of public health research at Johns Hopkins. In many respects, NIH-sponsored growth conformed schools of public health to a medical model, yet in the cases of biostatistics and chronic disease epidemiology, public health faculty succeeded in infusing some of the largest NIH institutes with distinctly prevention and population-based perspectives. As the largest sponsor of research at JHSPH from 1960 to 1980, the NIH profoundly influenced the size, structure, and agendas of the school's departments. Even in departments not traditionally oriented toward laboratory investigation, NIH R01 grants to individual researchers substantially expanded clinical and basic science activities. Prior to 1970, Mental Hygiene and Population Dynamics had received NIH grants for training programs but little for research; after 1970, the NIH became a major funding source for both departments.

NIH funding guided the outcome of administrative realignments within the school and pushed "soft science" departments such as Mental Hygiene and Population Dynamics toward basic science and clinical research. This shift in Population Dynamics was promoted by its new chair, W. Henry Mosley, who brought with him both cutting-edge knowledge of methods for conducting large-scale research projects in developing countries and the administrative skills to attract funding and build the department. In 1970, when Mosley was still in Dacca, Pakistan, a young EIS officer named Alfred Sommer (MHS 1973) joined his staff as a medical epidemiologist. Mosley and Sommer, who would later be named JHSPH dean in 1990, oversaw randomized controlled trials of the most widely used cholera vaccine in 280,000 patients and demonstrated that the vaccine then required by international quarantine regulations only protected about 50 percent of the patients for a period of less than six months. They published their findings in *The Lancet*, contending that for cholera control in Bangladesh, "mass vaccination programmes are an ineffective public-health measure. Under field conditions, vaccinating 5,000 individual village contacts of active cases requires a vaccinator to work full-time for 4 months, costs over $300, and prevents, at best, only 1 out of every 20 cases."[18]

Despite the unrest around them, Mosley and Sommer stayed to conduct the first epidemiological assessment of a major natural disaster, the devastating cyclone and tidal bore that decimated East Bengal in November 1970 and killed more than 224,000 people. Shortly after the cyclone hit, Mosley launched a rapid 18-site survey and "flew over the entire cyclone region daily, plotting affected areas with respect to remaining population and selecting sampling sites where there were sufficient survivors to warrant investigation." Sommer returned two and three months later to direct an in-depth survey of nearly 3,000 families, who lost 29 percent of their children under age 5. Sommer's team compiled detailed data on the loss of life, housing, and livestock; assessed post-cyclone morbidity, mortality, and nutritional status; evaluated the effectiveness of recovery programs; and established guidelines for further relief efforts. Sommer and Mosley's 1972 *Lancet* article, "Epidemiological Approach to Disaster Assessment," became a seminal paper that established the value of both initial assessments and in-depth follow-up surveys for long-term relief and recovery planning.[19]

In the midst of this chaos, Hume invited Mosley in January 1971 to apply for the chairmanship of Population Dynamics. Mosley was the hands-down favorite to succeed Paul Harper, even though, as noted in chapter 9, Mosley had essentially debunked the last decade of efforts to increase acceptance of family planning by the Pakistani government and, by extension, Harper's population research and planning unit. Mosley's extensive experience at the CDC and in Bangladesh ideally qualified him to head the multidisciplinary department, which included reproductive biology, basic sciences, social sciences, epidemiology, and programmatic work. Indeed, there were very few individuals who possessed the broad range of knowledge and experience sought by the search committee. Alex Langmuir, who had watched Mosley ascend through the EIS ranks, wrote him that "you are superbly prepared and could make the Hopkins Center into the leading university based population center in the country, if not the world."[20]

Remarkably, the political upheavals in South Asia did not stop or even seem to slow the momentum of USAID's population program. In a 1970 congressional hearing on aid for family planning, Harper's close collaborator, Pakistan's director of family planning Envir Adil, freely admitted that "the IUD device leads to excessive bleeding, a deadly factor in a population that suffers from anemia and undernourishment." But rather than dismiss new methods as too dangerous, Adil declared that "the crying need of the developing nations today in the field of family planning is for a technological breakthrough" that could do what the IUD then could not: provide safe, cheap, and effective birth control to the masses. In the same hearing, William Draper, national chairman of the Population Crisis Committee, averred that "particularly in countries like India and Pakistan, modern science, which created the population problem by checking disease and postponing death, has still to find those improved contraceptives which will be necessary for its solution." Draper emphasized that supporting both domestic and foreign scientific research to develop better contraceptive technology was "perhaps [the US government's] most important responsibility."[21]

Not only did Adil credit USAID's important role in establishing and evaluating Pakistan's family planning program, he also urged the US government to increase funding to develop "a far-ranging domestic family planning program" in *its own country*, which would, in turn, stimulate the USAID population programs in foreign countries. As the new chair of Population Dynamics at JHSPH, Mosley stood ready to answer this challenge.[22]

Almost immediately after his arrival at JHSPH in 1971, Mosley founded an interdisciplinary Hopkins Population Center. The center received a major grant from the National Institute of Child Health and Human Development (NICHD), which prioritized reproductive biology research geared, like all NIH grant programs, toward domestic problems. Large NIH research grants germinated the Population Center's labs for hormone assay and analytical cytology, as well as components for population information, data processing, mathematical and statistical service, field research, clinical research and training, and reproductive biology.

John Biggers established the Population Dynamics Laboratory of Reproductive Physiology in 1966, which expanded into a full division in 1972, headed by Larry L. Ewing, the Hopkins Population Center's associate director for biomedical programs. Cell biologist Barry Zirkin, whose research focused on mammalian spermatogenesis and fertilization, joined the faculty in 1971 and established the Core Electron Microscopy Lab, which he directed from 1978 to 1998. Whereas Population Dynamics had previously collaborated primarily with the departments of International Health and Behavioral Science, the reproductive biology labs fostered closer ties with the medical school on topics including human male sex differentiation and development, the etiology of male infertility and new methods of therapy, prostanoids produced by the pregnant uterus and their role in parturition, toxicological evaluation of chemical methods of tubal closure, regulation of spermatogenesis by the Sertoli cell, regulation of androgen secretion by mammalian testes, and development of a male contraceptive.[23]

Division of Reproductive Physiology faculty lectured in the JHSPH departments of Environmental Health Sciences, Pathobiology, and Maternal and Child Health. The division initiated a joint PhD program and joint faculty appointments with the medical school departments of Gynecology and Obstetrics, Pediatrics, and Urology, as well as the Arts and Sciences Department of Biology. In the 1970s under Mosley and his successor, John Kantner, Population Dynamics continued to receive major funding from NICHD and relatively little from USAID. Although research still addressed fertility regulation, the department moved well beyond its previous focus on the relationship between population growth and economic development overseas and embraced topics such as infertility, sex differentiation, and evaluating potential dangers of sterilization, as well as social and cultural determinants of reproductive behavior and health outcomes.[24]

One major effect of NIH research grants was to narrow the salary gap between medical and public health faculty and enable schools of public health to compete more successfully for scientific talent. In 1960, JHSPH faculty salaries were below average in comparison to both the School of Medicine basic science departments and the 11 US schools of public health. The university board of trustees and the School of Hygiene Visiting Committee had identified lagging faculty salaries as the school's number one problem, especially given "the keen competition for qualified research staff people and faculty members." In 1963, the school received $150,000 from the Ford Foundation to support faculty salary increases, which at least raised Hopkins salaries to the average for schools of public health but not to the level at Harvard or other peer universities. The JHSPH basic science faculty earned nearly the same compensation as basic scientists, but not clinical scientists, in the School of Medicine.[25]

Epidemiologist George Comstock was one of many JHSPH faculty to hold NIH Career Research Awards. Comstock held the award from the National Heart Institute for 40 years and remembered that when he first received the award in 1964, "it paid a significant part of my salary, and took some of the concern out of constant competition for research grants." While NIH programs such as career investigator awards contributed greatly toward equalizing public health salaries, the competition for grants also exacerbated divisions between research-oriented and practice-oriented schools of public health, as well as among departments within the schools, given the NIH's emphasis on basic science and clinical research. The main exception was in biostatistics, where NIH departmental training grants permitted faculty to focus on labor-intensive graduate teaching without pressure to bring in external research funding.[26]

As NIH funding bolstered faculty salaries and enabled JHSPH to hire more faculty, the traditionally tight limitations on granting tenure loosened. Until the mid-1950s, only department chairs had received tenure, but by 1967, 38 JHSPH faculty held tenure. On learning that the school intended to add five more tenured positions, JHU provost William Bevan alerted the president, Milton Eisenhower, "Serious attention should be given to the problem of funding tenured positions in [the School of Hygiene]." Since total salaries for tenured faculty exceeded the university's income from nonfederal sources, Bevan insisted that "serious consideration must be given to ways in which patterns of promotion can be kept in balance. We must be aware of the possible erosion of the tenure principle due to the possibility that the University might be unable to meet its tenure commitment."[27]

Increasing dependence on the NIH and other federal funding also pushed faculty hiring committees to pay more attention to applicants' ability to attract new grants. In 1975, the search committee for a chair of the new Department of Environmental Health Sciences had unanimously recommended Claude J. M. Lenfant, director of the National Heart and Lung Institute Division of Lung Diseases. Lenfant declined the offer because he "could not convince myself that the resources that could be committed by the Johns Hopkins University to meet the needs of this Department would be sufficient. I am mostly referring to the space and the financial support needed for the normal growth—if not the expansion of this Department." Despite his background as an NIH insider, Lenfant was distressed by "the expectation of the School that, eventually, a Chairman should provide his own salary support, if he wants to expand his Department."[28]

Chairs such as Fred Bang in Pathobiology and Abe Lilienfeld in Epidemiology had set the bar that Lenfant disparaged. NIH funding had made the Johns Hopkins Department of Epidemiology the largest and most active department of epidemiology in the world. By 1976, Epidemiology had 20 full-time faculty with primary appointments and over 70 graduate students, and the department's Training Center for Public Health Research in Hagerstown, Maryland, had published 56 scholarly articles since the center was established in 1962 under the direction of George W. Comstock. Ninety percent of the department's budget came from Lilienfeld's two core NIH grants in cancer and stroke, which over nearly two decades had together generated between $1 and $2 million of annual flexible support for research and education. But by the mid-1970s, each of the grants had declined to about $200,000 annually, and they were set to terminate in 1979. Since Epidemiology was "more active across divisional lines than any other department in this University" and this collaboration was largely unremunerated, Lilienfeld's successor as chair, Leon Gordis, wanted JHU President Steven Muller to designate Epidemiology a university-wide department that received general funds from the university budget. But, as Lenfant had surmised, the era of university or school sponsorship for core operating funds was over, at least on the Hopkins medical campus.[29]

Gordis was "optimistic that additional programmatic money can be generated, particularly in the environmental areas," but predicted "a period of several years without this major programmatic funding." Although Gordis correctly observed that "the Federal largesse which came essentially with few if any restrictions, is unlikely to be duplicated," the Department of Epidemiology continued as one of the NIH's largest grant recipients. Gordis established a cardiovascular epidemiology fellowship program in 1980 with an institutional grant from the National Heart, Lung and Blood Institute, and Moyses Szklo led an epidemiological investigation of aplastic anemia in Baltimore with NCI support. Lilienfeld's stroke grant was renewed for five years at $2.5 million, and he also received grants from the National Institute of Arthritis, Metabolic and Digestive Diseases for a study of familial aggregation of inflammatory bowel disease and from the National Institute of General Medical Sciences to research the public health aspects of chronic disease. Together, these grants not only maintained but increased the previous level of NIH funding.[30]

After Kerr White left Hopkins in 1974, the Department of Medical Care and Hospitals was renamed Health Care Organization, with Philip Bonnet as acting chair. On July 1, 1976, the JHSPH Advisory Board voted to merge the departments of Public Health Administration and Health Care Organization under a new Department of Health Services Administration, with Art Bushel as chair. The merger, like the mergers of Chronic Diseases and Epidemiology and of the three departments forming Environmental Health Sciences, was a fiscal conservation measure that was also intended to strengthen the integration of teaching and research and to foster communication among faculty members with related interests.[31]

The merger was also a reaction against the Johnson-era policies that had created outsized departments like Medical Care and Hospitals that could not sustain the loss of single-source funding, the founding director, or both. Paul White, chair of Behavioral Sciences in the 1970s, remembered that Kerr White "had his own world, he might as well have had his own school." Flagle recalled, "in a couple of conversations I had with Kerr, I got the impression he really wasn't interested in the Department of Public Health Administration, in the School of Public Health." In discussions of restructuring the school's administrative and departmental organization, the school's leadership supported a pared-down matrix of "basic disciplines" that "would be represented in units that would permit them to maintain a relevant spectrum of competencies, educate for their respective disciplines and provide relevant courses in the curricula of the professional programs. The structure should provide for representation of professional programs and basic disciplines." In a "matrix" structure, professional programs and basic disciplines "could be integrated in response to need. The structure would constrain programs from developing semi-autonomous 'mini-schools' with their own ancillary faculty representing the basic disciplines. The organization would integrate the units of the School and its curricula rather than creating pressures to build segregated 'empires.' "32

JHSPH's departmental structure had sprouted in the hothouse atmosphere of a bewildering jungle of federal health agencies. To unify these agencies, John Glenn Beall Jr., US senator from Maryland, had proposed in 1971 to elevate the National Health Services Research and Development Center to become an institute of the NIH, creating a new National Institute of Health Care Delivery. David E. Rogers, dean of medicine at Hopkins, questioned Beall's analogy between the impact of NIH research on medical practice and the potential of such an institute to transform the delivery of medical care. "The biomedical research advances supported by NIH," Rogers wrote Beall, "have directly influenced practice by changing approaches to specific disease because of new knowledge. This could be readily incorporated in the management of individual patients without changes in legislation or, in most instances, without any changes in attitudinal set of doctors. In general, new technology and new knowledge is rapidly embraced by and utilized as swiftly as possible by the profession."33

The field of health care delivery, however, posed much more complex problems. Rogers asserted, "There is already considerable evidence that the development of new information on ways of giving health care, or the shortcomings of the current system, or the shortcomings on our ways of paying for medical care, do not have much impact on the way health care is delivered." As proof, Rogers cited "the enormous problems we ran into in attempting to develop a comprehensive, prepaid practice program for the city of East Baltimore. The thing which came very much home to us was the incredible fractionation of health care programs within the state and federal sector." To be successful, a new NIH institute devoted to health care delivery would "need to have significant influence on decision making and legislation, and would probably need a considerable operational in-put—not just an observational or research one." Rogers insisted that continuing to increase research grants for more critiques of the existing health care delivery system was wrongheaded, since "much of what is wrong with the [system] relates to the categoric funding of programs such as Medicare, Medicaid, the Children's Bureau, etc." Rogers, Milton Eisenhower, Russell Nelson, and Robert Heyssel all supported a cabinet-level secretary of health as "a major need in this country . . . if we are to genuinely effect change in the health care system . . . and [not] continue to fail to pull all of our crazy quilt of funding for health care under a single roof." Neither a cabinet position nor an NIH institute devoted to solving the nation's health care problems ever overcame political opposition to become reality. But as the next chapter will show, JHSPH faculty would apply health services research to guide state and federal health finance policy in the 1980s and would help establish the PHS Agency for Health Care Policy and Research in 1989.[34]

Affirmative Action at JHSPH

Civil rights legislation required all federal employers, including universities, to develop affirmative action plans that demonstrated nondiscrimination in hiring and to initiate training programs for employees to improve their job skills. Eligibility for federal grants and contracts depended on having an approved affirmative action plan. In 1970, Baltimore City's population was 44 percent black. The proportion of blacks on the Johns Hopkins faculty was only 2 percent in the medical school, 1.4 percent in JHSPH, and 0.7 percent at Homewood. Black employees on the JHSPH staff included 12 percent of technicians and 60 percent of service workers, but none of the 14 administrative managers was black. The school had been most successful in increasing the diversity of its office and clerical staff, of whom African Americans had represented 8 percent in 1968 but 18 percent by 1970. Black women were a majority of the 29 part-time interviewers hired by the Hopkins Population Center Survey Research Unit to conduct a survey in East Baltimore, which, according to the unit's director, reflected the center's "concerted effort to hire members of this minority group."[35]

JHSPH established a committee on minority student recruitment in 1970 and a permanent affirmative action committee the next year. HEW had disapproved Hopkins' inaugural affirmative action plan twice before the third version was approved, which set specific goals for employment of women and minorities. Based on the medical school's self-study of problems in hiring women and minorities for faculty positions, the provost and vice-president for administration asked each university division to conduct a similar analysis. John Hume admitted, "For many reasons, there is 'under representation' of women and minority groups on our faculty." The School of Hygiene's affirmative action report had to be submitted in time to be included with the university's annual progress report to HEW on June 12, 1971. Hume told the faculty, "It is vital to the university that an acceptable progress report is submitted. . . . Since our demonstrable progress has been minimal during the past year, we are eager to have as much evidence of interest and concern available for inclusion in the report as may be possible."[36]

Pressure to abide by affirmative action policies continued to build as federal Equal Employment Opportunity Commission regulations required departments to open faculty records if a discrimination lawsuit was filed and to keep records and track statistics in promotion and hiring. Barbara Starfield in the Department of Health Services Administration was a key advocate for racial and gender equity and chaired the JHSPH Affirmative Action Committee. The Advisory Board had approved an affirmative action policy in April 1973, and by 1974, JHSPH job postings began to include the statement, "Other qualifications being equal, it is University policy to preferentially hire women and minorities." At Starfield's urging, Hume sent the department chairmen a report of a recent EEOC decision on a medical school that had shown sex bias in its tenure procedures and had excluded minorities and females from nonfaculty jobs.[37]

In January 1974, Starfield sent a letter to chairs of departments and active search committees requesting what specific actions their departments had taken to implement the school's policy. Roger Herriott, who had chaired Biochemistry since 1948, replied that he "probably would take a conservative approach which is not to say—unsympathetic. From my knowledge and experience the School has shown the highest regard for women. Long before affirmative action we had female Professors and acting heads of departments. I believe we have not appointed one head of a department because we haven't seen one as good as the male candidates. We do not have to take a back seat on this issue yet I don't feel we should be belligerent about it." When Herriott retired a few months later, Starfield asked Hume to provide documentation that qualified women and minority group members had received due consideration for the vacant position. Starfield wrote Paul Lemkau, who chaired the search committee, "Considering the relatively large number of highly qualified women in areas related to mutagenesis, immunotherapy, and biochemistry, I am puzzled and concerned that no women were actually recruited and considered for the position as chairman of the Biochemistry Department." She attached a news article about one such scientist, Bridgid G. Leventhal.[38]

Most faculty responses to Starfield's query emphasized progress toward hiring women but either did not mention minorities or admitted little success despite sincere efforts. In contrast, Carl Taylor, chair of International Health, overlooked sex as an affirmative action category. He boasted that "the policy adopted by the Board required little change in the recruitment methods of this department. Many years of performing research in the developing countries of Asia, Africa and Latin America, in close collaboration with the nationals of these countries, have long since made recruitment on 'affirmative action' basis a natural, fundamental part of all the department's activities. Thus, it is perhaps not surprising that the first black faculty member in the University to be elevated to the rank of professor was on the faculty of this department (Al Haynes), or that a substantial proportion of the department's employees have always been drawn from various minority groups."[39]

While the number of minorities appointed as public health faculty remained small, student bodies in schools of public health welcomed increasing numbers of racial and ethnic minorities, women, and younger students between 1960 and 1980. Minority recruitment was strongly supported by most JHSPH faculty and administrators, but in 1971, the Policy Committee had warned the Advisory Board, the administration, and the Committee on Minority Recruitment that "an active program to recruit more students from minority groups may well create difficult financial problems to the University," since most of these students would require financial aid "at a time when the number of available fellowships and traineeships is decreasing. Hence, many students may find themselves disappointed that no financial assistance is available after they have gone to the very considerable effort to apply for and gain admission to the School. All possible means should be explored to avoid this difficulty before the recruitment program is undertaken." Moreover, black public health professionals were even less likely than their white counterparts to be able to forego one year's income to pursue a full-time MPH degree program.[40]

An ideal opportunity to address these concerns came when the District of Columbia Community Health and Hospitals Administration approached JHSPH about providing graduate training for its employees. The agency and the school co-designed an extended MPH program for DC employees, based on an existing program at the University of North Carolina with key improvements. Between 1971 and 1974, the Johns Hopkins extended MPH program enabled 37 DC public health workers to retain their full-time status while earning the degree in two years by completing two short periods of full-time work in Baltimore and taking the remaining courses two or three half-days per week in Washington, DC. The program boosted enrollment of African-American students, who represented 43 percent of the DC extension cohort. Despite the Policy Committee's initial fears that minority recruitment might impose a financial strain on the university, proportionally more PHS traineeships were awarded to black students, who were less able to rely on family or personal savings to meet educational costs. By fall 1975, the proportion of students enrolled in schools of public health who identified themselves as black, Asian, Hispanic, or Native American reached a combined total of 18 percent. Two-thirds of enrolled students were under 30, whereas the median age for male and female recipients of graduate public health degrees during the 1960s was 32. The DC extension program was the first part-time MPH program ever offered at JHSPH.[41]

The increase in minority students at JHSPH helped draw the attention of faculty and students throughout the school to racial discrimination and disparities in health services and outcomes. While Edgar E. Roulhac (MPH 1975) was an MPH student and a member of the JHSPH Minority Recruitment Committee, he led the student committee charged with surveying student attitudes toward "an organized learning experience designed to enhance and facilitate all health professionals' understanding of problems and issues unique to the delivery of health care to minorities and the disadvantaged." Write-in survey respondents suggested that the course should be developed in conjunction with a Division of Minority Affairs in Public Health and should be "supplemented with field experience in agencies delivering care to minority populations." One respondent suggested that the topic should be "treated as any other important and significant area of public health without racial overtones." Other comments included the observation that disadvantaged groups were the primary recipients of government-sponsored medical care and public health services and therefore "the problems of administering health care to these groups should be seriously considered. It is about time that ivory tower medical care came down to the 'grass roots' problems faced by most of the world's population, be it India, Pakistan, or Appalacia [*sic*] USA." Another student disagreed, stating that "the problems of care delivery to minority groups should never be taught separately but only embraced within courses that consider the totality of care delivery to the public."[42]

In 1978, Roulhac's prior administrative experience as an educator, together with his firsthand knowledge of the school, led to his appointment as the first full-time dean of student affairs, with a faculty appointment in the Department of Health Services Administration Division of Health Education. With the able administrative assistance of Betty Addison, Roulhac instituted systemic changes in management, organization, and data processing that modernized admissions and financial aid, as well as the registrar's office. As coordinator for student services, Addison remembers that she "was the troubleshooter for all the problems the departments couldn't handle." She started the alumni career development network to help JHSPH students find jobs after graduation and also helped institute course evaluations in the late 1970s. She was the point person for the many international students at JHSPH and organized volunteers to help with language learning, shopping, and even field trips to the beach and Washington, DC.

Addison remembers that in 1978, there were very few black students, and she and Roulhac were the only African Americans employed at the school, other than the janitorial staff, one professor in Epidemiology, and one secretary in Maternal and Child Health. With support from Dean Donald A. Henderson, Roulhac and Addison established minority recruitment programs that promoted public health as a career option. They also inaugurated retention programs, including the first minority scholarships. These programs sparked improvements in student services across the board. For example, the new student orientation, which became an annual ritual at JHSPH, originated as an orientation for new minority students that was expanded to include the whole entering class. Roulhac, the first African-American to serve as an associate dean at JHSPH as well as at Johns Hopkins University, would join the JHU administration as vice provost in 1985.[43]

Conclusion

The 1960s surge in federal funding transformed schools of public health by increasing their size, numbers, and disciplinary scope, as well as introduced the first incentives and penalties to promote greater gender and ethnic diversity in hiring and admissions. Great Society initiatives contributed to the moral as well as the material economy of American public health. For example, the search for ways to make the health care system more equitable and efficient had helped launch the JHSPH Department of Medical Care and Hospitals and the university-wide Office of Health Care Programs. Yet these socially conscious programs proved vulnerable to political attack, leaving their academic offspring orphaned and fiscally unstable. Departments that emphasized collaborative teaching and research such as Biostatistics, Behavioral Sciences, and International Health served the school and the university, but by the end of the 1970s, all three were on the financial ropes. By contrast, large grants from the NIH made the departments of Chronic Diseases, Radiological Science, and Pathobiology funding dynamos that also rebuilt bridges to the medical school.

In the long run, federal research and training programs more than adequately sustained schools of public health, whose enrollments expanded fivefold between 1961 and 1978. Not a single school of public health closed its doors; instead, the number of US and Canadian schools rose during those years from 14 to 21. In 1977, Daniel F. Whiteside, director of the PHS Health Resources Administration Bureau of Health Manpower, analyzed the state of the health workforce and the impact of Great Society health professional training legislation. The schools were financially stable, and Whiteside concluded that "increasing student enrollment, a major reason for instituting the Health Professions Educational Assisting Program in 1963, is no longer a primary objective." More than $5 billion had been awarded through fiscal year 1976 under the Health Professions Educational Assistance Act (HPEA), and during the decade from academic years 1967 to 1976, the number of health professions schools, including medicine, public health, osteopathy, dentistry, nursing, and pharmacy, increased from 256 to 297. In 1978, the Hill–Rhodes formula grant program was replaced by capitation grants under the Comprehensive Health

Manpower Training Act, which reimbursed schools of public health for approximately 22 percent of educational costs.[44]

The most obvious result of the dramatic increase in federal support for graduate public health education was that the annual production of public health degrees dramatically increased. In higher education generally, public health and nursing programs were among the fastest growing fields. Federal aid also helped to concentrate one-third of all public health students in the three largest state schools: the University of Michigan, University of North Carolina, and University of California, Los Angeles.[45]

CHAPTER THIRTEEN

Days of Reckoning and Renewal

Johns Hopkins public health faculty had always firmly believed that statistically and methodologically rigorous research offered the best hope for solving the dire health crises facing the populations they studied in Baltimore and around the world. From the 1940s onward, they developed exceptionally sophisticated research methods in an era when public health programs often lacked means of effective evaluation. In the 1970s, however, critics from many quarters demanded a higher level of accountability from the public health profession and government health agencies. A brief overview of three major challenges to the credibility of public health, one domestic and two international, illustrates the looming obstacles that faced the School of Hygiene and Public Health in 1977, when Donald A. Henderson succeeded John Hume as dean. The remainder of the chapter outlines the initiatives launched under Henderson that built on the school's past work in the fields of health services research, global health, and environmental health, while also responding to new challenges with innovative programs in areas such as computing, public–private partnerships, and tissue culture research.

The Risks of Intervention and Hope for Change

As noted in chapter 1, US Public Health Service researchers had committed egregious ethical violations against human subjects in both Macon County, Alabama, and Guatemala (the focus here is on Tuskegee, since the Guatemala research was not made public until 2010 through an investigation by historian Susan L. Reverby). The findings of the PHS Tuskegee Study of Untreated Syphilis in the Negro Male had been published in medical journals for decades, but the general public first learned of the study in an article by Jean Heller published by the *New York Times* in 1972. The article was the catalyst for congressional hearings as well as an Ad Hoc Advisory Panel on the Tuskegee Study convened by the US Department of Health, Education, and Welfare, which declared the study "ethically unjustified" in April 1973. One of the HEW advisory panel's members was JHSPH alumnus Reginald James, who, as one of the earliest African-American PHS physicians, had staffed the syphilis control program in Macon County, Alabama, before studying at Hopkins and then becoming a career PHS officer. Each of these investigations explained in detail how the PHS physicians in charge of the study had selected a group of African-American men with positive blood tests for syphilis in 1932 and then conducted annual follow-up testing and physicals, including painful spinal tap procedures without any type of anesthesia, over a 40-year period. The researchers overtly deceived the men to make them believe they were receiving treatment for their "bad blood" when, in fact, the study's administrators intervened (although not always successfully) to prevent the men from receiving penicillin through either military or civilian treatment programs.[1]

The PHS conducted the Tuskegee Study openly and it endured for four decades with virtually no opposition from within the PHS. Neither did the Tuskegee Study attract external criticism from local health officers, physicians who read about the study in medical journals, or even the black clinicians and administrators at the Tuskegee Institute who assisted the PHS. The PHS also oversaw the Indian Health Service, which sterilized an estimated 25 percent of Native American women between the ages of 15 and 44 during the 1970s, often without obtaining informed consent and in some cases without their knowledge. In both these examples, government health officials (virtually all of whom were white male physicians) persuaded or coerced participation without obtaining informed consent or engaging in dialogue about the purposes, benefits, and risks of these programs with the politically and economically marginalized minority groups from which the subjects were drawn.[2]

In 1972, the same year the Tuskegee scandal broke, Mahmood Mamdani published *The Myth of Population Control: Family, Caste, and Class in an Indian Village.* While Mamdani was still a Harvard graduate student in anthropology, he had obtained permission from John Wyon, principal investigator of the Harvard Khanna Study (discussed in chapter 7) to access the study's original documents and interview its principal staff. Mamdani had returned in 1970, a decade after the study's completion, to conduct his own investigation in one of the study's villages, Manupur. He claimed that respondents had lied to Harvard investigators because their culture's veneration of visitors required them to express a polite interest in and acceptance of contraceptive information and materials. As a matter of village pride, they respected outsiders but masked their conviction that, according to Mamdani, "to practice contraception would have meant to willfully court economic disaster."[3]

Mamdani, who was born in India and grew up in East Africa, focused on what he viewed as the Khanna Study's ethnographic shortcomings and discounted its public health strengths as a large-scale epidemiological field trial. He charged that the Harvard researchers had pushed the Western agenda of family planning in disregard of villagers' local values and culture. Carl Taylor, who like Mamdani was a native of India but born to American parents, defended the study's field work methods as "especially sensitive to what people in the villages were thinking." Writing in 1983, Taylor, who was well versed in sociology and incorporated comparative perspectives into his approach to primary health care, insisted that Khanna's "style of research and published reports stressed sociocultural and economic considerations and the need for sympathetic understanding of the way village people think about problems of fertility and the value of children." Mamdani's critique of the Khanna Study later attracted a variety of rebuttals on scholarly and ideological grounds, including feminists who faulted him for privileging male patriarchs' perspectives. Yet *The Myth of Population Control* gained traction at the same charged cultural moment when the Tuskegee Syphilis Study came to light and when Marxist and Afrocentric scholars were analyzing the combined toll of racism, capitalism, and colonialism across the African diaspora. The Khanna and Tuskegee studies remain two of the most widely cited indictments of ethnocentrism in public health research.[4]

The spectacular collapse of India's population control program in the late 1970s also stemmed in part from ethnocentrism, but in this case it was based on caste rather than race or nationality. During the period of national emergency declared by Prime Minister Indira Gandhi from 1975 to 1977, the Indian central government instituted a coercive sterilization program. Historian Matthew Connelly concisely summarized the episode as "emblematic of everything that can go wrong in a program premised on 'population control' rather than on reproductive rights and health. This included time-bound performance targets; a preference for methods that minimized the need for sustained motivation; disregard for basic medical standards; incentive payments that, for the very poorest, constituted a form of coercion; disincentives that punished non-participation; and official consideration of compulsory sterilization, which, even if never enacted into law, signaled that achieving national population targets might override individual dignity and welfare." In a single year, more than 8 million Indian men and women were sterilized, tripling the number in the preceding year. In September 1976 alone, over 1.7 million sterilizations were performed. Within a matter of months, the proportion of Indian couples estimated to be practicing modem contraception increased by nearly 50 percent. But the intensive, top-down application of political will to implement the program caused millions to suffer harassment—and hundreds to die—at the hands of government officials. As soon as the country held open elections, Indian voters overwhelmingly rejected the political leaders who had supported the sterilization drive. Indira Gandhi fell from power amid a rising chorus of developing-world denunciations of national family planning programs as a plot of white Western elites.[5]

The controversies over the Tuskegee Study and those surrounding family planning in India—whether in Western-led research or government-driven mass sterilizations—were but a few examples of debates over the soul of public health that already had been brewing within the profession but became more public during the 1970s. As support for population control accelerated in the 1960s, the methods and leadership that had distinguished the WHO malaria eradication campaign were losing support within the international development community, even in public health circles. In 1948, Fred Soper had predicted that 90 percent of malaria worldwide could be eradicated within 10 years, at a cost of $280 million. Tim Baker, as a top official in the US International Cooperation Administration health mission in India in the mid-1950s, had told the minister of finance that if the Indian government sponsored half the cost, ICA would do the rest and eradicate malaria within 10 years, making further spending unnecessary.[6]

Yet as the malaria control program unfolded, human, political, biological, and environmental factors had often wreaked havoc with the best-laid plans of technical advisers. Monsoons in Asia and sand in Africa rendered vehicles and other equipment useless, and mosquitoes' growing resistance to insecticide everywhere mocked the dream of disease eradication. WHO's epidemiological paradigm posited static, measurable populations, but mass migration rendered large groups of people more susceptible to disease yet less accessible to public health outreach efforts. In many newly independent Asian and African countries, migration was dramatically accelerated by poverty, inadequate food production, and political insurrections. US policy priorities also played a role. Officials at USAID preferred to focus on bilateral economic development and population control programs rather than cooperate with WHO and other multilateral agencies to expand communicable disease control programs beyond the existing malaria campaign.[7]

Petty politics and charges of mismanagement dogged international health efforts to control malaria. For example, in 1965, USAID officials had resisted the proposal of D. A. Henderson, then head of the CDC's Smallpox Surveillance Unit, to save money and increase coverage by combining the WHO and USAID malaria control and smallpox vaccination programs and expanding them throughout 18 countries in West and Central Africa. Since Nigeria was already receiving substantial economic assistance from USAID, the agency was particularly opposed to expanding its own proposed stand-alone measles vaccination program to include Nigeria's large population, which would have represented half of the total number of immunizations to be completed under the combined program proposed by Henderson. WHO director-general M. G. Candau also initially opposed the new smallpox campaign because he feared that it would siphon resources and personnel away from the flagging antimalaria program. He remained skeptical of the chances for achieving the full eradication of smallpox and wanted to avoid embarrassing the organization at an already delicate point in its history. Many delegates at the World Health Assembly also opposed the program, in part because they erroneously believed that eradication would require vaccinating everyone living throughout the world.

After the World Health Assembly approved a global smallpox eradication program in 1966 by a narrow two-vote margin, Candau tapped Henderson to head it because he wanted an American to take responsibility in the event of failure. When James Watt, who was now director of the PHS Office of International Health, called Henderson to PHS headquarters and told him that Candau had asked for him by name, Henderson balked at first. Not only was Henderson committed to his current assignment to eliminate smallpox from West Africa, he viewed WHO as "a dysfunctional bureaucracy that was incapable of managing a global disease eradication campaign—particularly given the director-general's obvious lack of commitment to that goal." Despite the fact that Candau, Watt, and Henderson were all JHSPH alumni who had each enjoyed considerable success in their respective international health leadership roles, their lack of consensus on the feasibility of smallpox eradication at the campaign's outset underlined the hard times on which their field had fallen.[8]

Although the WHO malaria campaign had reduced mortality in endemic regions, especially India and much of Asia, it had failed to consolidate its initial gains to fully eradicate all remaining cases, particularly among the scattered rural poor. International health and development agencies, foreign investors, and the emerging bourgeoisie of developing nations all concentrated their efforts on urban and industrial centers to the detriment of rural areas, where substandard living conditions, malnutrition, and inadequate or nonexistent local health services perpetuated malaria transmission and allowed its resurgence. In 1969, just two years into the smallpox campaign, WHO formally abandoned the global malaria eradication campaign first proposed by Soper and advanced by a generation of JHSPH parasitologists. International health insiders began to joke that the WHO malaria campaign had not eradicated malaria—just malariologists, referring to the widespread assumption among public health graduates that working in malaria control would be a career dead end. Over the twentieth century, the global mortality burden of malaria had declined dramatically from its 1930 peak of approximately 3.5 million annual deaths to a low point of 578,000 annual deaths in 1970. But without vigilant treatment and vector control efforts, and with the rise of insecticide-resistant mosquitoes and chloroquine-resistant *P. falciparum* (the most deadly type of malaria), the death rate began a steady upward climb that would continue for the rest of the century, once more exceeding 1 million annual deaths by 1997.[9]

The contemporary criticisms of the WHO malaria eradication program, the PHS Tuskegee Syphilis Study, and population control programs cited a range of reasons for their failures, ranging from Tuskegee's unethical and unscientific methods, to the logistical failures of the malaria campaign, to the cultural insensitivity of USAID and developing country officials in national family planning programs. Yet a common thread of fatalism ran through all these criticisms. Separately but especially taken together, these examples could be used to argue that inaction is better than intervention. Any public health intervention carries the risk of failing to achieve lasting positive change and the potential, even if inadvertent, to cause negative outcomes for at least some participants. Such metaphysical questions underlay a sense of defeatism and existential crisis in the public health profession in the 1970s. At Johns Hopkins, the School of Hygiene and Public Health was buffeted by a severe university budget shortage that paralleled the instability and retrenchment in federal health programs, as well as double-digit inflation and sky-high oil prices.

John Hume had served as dean of JHSPH since 1967 and announced that he would retire at the end of the 1976–1977 academic year. The search committee, which included Abe Lilienfeld and Edyth Schoenrich (MPH 1971), had heard from their colleague Kerr White, former chair of Medical Care and Hospitals. White had written JHU President Steven Muller to encourage the selection of a leader who would fulfill "Welch's dream, 'the integration of medicine and public health.'" White, with his typical combination of insistence and vision, told Muller, "I want to urge, once more, consideration of organizational and structural changes, and not more of the 'old-time public health religion.' Hopkins now has a great opportunity to change the course of public health and of medicine."[10]

TABLE 13.1
JHSPH Leadership Transitions, 1970–1985

Served under Hume 1967–1977			Appointed under Henderson 1977–1990		
Chair name	Years Served	Department	Chair name	Years Served	
Sol Levine	1967–1972	Behavioral	Abraham Lilienfeld	1982–1984	
Paul E. White	1972–1981	Sciences	Frank Baker	1984–1987	
Roger Herriott	1948–1975	Biochemistry	Lawrence Grossman	1976–1989	
Alan Ross	1967–1981	Biostatistics	Charles A. Rohde	1981–1996	
Cornelius Kruse	1961–1976	Environmental	Gareth M. Green	1977–1990	
Richard L. Riley	1961–1976	Health Sciences			
Russell Morgan	1961–1971				
Abraham M. Lilienfeld	1970–1974	Epidemiology	Leon Gordis	1975–1993	
Arthur Bushel	1969–1983	Health Policy and	Karen Davis	1983–1992	
Kerr L. White	1969–1971	Management			
Philip D. Bonnet	1971–1973				
Frederik B. Bang	1953–1981	Immunology and Infectious Diseases	Noel R. Rose	1982–1993	
Carl E. Taylor	1962–1982	International Health	Robert E. Black	1985–2013	
Donald Cornely	1970–1989	Maternal and Child Health	Bernard Guyer	1989–1998	
Paul Lemkau	1962–1975	Mental Hygiene	Ernest Gruenberg	1975–1981	
			Sheppard G. Kellam	1982–1993	
W. Henry Mosley	1971–1977	Population Dynamics	John Kantner	1978–1985	
			W. Henry Mosley	1985–1998	

Stebbins and Hume had collaborated closely to lead the school since just after the end of World War II. The decade of Hume's deanship was characterized by the most rapid growth and greatest organizational changes in JHSPH history to date. The school underwent a monumental leadership transition from 1972 to 1985, when search committees were appointed to select 14 department chairs and the deanship (table 13.1). In addition to finding chairs for the newly established departments of Behavioral Sciences, Environmental Health Sciences, and Medical Care and Hospitals, Dean Hume appointed a series of younger successors for chairs who had been serving since the 1940s and 1950s. In 1940, the school's departmental structure had been heavily weighted toward the basic sciences, with a single, small Department of Public Health Administration. Over the next four decades, PHA birthed 13 new divisions, of which six became independent departments, while the basic and environmental

TABLE 13.2
Evolution of JHSPH Science Departments

Established	Department	Change	Result
1930	Biology	Chair died, Rockefeller Foundation grant terminated.	Department dissolved in 1940.
1917	Biochemistry	In 1950s, department shifted from sole focus on nutrition to cellular and molecular biology. Some biophysics faculty from Radiation Science transferred to Biochemistry.	Department renamed Biochemical and Biophysical Sciences in 1971.
1917	Immunology	Chair died.	Department merged with Bacteriology in 1947.
1917	Bacteriology	Renamed Microbiology in 1951, chair became dean of Medicine in 1957, Microbiology was joint department until 1962.	Remaining faculty transferred to Pathobiology in 1962.
1927	Helminthology Protozoology and Medical Entomology	Merged to form Parasitology in 1942, renamed Pathobiology in 1955.	Under new chair, Pathobiology was reoriented and renamed Immunology and Infectious Diseases in 1982.
1917 1937	Physiological Hygiene Sanitary Engineering	Reorganized as Environmental Medicine in 1950. Renamed Environmental Health in 1961.	Environmental Medicine and Environmental Health merged in 1976 to form Environmental Health Sciences.
1962	Radiological Science	Chair became dean of Medicine in 1971, department became division of Environmental Health.	

science departments underwent periodic mergers as funding tightened and research agendas shifted. What had been eight basic and applied science departments had become three by 1976 (table 13.2). Pathobiology was still chaired by Fred Bang, Lawrence Grossman succeeded longtime Biochemistry chair Roger Herriott in 1975, and Gareth Green chaired the new Department of Environmental Health Sciences.

The search committee chose Donald A. Henderson as the eighth dean of JHSPH. Of the 10 deans who have led JHSPH from 1916 to 2016, Stebbins and Henderson are the only two who were appointed after serving in high-level public health practice positions with no prior academic leadership experience;

they are also the only two who had been recruited from outside Johns Hopkins University, although both were JHSPH alumni. Stebbins had led the New York City Health Department through World War II, while Henderson had just returned to the United States after directing the WHO campaign to eradicate smallpox from 1966 to 1977. When WHO certified in 1980 that no more cases had been reported since the last patient had been diagnosed in 1977 in Somalia, smallpox became the first disease in world history to be eradicated.[11]

Henderson stepped into the deanship in August 1977, just shy of his 49th birthday. While Hume had been consumed and worn down by the erratic twists and turns of federal public health policy in the 1970s, Henderson had been operating in an entirely different sphere of global disease eradication, working not only on smallpox but also playing a key role in initiating WHO's Expanded Program on Immunization in 1974. The WHO smallpox campaign, and by extension Henderson's career, was upheld as an example of what was going right in public health at a time when so much seemed to be going wrong.[12]

Henderson prided himself on being a disciple of Alex Langmuir, his direct superior in the CDC Epidemiology Branch and a fellow shoe-leather epidemiologist who went out and talked to people on the ground to find the causes of epidemics. Like Langmuir, Henderson had no use for "paper pushers" or "shiny pants epidemiologists," so named because they spent most of their time sitting down behind a desk. Henderson's frame of reference and unsinkable philosophy are well illustrated in a 1980 speech to the American Academy of Pediatrics titled "Expanding Horizons on a Diminishing Planet." He blamed the rapid pace of social change and the mass media's "documentation of catastrophes, instantly communicated around the world," for "eroding a public confidence that either individuals or institutions have the capacity or ability to intelligently guide their futures." As an antidote, Henderson pointed to the final stage of the smallpox campaign in India, the last endemic country, where more than 120,000 health workers had visited each house in the whole country for one week each month to ferret out cases. Henderson used independent confirmation to ensure that more than 90 percent of Indian households were indeed being visited each month. Using eight tons of forms, the "perennially maligned Indian Ministry of Health had made a vigorous commitment to the apparently impossible task of smallpox eradication." In 1974, when India's number of reported smallpox cases had been the highest in 15 years, due in part to the intensifying eradication campaign and better surveillance, the headlines trumpeted the bad news week after week. Yet when the country declared its freedom from smallpox one year later, Henderson told the audience, "The event was reported in a terse article on the fifth page of New Delhi's principal paper." Henderson concluded triumphantly, "The capacity of the Indian national health service to effect rapid change was and is vastly greater than any had imagined," and the same was true, he averred, of other countries' health agencies during the smallpox campaign. For Henderson, smallpox eradication had "reinforced a personal optimism that we [in public health] have the capacity to meet the challenges of the coming decades. Our problems are three—to decide which are the essential issues, to make necessary political and moral commitments and to identify and support the necessary leadership."[13]

In a March 1978 letter to the faculty outlining his priorities and goals, Henderson, who had been living outside the United States for most of the past decade, echoed Thomas Turner's unflattering assessments of American public health in the 1950s. In Henderson's view, American public health professionals had been "relegated to the periphery by the evolution of medical and health practice." Like Turner, Henderson also viewed most schools of public health as out of touch and insufficiently involved in practical problem solving. Emphasizing their role as professional schools more than as graduate schools, Henderson vowed to make JHSPH "fully relevant to the work-place." A born leader, Henderson was impatient for the coming of a new and better age and scoffed at doomsayers. "We accept the principle uncritically that social change is inevitably slow," he observed, but then voiced his suspicion that this was, "in fact, a rationalization for uninspired leadership or an excuse for inaction." Henderson prized the art and science of management and wanted to apply business administration principles to both the health care sector and the school. He proposed to increase JHSPH's involvement in health and social policymaking at the state and local levels, especially in the development of comprehensive health care programs.[14]

Echoing concerns that Alan Gittelsohn, Charles Flagle, and others had voiced since the early 1960s, Henderson observed that "measurement in the health sector has lagged far behind that in other sectors of the economy. There has been little motivation to collect and analyze such community-based data as disease prevalence, utilization and costs of service, and environmental and behavioral risk factors. As yet, the data are only marginally employed in health policy formulation." In complex ways, the threads of bioethics, technology, advocacy, and management would define Henderson's deanship and transform the interface of public health with the health care system in the 1980s. As discussed in chapter 8, the founding in 1969 of the Department of Medical Care and Hospitals under Kerr White and the Health Services Research and Development Center had stimulated the school's research on health care financing, organization, and staffing, as well as their impact on the utilization, cost, and quality of health services. All these activities were shaped in important ways by both the development of health information technology and the context of urban health problems and community activism.

The school's leadership recognized that computer literacy was becoming a critical basic skill for public health professionals. Advised by the chairs of Biostatistics and Epidemiology, Henderson expanded computing infrastructure and access throughout the school and pursued private grants to help recruit additional faculty who would elevate research and teaching in the field later known as Big Data. Until the mid-1970s, computer access had been restricted to trained professionals using punched cards and a mainframe. Beginning in the early 1980s, evolving technology gave users more universal access, first with a terminal and keyboard that provided networked mainframe access, then via personal computers. Henderson established the university's first computer laboratory with individual terminals for student use and continued to upgrade the computer infrastructure.

Computer literacy was also a goal of new summer programs. To improve continuing education offerings and to better use the school building, which stood empty throughout the summer months, Henderson enlisted Leon Gordis and Moyses Szklo to organize the school's first summer session in June 1983. The Graduate Summer Institute of Epidemiology enrolled more than 100 public health professionals for short, intensive courses in epidemiology, biostatistics, and computing. After the summer institute became a joint venture of the departments of Epidemiology and Biostatistics in 1999, it was accordingly renamed and, by 2015, had trained more than 10,000 students worldwide.[15]

Alongside the computer revolution of the 1980s, two of the school's most far-reaching contributions to health reform were (1) the application of health services research and the framework of primary care to shape policy and (2) the initiation of one of the first university-based bioethics programs. The national urban unrest leading up to and including the 1968 Baltimore riots had provided the political atmosphere of crisis that enabled East Baltimore community activists to convince city officials and Johns Hopkins administrators to establish prepaid primary health care programs. The East Baltimore Health Plan built on the Baltimore City Medical Care Program that JHSPH had helped establish in the 1940s. Based on their intensive involvement with and understanding of local health needs, JHSPH faculty, including Paul Lemkau, Paul Harper, Wallace Mandell, Ernest Stebbins, John Hume, Kerr White, Vicente Navarro, Barbara Starfield, Sam Shapiro, Matthew Tayback, Sol Levine, Eugene Feinblatt, and many others, had helped the city and state health departments to improve their responsiveness and efficiency on issues such as Medicaid financing, nursing home and hospital patient safety, and community-based health services for psychiatry, substance abuse, and maternal and child health. By providing a catalyst that moved the university to listen and address community concerns about health care access, the 1968 riots also helped to create an atmosphere in which the School of Hygiene and Public

Health's survey research could be conducted with the support and cooperation of East Baltimore residents. Out of the school's efforts to both conduct high-quality community-based epidemiological research and shape state and local health policy came much of the framework for the advancement of primary care in the United States and abroad, a chief goal of which was to develop population-level, evidence-based methods to close racial and socioeconomic gaps in the quality and accessibility of health care.

Johns Hopkins was the first university to train interdisciplinary health services researchers, incorporating sociology, economics, epidemiology, biostatistics, operations research, and clinical medicine. The Health Services Research and Development Center at Johns Hopkins had been started in 1969 within the Office of Health Care Programs with a grant from the National Center for Health Services Research and Development, which remained its main funder during the center's first decade. In early 1971, the *NBC Evening News* featured a story on how President Nixon's new plan to curb health care inflation had been inspired by prepaid health plans developed by Johns Hopkins. The Johns Hopkins–affiliated health maintenance organizations (HMOs) were among the early models that helped convince Congress to pass the Health Maintenance Organization Act of 1973, which became another important source of funding for health services research at JHSPH and other universities.[16]

A cornerstone of health services research at JHSPH was the Johns Hopkins Adjusted Clinical Groups (ACGs) System developed in the 1970s by Barbara Starfield (MPH 1963), Sam Shapiro, and Donald Steinwachs (PhD 1973), who succeeded Shapiro as director of the Health Services Research and Development Center in 1982. Starfield's clinical observations in pediatric populations led to her research with colleagues in the early 1980s that showed that children with multiple, seemingly unrelated conditions used the most health care resources, not patients with a single chronic illness. Starfield's work complemented the work of HPM colleagues, including Karen Davis and Laura Morlock on the organization and financing of state programs designed to expand medical care for children. Starfield and her protégé Jonathan Weiner (DrPH 1981) extended these findings to all patients, ultimately demonstrating that the clustering of morbidity is a better predictor of health services utilization than the presence of specific diseases.[17]

The ACG acronym, which originally stood for Ambulatory Care Group, denoted the system developed by JHSPH faculty to provide a simple, statistically valid, clinically relevant method for predicting the utilization of ambulatory health services within a particular population group. Kerr White, chair of Medical Care and Hospitals, also chaired the National Committee on Vital and Health Statistics, which issued national recommendations for minimum data sets in billing and discharge records management for ambulatory care, hospitals, and nursing homes. As Steinwachs recalled, "These became the building blocks for information systems and defined key aspects of care delivery and information that you'd like to capture in data systems, as well as the information that should be captured in medical charts." The Health Services Research and Development Center was responsible for developing and operating the computer system used to administer the two local prepaid health plans established by Johns Hopkins, discussed in chapter 9. The ACG system tracked a patient's demographic characteristics and pattern of disease over a year, using ICD-9 diagnoses assigned during patient–provider encounters. By using collected data to create broad clusters of diagnoses and conditions in a patient population, such as a managed care program, the system predicted the presence or absence of each disease cluster. This information, combined with age and sex, was then used to classify each member of the group into one of 51 ACG categories.[18]

JHSPH faculty developed the ACG system by using computerized encounter and claims data from more than 160,000 continuous enrollees in the East Baltimore and Columbia HMOs, as well as the Maryland Medicaid program. By determining the length and frequency of episodes of care within the system and then tracking whether or not patients returned for subsequent care, researchers could begin to determine reasons for variation in the patterns, such as treatment effectiveness or patients not adhering to a plan of care. The ACG system was capable of explaining more than 50 percent of the variance in ambulatory care utilization if used retrospectively and more than 20 percent if applied prospectively. Only 6 percent of the variance was explained by age and sex alone. The ACG system was also expanded to include provider payment, quality assurance, utilization review, and health services research, particularly for capitated health care programs. Although initially used to set insurance rates, patterns from the data could also reveal the scope of specific conditions and point to their causes, help to identify patients at high risk for certain types of illness, or elucidate relationships among different types of disease, such as diabetes and heart disease.[19]

The ACG system was revolutionary because it combined the previously separate functions of health care management with high-volume data collection and analysis for academic research and policymaking. This detailed information could not only drive the business objectives of cost analysis and quality control but also be used to guide health policy and advocate for reform. In its early years, the ACG system was adopted in settings ranging from military health care to insurers such as Aetna, and by 2015, it was operating in 20 countries as the world's most widely used population case-mix system. It would lay the foundation for the adoption of electronic medical records and generate knowledge that contributed to the fields of primary care, health outcomes research, and patient safety. In 1981, Shapiro and Steinwachs were among the founders of the Association for Health Services Research, the field's first professional organization. Steinwachs, as president of the association, and Karen Davis would later play integral roles in establishing the federal Agency for Health Care Policy and Research in 1989.[20]

Steinwachs remembers that, even within the managed care environment, he quickly realized that information by itself was not enough to lead to action. "Information systems could be very valuable," he recalled, "in trying to understand problems and characterize patterns of care and some indicators of outcome." One of the examples where information *did* lead to action was the NIMH Epidemiological Catchment Area Study, which brought Steinwachs and Shapiro in to collaborate with faculty in Mental Hygiene, including department chair Ernest Gruenberg, Mort Kramer, and Paul McHugh, chair of the Department of Psychiatry. Steinwachs became an expert on the relationships between psychiatric illness, particularly severe conditions such as schizophrenia, and medical care utilization for both mental and physical illness.[21]

Shortly after Jimmy Carter took office as president in 1977, he established the President's Commission on Mental Health, chaired by First Lady Rosalyn Carter. The commission issued a report calling for expanding research to accurately determine the prevalence and incidence of mental disorders. NIMH created the Epidemiologic Catchment Area Program (ECA) to measure the prevalence of mental illness in the general population in sites around the United States. The agency recruited William W. Eaton from his position at McGill to coordinate the ECA program. Johns Hopkins received a grant to establish Baltimore as one of five ECA research sites. The ECA survey would measure and quantify the unmet care needs for people with mental and emotional problems. Steinwachs noted, "It was a bellwether study in using a variety of criteria to define whether someone had a mental health problem or a need for mental health care, and then using criteria to look at different ways about was that need being met, at least in health care." The survey employed lay interviewers who underwent an intense two-week training program to administer the complex survey instrument. To determine incidence, or the rate at which new cases form, as well as the overall prevalence of mental illness, the study required sites to conduct an initial survey and a follow-up survey one year later. The newly revised *Diagnostic and Statistical Manual of Mental Disorders* (*DSM-III*) introduced explicit diagnostic criteria and classifications of mental illness. The ECA survey operationalized these classifications and generated psychiatric diagnoses by incorporating the clinical diagnosis criteria for the most prevalent conditions, including depression, schizophrenia, panic disorder, obsessive–compulsive disorder, and substance abuse and dependence. Once the survey identified individuals with a definite or probable psychiatric disorder, follow-up questions asked about utilization of mental health services, including what types of obstacles may have interfered with seeking treatment. Eaton noted that "the degree of psychological introspection in the culture had changed a lot by 1980. You could come and ask people, basically, have they ever heard voices and they won't be completely offended or turn you out the door." The ECA studies revealed that about one-third of Americans would suffer from at least one type of mental illness during their lifetimes and that mental disorders went untreated in many cases.[22]

Carolyn L. Gorman, who worked as an interviewer for the ECA study from its inception in 1979, loved going door to door in East Baltimore. Few residents refused to participate, despite the personal nature and length of the survey, which took about one and a half hours to complete. Gorman recalled that the questions on mental illness were less likely to offend respondents than those on drug use. Gorman could usually predict whether the inhabitant would participate based on the house's exterior appearance: well-kept and painted houses with toys and flowers in the yard usually meant yes. She had a collection of Polish dolls and would take a doll with her on interviews. When one of the many Polish women in the neighborhood saw her doll, they would always agree to take the survey. At the Survey Research Associates office on 23rd Street, Gorman trained most of the 30 interviewers who conducted the ECA survey.[23]

At NIMH, Bill Eaton helped to guide the Baltimore study's design and argued to include its clinical reappraisal component in all the ECA study sites. After winning an ADAMHA Administrator's Award for his implementation of the ECA Program, Eaton joined the Department of Mental Hygiene faculty in 1983 and would serve as chair from 2004 to 2014. The Baltimore study was unique among the ECA sites for conducting additional follow-up surveys beyond the one-year mark. After the first two surveys in 1981 and 1982, the Baltimore study reinterviewed the participants in 1993 and again in 2004. One of the most remarkable findings was the degree to which major depressive disorder was predictive of the new occurrence of important physical conditions such as type 2 diabetes, heart attack, stroke, and breast cancer.[24]

Henderson would consolidate and enhance the school's work in primary care by reorganizing its programs in health services research, administration, and policy. He began with the teaching programs, since by 1978, Congress had narrowed and more explicitly defined the purposes of federal support for public health training to prescribe that training in health administration, the most popular public health subspecialty, should focus on meeting "the shortage of appropriately trained managers throughout the health system and the inadequacy of current training resources to solve that problem." The program continued public health special project grants to support "accredited graduate programs in health administration, health planning, or health policy analysis and planning to meet the costs of developing programs in four areas: (a) biostatistics or epidemiology; (b) health administration, health planning, or health policy analysis and planning; (c) environmental or occupational health; or (d) dietetics and nutrition." Moreover, the legislation specified the share of public health traineeships to be awarded in these areas, increasing from a combined total of at least 45 percent in fiscal year 1978 to 65 percent by fiscal year 1980. Federal funding for traineeships at JHSPH, therefore, was targeted toward the departments of Biostatistics, Epidemiology, Health Services Administration, and Environmental Health Sciences. These departments were also, along with Mental Hygiene and Maternal and Child Health, those most deeply involved with the MPH program.[25]

In 1979–1980, the Curriculum Committee conducted a year-long study of the MPH program and made five recommendations, including nomination of a faculty member as director of the MPH program. Abe Lilienfeld was appointed director of the MPH program beginning April 1, 1980, for a three-year, renewable term. With a new MPH program budget of $100,000, the director was accorded equal status with the department chairs, including membership on the school's Advisory Board. Lilienfeld appointed an MPH program committee of six faculty members to revise the existing MPH program and oversee its progress. He wrote Henderson,

> The MPH program is what makes a school of public health the unique type of institution that it is. . . . It should be understood that the MPH Program requires considerable substantive changes. . . . Frankly, our MPH program as well as those in all of the other schools of public health have not changed materially over the past 20–30 years. Many have been floundering in attempting to revitalize these programs. . . . I think that our School, with its unparalleled resources, has a real opportunity to make a markedly innovative contribution to graduate education in public health in restructuring the MPH program.[26]

After Arthur Bushel retired as chair of Health Services Administration in 1983, his successor, Karen Davis, became the first woman chair at JHSPH. Davis had served as chief health policy adviser to President Jimmy Carter, and she changed the department's title to Health Policy and Management to reflect Henderson's and her own plans to strengthen the department in the areas of effective health services leadership and influencing health care legislation. In 1984, HPM assumed administrative oversight of the previously independent Health Services Research and Development Center. In 1987, the Department of Behavioral Sciences and Health Education also became a division of HPM.[27]

In addition to the development of primary care and health services research, bioethics was the second gift that crisis bestowed on JHSPH. National outcry over the Tuskegee Syphilis Study came at the height of the Black Power movement and just before the Watergate scandal further undermined public trust in the federal government. Congress responded in 1974 by creating the National Commission for the Protection of Human Subjects of Biomedical and Behavioral Research. The commission's Belmont Report, issued in April 1979, was the basis for the development and implementation of modern human subjects research protections, including the establishment of institutional review boards (IRBs) at universities and federal agencies. At JHSPH, the school's Advisory Board had first required approval for research involving human subjects in 1952 and established a formal IRB in 1975 under the direction of Roger Herriott. IRB members were tasked with evaluating proposed research to ensure that the rights and well-being of human volunteers were protected and that investigators obeyed federal and institutional guidelines for ethical research. Ruth R. Faden, who joined the Public Health Administration faculty in 1975, and her husband Tom L. Beauchamp, principal author of the Belmont Report, published one of the founding texts of bioethics, *A History and Theory of Informed Consent* (1986). Faden would go on to found the Berman Bioethics Institute in 1995, endowed with a gift from philanthropist Phoebe R. Berman.[28]

Like the Health Services Research and Development Center and the ECA Catchment Study, Carl Taylor's Narangwal Experiment illustrates how the school learned to combine good science with sound ethics and how these goals complemented each other. The Narangwal Experiment involved more than 150 Indian staff members and four Hopkins staff who conducted projects in five rural areas with a population of about 25,000 in the Indian state of Punjab. Taylor wrote to D. N. Chaudhuri, deputy secretary of Health and Family Planning, "We have worried more than any one else about ensuring that our research be relevant to India. Being a villager myself I have an abhorrence of esoteric research that does not reach the village." But by "taking sophisticated scientists to the village to live," Taylor had been able to generate "vastly greater research outputs resulting from their proximity to their work and the clear change in orientation and understanding that comes from close personal association with our wonderful village friends." Taylor also justified the study's use of randomized subjects and a control group, which tested health, nutritional, and family planning services in isolation and in different combinations to determine what "produces the greatest results for the least cost."[29]

The nutrition and infection component of the Narangwal Study, conducted over a seven-year period, demonstrated that community health workers could reduce child mortality in all three trial groups (health services only, nutrition services only, and integrated health and nutrition services) by as much as 45 percent, which was much greater than in the traditional government health centers that served as the control. Moreover, the integrated services were five times more cost-effective than the stand-alone services. Further studies comparing the provision of family planning, nutrition, and basic maternal and child health services alone and in combination achieved similar results, including the doubling or tripling of rates of contraceptive use by couples who had not previously used modern family planning.[30]

In countries such as India, USAID's international health programs focused on maternal and child health but with a greater (sometimes competing) emphasis on family planning. Despite strong pressure from the USAID Office of Population, International Planned Parenthood Federation, and other groups that focused primarily on curbing population growth, most countries by the late 1970s followed India's example of administering family planning programs through the Ministry of Health rather than in stand-alone programs, which reflected to no small degree the influence of JHSPH faculty and alumni in those countries. The Narangwal Study was a major turning point that helped international public health workers to recognize the disadvantages of traditional vertical public health campaigns and the ethnocentric approach that often accompanied them. The study also built on the longstanding commitment of Taylor and Indian Minister of Health Sushila Nayar to integrating family planning into a comprehensive public health and medical care program. They emphasized both the ethical and practical importance of cultural sensitivity to patients' preferences.[31]

In May 1974, the Indian government forced Taylor to shut down the Narangwal Rural Health Research Center, which had survived for the past year as the last USAID project left in India. Yet even after the field operations closed, Taylor's close relationship with Indian medical schools and the Indian Council on Medical Research ensured that the Narangwal model was built directly into India's new Fifth Five-Year Plan. The study's influence would soon expand beyond India. On the return flight from India back to the United States, Taylor received a random upgrade to first class and found himself seated next to Robert McNamara, president of the World Bank. Taylor urged McNamara, the world's leading foreign development official, to embrace Narangwal's holistic approach to reproductive health and to broaden loan programs to support "human capital" through health, nutrition, education, and family planning.[32]

In addition to advocating for a horizontal approach to primary care and reproductive health services among Western-led development agencies, Taylor also played a pivotal role in organizing the 1978 Alma Ata World Conference on Primary Health Care, where representatives of medicine and public health from around the world met in the Soviet Union to declare that equity should be central to primary health care, with the slogan "Health for All by the Year

2000." The two key principles to which Taylor and his fellow delegates dedicated themselves at Alma Ata were the need to abandon vertical models of disease control and family planning in favor of integrated services, as well as the desirability of "community-based primary health care in which a primary responsibility of health workers is to empower people to solve their own problems rather than to promote dependency." The Alma Ata Declaration has since served as the touchstone of the global health equity movement.[33]

The ideals of Narangwal and Alma Ata would be taken up by the WHO under director-general Halfdan T. Mahler, an ally of D. A. Henderson. But at a 1979 conference in Bellagio, Italy, sponsored by the Rockefeller Foundation, McNamara, UNICEF executive secretary James P. Grant, and representatives of USAID and the Ford Foundation formulated what they believed to be a more practical and achievable strategy for reducing global mortality among children under age 5. Instead, they pursued selective primary health care, which focused on applying a set of low-cost but highly effective interventions that could be easily monitored and evaluated on a mass scale. Selective primary health care endeavored to capitalize on the best of both primary health care and the most successful vertical campaigns, namely WHO's global smallpox eradication and Expanded Program on Immunization.[34]

The Child Survival Revolution

The Narangwal research and the Alma Ata conference had made Carl Taylor one of the world's most respected global health experts, but his Department of International Health was in financial trouble. As early as 1973–1974, Hume and Taylor had been forced to lay off 12 International Health faculty and staff. By 1977, USAID funding for the department was rapidly drying up, especially after Daniel Patrick Moynihan, as US Ambassador to India, had convinced President Nixon and his foreign policy advisers that the best way to prevent further instability in South Asia was to forgive the entire rupee debt that India owed under the P.L. 480 program. Taylor told Vicente Navarro (DrPH 1968), editor of the *International Journal of Health Services*, that the Department of International Health would have to terminate its annual support of $9,000 for the journal because the department's current USAID grant term had ended and its faculty was "having a very difficult time and are having to survive on carry-over funds. The new grant will be much more targeted to specific activities. It will not permit the flexibility that we have enjoyed under 211-d. I am extremely sorry but again I hope that the Journal is sufficiently mature that it does not need to depend on this support." Taylor also expressed to Henderson the department's "tremendous need for financing for the residency programs. Because we have had no financing for the international health residencies we have had to grab funds from wherever they became available."[35]

Henderson and Taylor had spent their careers pursuing many of the same goals for improving the health status of populations in low-income, underresourced countries; both men highly valued scientific data collection and the practical application of research, and both had logged extensive field experience in India and across the globe. But what set them apart was Taylor's principled insistence that primary health services, including reproductive health and family planning, should be horizontally organized. Taylor saw the vertical health campaign as a fundamentally flawed model, while Henderson was cognizant of the lessons of the malaria eradication campaign but believed that smallpox eradication was irrefutable proof that vertical campaigns could be not only redeemed but also taken to new levels. Taylor and Henderson would frequently debate each other on the merits of their respective strategies.[36]

For most of the twentieth century, birthrates and infectious disease mortality in Africa, Asia, and Latin America had remained tragically high, with women of childbearing age and children under age 5 at highest risk from complications of pregnancy and the combined effects of prematurity, malnutrition, and infectious disease. During the 1970s, both USAID and the World Bank began to move beyond "gross economic goals" such as increasing gross domestic product and also began to pursue the equitable distribution of development's benefits within recipient nations. Taylor leveraged his Narangwal research on the cost-effectiveness and efficacy of integrated primary health and family planning services to influence Robert McNamara at the World Bank to broaden loan programs to strengthen health, nutrition, education, and family planning programs in borrower nations. The Narangwal Study would become one of the bases for the 1994 Cairo World Population Conference's endorsement of the reproductive health model that stressed the full integration of family planning and maternal and child health services. Under McNamara's influence, international development agencies, including USAID, began to focus on alleviating poverty as a central objective. By 1982, half of USAID's health budget supported delivery of basic health services in the less developed countries via direct payments to national governments, and population control receded in importance under pressure from both domestic pro-life activists and developing-world advocates of self-determination. In 1983, the Reagan administration defined USAID's top priorities as raising the life expectancy in all developing countries above 60 years, reducing infant mortality to less than 75 per 1,000, and increasing literacy rates to 70 percent.[37]

Building on the foundation of the polio vaccine and pregnancy and prematurity research of the 1950s, the epidemiological studies of developmental disabilities in the 1960s, and the research on diarrheal diseases, pediatric malnutrition, family planning, and primary health care of the 1970s, JHSPH researchers would target each of these factors one by one and then in combination, carefully amassing the scientific basis for what would become known in the 1980s as the "global child survival revolution." Nathaniel F. Pierce (who would later join the JHSPH International Health faculty), Brad Sack, Charles Carpenter, and their colleagues, drawing from their work in Calcutta with the Johns Hopkins Center for Medical Research and Training cholera program and in other countries, helped to establish oral rehydration therapy (ORT) as the standard pediatric treatment for cholera and other diarrheal illnesses. They also worked hard and effectively to convince US physicians to adopt ORT in place of traditional intravenous therapy requiring hospitalization.[38]

Henry Mosley, who had served as chair of Population Dynamics from 1971 to 1977, was at the confluence of the family planning, diarrheal disease, and nutrition streams of the child survival river. He had returned to Dhaka in 1977 to lead the reorganization of the SEATO–Pakistan Cholera Hospital to become the independent International Centre for Diarrheal Disease Research, Bangladesh. Since the 1960s, the center has been a research and training base for many JHSPH faculty working on cholera therapy and vaccine research. When Jim Grant, John Black Grant's son who was director of UNICEF, launched its historic child survival initiative in 1980, he asked Mosley to advise a range of agencies, including the Population Council and Ford Foundation, to develop the framework for child survival programs in Kenya and Indonesia. In 1984, Mosley and his former student Lincoln Chen (MPH 1973) published *Child Survival: Strategies for Research*, which became a master plan for child survival similar to what the proximate determinants framework, developed in 1956 by Kingsley Davis and Judith Blake, had been for population and family planning.[39]

Since Henderson became dean, he had been trying to recruit Mosley back to JHSPH. He finally succeeded in 1985, when Mosley was appointed chair of the Department of Population Dynamics. Meanwhile, Mosley's former EIS colleague at the International Center for Diarrheal Disease Research, Al Sommer, had returned to the Johns Hopkins medical faculty in Ophthalmology with a joint appointment in Epidemiology. With Henderson's support, Sommer established the Dana Center for Preventive Ophthalmology as a collaboration between the schools of Medicine and Hygiene that included a year-long MPH program in public health ophthalmology for 10 to 20 students. The center drew on faculty from the JHSPH departments of Biostatistics, Epidemiology, Environmental Health Sciences, and International Health, and three of the center's faculty who transferred their primary appointments from Medicine to Hygiene in 1994 (Keith West, Joanne Katz, and Jim Tielsch) have become, like Sommer, senior leaders at JHSPH. In 1983, Sommer published the first in a series of articles on his landmark epidemiological field trials on the causes and consequences of vitamin A deficiency. Sommer's research, after steep initial resistance, would eventually lead WHO and UNICEF to adopt large-scale distribution of high-dose oral vitamin A supplementation in developing countries as a cost-effective method to prevent blindness and cut child mortality rates by 34 percent. UNICEF, WHO, and other international agencies and NGOs combined micronutrient supplementation with oral rehydration, breastfeeding, and immunization to launch mass child survival campaigns throughout the developing world. The implementation of these child survival methods, which later included family planning, resulted in halving the global mortality rate among children under age 5 between 1980 and 2010.[40]

Taylor had resigned in 1983 to become the UNICEF representative in China, just as the philosophy of universal free access to primary health care from the Alma Ata movement was encountering competition from the selective primary health care model advocated by UNICEF. Taylor's departure meant that Henderson was faced with another critical hiring decision: finding a suitable successor. The search did not progress quickly, but in 1985, Henderson appointed Robert E. Black as the second chair of International Health. Black, like Henderson, Sommer, Mosley, and so many other leaders at JHSPH and in public health generally, had served in both the Epidemic Intelligence Service and at the ICDDR,B in Dacca. The EIS was well known as a high-quality training ground for international health physicians and also represented a much more attractive option to most physicians than serving in Vietnam, leading to the nickname "the Yellow Berets." Black, however, did not join the EIS until 1975, when he went to Dacca to work on solutions to the problems of extremely severe pediatric diarrhea, a major source of developing-world child mortality. He tested the effectiveness of oral rehydration therapy against different causes of diarrhea, including rotavirus, toxic *E. coli*, and other newly discovered pathogens.[41]

When Black arrived at JHSPH in 1985, only one faculty member in International Health, George Graham, was studying nutrition. Likewise, at USAID and UNICEF, immunization and oral rehydration therapy were considered the "twin engines" of child survival, with little attention to nutrition. Black had to overcome significant resistance to convince the agencies that nutrition was an equally important factor in preventing mortality in young children. Mosley returned to JHSPH just as Black arrived, and the two chairs would work to develop a new agreement with USAID to support child survival research at JHSPH. Henderson often convened Mosley, Black, and Sommer to strategize in the dean's office. As Sommer's work on vitamin A in the medical school and Department of Epidemiology grew alongside Black's in International Health and Mosley's in Population Dynamics, they were able to take advantage of a powerful synergy at JHSPH to promote micronutrient supplementation as a centerpiece of child survival research and policy. Black began to study the links between nutrition and susceptibility to infections, first hinted at in Gilbert Otto's long-ago studies of hookworm in southern children, and Black built on Taylor's description in Narangwal of the weaning syndrome, especially in areas where food availability was irregular. JHSPH faculty took advantage of the new analytic methods that had arisen from biocomputing and large-scale cohort studies and clinical trials to develop deeper, more quantified understandings of the dynamics among nutrition, infectious disease, and social and environmental factors. With Republicans in Congress heavily backing child survival funding during the Reagan administration, funding from USAID resumed and increased, and the department won child survival grants from the Ford, Rockefeller, and Carnegie foundations.[42]

While on the faculty at the University of Maryland School of Medicine, Black had worked closely with the Center for Vaccine Development and tested vaccines for diarrheal and respiratory viruses. He began to see connections emerging between the treatment of both types of disease with micronutrient supplementation and, in the early 1990s, began landmark large-scale clinical trials of zinc to treat diarrhea in children in Peru, Bangladesh, Chile, and other countries. The work on the interrelated issues of vaccines, nutrition, diarrheal and respiratory disease, and low birth weight by Henderson, Sack, Pierce, Mosley, Sommer, Taylor, Mathuram Santosham (MPH 1975), Robert Gilman, Keith West (DrPH 1986), and many other JHSPH faculty has been such a crucial factor in the success of the child survival revolution that they are rightly considered to be among its architects. Even after so much progress, however, two-thirds of the nearly 7 million child deaths in developing countries each year are directly caused by infectious diseases such as pneumonia, diarrhea, and malaria, with undernutrition contributing to one-third of under-5 mortality.[43]

D. A. Henderson and the Rise of Academic Centers

Henderson urged the school's leaders to proactively set their own goals and parameters for research and training programs, instead of chasing after the constantly moving targets of federal granting agencies. This was easier said than done, however. During the 1970s, major shifts in the political economy of public health research added new layers of accountability and transparency for investigators, which instituted critically important protections for human subjects but also introduced new challenges, costs, and uncertainties into the research enterprise. Stand-alone centers that focused on specific health problems gained popularity as both a policymaking tool and a tactic for universities to secure additional funding for program expansion. But Hume had been wary of them. JHSPH participation in the Center for Urban Affairs, for example, had only lasted four years before its founding director, Sol Levine, left Johns Hopkins and the university's new president, Steven Muller, relocated the center from East Baltimore to the Homewood campus. Three other JHSPH-led centers had proven more lasting and fruitful: the Training Center for Public Health Research in Hagerstown, the Health Services Research and Development Center, and the Hopkins Population Center. Some biostatistics and epidemiology faculty were also involved with the medical school's Oncology Clinical Center, essentially a dedicated cancer hospital funded by a large NCI grant.

Hume wrote in 1974 that, while centers offered "tremendous opportunities" for attracting major funding and applying diverse expertise to solve key problems, they were also expensive and often ephemeral, due to "the evanescent societal interest in any given problem." Hume worried that departments would become dependent on center funding that could, if it disappeared, jeopardize primary teaching functions. His caution was well taken, given the school's frustrating experience with federal funding for public health. "The perennial fluctuation in federal policy," Hume complained, "the inability to plan for the future even for the short range caused by fiscal uncertainties, to say nothing of the more general problems of inflation and lack of direction in the government, create a sense of insecurity among the faculty which becomes most wearing and . . . leads to the erosion of the satisfaction which most faculty members have derived from their work over the years." Yet during Hume's deanship, federal funding would drive the school's expansion from direct expenditures of $8.2 million in fiscal year 1967 (74 percent for sponsored research) to $20 million in fiscal year 1977 (70 percent for sponsored research).[44]

Henderson, by contrast, embraced centers as a way of "promoting meaningful collaboration between a multidisciplinary group of faculty and professionals [who] will generate new policies, new strategies, and new tactics in public health far sooner than through any other approach." In his initial letter to the faculty, Henderson stated his intention to strengthen programs that integrated disciplines, departments, and university divisions, as well as those that promoted collaboration between the school and both the public and the private sectors. The number of centers at JHSPH would grow from four when Henderson arrived in 1977 to 19 when he stepped down in 1990.[45]

Like the mid-1930s and the late 1950s, the late 1970s were years of financial reckoning for JHSPH, when both the school and the university were merging departments to streamline administration and reduce costs. In 1976, the departments of Environmental Health and Environmental Medicine (which had absorbed Radiological Science as a division after Russell Morgan was appointed dean of medicine in 1971) had merged to form the Department of Environmental Health Sciences (EHS). The idea had been proposed in a letter written by Gareth Green after he interviewed for the chairmanship of Environmental Health. In 1978, Green invited faculty to serve on a committee to review the field of Environmental Health Engineering, since Cornelius Krusé was retiring as head of the division. Green wrote that the need to regulate and control chronic diseases caused by the environmental hazards of industrial civilizations posed the greatest challenges for environmental health engineering since the early twentieth century, when sanitary engineering first developed methods for the mass control of infectious disease. Green believed that JHSPH and the Division of Environmental Health Engineering in particular were "at a major turning point in the history of public health practice" but were "ill prepared to respond to the demands in air pollution control, industrial hygiene and safety, occupational health, toxic substances control, accident prevention and safety management, solid waste disposal and waste water management, and related areas where control technology might conceivably reduce the burden of accident and illness, morbidity and mortality in industrialized civilizations." The merger made EHS the largest department of its kind in the country, with more faculty and students than many entire schools of public health. The EHS budget grew from $4.6 million in 1980 to $11.6 million by 1990.[46]

Several national trends in the late 1970s supported the decision by Henderson and other JHSPH leaders to establish a novel research partnership with industry that began with a focus on environmental issues and later extended across the spectrum of public health issues. First, federal agencies aimed to encourage universities and industry to reestablish mutually beneficial relationships. In the 1980s, universities and private industry groups established a variety of successful cooperative research programs. Second, both universities and the cosmetics industry faced increasing pressures to fundamentally change the way they treated animals. The Congressional Office of Technology Assessment estimated that about 22 million animals died annually in academic and industrial research testing labs, and other estimates placed the figure as high as 70 million. Three-quarters of these animals were used in biomedical research on animal models to benefit humans, for which Johns Hopkins had helped set the international standard. But as Ellen Silbergeld, an EHS postdoctoral fellow and future faculty member, recalled, "We had horrible attitudes towards the treatment of animals [in the 1970s]. You didn't have to justify animal use for research, you could just order some animals and there was no sense of the sanctity of life of animals and their experience."[47]

Between 2 and 5 million animals died annually in consumer product safety testing alone. Two standard animal tests had long been used to satisfy FDA requirements to provide proof that products were not harmful to humans: the Draize eye test, introduced in 1944 by John Draize, and the Lethal Dose 50 test (known as LD 50) in use since the 1920s, which measures a substance's toxicity by determining the dosage required to kill half of the test group of animals, which are injected, force-fed, or forced to inhale the substance.[48]

American researchers had balked at having restrictions placed on animal use to promote ethical treatment and assumed that such guidelines would cause expensive delays that would affect the quality of their science. But during her first experience doing research in Sweden, Silbergeld was struck by the differences she observed "in very productive labs doing the best work and treating the animals with respect." In response to a clash between the cosmetics industry and the animal rights movement, environmental toxicologist Alan Goldberg founded the Center for Alternatives to Animal Testing (CAAT) at JHSPH. In 1980, animal rights activist Henry Spira had formed the Coalition to Abolish the LD 50 and Draize Tests, which included more than 400 animal welfare organizations. The coalition urged cosmetics companies such as Revlon and Avon to find humane alternatives to the tests and took out a full-page *New York Times* ad showing a white rabbit with tape across both eyes, with the caption, "How many rabbits does Revlon blind for beauty's sake?" In the immediate fallout from the ad, Revlon and Avon responded by contributing hundreds of thousands of dollars to an alternative testing program at Rockefeller University. But at JHSPH during the 1950s, polio and defense research had led to major advances in tissue culture methods and in vitro toxicity testing. Goldberg wanted to use this commanding knowledge to develop alternative testing methods that were not only humane but would greatly improve on the precision and scientific validity of existing animal tests.[49]

Goldberg called the LD 50 test "grossly unreliable" because various animal species produced divergent results, and even among the same species, results varied from lab to lab. According to Goldberg, "The change in a cell culture can be measured with assurance after it has been treated with a toxic substance," whereas it was not always certain whether an animal's metabolism was responding to the toxic substance or an unknown stimulus. He acknowledged that "we have an obligation and a necessity to use animals, but I think we have to do that with great care and justification." Rather than a standard in-house research center, Goldberg set up CAAT in 1981 as an international clearinghouse for non–animal testing research, with an extramural grants program to independent researchers. He established an advisory board with scientists from academics, industry, and regulatory agencies, which dovetailed with the new emphasis on public–private research partnerships under Henderson.[50]

The Cosmetics, Toiletry, and Fragrance Association trade group also considered in vitro testing with test tubes the most viable alternative to live animal (in vivo) testing. The cosmetics trade group became CAAT's top funding source, with substantial contributions from Noxell and Avon as well as from Bristol-Meyers, Exxon, Clorox, and Bausch and Lomb. Corporations recognized that in vitro testing would be less expensive and might even represent a new industry itself. Commercial breeders who produced rats, mice, rabbits, and other animals used for testing earned annual profits totaling $1 billion. Alternative testing labs hoped to take advantage of the new market, but alternatives to the Draize test on rabbits had to be intensely evaluated for reliability, reproducibility, and sensitivity, which could take up to eight years for FDA and EPA approval.[51]

In 1983, Goldberg convened a CAAT symposium that convinced FDA and EPA officials to urge the cosmetics industry to reduce the number of animals it used. Many companies responded by reducing the number of animals used for LD 50 testing or abandoning the test entirely. CAAT-sponsored research also helped pass amendments to the 1985 Animal Welfare Act to require personnel who conduct animal tests to use methods that minimize or eliminate the use of animals and limit their distress. CAAT influenced the FDA to invest in research on in vitro alternatives, which by 1986 accounted for $10 million of the FDA's total $70 million budget. By 1992, CAAT's budget had risen to $1.5 million and was a mainstay of the EHS departmental budget, which validated Goldberg and Henderson's twin funding strategies of establishing department-based research centers and building public–private partnerships with private industry, corporations, and government agencies (table 13.3).[52]

Fred Bang's empire in the Department of Pathobiology also had involved animal research in both the laboratory and ecological fieldwork that closely aligned the department's faculty with their colleagues in EHS. From 1953 until his death in 1981, Bang had broadened the scope of basic science far beyond the laboratory and outward all the way to both poles, while establishing and retaining high-quality research in tropical diseases (notably malaria, leprosy, and schistosomiasis). William Sladen, G. Carleton Ray, and their likeminded colleagues had taken Rachel Carson's gospel of biodiversity and run with it, but some faculty had criticized their vertebrate ecology research as peripheral to public health. In their heyday, the population biology programs had helped to make Pathobiology the school's best-funded department, but by the early 1980s, the tide of support had receded. Space in the school was at a premium, and the Pathobiology menagerie, including the 5,000-gallon seal tank and freezers containing penguin excrement of unknown vintage, occupied most of the basement. Henderson, under budgetary pressures and eager to revive the school's storied programs in infectious disease and bench science, knew exactly what kind of candidate he wanted to take the helm of Pathobiology.[53]

One of the last papers that Isabel Morgan published before she left JHSPH had foreshadowed the department's new direction. She had described the pathogenesis of experimental allergic encephalomyelitis, or virus-induced encephalitis, one of the first experimentally induced autoimmune diseases. In 1982, Henderson appointed Bang's successor, Noel R. Rose, an immunologist at Wayne State University. Rose's pioneering studies in the 1950s on autoimmune

TABLE 13.3
Growth of Centers at JHSPH, 1932–1990

Name	Founding Director	Year Founded	Notes
Eastern Health District	Harry S. Mustard	1932	Teaching and research field study district administered jointly with the Baltimore City Health Department, dissolved 1964.
Center for the Study of Infantile Paralysis and Related Viruses	Kenneth F. Maxcy	1942	Founded with grant from National Foundation for Infantile Paralysis, dissolved 1960.
Center for Medical Research and Training	Frederik B. Bang	1960	Founded in Calcutta, India; later relocated to Dacca, Bangladesh, and renamed Tropical Medicine Center; dissolved 1978.
Johns Hopkins Training Center for Public Health Research	George W. Comstock	1962	Located in Hagerstown, Maryland.
Narangwal Rural Health Research Center	Carl E. Taylor	1962	Located in Narangwal, India, closed by Indian government in 1974.
Center for Urban Affairs	Sol Levine	1968	Moved to Homewood campus and renamed the Center for Metropolitan Planning and Research in 1970, renamed Institute for Policy Studies in 1985, moved to HPM in 2009 and renamed Institute for Health and Social Policy.
Health Services Research and Development Center	Malcolm Peterson	1969	Based in JHMI Office of Health Care Programs 1969–1973; free-standing center 1973–1984; administered under HPM since 1984.
Hopkins Population Center	W. Henry Mosley	1971	University-wide center.
Center for Hospital Finance and Management	Carl J. Schramm	1977	
Dana Center for Preventive Ophthalmology	Alfred Sommer	1980	Based in the SOM Wilmer Eye Institute with JHSPH collaboration.
Center for Alternatives to Animal Testing	Alan Goldberg	1981	
Prevention Research Center	Sheppard G. Kellam	1983	
Center for the Advancement of Radiation Education and Research	Henry Wagner	1983	

(*continued*)

TABLE 13.3 *(continued)*
Growth of Centers at JHSPH, 1932–1990

Name	Founding Director	Year Founded	Notes
Center for Immunization Research	Mary Lou Clements-Mann	1985	
Institute for International Programs	W. Henry Mosley	1985	
Occupational Safety and Health Education and Research Center	Morton M. Korn	1985	
Johns Hopkins Injury Prevention Center	Susan P. Baker	1987	
Johns Hopkins– University of Maryland Center for Research on Services for Severe Mental Illness	Donald Steinwachs	1987	
Center for Communication Programs	Phyllis Piotrow	1988	Piotrow brought the Population Information Program to JHSPH in 1979 and added the Population Communication Services project in 1982.
Fogarty Epidemiology of AIDS International Training and Research Program	Harvey Fischman	1989	
Welch Center for Prevention, Epidemiology and Clinical Research	Paul Whelton	1989	Joint center with SOM.
Center for American Indian Health	Mathuram Santosham	1990	
Center for Human Nutrition	Benjamin Caballero	1990	

Note: Entries shaded in gray denote centers that no longer exist.

thyroiditis, one of more than 80 conditions identified by the autoimmune disease criteria published in 1957 by Rose and Ernst Witebsky, established him as the father of autoimmune research. His subsequent work revealed the genetic, infectious, and environmental factors that increase risk of autoimmune diseases such as multiple sclerosis and trigger their onset. Rose edited the field's first textbook, *The Autoimmune Diseases*, with Ian McKay in 1985.[54]

Rose acknowledged the contributions of Bang and his predecessors, who had "created a whole new field of study in this country, medical zoology, and put medical protozoology, helminthology and entomology on the academic map." Yet in the two decades since the joint Medicine–Hygiene Department of Microbiology had been dissolved in 1961, bench science work in microbiology had faded and the department had abandoned its once-prodigious work on malaria. Rose was also influenced by the work of Manfred Mayer, who, after leaving Hygiene with Turner and David Bodian, had gone on to chair the medical school's Department of Molecular Biology and Genetics. Mayer's lab had helped to usher in a renaissance in molecular-level complement research in the 1960s and 1970s. By renaming the department Immunology and Infectious Diseases, Rose reclaimed the Welchian legacy of Turner, Bodian, and Mayer. Rose increased the size and quality of the graduate program by landing an NIH training grant on the Molecular Basis of Infectious Disease. The department's research emphasized protective immunity in infectious disease and immune-mediated disorders, including HIV/AIDS, hantavirus, human papillomavirus, and tuberculosis.[55]

Conclusion

During the quarter century following World War II, the Cold War had inflamed US policymakers' concerns about national security and global political stability, which had in turn accelerated the growth of academic public health in the United States. But in the 1960s and 1970s, Cold War tensions eased while Great Society health and education funding rapidly rose and then evaporated. These events prompted Johns Hopkins and other schools of public health to reduce their reliance on defense-related funding and diversify their programmatic scope and funding base. Examples of this at JHSPH included the NIH-funded expansion of chronic disease epidemiology, reproductive biology, and methods to prevent and treat substance abuse and addiction, as well as the establishment of academic research centers such as the Health Services Research and Development Center and the privately funded Center for Alternatives to Animal Testing. As this chapter has shown, under D. A. Henderson, JHSPH also capitalized on its existing strengths and built new capacity in international and environmental health, which have been two of the top public health growth fields of the last half century in terms of available funding and numbers of graduates. Under Henderson, these two fields drove the school's unprecedented expansion: the JHSPH budget nearly quadrupled from $20 million in 1977 to $94 million in 1990.

Although constantly shifting funding sources undeniably shaped the development of the school's departmental structure and research programs, this chapter has also demonstrated the faculty's core humanitarian commitment to the mission of improving the health of people everywhere, from East Baltimore to the Punjab. Both Barbara Starfield and Carl Taylor, along with their many colleagues, devoted their careers to expanding primary health care access for all. Starfield and Taylor wrestled at close range with the devastating effects of poverty and isolation from basic health services, and their achievements illustrate the intricate and powerful ways that the very best public health research melds high ethical and scientific standards. They were also instrumental in reorienting the Preventive Medicine Residency at JHSPH from a program administered by separate departments to a single General Preventive Medicine Residency.

Taylor and Starfield served with Edyth Schoenrich, Gareth Green, and Don Cornely as Hygiene representatives on the JHMI Committee on Primary Care, chaired by Cornely in the mid-1970s. The committee was concerned that the current Preventive Medicine Residency was too specialized and departmentally focused, and was not adequately preparing candidates for either certification by the American Board of Preventive Medicine or careers as administrators in programs to provide comprehensive health services. Schoenrich, who then headed the Division of Public Health Administration in the Department of Health Care Organization, proposed creating a post-MPH residency program with six months in Health Care Organization, six in Maternal and Child Health and Population Dynamics, six in Epidemiology, and six in Environmental Health, which would provide "depth and breadth that would qualify a resident for a fairly high level health administration role in society." Central to the committee's proposed changes to the residency was adding a clinical primary care component, which inculcated residents with the values and methods that Taylor, Starfield, Cornely, and Green had championed in their own research and advocacy on various aspects of primary care, whether in domestic, international, environmental, or maternal and child health. After Henderson appointed Schoenrich Associate Dean for Academic Affairs in 1977, she led in implementing these reforms in the early 1980s.[56]

Epilogue

In 1916, Johns Hopkins became the world's first university to establish an independent graduate school of public health. Although the federally funded growth of enrollments from 1960 to 1975 was impressive, it pales in comparison to that of the past 40 years. In 1975, there were 21 schools of public health in the United States with a total graduate enrollment of 5,821 and no programs outside these schools. By 2016, the Council for Education in Public Health (CEPH) had accredited 55 schools and 45 programs in the United States, with an enrollment of 53,000 (34,000 graduate students). In 2015, these institutions awarded nearly 13,000 master's and doctoral degrees in public health.[1]

From 1975 to 2015, the increase in the number of schools and the size of enrollments in public health was exponentially greater than in any other health science field (by comparison, no new medical schools were accredited between 1980 and 2005) and far greater than in most other higher education fields. This expansion has intensified especially in the past 15 years, despite the severe economic downturn that began in 2008, due to the influx of both federal and philanthropic funding as well as intensifying interest in global health, AIDS research, and the value of social and behavioral science methodology for advancing public health.

The career of David Celentano (MHS 1975, ScD 1977) illustrates how many of the themes discussed in this book have played out into the twenty-first century, particularly the profound influence of social and behavioral science methods on the development of risk factor epidemiology. After earning a bachelor's degree at Hopkins in the early 1970s, Celentano had taken a year off to work in the University of Maryland's methadone maintenance program "in the deepest, most horrible part of Baltimore, really getting to see what human suffering and misery were all about." He had planned to apply to medical school, but his experiences with substance abuse treatment made him realize that "I'm never going to save them one at a time." Celentano instead enrolled at JHSPH in Wallace Mandell's 11-month alcoholism counseling MHS program, which included rotations at different inpatient and outpatient treatment centers in Baltimore. The students discussed their field experiences and learned new methods for program evaluation. At the time, substance abuse treatment programs were rarely expected to show proof of their effectiveness. Even the Baltimore City Health Department program was small and had no coordinated data.[2]

After completing the counseling training program, Celentano received an NIAAA fellowship to pursue a doctorate in Behavioral Sciences. His dissertation with Mandell and epidemiologist George Comstock addressed the epidemiology of alcoholism at a community level in Hagerstown, Maryland. Celentano learned to compare different ways of estimating the prevalence and risk factors for alcoholism. His doctoral training combined "the strengths of epidemiological methods and the theoretical rigor of the social sciences," which developed Celentano's "entire approach to looking at risk factors and [their] immutability for different kinds of health conditions." The school had evolved from its early narrow focus on the infectious diseases of poverty, such as hookworm, malaria, and syphilis, and faculty such as Mandell and Comstock applied the social epidemiology principles developed by Frost, Maxcy, and Lilienfeld to study noncommunicable diseases, both mental and physical.[3]

In addition to social and behavioral science becoming a methodological pillar of public health equal to biostatistics and epidemiology, the social and political ferment of the 1960s and 1970s had also elevated advocacy as a positive good rather than a professional liability. Laurie Schwab Zabin remembered that when she first joined the faculty in the early 1980s, there was "a much larger separation between the notion of advocacy, of public health practice, and academia. And there was a great attempt to keep academia pure. The emphasis was therefore on keeping advocacy out of your CV." Zabin and Celentano's generation of JHSPH faculty who were applying for tenure in the 1980s and 1990s paved the way for making advocacy a legitimate category for promotion and tenure at the school.[4]

Celentano joined the Behavioral Sciences faculty in 1978. He met B. Frank Polk in 1982, who had come to Johns Hopkins from the Channing Laboratory at Harvard Medical School to head the infectious disease program in the Department of Epidemiology. Celentano remembered Polk as a "great, big Texan" who introduced himself by saying, "I hear you're the questionnaire guy. I need a questionnaire on how gay men have sex. I know you know all about sex." Celentano replied, "Well, I'm doing studies on cervical cancer, so I know how to take sexual history from women. But I don't know anything about gay men." The AIDS epidemic provided the opportunity for JHSPH to incorporate all the major elements of mental hygiene, behavioral science, and health education research that had crystalized over the previous two decades. Celentano and Mandell applied their expertise in epidemiology and substance abuse prevention and treatment to address the AIDS epidemic.[5]

Polk assembled groups of six to eight gay men, who met for focus groups with Celentano at a downtown Baltimore hotel. With a tape recorder and a list of 15 questions, Celentano conducted "eight or ten sessions of two to three hours, in about a three-week period. And it was very camp and very funny and very graphic." The secretary who initially transcribed the sessions quit in disgust, but Celentano's questionnaire became the baseline for the Multicenter AIDS Cohort Study (MACS), the longest-running HIV study in the world. The National Institute of Allergy and Infectious Diseases funded the study in Baltimore, Pittsburgh, Chicago, and Los Angeles, where researchers visited HIV patients every six months and conducted a physical exam and a blood test, after the HIV diagnostic test was developed in 1985. The study determined risk factors for infection, the importance of opportunistic infections, and the natural course of the disease, which in turn revealed critical information for developing effective HIV therapies.

Celentano remembered the first decade of the AIDS epidemic as "one of the most exciting times I've had here [at Hopkins], where we didn't know what was going on. We were learning all about immunology and virology. We were learning about these strange bugs, about all different mechanisms of acquisition and transmission." The school's collective experience over the past half-century—laying the epidemiological and statistical foundations for large-scale cohort studies and clinical trials, helping to develop the Salk polio vaccine and vaccine evaluation methods generally, and forging the survey research and computerized data analysis capacity to produce scientifically sound policy recommendations—everything that came before had positioned JHSPH to meet the challenge of AIDS.[6]

Behavioral science theory and methodology transformed the fields of sexually transmitted diseases, which had fallen out of academic fashion, and drug addiction, which had never been in fashion, into highly attractive options for both research careers and as sources of grant funding. During World War II, Thomas Turner had briefly opened the window for advocating condom use in the military, but in the long interim since then, the word "condom" had disappeared from the public health lexicon. Celentano observed that "AIDS allowed us to really talk in public about sex and condom use, protection, risk avoidance. In a perverse way, HIV legitimized the field of sexually transmitted infections." In 1987, Polk, Celentano, and other researchers who had been involved with MACS received funding from NIDA for the ALIVE (AIDS linked to the intravenous experience) study of HIV infection among 3,000 intravenous drug users in Baltimore. Of the study's living participants who returned for at least one visit, 95 percent remained involved in the study, with some logging up to 40 visits. The MACS and ALIVE studies continue to the present day, and their staffs have been highly effective at building rapport with participants, using techniques that in part originated in the Kinsey Institute's interviewing methods for collecting sexual histories.[7]

Using baseline data from the ALIVE study, Celentano's group demonstrated that users who bought drugs or syringes at shooting galleries (clandestine locations to buy and use drugs, usually in abandoned housing) were at much higher risk of acquiring HIV from using dirty needles. This insight led to further research on who used the shooting galleries and why, which addressed the upstream factors rather than just the route of the infection. With the cooperation of Baltimore mayor Kurt Schmoke and Epidemiology faculty David Vlahov, Steffanie Strathdee, and Susan Sherman, Celentano marshalled data from the ALIVE study to overcome the resistance of the Baltimore City Council and Maryland General Assembly, resulting in the establishment of the largest needle-sharing program in the country.[8]

Needle-sharing programs have become a prime example of how public health interventions must address social and behavioral factors to be effective— an insight that first began to affect the JHSPH curriculum and research agenda in the early 1960s. The AIDS epidemic bolstered the legitimacy of social and behavioral science methodologies and promoted their widespread adoption as indispensable tools for public health research and practice. In 2009, Celentano became the first nonphysician in JHSPH history to chair the Department of Epidemiology. He joined social and behavioral scientists who headed the present-day departments of Mental Health and of Health, Behavior and Society, so that three of the school's 10 departments reflected Lowell Reed's observation from 60 years before: "There is ample evidence that public health is becoming more and more a social science."[9]

Alongside the dramatic expansion of public health degree programs and the rise of social science in the age of AIDS, during the second half of the twentieth century, the funding pendulum in academic public health swung away from private funders such as the Rockefeller Foundation and the National Foundation for Infantile Paralysis and sharply toward federal grants from a variety of government agencies. In 2001, the pendulum began to swing back toward philanthropy as the School of Hygiene and Public Health was renamed the Johns Hopkins Bloomberg School of Public Health, in honor of Michael R. Bloomberg's significant commitment to the school and the university. Bloomberg, an alumnus of Johns Hopkins and member of the Board of Trustees, had made his fortune as the founder of the Bloomberg Financial Network. While serving as mayor of New York City from 2002 to 2013, he sought the advice of JHSPH faculty on key health policy issues, most famously in passing the first municipal indoor smoking ban, including bars and restaurants, in a major US city. The research of Jonathan Samet, chair of Epidemiology, and Scott Zeger, chair of Biostatistics, on secondhand smoke helped convince Bloomberg to pursue the legislation. The mayor called the law, which took effect on March 30, 2002, one of the most important things he has done in his life, because it would save "literally tens of thousands of lives." In 2004, the Bloomberg School of Public Health would adopt the tagline "Saving Lives, Protecting Health—Millions at a Time."[10]

The Bloomberg Philanthropies has continued to provide essential support for the school, particularly for new research initiatives in crucial areas such as malaria. Fred Soper's original price tag for eradicating 90 percent of global malaria—equal to about $2.8 billion in 2016—matched total global spending on malaria control in 2013. Although this represented a threefold increase since 2005, it still fell far short of the $5.1 billion estimated to be required annually to achieve global targets if malaria is to be completely eradicated—*in 2030*.

At JHSPH, malaria research had reemerged under Noel Rose and became central to the immunology program under Diane E. Griffin, chair of the Department of Molecular Microbiology and Immunology from 1994 to 2015. Griffin, like Rose and Bang before her, renamed the department to reflect increased attention to the molecular mechanisms underlying infectious and immunologic disease. By the late 1990s, an estimated 300 million to 500 million people were infected with malaria worldwide, and in 1998, WHO launched the Roll Back Malaria initiative, a partnership among WHO, UNICEF, the UN Development Program, and the World Bank to mount a coordinated global response to the disease.[11]

In the early 2000s, the Bloomberg Philanthropies and the Bill and Melinda Gates Foundation initiated privately funded campaigns against malaria that energized the existing programs of national and international health agencies and nongovernmental organizations. Bloomberg supported the expansion of research on malaria treatment and prevention methods, while Gates focused on bed nets and other prophylactic measures. Of more than 1 million malaria deaths each year, 90 percent were in Africa, and the vast majority were among children. In 2001, Griffin spearheaded the establishment of the Johns Hopkins Malaria Research Institute, founded with a $100 million gift from Bloomberg. Some of the twenty-first-century solutions that the institute is working to develop include enhancing mosquitoes' natural defenses and building a "better mosquito" through genetic engineering that can block transmission and displace malarial mosquitoes.[12]

During its century of existence, the Johns Hopkins Bloomberg School of Public Health has dramatically broadened the scope of public health, strengthened its scientific evidence base, and trained a global network of public health leaders from the village to the international level. The school's founders proposed an intimate link between research, teaching, and practice—insisting that attempts to apply new public health techniques were destined to fail without constant testing and evaluation to determine what worked and what did not. Perhaps the simplest yet most profound measure of the power of public health is that 100 years ago, morbidity and mortality statistics were measured in units per *thousand*, and today they are measured in units per *hundred thousand*. May we one day measure death and disease as a one-in-a-million occurrence.

JHSPH Leadership and Budgets

Years are fiscal years. Budgets include all direct expenditures, from general, restricted, and unrestricted funds.

	1940	
JHSPH	Lowell J. Reed	$227,030
Bacteriology	Thomas B. Turner	25,747
Biochemistry	E. V. McCollum	26,289
Biostatistics	Lowell J. Reed	16,545
Epidemiology	Kenneth F. Maxcy	17,622
Helminthology	William W. Cort	15,655
Immunology	Roscoe Hyde	27,470
Protozoology and Medical Entomology	Robert W. Hegner	20,250
Physiological Hygiene	Abel Wolman (interim)	6,706
Public Health Administration	Allen W. Freeman	14,268
Sanitary Engineering	Abel Wolman	2,800

	1950	
JHSPH	Ernest L. Stebbins	$1,132,825
Bacteriology	Thomas B. Turner	179,332
Biochemistry	Roger Herriott	125,189
Biostatistics	William G. Cochran	85,290
Environmental Medicine[1]	Joseph Lilienthal	102,714
Epidemiology	Kenneth F. Maxcy	169,156
Parasitology	William W. Cort	73,815
Public Health Administration	Ernest L. Stebbins	257,811
Sanitary Engineering	Abel Wolman	12,780

[1] Formerly Physiological Hygiene.

	1960	
JHSPH	Ernest L. Stebbins	$2,894,905
Microbiology (joint with Medicine)	Thomas B. Turner	20,413
Biochemistry	Roger Herriott	211,183

(*continued*)

	1960	
Biostatistics	Jerome Cornfield	78,072
Environmental Medicine	Richard L. Riley	291,136
Epidemiology	Philip Sartwell	244,041
Pathobiology	Frederik B. Bang	695,125
Public Health Administration	Ernest L. Stebbins	659,517
Sanitary Engineering	Abel Wolman	24,866

	1970	
JHSPH	John C. Hume	$12,361,428
Behavioral Science	Sol Levine	153,518
Biochemistry	Roger Herriott	448,897
Biostatistics	Alan Ross	250,618
Chronic Diseases	Abraham Lilienfeld	909,267
Environmental Health	Cornelius Kruse	93,322
Environmental Medicine	Richard L. Riley	913,325
Epidemiology	Philip Sartwell	572,214
Health Services Research and Development Center	Malcolm Peterson	29,900
International Health	Carl E. Taylor	780,042
Maternal and Child Health	Donald Cornely	Not listed
Medical Care and Hospitals	Kerr L. White	1,048,188
Mental Hygiene	Paul V. Lemkau	298,140
Pathobiology	Frederik B. Bang	1,347,401
Population Dynamics	W. Henry Mosley	1,057,663
Public Health Administration	Arthur Bushel	464,101
Radiological Science	Russell H. Morgan	983,052

	1980	
JHSPH	Donald A. Henderson	$24,567,497
Behavioral Sciences	Paul White	281,116
Biochemistry and Biophysical Sciences	Larry Grossman	2,883,551
Biostatistics	Alan Ross	468,862
Environmental Health Sciences	Gareth M. Green	4,639,345
Epidemiology	Leon Gordis	3,548,024
Health Services Administration	Arthur Bushel	3,087,322
Health Services Research and Development Center	Sam Shapiro	1,489,333
International Health	Carl E. Taylor	846,868
Maternal and Child Health	Donald Cornely	1,849,301
Mental Hygiene	Ernest Gruenberg	962,356
Pathobiology	Frederik B. Bang	1,917,450
Population Center	John Kantner	1,757,650
Population Dynamics	John Kantner	1,558,955

	1990	
JHSPH	Donald A. Henderson	$94,179,579
Biochemistry and Biophysical Sciences	Roger McMacken	4,190,926
Biostatistics	Charles A. Rohde	1,213,565
Center for Alternatives to Animal Testing	Alan Goldberg	294,557

(continued)

	1990	
Environmental Health Sciences	Gareth M. Green	11,291,442
Epidemiology	Leon Gordis	13,996,284
Health Policy and Management	Karen Davis	9,727,976
Health Services Research and Development Center	Donald Steinwachs	20,713
Immunology and Infectious Diseases	Noel R. Rose	4,052,526
Institute for International Programs	W. Henry Mosley	3,025,040
International Health	Robert E. Black	10,873,853
Maternal and Child Health	Bernard Guyer	1,695,034
Mental Hygiene	Sheppard Kellam	2,132,290
Center for Communication Programs	Phyllis Piotrow	11,341,399
Population Dynamics	W. Henry Mosley	4,690,166

Publications from Research on the Eastern Health District of Baltimore

1937	Ruth E. Fairbank, "Mental Hygiene Component of a City Health District," *AJPH* 27.3, 247–52.
1938	Bernard M. Cohen and Ruth E. Fairbank, "Statistical Contributions from the Mental Hygiene Study of the Eastern Health District of Baltimore: I. General Account of the 1933 Mental Hygiene Survey of the Eastern Health District," *American Journal of Psychiatry* 94, 1153–61.
1938	Bernard M. Cohen and Ruth E. Fairbank, "Statistical Contributions from the Mental Hygiene Study of the Eastern Health District of Baltimore: II. The Incidence and Prevalence of Psychosis in the Eastern Health District," *American Journal of Psychiatry* 94, 1377–95.
1938	W. H. Frost, "The Familial Aggregation of Infectious Diseases," *AJPH* 28.1, 2–13.
1939	Bernard M. Cohen, Christopher Tietze, and E. Greene, "Statistical Contributions from the Mental Hygiene Study of the Eastern Health District of Baltimore: III. Personality disorder in the Eastern Health District in 1933," *Human Biology* 11.1, 112–29.
1939	Bernard M. Cohen, Christopher Tietze, and E. Greene, "Statistical Contributions from the Mental Hygiene Study of the Eastern Health District of Baltimore: IV. Further Studies on Personality Disorder in the Eastern Health District in 1933," *Human Biology* 11.1, 485–512.
1939	Thomas B. Turner, A. Gelperin, and J. R. Enright, "Results of Contact Investigation in Syphilis in an Urban Community," *AJPH* 29, 768–76.
1940	P.M. Densen, "Family Studies in the Eastern Health District II: The Accuracy of Statements of Age on Census Records," *American Journal of Hygiene* 32.1, 1–38.
1940	Jean Downes and Selwyn D. Collins, "A Study of Illness among Families in the Eastern Health District of Baltimore," *Milbank Memorial Fund Quarterly* 18.1, 5–26.
1942	E. Gurney Clark and T.B. Turner, "Studies on Syphilis in the Eastern Health District of Baltimore City III: Study of the Prevalence of Syphilis Based on Specific Age Groups of an Enumerated Population," *AJPH* 32.3, 307–13.
1942	Jean Downes, "Illness in the Chronic Disease Family," *AJPH* 32.6, 589–600.
1942	Christopher Tietze and Paul V. Lemkau, "Personality Disorder and Spatial Mobility," *American Journal of Sociology* 48, 29.

1943 Lowell J. Reed, W. Thurber Fales, and G. F. Badger, "Family Studies in the Eastern Health District I: General Characteristics of the Population," *American Journal of Hygiene* 37.1, 37–52.

1943 R. V. Rider and G. F. Badger, "Family Studies in the Eastern Health District III: A Consideration of Issues Involved in Determining Migration Rates for Families," *Human Biology* 15.2, 101–26.

1944 Jean Downes and Anne Baranovsky, "Food Habits of Families in the Eastern Health District of Baltimore in the Winter and Spring of 1943," *Milbank Memorial Fund Quarterly* 22.2, 161–92.

1944 Jean Downes, "Findings of the Study of Chronic Disease in the Eastern Health District of Baltimore," *Milbank Memorial Fund Quarterly* 22.4, 337–51.

1944 Marcia Cooper, "Report of an Experiment in Mental Hygiene," *Public Health Nursing* 36, 80.

1947 G. M. Leiby and T. B. Turner, "Studies on Syphilis in the Eastern Health District of Baltimore City: Syphilis among Parturient Women as an Index of the Trend of Syphilis in the Community," *American Journal of Hygiene* 46.2, 26.

1947 H. M. C. Luykx, "Family Studies in the Eastern Health District IV: Permanence of Residence with Respect to Various Family Characteristics," *Human Biology* 19, 91–132.

1949 J. Downes, S. D. Collins, and E. H. Jackson, "Characteristics of Stable and Non-Stable Families in Morbidity Study in Eastern Health District," *Milbank Memorial Fund Quarterly* 27, 200–82.

1950 Selwyn D. Collins, F. Ruth Phillips, and Dorothy S. Oliver, "Specific Causes of Illness Found in Monthly Canvasses of Families: Sample of the Eastern Health District of Baltimore, 1938–43," *Public Health Reports* 65.39, 1235–64.

1950 Lillian Guralnick and W. Thurber Fales, "Family Studies in the Eastern Health District V: Job Stability for White Men, 1939 to 1947," *Milbank Memorial Fund Quarterly* 28, 355–406.

1950 Elizabeth H. Jackson, "Morbidity among Males and Females at Specific Ages: Eastern Health District of Baltimore," *Milbank Memorial Fund Quarterly* 28.4, 429–48.

1951 Jean Downes and Elizabeth H. Jackson, "Medical Care among Males and Females at Specific Ages: Eastern Health District of Baltimore, 1938–1943," *Milbank Memorial Fund Quarterly* 29.1, 5–30.

1951 Selwyn D. Collins, F. Ruth Phillips, and Dorothy S. Oliver, "Age Incidence of Specific Causes of Illness Found in Monthly Canvasses of Families: Sample of the Eastern Health District of Baltimore, 1938–43," *Public Health Reports* 66.39, 1227–45.

1951 Selwyn D. Collins, F. Ruth Phillips, and Dorothy S. Oliver, "Disabling Illness from Specific Causes among Males and Females of Various Ages: Sample of White Families Canvassed at Monthly Intervals in the Eastern Health District of Baltimore, 1938–43," *Public Health Reports* 66.50, 1649–71.

1951 William Thurber Fales, "Matched Population Records in the Eastern Health District, Baltimore: A Base for Epidemiological Study of Chronic Disease," *AJPH* 41.8 pt. 2, 91–100.

1951 Elizabeth H. Jackson, "Duration of Disabling Acute Illness among Employed Males and Females: Eastern Health District of Baltimore, 1938–1943," *Milbank Memorial Fund Quarterly* 29.3, 294–330.

(continued)

1952	Margaret Merrell, "The Family as a Unit in Public Health Research," *Human Biology* 24.1, 1–11.
1953	Selwyn D. Collins, F. Ruth Phillips, and Dorothy S. Oliver, "Accident Frequency by Specific Cause and by Nature and Site of Injury: Sample of White Families Canvassed at Monthly Intervals Eastern Health District of Baltimore 1938–43," *Public Health Monograph* 14, 1–22.
1953	Selwyn D. Collins, "Risk of Accident at Home, in Public Places and at Work: Sample of White Families Canvassed at Monthly Intervals Eastern Health District of Baltimore 1938–43," *Public Health Monograph* 14, 23–42.
1953	Selwyn D. Collins, "Relation of Chronic Disease and Socioeconomic Status to Accident Liability: Sample of White Families Canvassed at Monthly Intervals Eastern Health District of Baltimore 1938–43," *Public Health Monograph* 14, 43–65.
1953	Selwyn D. Collins and F. Ruth Phillips, "Dental, Eye, and Personal Preventive Services Received by an Observed Population; Sample of White Families Canvassed at Monthly Intervals Eastern Health District of Baltimore 1938–43," *Public Health Monograph* 16, 1–25.
1953	Marguerite Keller, "Progress in School of Children in a Sample of Families in the Eastern Health District of Baltimore, Maryland," *Milbank Memorial Fund Quarterly* 31.4, 391–410.
1954	Matthew Tayback, "Family Studies in the Eastern Health District VI: Family Structure and Its Changing Pattern," *Milbank Memorial Fund Quarterly* 32, 343–82.
1955	Martha Rogers, Abraham M. Lilienfeld, and Benjamin Pasamanick, *Prenatal and Paranatal Factors in the Development of Childhood Behavior* (Acta Psychiactric Neurology Supplement No. 102), 12–18.
1955	Matthew Tayback, "Family Studies in the Eastern Health District VI: Family Structure and Its Changing Pattern. Part II. Matched Cohort Studies, Evaluation of Time Study Methods in Family Sociology, Summary, and Conclusions," *Milbank Memorial Fund Quarterly* 33, 5–49.

Prologue

1. Barbara Rosenkrantz, *Public Health and the State: Changing Views in Massachusetts, 1842–1936* (Harvard University Press, 1972); John Duffy, *The Sanitarians: A History of American Public Health* (University of Illinois Press, 1990), 223–57.

2. Nancy Tomes, *The Gospel of Germs: Men, Women, and the Microbe in American Life* (Harvard University Press, 1999); Elizabeth Fee and Roy Acheson, "Introduction," 12, and Elizabeth Fee, "Designing Schools of Public Health for the United States," 161, both in Elizabeth Fee and Roy Acheson, eds., *A History of Education in Public Health: Health That Mocks the Doctors' Rules* (Oxford University Press, 1991); Saul Benison, "Poliomyelitis and the Rockefeller Institute: Social Effects and Institutional Response," in Gert H. Brieger, ed., *Theory and Practice in American Medicine* (Science History Publications, 1976), 85–86, 95–103.

3. Paul Starr, *The Social Transformation of American Medicine* (Basic Books, 1982), 115–16; E. Richard Brown, *Rockefeller Medicine Men: Medicine and Capitalism in America* (University of California Press, 1979), 102–13.

4. Robert E. Kohler, *From Medical Chemistry to Biochemistry* (Cambridge University Press, 2008), 277–79, quote p. 279; Rosemary Stevens, *In Sickness and in Wealth: American Hospitals in the Twentieth Century* (Basic Books, 1989), 55–59.

5. John Ettling, *The Germ of Laziness: Rockefeller Philanthropy and Public Health in the New South* (Harvard University Press, 1981), Ferrell qtd. p. 203.

6. Ettling, *Germ of Laziness*, chaps. 2 and 5; William A. Link, " 'The Harvest Is Ripe, but the Laborers Are Few': The Hookworm Crusade in North Carolina, 1909–1915," *North Carolina Historical Review*, 67 (January 1990), 1–27.

7. Welch–Rose Report, p. 1.

8. US Department of the Interior, Bureau of Education, *Statistics of Universities, Colleges, and Professional Schools 1917–1918*, Bulletin No. 34 (Washington, DC: GPO, 1921).

9. Welch–Rose Report, p. 1.

10. Fee 75th Anniversary of JHSHPH; Rockefeller Foundation, 1917 Annual Report (Sleepy Hollow, NY: 1918), 34–35; Rockefeller Foundation, 1919 Annual Report (Sleepy Hollow, NY: 1920).

11. Elizabeth Fee, *Disease and Discovery: A History of the Johns Hopkins School of Hygiene and Public Health, 1916–1939* (Johns Hopkins University Press, 1987), 75–76; Ferrell qtd. in Ettling, *Germ of Laziness*, 203.

12. Fee, *Disease and Discovery*, 66–68; Starr, *Social Transformation of American Medicine*, 122–23.

13. Rockefeller Foundation, 1924 Annual Report (Sleepy Hollow, NY: 1925), 18–19.

14. Simon Flexner and James Thomas Flexner, *William Henry Welch and the Heroic Age of American Medicine* (Baltimore, MD: Johns Hopkins Press, 1941); Winslow, 1949 APHA accreditation report, 6; "Report of the Dean of the School of Hygiene and Public Health," *JHU Circular* (1939–40), 109–16; 1936–37 JHSPH Catalog, 35–37; Thomas B. Turner, *Heritage of Excellence: The Johns Hopkins Medical Institutions 1914–1947* (Johns Hopkins University Press, 1974), 365; Noel R. Rose, "America's First Department of Immunology: An Informal History," *Journal of Immunology* 47 (2010), 240–47; "Expansion of Harvard University's Graduate School of Public Health," *Science* 104.2710 (1946), 541–42. MIT was the only other university that offered science degrees in public health in the 1920s and 1930s, but it did not have an independent school.

15. Starr, *Social Transformation of American Medicine*, 194–96; Fee, *Disease and Discovery*, 179, 184–214.

16. Lowell J. Reed and Huntington Williams, "The Unique Nature of the Eastern Health District Studies and Census Surveys," *Baltimore Health News* 25.9 (Sept. 1948), 57–62; "Report on the Eastern Health District to the IHD," 1941, 1942, 1943, 3a O. D. Corres., box 502037, "Rockefeller Foundation" folder, Alan Mason Chesney Medical Archives of the Johns Hopkins Medical Institutions, Baltimore, MD (AMC); "Eastern and Western Health Districts Enlarge," *Baltimore Health News* 15.10 (Oct. 1938), 76–77; Turner, *Heritage of Excellence*, 367; Huntington Williams to Mayo L. Emory, Mar. 3, 1949, Huntington Williams papers, box 505733, "Eastern Health District correspondence 1948–1949" folder, AMC.

17. Turner, *Heritage of Excellence*, 367, 359–62; Fee, *Disease and Discovery*, 143–46; JHSPH Advisory Board Minutes, Mar. 27, 1930, vol. 2, p. 325.

18. Turner, *Heritage of Excellence*, 359, 362; Lowell J. Reed bio file, AMC; "Dr. L. J. Reed Is Appointed," *Baltimore Sun*, Nov. 15, 1950; "APHA Past Presidents" (http://www.apha.org/about/aphapastpresidents.html); "Report of the Dean of the School of Hygiene and Public Health," *JHU Circular* (1939–40), 111; Fee, *Disease and Discovery*, 138–46.

19. Alan Derickson, *Health Security for All: Dreams of Universal Health Care in America* (Johns Hopkins University Press, 2005), 79; William Shonick, *Government and Health Services: Government's Role in the Development of U.S. Health Services, 1930–1980* (Oxford University Press, 1995), 20–21; Duffy, *The Sanitarians*, 229–30, 257; Frederick D. Mott and Milton I. Roemer, *Rural Health and Medical Care* (McGraw-Hill Book Co., 1948), 50–51; National Office of Vital Statistics, US Public Health Service, "Births and Deaths by Specified Race, United States, Each Division and State, 1944," *Vital Statistics—Special Reports* 25.11 (Oct. 3, 1946), 199; George Rosen, *A History of Public Health* (Johns Hopkins University Press, 1993), 446–52.

20. JHSHPH Executive Committee Minutes, Jan. 31, 1950, p. 149; Public Health in Maryland 1950.

21. Reed and Williams, "The Unique Nature of the Eastern Health District Studies," 60–61.

22. 1936–37 JHSHPH Catalog, 32; Lowell Reed, "Department of Biostatistics," Oct. 24, 1939, 3a D.O. correspondence, box 502103, "Department Reports (Biostatistics)" folder; Halbert L. Dunn, "Record Linkage," *AJPH* 36.12 (1946), 1412–16.

23. Fee, *Disease and Discovery*, 69–70, 132–46; "Report of Sub-Committee of Applications and Curriculum Committee on Alumni and their MPH Curriculum Suggestions,"

12–13; Fee and Rosenkrantz, "Professional Education for Public Health in the United States," 242–46; 1936–37 JHSPH Catalog, 31–32; Lowell Reed, "Department of Biostatistics"; 1944–45 JHSPH Catalog, 32–33; 1948–49 SOM Catalog, 115–16; 1954–55 SOM Catalog, 124; Lydia Edwards, *Life as a Doctor: A Pesky Darling Grows Up*, unpublished manuscript, 2001, Lydia B. Edwards papers, AMC, 28.

24. Reed and Williams, "The Unique Nature of the Eastern Health District Studies," 60–61; *City of Baltimore 125th Annual Report of the Department of Health, 1939*, 20.

25. Lowell J. Reed bio file, AMC.

26. Halbert L. Dunn, "Recent Developments in the Field of Public Health Statistics," *AJPH* 40.6 (June 1950), 659–69.

27. John A. Ferrell and Pauline A. Mead, *History of County Health Organizations in the United States, 1908–1933*, Public Health Bulletin No. 22 (GPO: 1936), 10–20; Ettling, *The Germ of Laziness*, 118–21; Fee, *Disease and Discovery*, 217, 224; William P. Shepard, "Professional Education," *AJPH* 33 (Apr. 1943), 425–27; "Educational Qualifications of Health Officers," *AJPH* 29 (July 1939), 787–88.

28. Fee, *Disease and Discovery*, 30–31, 168, 177–79; JHSPH Budgets 1924–67, box 506105, AMC; JHSPH Salary Lists, 3b O. D. Financial, box 502108, "History of Endowment Consolidation" folder; "Memorandum for the Finance Committee of the Board of Trustees on the Proposed 'Consolidation of Investments' as It Affects the School of Hygiene and Public Health," April 15, 1935, "History of Endowment Consolidation" folder, AMC.

29. Fitzhugh Mullan, *Plagues and Politics: The Story of the United States Public Health* Service (Basic Books, 1989), 104–7; Thomas Parran, "The Health of the Nation," *AJPH* 28 (Dec. 1938), 1376–77 (quotes).

30. Shonick, *Government and Health Services*, 93; Fee, *Disease and Discovery*, 180–81, 220.

31. Fee, *Disease and Discovery*, 222–23.

32. Thomas Parran and Livingston Farrand, *Report to the Rockefeller Foundation on the Education of Public Health Personnel* (1939), Rockefeller Foundation Archives, RG 1.1, Series 200, box 185, "200 L Institutes of Hygiene–Reports INS-1 'The Education of Public Health Personnel' 1939" folder, pp. 34, 38, 90, Rockefeller Archives, Sleepy Hollow, NY.

33. A. W. Freeman to Fred T. Foard, May 11, 1936, 3a O.D. Corres., box 502041, "U.S. Public Health Service May 1936–Feb 1940" folder, AMC; JHSPH Registrar's Office enrollment reports; "1938–39 Report of the Dean of the School of Hygiene and Public Health," *JHU Circular* (1939), 142–46.

34. Beardsley, *History of Neglect*, 120, 146–49; Link, "The Harvest Is Ripe," 3–4; Fee, *Disease and Discovery*, 17–18, 68–70, 75–76.

35. "John A. Ferrell: Humanitarian," *Southern Medical Journal* 37.9 (Sept. 1944), 527–28; Korstad, *Dreaming of a Time*, 18–26, 37; "University of Michigan School of Public Health," *AJPH* 31 (Oct. 1941), 1110; "A California School of Public Health," *AJPH* 33 (July 1943), 916; "The Mayo Professorship in Public Health," *AJPH* 36 (Mar. 1946), 311.

36. UNC University Archives, Finding aid for Records of the School of Public Health.

37. JHSPH Advisory Board Minutes, Apr. 25, 1939, vol. 3, pp. 416–17.

38. E. B. Wilson to Reed, Dec. 11, 1941, Dean's Office Corres., box 502032, "Harv-Hay Feb 1941–Aug 1943" folder.

39. Turner, *Heritage of Excellence*, 372; "Report of the Dean of the School of Hygiene and Public Health," *JHU Circular* (1940–41), 94; W. P. Shepard, "Work of the Committee on Professional Education," *AJPH* 30 (Dec. 1940), 1443–46; "Accreditation of Schools of

Public Health," *AJPH* 35 (Sept. 1945), 953–55. For examples of planning new schools, see Reed's correspondence with Milan Novak of the University of Illinois ("Nor-Nov Jun 1942–May 1944" folder) and officials at the University of Oklahoma ("Obi-Oli Apr. 1941– Feb. 1944" folder) in 3a: Dean's Office corresp., box 502036.

Chapter 1 · The Southern Roots of Public Health at Johns Hopkins

1. Fitzhugh Mullan, *Plagues and Politics: The Story of the United States Public Health Service* (Basic Books, 1989), 116, 122; Alexander D. Langmuir, "The Surveillance of Communicable Diseases of National Importance," *New England Journal of Medicine* 268.4 (1963), 182–92.

2. Marcos Cueto, *The Value of Health: A History of the Pan American Health Organization* (Pan American Health Organization Scientific and Technical Publication No. 600, 2007), 88–89; Alan Derickson, *Health Security for All: Dreams of Universal Health Care in America* (Johns Hopkins University Press, 2005); on the racial and regional dimensions of American attempts to pass comprehensive health reform, see Karen Kruse Thomas, *Deluxe Jim Crow* (University of Georgia Press, 2011), 113–15, 158–59, 180–83, 228–29.

3. Isaiah Bowman to B[enjamin] Howell Griswold Jr., Jan. 27, 1938, Records of the Office of the President, box 184, "745 (1938–1939)" folder, JHU Hamburger Archives.

4. Turner, *Heritage of Excellence*, 359, 362; Lowell J. Reed bio file, AMC; "Dr. L. J. Reed is Appointed," *Baltimore Sun*, Nov. 15, 1950; "APHA Past Presidents" (http://www.apha.org/about/aphapastpresidents.html, accessed Nov. 19, 2009); "Report of the Dean of the School of Hygiene and Public Health," *JHU Circular* (1939–40), 111; Fee, *Disease and Discovery*, 138–46.

5. Abel Wolman bio file, AMC; Abel Wolman papers finding aid, JHU Hamburger Archives; M. Gordon "Reds" Wolman interview, Sept. 25, 2008, conducted by Brian Simpson and Karen Kruse Thomas.

6. Kenneth Maxcy bio file, AMC.

7. A. McGehee Harvey, *Adventures in Medical Research*, 252; bio files for Lowell J. Reed, Abel Wolman, Kenneth F. Maxcy, and Thomas B. Turner, AMC.

8. Thomas Parran, qtd. in Alva W. Taylor, "Health Deficit Limits Southern Manpower," *Southern Patriot* 1 (Aug. 1943), 3.

9. W. Barry Wood and Mary Lee Wood, "Kenneth Fuller Maxcy, 1889–1966," *Biographical Memoirs*, vol. 42 (Columbia University Press, 1971), 161–73, quote p. 162.

10. Maxcy bio file; John E. Gordon, "The Twentieth Century—Yesterday, Today, and Tomorrow," in Franklin H. Top, ed., *The History of American Epidemiology* (C. V. Mosby Company, 1952), 119–20.

11. Robert E. Kohler, *Landscapes and Labscapes: Exploring the Lab-Field Border in Biology* (University of Chicago, 2002), 3; Kenneth F. Maxcy, "Epidemiological Principles Affecting the Distribution of Malaria in the Southeastern U.S.," *Public Health Reports* 39 (1924), 1113–27; Wood and Wood, "Kenneth Fuller Maxcy"; "Typhus Fever in the United States," 1929, in Nicholas Hahon, ed., *Selected Papers on the Pathogenic Rickettsiae* (Harvard University Press, 1968), 91–100; Francis G. Blake, Kenneth F. Maxcy, Joseph F. Sadusk Jr., Glen M. Kohls, and E. John Bell, "Tsutsugamushi Disease (Scrub Typhus, Mite-borne Typhus) in New Guinea," *AJPH* 35.11 (Nov. 1945), 1121–30.

12. Kenneth Maxcy, "Epidemiological Principles Affecting the Distribution of Malaria in the Southeastern U.S.," *Public Health Reports* 39 (1924), 1113–27, quote p. 1117; Kenneth

Maxcy, Wilson G. Smillie, and W. A. Plecker, "Malaria Statistics," *Southern Medical Journal* 18 (1925), 449–52.

13. Maxcy, "Spleen Rate of School Boys in the Mississippi Delta," *Public Health Reports* 38 (1923), 2466–72; Margaret Humphreys, *Malaria: Poverty, Race, and Public Health in the United States* (Johns Hopkins University Press, 2003), 51–65; Randall M. Packard, *The Making of a Tropical Disease: A Short History of Malaria* (Johns Hopkins University Press, 2007), 72–75.

14. Ruth Rice Puffer, "Measurement of Error of Death Rates in the Colored Race," *AJPH* 27.6 (June 1937), 603–8, quote p. 607.

15. Martin D. Young, "In Memoriam: Justin M. Andrews (1902–67)," *Journal of Parasitology* 56.6 (1970), 1278–79; Lloyd E. Rozeboom, *Medical Zoology at the Johns Hopkins University School of Hygiene and Public Health* (JHSPH Department of Immunology and Infectious Diseases, 1990), quote p. 6.

16. Richard Carter and Kamini N. Mendis, "Evolutionary and Historical Aspects of the Burden of Malaria," *Clinical Microbiology Reviews* 15.4 (2002), 564–594; Fred L. Soper, D. Bruce Wilson, Servulo Lima, and Waldemar Sa Antunes, *The Organization of Permanent Nation-wide Anti-Aedes Aegypti Measures in Brazil* (New York: The Rockefeller Foundation, 1943); Fred L. Soper and D. Bruce Wilson, *Anopheles gambiae in Brazil, 1930 to 1940* (New York: The Rockefeller Foundation, 1943).

17. Justin Andrews, review of *Studies on Brazilian Anophelines from Northeast and Amazon Regions, AJPH* 36.10 (1946), 1170–71; "1938–39 Report of the Dean of the School of Hygiene and Public Health," *JHU Circular* (1939), 110; "1939–40 Report of the Dean of the School of Hygiene and Public Health," *JHU Circular* (1940), 96; Rozeboom, *Medical Zoology at JHSPH*, 7.

18. Ernest L. Stebbins interview by Elizabeth Fee, Oct. 15, 1979, Fee papers; Nancy Elizabeth Gallagher, *Egypt's Other Wars: Epidemics and the Politics of Public Health* (Syracuse University Press, 1990), 20–31.

19. "Scientific Developments and the War," *Marine Corps Gazette* 29.4 (Apr. 1945), 36; H. L. Haller and Stanley J. Cristol, "The Development of New Insecticides," in E. C. Andrus, ed., *Advances in Military Medicine, by American Investigators, Vol. II* (Little, Brown and Company, 1948), 621–26; F. L. Soper, W. A. Davis, F. S. Markham, and L. A. Riehl, "Typhus Fever in Italy, 1943–1945, and Its Control with Louse Powder," *American Journal of Hygiene* 45.3 (May 1947), 305–34.

20. Justin M. Andrews, "What's Happening to Malaria in the U.S.A.?" *AJPH* 38.7 (1948), 931–42; Justin M. Andrews, Griffith E. Quinby, and Alexander D. Langmuir, "Malaria Eradication in the United States," *AJPH* 40.11 (1950), 1405; Chad H. Parker, "Controlling Man-Made Malaria: Corporate Modernisation and the Arabian American Oil Company's Malaria Control Program in Saudi Arabia, 1947–1956," *Cold War History* 12.3 (2012), 473–94. For an in-depth discussion of the history of debates over the relationship between malaria control and economic development, see Randall M. Packard, " 'Roll Back Malaria, Roll in Development'? Reassessing the Economic Burden of Malaria," *Population and Development Review* 35.1 (2009), 53–87.

21. Leo Slater, *War and Disease: Biomedical Research on Malaria in the Twentieth Century* (Rutgers University Press, 2009), 41, 50–52.

22. Ibid.; W. H. Taliaferro to Kenneth F. Maxcy, Apr. 17, 1951, Records of the Office of the JHU President, series 1, box 185, 745 (1952) folder.

23. Slater, *War and Disease* 8, 123–55, 170–71; Packard, *The Making of a Tropical Disease*, 140–41; Donald Burke and David Sullivan, "A Brief History of Malaria Research at Johns Hopkins," Johns Hopkins Malaria Research Institute, Malaria: Progress, Problems and Plans in the Genomic Era conference proceedings, Jan. 27–29, 2002, Baltimore, MD.

24. "Naval Medical Research Unit 2, Phnom Penh" (http://www.med.navy.mil/sites /namru2pacific, accessed July 1, 2014).

25. W. W. Cort, "The Development of the Subject of Helminthology in the SHPH of the Johns Hopkins University," 1939, 3a D.O. Correspondence, box 502103, "Department Reports (Helminthology)" folder; Fee, *Disease and Discovery*, 104–9; Malcolm S. Ferguson, "Norman Rudolph Stoll: Scientist, Teacher, Friend: An Appreciation," *Experimental Pathology* 41.2 (1977), 253–71; E. H. Loughlin and N. R. Stoll, "Fomite-Borne Ancylostomiasis," *American Journal of Hygiene* 45.2 (1947), 191–203; E. H. Loughlin and N. R. Stoll, "Hookworm Infections in American Servicemen with Reference to the Establishment of Ancylostoma Duodenale in the Southern United States," *JAMA* 136.3 (1948), 157–61.

26. WHO, "Health Topics: Filariasis" (http://www.who.int/topics/filariasis/en, accessed Jan. 7, 2011).

27. Norman R. Stoll, "This Wormy World," *Journal of Parasitology* 33 (1947), 1–18; Eric S. Loker, "This De-Wormed World?" *Journal of Parasitology* 99.6 (2013), 933–42.

28. Turner, *Heritage of Excellence*, 543–44; 1935–36 Report of the Dean of the JHSPH, 179–84; 1936–37 JHSPH Catalog, 32–37; Rozeboom, *Medical Zoology at the JHSPH*, 133–36; William W. Cort, "Annual Report of the Department of Parasitology 1942–43," 3a O. D. Corres., box 502031, "Department Reports to the Dean 1942–1943" folder, AMC.

29. Ruy Laurenti, "Ruth Rice Puffer," *AJPH* 93.6 (2003), 865–66.

30. Parran–Farrand Report, 34; "Report on the Mental Hygiene Study to the IHD 1941," "Rockefeller Foundation" folder; Allen Freeman, "Annual Report of the Department of Public Health Administration 1942–43," 3a O. D. Corres., box 502031, "Department Reports to the Dean 1942–1943" folder; Nov. 1, 1943 EHD Committee minutes, Huntington Williams papers, box 505733, "Eastern Health District Committee Meetings 1933–1955" folder.

31. Antero Pietila, *Not in My Neighborhood: How Bigotry Shaped a Great American City* (Ivan R. Dee, 2010), 131–34; Thomas, *Deluxe Jim Crow*, 208–11.

32. Neil Smith, *American Empire: Roosevelt's Geographer and the Prelude to Globalization* (University of California Press, 2003), 246–48; "Deaths," *Time* 25.7 (Feb. 18, 1935), 79; Thomas M. Daniel, *Wade Hampton Frost, Pioneer Epidemiologist 1880–1938: Up to the Mountain* (University of Rochester Press, 2004), 1–2; Eric Foner, *Reconstruction: America's Unfinished Revolution, 1863–1877* (Harper & Row, 1988), 574–55. The following JHSPH Advisory Board Minutes record the decisions regarding black applicants: vol. 1: Mar. 2, 1922 p. 156 and vol. 2: Sept. 30, 1926 p. 157, Mar. 27, 1930 p. 325, and Dec. 18, 1930 p. 368. The Advisory Board even denied admission to a black physician preparing for service in the Ethiopian Ministry of Health. The single exception to the pre-1945 exclusion of blacks from JHSPH was in 1933, when Marjorie A. Forte and Myrtle M. Patton, the only two black public health nurses practicing in Maryland, joined 50 white nurses at a one-day Institute of Hygiene hosted by JHSPH ("Taking Course at Johns Hopkins," *Baltimore Afro-American,* Jan. 31, 1933). In 1912, Johns Hopkins received a state appropriation of $600,000 to construct buildings for a new School of Engineering and thereafter received $50,000 annually for operating funds (*Report of the Johns Hopkins University to the Governor and to*

the General Assembly of Maryland on the School of Engineering: Its Organization, Operation, Accomplishments, and the Award of Scholarships [Baltimore, 1939], 9).

33. C. H. Epps Jr., D. G. Johnson, and A. L. Vaughan, "Black Medical Pioneers: African-American 'Firsts' in Academic and Organized Medicine. Part Two," *Journal of the National Medical Association* 85.9 (Sept. 1993), 707.

34. Thomas, *Deluxe Jim Crow*, 209, 56, 66–67; Isaiah Bowman, Memorandum, Apr. 23, 1938, Records of the Office of the President of JHU, box 184, "745 (1938–1939)" folder; Fee, *Disease and Discovery*, 81.

35. Thomas, *Deluxe Jim Crow*, 104–5.

36. "Johns Hopkins Teacher Would Let Down Bars," *Baltimore Afro-American*, Dec. 24, 1938; Broadus Mitchell, "Hopkins Jim Crow Flayed," *Baltimore Afro-American*, Jan. 13, 1940.

37. *City of Baltimore 125th Annual Report of the Department of Health, 1939*, 20; Frederick N. Rasmussen, "Pioneering Doctor Helped Black Residents of Baltimore," *Baltimore Sun*, Feb. 19, 2011; Edward H. Beardsley, *A History of Neglect: Health Care for Blacks and Mill Workers in the Twentieth-Century South* (University of Tennessee Press, 1987), 91–93; Mullan, *Plagues and Politics*, 122; Thomas, *Deluxe Jim Crow*, 11–19.

38. Isaiah Bowman to Howard W. Jackson, Dec. 1, 1938, and Lowell Reed, Memorandum on Eastern Health District Building, Records of the Office of the JHU President, box 184, "745 (1938–1939)" folder.

39. Huntington Williams to Isaiah Bowman, May 29 and 31, 1944, Records of the Office of the JHU President, box 184, "745 (1944–1945)" folder; *City of Baltimore 125th Annual Report of the Department of Health, 1939*, 9; "Somerset Health Center Is Dedicated," *Baltimore Health News* 21.7 (July 1944), 49–50.

40. "High V.D. Rate Among Soldiers Prompts 3-Front Campaign to Prevent Spread," *Baltimore Afro-American*, Dec. 14, 1943; D. N. Scheck and Edward Hook, "Neurosyphilis," *Infectious Disease Clinics of North America* 8 (1994), 769–95.

41. Parran, "The Health of the Nation," 1377–78; Paul Starr, "The Boundaries of Public Health," chap. 5 in *The Social Transformation of American Medicine* (Basic Books, 1982), 180–97; Rosemary Stevens, *In Sickness and in Wealth: American Hospitals in the Twentieth Century* (Basic Books, 1989), 220–21; Daniel M. Fox, *Health Policies, Health Politics: The British and American Experience, 1911–1965* (Princeton University Press, 1986), 117–31.

42. Allan Brandt, *No Magic Bullet: A Social History of Venereal Disease in the United States since 1880* (Oxford University Press, 1987), 40–41. The term "venereal disease" or abbreviation "VD" was in common use during the era under discussion and is used here rather than the more contemporary terms "sexually transmitted disease" or "sexually transmitted infection."

43. Ibid.

44. "'Shadow on the Land': Thomas Parran and the New Deal," chap. 4 in Allan M. Brandt, *No Magic Bullet*, 122–60; Harry M. Marks, *Progress of Experiment: Science and Therapeutic Reform in the United States, 1900–1990* (Cambridge University Press, 2000), 54–57, quote p. 57.

45. JHSPH Advisory Board minutes, Oct. 1, 1936; "Conference at Rockefeller Institute," June 13, 1936, and McIver to Allen W. Freeman Aug. 28, 1936, RG 100.1, series 200, box 28, folder 319, Rockefeller Foundation Archives, Sleepy Hollow, NY (RFA).

46. A. McGehee Harvey, *Adventures in Medical Research: A Century of Discovery at Johns Hopkins* (Johns Hopkins University Press, 1976), 252; "Report of the Dean of the

Medical Faculty," *JHU Circular* (1957–58), 71; Rockefeller Foundation 1937 Annual Report, 101–2; Marks, *Progress of Experiment*, 53–59 (Parran qtd. 57), 98–103; Thomas Parran and Raymond A. Vonderlehr, *Plain Words about Venereal Disease* (Reynal & Hitchcock, 1941), 25; Susan M. Reverby, *Examining Tuskegee: The Infamous Syphilis Study and Its Legacy* (University of North Carolina Press, 2009), 136–39. The Alan Mason Chesney Medical Archives at Johns Hopkins contain extensive correspondence between Parran and Hopkins faculty.

47. Thomas Turner, "Memo to Dean Reed Concerning the Division of Venereal Diseases," JHSPH Advisory Board Minutes, vol. 4, Jan. 27, 1942, pp. 76–77; "Conference at Rockefeller Institute," June 13, 1936, McIver to Allen W. Freeman Aug. 28, 1936, Thomas Parran to Wilbur A. Sawyer Jan. 22, 1938, RG 100.1, series 200, box 28, folder 319, RFA; Fee, *Disease and Discovery*, 210–12.

48. John A. Ferrell to Thomas B. Turner, Feb. 2, 1938, Turner to Ferrell, Feb. 4, 1938, Parran to Ferrell, Feb. 15, 1938, folder 319.

49. Turner, *Heritage of Excellence*, 370; "Report of the Dean of the Medical Faculty," *JHU Circular* (1939–40), 72; "Report of the President," *JHU Circular* (1939–40), 15–16; J. E. Moore to Thomas Parran, June 12, 1939, and Moore to Lowell Reed, June 13, 1939, 3a O. D. Corres., box 502039, "Treasurer's Office-Turner Correspondence Jun 1939–March 1941" folder, AMC; Alonzo F. Brand, "The Part of the Johns Hopkins Hospital in the Campaign Against Syphilis," *The Johns Hopkins Nurses Alumnae Magazine* 37.1 (Jan. 1938), 24–26.

50. J. E. Moore to Thomas Parran, May 26, 1936, Parran to Michael M. Davis, May 28, 1936, Davis to Moore, June 4, 1936, Thomas Parran papers, series 90/F-14, FF3, University of Pittsburgh; "Postgraduate Training of Negro Physicians in the Clinical Management and Public Health Control of Syphilis," *Journal of the National Medical Association* 29.4 (Nov. 1937), 171; J. R. Heller to Lowell Reed, Nov. 26, 1941, Reed to Heller, Dec. 4, 1941, JHSPH records, 3a O. D. Corres., box 502041, "U.S. Public Health Service Dec 1941–Feb 1942" folder, AMC; "Lt. Fawcett at WAC Confab," *Baltimore Afro-American,* July 17, 1943.

51. Brandt, *No Magic Bullet*, 165–70; Thomas Parran to Lowell J. Reed, Mar. 28, 1940, 3a O. D. Corres., box 502041, "U.S. Public Health Service Feb 1940–June 1941" folder, AMC; Thomas B. Turner, "Qualifications of a Venereal Disease Control Officer," *AJPH* 28.5 (May 1938), 559–65; Thomas H. Sternberg, Ernest B. Howard, Leonard A. Dewey, and Paul Padget, "Chapter X Venereal Diseases," in John Boyd Coates, ed., *Preventive Medicine in World War II, Volume V: Communicable Diseases Transmitted through Contact or by Unknown Means* (Office of the Surgeon General, Department of the Army, 1960), 139–331, quote p. 156; Thomas B. Turner, "Immediate Wartime Outlook and Indicated Post-War Conditions with Respect to the Control of the Venereal Diseases," *AJPH* 33.11 (Nov. 1943), 1312.

52. Brandt, *No Magic Bullet*, 164–65; Anahad O'Connor, "Thomas Turner, 100, Hopkins Medical Dean" (obituary), *New York Times*, Oct. 2, 2002 (quote).

53. Turner, *Heritage of Excellence*, 509–12.

54. Ibid., 509–12; 1947–48 Johns Hopkins School of Medicine Catalog, 63; Maryland State Department of Health, *Public Health in Maryland* (Maryland State Department of Health, 1952); "Open Fight on T.B., Syphilis at Forum," *Baltimore Afro-American,* Mar. 27, 1943.

55. JHSPH Student Photos, boxes 507941–46, AMC; JHSPH Directory of Alumni, 1919–1975; Louise Cavagnaro, "A History of Segregation and Desegregation at the Johns Hopkins Medical Institutions," February 18, 1992, updated April 26, 2002, in the Louise

Cavagnaro Collection, AMC; Robert Rodgers Korstad, *Dreaming of a Time: The School of Public Health: the University of North Carolina at Chapel Hill, 1939–1989* (University of North Carolina School of Public Health, 1990), 49–53. Neither of the historically black medical schools at Howard University or Meharry Medical College offered public health degrees, although Cornely chaired the Department of Bacteriology, Preventive Medicine and Public Health at Howard. Paul B. Cornely, "The Howard Department of Preventive Medicine and Public Health," *Journal of the National Medical Association* 59 (Nov. 1967), 435–40.

56. J. E. Moore to Thomas Parran, June 12, 1939 and Moore to Lowell Reed, June 13, 1939; Thomas Parran to Lowell J. Reed, Mar. 28, 1940; Turner, "Memorandum to Dean Reed"; "1940–41 Report of the Dean of the School of Hygiene," *JHU Circular* (1941), 97; "1941–42 Report of the Dean of the School of Hygiene," *JHU Circular* (1942), 96; Maryland State Department of Health, *Public Health in Maryland* (Maryland State Department of Health, 1942), 13–14; "Changes in Health Personnel in Maryland," *AJPH* 37.1 (Jan. 1947), 136; John Hume bio file, AMC; Lawrence K. Altman, "Leroy Burney, 91, Early Critic of Effects of Cigarette Smoking," *New York Times,* August 4, 1998.

57. EHD Committee minutes Dec. 6, 1943, Jan. 24, 1944, Mar. 6, 1944, and June 5, 1944, "Plans for Patterson Park High School Serological Survey," Apr. 10, 1944, Huntington Williams papers, box 505733, "Eastern Health District Committee Meetings 1933–1955" folder, AMC; Fee, *Disease and Discovery,* 213.

58. Marks, *Progress of Experiment,* 53–59; "Annual Report of the President, 1945–46," *JHU Circular* (1946), 65–75, 90–92; Johns Hopkins Syphilis Study Rockefeller Foundation grant action form, Sept. 19, 1936, folder 318; "Dr. Thomas B. Turner," W. A. Sawyer diary entry June 17, 1936, folder 319; Johns Hopkins Syphilis Study Rockefeller Foundation grant action form, Dec. 6, 1937, folder 318; Thomas Turner to John Ferrell Oct. 18, 1938, folder 319; "Accounts of Grant Money Received and Spent," 1–2, 12, 14–15, 44, 76–77; Fee, *Disease and Discovery,* 210–12; Turner, "Memo to Dean Reed."

59. Fee, *Disease and Discovery,* 64, 146.

60. George Comstock, "In Memoriam: Carroll Edwards Palmer, 1903–1972," *American Journal of Epidemiology* 95.4 (Apr. 1972), 305–7, quote p. 307.

61. "Spirochete's Return," *Time* 49.22 (June 2, 1947), 78; Scheck and Hook, "Neurosyphilis."

62. Starr, *Social Transformation of American Medicine,* 335–44; Marks, *Progress of Experiment,* 105–28, 98–135; Turner, *Heritage of Excellence,* 363–64, 478, 496–98; Joseph Earle Moore, J. F. Mahoney, Walter Schwartz, Thomas Sternberg, and W. Barry Wood, "The Treatment of Early Syphilis With Penicillin: A Preliminary Report of 1,418 Cases," *JAMA* 126 (1944), 67–72; Joseph Earle Moore, *Penicillin in Syphilis* (Springfield, IL: Charles C Thomas, 1947), 4; C. A. Sargent and Margaret Merrell, "Method of Measuring the Effectiveness of Preventive Treatment in Reducing Morbidity," *AJPH* 30.12 (Dec. 1940), 1431–35; John J. Phair, Margaret Merrell, and Emanuel B. Schoenback, "Chemoprophylaxis in the Prevention of Disease with Especial Reference to Meningococcal Infections 1. A Comparative Study of the Absorption, Persistence and Excretion of Four Sulfonamide Compounds," *Human Biology* 18.4 (1946), 171–203; E. K. Marshall Jr. and M. Merrell, "Clinical Therapeutic Trial of a New Drug," *Bulletin of the Johns Hopkins Hospital* 85.3 (Sep. 1949), 221–30; M. Merrell, "Results of the Nationwide Study of Penicillin in Early Syphilis; Amorphous Penicillin in Aqueous Solution," *American Journal of Syphilis, Gonorrhea, and Venereal Diseases* 33.1 (Jan. 1949), 12–18; Margaret Merrell, "Discussion," *AJPH,* 41 (Aug. 1951), quote p. 76.

63. "Report of the Dean of the Medical Faculty," *JHU Circular* (1939–40), 72; "Report of the President," *JHU Circular* (1939–40), 15–16; "1941–42 Report of the Dean of the School of Hygiene," *JHU Circular* (1942), 75–77; Turner to Ferrell, Nov. 2, 1937, and Ferrell to Huntington Williams, Nov. 3, 1937, folder 319.

64. Wade Hampton Frost, "The Familial Aggregation of Infectious Diseases," *AJPH* 28.1 (Jan. 1938), 2–13; Wade Hampton Frost, "The Importance of Epidemiology as a Function of Health Departments," *Medical Officer* 29 (1923), 113–14 (quote).

65. James H. Jones, *Bad Blood: The Tuskegee Syphilis Experiment* (Basic Books, 1981), 121–23, 179–80; Reverby, *Examining Tuskegee*, 136–39.

66. Ruth R. Faden and Tom L. Beauchamp, *A History and Theory of Informed Consent* (Oxford University Press, 1986), 165–67; R. Brookmeyer, N. E. Day, and S. Moss, "Case-Control Studies for Estimation of the Natural History of Preclinical Disease from Screening Data," *Statistics in Medicine* 5.2 (1986), 127–38; R. Brookmeyer, "Statistical Problems in Epidemiologic Studies of the Natural History of Disease," *Environmental Health Perspectives* 87 (1990), 43–49.

67. Susan M. Reverby, "Ethical Failures and History Lessons: The U.S. Public Health Service Research Studies in Tuskegee and Guatemala," *Public Health Reviews* 34.1 (2012), 1–18.

68. Ibid.

69. Donald G. McNeill Jr., "U.S. Apologizes for Syphilis Tests in Guatemala," *New York Times,* October 1, 2010; Susan M. Reverby, "Normal Exposure and Inoculation Syphilis: A PHS Tuskegee Doctor in Guatemala, 1946–1948," *Journal of Policy History* 23 (2011), 6–27; Presidential Commission for the Study of Bioethical Issues, *"Ethically Impossible": STD Research in Guatemala from 1946 to 1948* (2011).

70. John C. Cutler, "A Review of the National Venereal Disease Control Program," in University of North Carolina School of Public Health et al., *Working Conference for Nurses on the Public Health Aspects of Venereal Disease Control,* typescript of 1954 conference proceedings, North Carolina Collection in Wilson Library at the University of North Carolina at Chapel Hill, p. 10; Reverby, "Normal Exposure and Inoculation Syphilis."

71. Reverby, "Ethical Failures and History Lessons," 14.

72. Ibid., quote p. 5.

Chapter 2 · School at War

1. US Government Printing Office, Budget of the United States Government: Historical Tables Fiscal Year 2005, Table 1.1—Summary of Receipts, Outlays, and Surpluses or Deficits: 1789–2009 (www.gpoaccess.gov/usbudget/fy05/hist.html); Daniel M. Fox, "Health Policy and the History of Welfare States: A Reinterpretation," *Journal of Policy History* 10.2 (1998), 239–56; Starr, *Social Transformation of American Medicine,* 344–45.

2. Rockefeller Foundation, *1919 Annual Report* (Sleepy Hollow, NY: 1920); 1944–45 JHSPH Catalog, 21–22; "1939–40 Report of the Dean of the School of Hygiene and Public Health," *JHU Circular* (1940), 109–16; JHSPH Advisory Board Minutes, vol. 3, April 30, 1940, p. 465; "1940–41 Report of the President," *JHU Circular* (1941), 6; "1941–42 Report of the Dean of the School of Hygiene and Public Health," *JHU Circular* (1942), 99; "1943–44 Report of the Dean of the Medical Faculty," *JHU Circular* (1944), 37; "1943–44 Report of the Dean of the School of Engineering," *JHU Circular* (1944), 56; Turner, *Heritage of Excellence,* 372.

3. E. C. Andrus, ed., *Advances in Military Medicine, Made by American Investigators* (Boston: Little, Brown and Co., 1948).

4. "LaGuardia Elected to NAACP Board," Kansas City, MO *Call*, Jan. 18, 1946; "Disease in Europe Hits Epidemic Proportions," *Denver Rocky Mountain News*, July 14, 1946; "Stebbins Named ARC Official," *Baltimore Sun*, Aug. 27, 1947; "Unitarians Add German Mission to Health Groups," *Boston Globe*, June 14, 1951.

5. Bio files for Cornelius Kruse, Manfred Mayer, Abraham Schneidmuhl, and Ernest Bueding, AMC; Lemkau quoted in Rockefeller Foundation 1946 Annual Report, 1.

6. Alberta Szalita-Pemow bio file, AMC; "Humanitarian Service to Displaced Persons," *San Antonio Express*, July 11, 1948; Szalita-Pemow, qtd. in Gail A. Hornstein, *To Redeem One Person Is to Redeem the World: A Life of Frieda Fromm-Reichmann* (Simon and Schuster, 2002), 181.

7. Kenneth Maxcy, "A Review of the Activities of the Department of Epidemiology," 1939, JHSPH Departmental Reports, "Department Reports (Epidemiology)" folder; Reed to William M. McKay, Apr. 16, 1941, 3a O. D. Corres., box 502037, Positions P.H., June 1940–May 1941; JHSPH Advisory Board Minutes, vol. 5, Sept. 25, 1945, p. 1.

8. Reed to Ferrell, June 30, 1943, "Rockefeller Foundation Sept 1941–Mar 1942" folder; Reed to Ferrell, June 30, 1943, "Rockefeller Foundation Sept 1941–Mar 1942" folder; "The American Public Health Association," *AJPH* 37 (Nov. 1947), 1470; Fee and Rosenkrantz, "Professional Education for Public Health in the United States," 235–40.

9. Emerson, *Local Health Units for the Nation*, 5–6, 12–18.

10. Josephine R. Campbell and Kathryn J. Connor, *Variations in State Public Health Programs During a Five-Year Period* (US Public Health Service, 1952), 6–7, 12, 39, 110, 126, 128; Lowell J. Reed to Milan Novak, May 17, 1944, 3a O. D. Corres., box 502036, "Nor–Nov Jun 1942–May 1944"; Fee and Rosenkrantz, "Professional Education for Public Health in the United States," 235–36; Fee, *Disease and Discovery*, 170, 182; "Public Health Degrees Granted in 1932," *AJPH* 25 (1934), 341–43; "Public Health Degrees and Certificates Granted in the United States and Canada during the Academic Year, 1947–1948," *AJPH* 39 (Jan. 1949), 71; Leroy Burney, "Public Health Degrees and Certificates Granted in the United States and Canada during the Academic Year, 1952–1953," *AJPH* 44 (May 1954), 662–63. The 940 graduate public health degrees awarded in 1953 included 135 nurses and 175 sanitary engineers.

11. "Too Many Degrees," *AJPH* 35 (Sept. 1945), 163–64.

12. H. C. Cranford, "A Formula that Gets Hospitals into Rural Areas," *Hospitals: The Journal of the American Hospital Association* 22.12 (1948), 33.

13. US Department of Health, Education, and Welfare, Office of Education, *Earned Degrees Conferred, 1956–57* (1958), 132.

14. Marilyn Thornton Williams, *Washing "The Great Unwashed": Public Baths in Urban America, 1840–1920* (Ohio State University Press, 1991), 22–23.

15. Janet Farrar Worthington, "When Psychiatry Was Very Young," *Hopkins Medicine* (Winter 2008); Turner, *Heritage of Excellence*, 368. For an in-depth treatment of Adolf Meyer and the Phipps Clinic, see Susan D. Lamb, *Pathologist of the Mind: Adolf Meyer, Psychobiology and the Phipps Psychiatric Clinic at the Johns Hopkins Hospital, 1908–1917* (2010 dissertation in History of Medicine, Johns Hopkins University).

16. JHSPH Advisory Board Minutes, vol. 4, May 27, 1941, p. 46; Leo Kanner to Lowell Reed, May 22, 1941, 3a O. D. Corres., box 502034, Kahn-Kar, May 1941–Jun 1944; Leo

Kanner Collection finding aid, AMC; Christopher Payne, *Asylum: Inside the Closed World of State Mental Hospitals* (MIT Press, 2009), 7.

17. Paul V. Lemkau bio file, AMC; Hans Pols, "Divergences in Psychiatry during the Depression: Somatic Psychiatry, Community Mental Hygiene, and Social Reconstruction," *Journal of the History of the Behavioral Sciences* 37 (Fall 2001), 369–88.

18. Ford qtd. in Kenneth Maxcy, "A Review of the Activities of the Department of Bacteriology," 1939, JHSPH Departmental Reports, "Department Reports (Bacteriology)" folder.

19. Lowell J. Reed to Victor Vogel, June 5, 1941, and Vogel to Reed, June 6, 1941, 3a O. D. Corres., box 502041, US Public Health Service, Feb 1940–June 1941; 1944–45 JHSPH Catalog, 21–24.

20. Shonick, Government and Health Services, 95; Starr, *Social Transformation of American Medicine*, 343–46; Fee and Rosenkrantz, "Professional Education for Public Health in the United States," 236–37; Thomas Parran, "Surmounting Obstacles to Health Progress," *American Journal of Public Health* 38.1 (1948), 168–72.

21. Federal Works Agency, Fourth Annual Report (Washington, DC, 1943), 61; "Federal Services Require Sanitary Engineers," *AJPH* 34.9 (Sept. 1944), 1042.

22. 1936–37 JHSPH Catalog, 35–37; 1944–45 JHSPH Catalog, 36–39; 1948–49 JHSPH Catalog, 41–42; "Hopkins Announces New One Year Graduate Course in Sanitary Engineering," *AJPH* 36.8 (Aug. 1946), 952.

23. 1946–47 Report of the Dean of the JHSPH, *JHU Circular* 66 (1947), 95, 97; quotation from Kazuyoshi Kawata to Elizabeth Fee, June 11, 1988, Elizabeth Fee papers, "Sanitary Engineering" folder; Cornelius Kruse, "Course of Curriculum Plan and Supporting Data, Community Air Pollution Training Grants Program," Nov. 13, 1956, and Cornelius Wolfram Kruse curriculum vita c. 1961, box 504582, "Department of Environmental Health" folder.

24. Carl M. Peterson to Reed, May 25, 1942, 3a O. D. Corres., box 502028, "American Medical Assn. Mar. 1941–Aug. 1943" folder; Anna M. Baetjer, 1941–42 Report of the Department of Physiological Hygiene, 3a O. D. Corres., box 502031, "Departmental Reports" folder; Susan P. Baker, oral history interview, Dec. 22, 2008; "News from the Field," *AJPH* 40.8 (Aug. 1950), 1063.

25. Fee, *Disease and Discovery*, 122–26, 172–76; Reed to Baetjer, March 7, 1942, and Baetjer to Reed, April 13, 1942, 3a O. D. Corres., box 502028, "Baetjer, Dr. Anna M. Oct. 1940–Mar. 1943," folder Michael Purdy, "Occupational Health's Dynamo," *Johns Hopkins Public Health Magazine*, Fall 2001.

26. Christian Warren, *Brush with Death: A Social History of Lead Poisoning* (Johns Hopkins University Press, 2000), 142–43, 156–57, 163–67, 173–74.

27. Williams, *Washing "The Great Unwashed,"* 28–29, 36–38, 115–24.

28. David Oshinsky, *Polio: An American Story* (Oxford University Press, 2005), 28–31.

29. Turner, *Heritage of Excellence*, 292; George W. Corner, *A History of the Rockefeller Institute: 1901–1953, Origins and Growth* (New York: The Rockefeller Institute Press, 1964), 429–33. Another early center of virology was the University of California at Berkeley, where Wendell M. Stanley left the Rockefeller Institute for Medical Research in 1948 to organize and direct the Virus Laboratory, which became a full department in 1958. University of California History website, "Berkeley Departments and Programs" (http://sunsite.berkeley.edu/~ucalhist/general_history/campuses/ucb/departments_m.html, accessed Feb.

4, 2015). Other former Rockefeller researchers were in the Department of Biochemistry: Bacon F. Chow, Winston H. Price, and Roger Herriott.

30. Kenneth F. Maxcy, "Hypothetical Relationship of Water Supplies to Poliomyelitis," *AJPH* 33 (Jan. 1943), 41–45; Philip E. Sartwell, "Why We Are Here: A Tribute Presented at the Dedication of the Kenneth F. Maxcy Laboratories," *American Journal of Epidemiology* 89 (1969), 505. The widespread impact of Maxcy's paper on polio at the APHA in 1942 is noted in "Highlights of the 71st Annual Meeting," *AJPH* 32 (Dec. 1942), 1388–89; "DDT Fly Spray Seen as Polio Curb Weapon," *Oklahoma City Times*, Dec. 15, 1949.

31. Turner, *Heritage of Excellence*, 356–58; Fee and Perry, "David Bodian," 168–69; George L. Radcliffe to Bowman, July 20, 1942, Records of the Office of the President, box 184, 745 (1940–1943) folder, Hamburger University Archives, JHU; Kenneth Maxcy bio file, AMC.

32. Saul Benison, *Tom Rivers: Reflections on a Life in Medicine and Science, An Oral History Memoir* (MIT Press, 1967), 241–49; Fee and Perry, "David Bodian," 169–70; A. McGehee Harvey and Susan L. Abrams, *For the Welfare of Mankind: The Commonwealth Fund and American Medicine* (Johns Hopkins University Press, 1986), 530.

33. Turner to Reed, Mar. 7, 1941, 3a: O. D. Corres., box 501039, "Treasurer's Office—Turner Correspondence Jun 1939–March 1941" folder, AMC; Turner, "Annual Report of the Department of Bacteriology 1942–43."

34. Elizabeth Fee and Manon Perry, "David Bodian. 15 May 1910–18 September 1992," *Proceedings of the American Philosophical Society* 150 (2006), 168–72, quote p. 168; Lewis H. Weed to Basil O'Connor, Nov. 28, 1941, Lewis H. Weed papers, Correspondence: National Foundation for Infantile Paralysis 1927–1946 folder, AMC (emphasis added).

35. Howard Howe to David Bodian, January 23, 1942, and January 29, 1942, David Bodian papers, Box 505280, AMC.

36. "Poliomyelitis Study Grant Awarded to Johns Hopkins," *AJPH* 32 (Sept. 1942), 1082; O'Connor qtd. in "Poliomyelitis," *Journal of Nervous & Mental Diseases* 96.3 (1942), 366–68.

37. "Poliomyelitis."

38. 1941–42 *Report of the President*, 99; Maxcy, "Annual Report of the Department of Epidemiology 1942–43," 3a: O. D. Corres., box 501031, "Department Reports to the Dean 1942–1943" folder, AMC.

39. Lewis H. Weed Collection finding aid, AMC; Lewis H. Weed to Isaiah Bowman, Aug. 7, 1944, Francis Schwentker to Edwards Park, Aug. 17, 1944, and Park to Bowman, Aug. 22, 1944, Records of the Office of the President, box 184, 745 (1944–1945) folder; Park et al., *The Harriet Lane Home: A Model and a Gem*, 191, 226, 238–40; Turner to Reed, June 13, 1940, 3a O. D. Corres., box 502039, "Treasurer's Office–Turner Correspondence Jun 1939–March 1941" folder.

40. Bowman to Park, Aug. 29, 1944, Bowman to Maxcy Aug. 28, 1944, Records of the Office of the President, 745 (1944–1945) folder; Lewis H. Weed to Henry R. Viets, June 25, 1946, and Viets to Weed, July 29, 1946, Lewis H. Weed papers, National Foundation for Infantile Paralysis 1927–1946 folder; Greer Williams, *Virus Hunters* (Alfred A. Knopf, 1967), 276.

41. Thomas B. Turner to Lewis H. Weed, Dec. 12, 1945, Lewis H. Weed papers, Correspondence, "Organization and Policy Committee Nov 1945–Jan 1946" folder, AMC.

42. "Memorandum Embodying A Statement by President Bowman on the Work of the Special Committee on Organization and Policy," revised draft Dec. 18, 1944, Records of

the Office of the President, series 1, box 13, "28.1 Organization and Policy, School of Medicine, 1944–46" folder, JHU Hamburger Archives.

43. JHSPH Advisory Board Minutes, vol. 5, Feb. 26, 1946, p. 36, AMC; Thomas B. Turner to Lewis H. Weed, Dec. 12, 1945, Kenneth Maxcy to Lewis H. Weed, Dec. 22, 1945, and J. E. Moore to Isaiah Bowman, Jan. 9, 1946, Lewis H. Weed papers, Correspondence, "Organization and Policy Committee Nov 1945–Jan 1946" folder, AMC.

44. William Henry Welch, "Duties of a Hospital to the Public Health," in *Papers and Addresses by William Henry Welch: Vol. 1, Pathology-Preventive Medicine* (Johns Hopkins Press, 1920), 621–28, quote p. 628; Fee, *Disease and Discovery*, 42, 68–70, 75–76.

45. Thomas B. Turner to Lewis H. Weed, Dec. 12, 1945, Lewis H. Weed papers, Correspondence, "Organization and Policy Committee Nov 1945–Jan 1946" folder, AMC.

46. Starr, "The Boundaries of Public Health," chap. 5 in *Social Transformation of American Medicine*, 180–97; Stevens, *In Sickness and in Wealth*, 220–21; Daniel M. Fox, *Health Policies, Health Politics: The British and American Experience, 1911–1965* (Princeton University Press, 1986), 117–31.

47. Viseltear, "Emergence of the Medical Care Section of the American Public Health Association"; Starr, *Social Transformation of American Medicine*, 136–39.

48. US Senate, Committee on Labor and Public Welfare, Subcommittee on Health, 93 Cong., 1 Sess., Hill–Burton Hospital Survey and Construction Act: History of the Program and Current Problems and Issues (Comm. Print, 1973), 11–13; Thomas, *Deluxe Jim Crow*, 177; Edward Berkowitz, "Historical Insights into the Development of Health Services Research: A Narrative Based on a Collection of Oral Interviews," National Library of Medicine (www.nlm.nih.gov/hmd/nichsr/intro.html#w31-3, accessed May 5, 2014).

49. US Public Health Service, Coordinated Hospital Service Plan (1945); US Public Health Service, 1945 Annual Report, 293; Isadore Rosenfield, *Hospitals—Integrated Design* (Reinhold, 1947), 222–26; Leonard A. Scheele, "Medical Education in Programs of the Public Health Service," JAMA 140.1 (May 7, 1949), 5–8, quote p. 5.

50. Abel Wolman to Lowell J. Reed, Mar. 17, 1947, MPDC Reference Book No. 1, box 507841.

51. J. E. Moore to Isaiah Bowman, Jan. 9, 1946; Kenneth Maxcy to Lewis H. Weed, Dec. 22, 1945.

52. JHSPH Advisory Board Minutes, vol. 5, Feb. 26, 1946, p. 36, AMC; Medical Planning and Development Committee subject file, "Founding of MPDC" folder, AMC.

53. 1936–37 JHSPH Catalog, 27–37; "Annual Report of the President, 1945–46," *JHU Circular* (1946), 65–75, 90–92; 1954–55 JHSPH Catalog, 41–67; RFA Grant Action Form, Mar. 22, 1948.

54. Grant Action Form, Mar. 22, 1948, "Johns Hopkins University–School of Hygiene and Public Health-Request to Foundation for Further Support," RG 1.1, Series 200, box 186, folder 2234, pp. 10–18, RFA.

55. Rockefeller Foundation 1951 Annual Report, 16–35.

56. Ibid.

57. Grant Action Form, Mar. 22, 1948, "Johns Hopkins University–School of Hygiene and Public Health-Request to Foundation for Further Support," pp. 13–14; Hugh H. Smith diary, Jan. 15, 1948, RG 1.1, Series 200, box 186, folder 2235, RFA; Rockefeller Foundation 1951 Annual Report, 16–35.

58. "Pittsburgh's New School of Public Health," *AJPH* 38 (Nov. 1948), 1618–19; Reed bio file.

59. Justin M. Andrews, "Influence of National Malaria Society on Malaria Eradication," *American Journal of Tropical Medicine and Hygiene* 1 (1952), 100–11.

Chapter 3 · Postwar Public Health Science

1. Richard G. Hewlett and Oscar E. Anderson Jr., *The New World: A History of the United States Atomic Energy Commission, Volume 1, 1939/1946* (Oak Ridge, TN: US AEC Technical Information Center, 1972), 723–24, cited on the Brookings Institution website, "The Costs of the Manhattan Project" (http://www.brookings.edu/about/projects/archive /nucweapons/manhattan, accessed Feb. 19, 2015).

2. Vannevar Bush, *Science: The Endless Frontier* (GPO, 1945), retrieved from the National Science Foundation website (https://www.nsf.gov/od/lpa/nsf50/vbush1945.htm, accessed Feb. 19, 2015).

3. Ibid.

4. "Medicine: Polluted Reservoir," *Time* 51.21 (May 24, 1948), 64.

5. Robert Cook-Deegan and Michael McGeary, "The Jewel in the Federal Crown? History, Politics, and the National Institutes of Health," chap. 8 in Rosemary A. Stevens, Charles E. Rosenberg, and Lawton R. Burns, eds., *History and Health Policy in the United States* (Rutgers University Press, 2006), 176–81.

6. Mullan, *Plagues and Politics*, 128–29, 146–49.

7. Cook-Deegan and McGeary, "The Jewel in the Federal Crown?" 180–81.

8. Kenneth F. Maxcy and Thomas B. Turner bio files, AMC.

9. Turner, Heritage of Excellence, 546 (quote); Harry M. Marks, *The Progress of Experiment: Science and Therapeutic Reform in the United States, 1900–1990* (Cambridge University Press, 2000), 45; Shonick, *Government and Health Services*, 414.

10. Marks, *Progress of Experiment*, 46–47, quote p. 47; Starr, *Social Transformation of American Medicine*. Martin Frobisher in Bacteriology, Isabel Morgan in Epidemiology, Frederik Bang in Pathobiology, and Reginald Archibald, Roger M. Herriott, and Bacon F. Chow in Biochemistry came to JHSPH from the Rockefeller Institute.

11. Fee, *Disease and Discovery*, 173; JHSPH Executive Committee Minutes, Sept. 25, 1950, p. 158; JHSPH Catalog 1957–58; Margaret Merrell to Ernest L. Stebbins, Nov. 6, 1957, Margaret Merrell papers, box 505378, "Office of the President" folder, AMC; Florence R. Sabin papers finding aid, AMC. The six associate professors were Janet Howell Clark (1923 in Physiological Hygiene), Linda B. Lange (1927 in Bacteriology), Margaret Merrell (1942 in Biostatistics), Ruth Freeman (1950 in PHA Division of Public Health Nursing), Anna Baetjer (1952 in Environmental Medicine), and Miriam Dorothy Pauls (1956 in Environmental Medicine, Division of Audiology and Speech). Baetjer and Freeman were made full professors in 1962. "1961–62 Report of the Dean of the JHSPH," *JHU Circular* 81 (1962), 103.

12. Oshinsky, *Polio*, 130; "Against Polio," *Time* 49.26 (June 30, 1947), 81.

13. Fee and Parry, "David Bodian," 170–72; Oshinsky, *Polio*, 130–33; Benison, *Tom Rivers*, 411.

14. Robert M. McAllister, "Viruses in Cancer," *California Medicine* 102.5 (May 1965), 344–52; Benison, *Tom Rivers*, 513; Oshinsky, *Polio*, 130–31; Greer Williams, *Virus Hunters* (Knopf, 1967), 283; Richard Carter, *Breakthrough: The Saga of Jonas Salk* (Trident Press,

1966), 100, 108–9; "Special Grants—Expense Accounts," JHSPH 1948–49 Budget, 3b O. D. Financial, Box 506105.

15. Carter, *Breakthrough*, 78–79; Jeffrey Kluger, *Splendid Solution: Jonas Salk and the Conquest of Polio* (G. P. Putnam's Sons, 2004), 102–4.

16. Oshinsky, *Polio*, 134; quote from David M. Oshinsky, "The Unsung Women in the Race for the Polio Vaccine," *Los Angeles Times*, Apr. 10, 2005; Autumn Stanley, *Mothers and Daughters of Invention: Notes for a Revised History of Technology* (Rutgers University Press, 1995), 159; personal communication from Noel R. Rose, Nov. 15, 2011.

17. Muriel Lederman, entry on "Thomas Hunt Morgan," in Marc Rothenberg, ed., *History of Science in the United States: An Encyclopedia* (Routledge, 2012), 357–59; Isabel Morgan Mountain finding aid, AMC; list of publications for Isabel Morgan Mountain retrieved on Oct. 1, 2015, from MedlinePlus www.nlm.nih.gov/medlineplus (National Library of Medicine); Maryalice Yakutchik, "Science of the Sexes," *Johns Hopkins Public Health Magazine*, Spring 2011.

18. John Rodman Paul, *A History of Poliomyelitis* (Yale University Press, 1971), 261–62.

19. Paul, *History of Poliomyelitis*, 237; Carter, *Breakthrough*, 63, 145, 170–71, 234–36; Kluger, *Splendid Solution*, 194, 273–74. Bodian's activities on these committees and projects are amply documented in the David Bodian papers in the Alan Mason Chesney Medical Archives at Johns Hopkins. For general background on the NFIP cooperative typing program, see Paul, *History of Poliomyelitis*, 233–39. For the gamma globulin trials, see Charles R. Rinaldo Jr., "Passive Immunization against Poliomyelitis: The Hammon Gamma Globulin Field Trials, 1951–1953," *AJPH* 95 (2005), 790–99. Rinaldo does not adequately convey the extent of skepticism in the polio research community about Hammon's results. For the Salk polio vaccine trials, see Harry M. Marks, "The 1954 Salk Poliomyelitis Field Trial," *Clinical Trials* 8 (2011), 224–34.

20. 1956–57 JHSPH Catalog, 141; Langmuir, "The Surveillance of Communicable Diseases of National Importance"; Marks, "The 1954 Salk Poliomyelitis Field Trial"; Oshinsky, *Polio*, 214–36; Paul A. Offit, *The Cutter Incident: How America's First Polio Vaccine Led to the Growing Vaccine Crisis* (Yale University Press, 2005).

21. "Formula to Determine the Total Cost of Conducting a Program of Research as Applied to the National Foundation for Infantile Paralysis and the Johns Hopkins University School of Hygiene and Public Health," May 25, 1949, Records of the JHU President, box 185, "745 (1949)" folder; JHSPH Budgets 1949–50 and 1955–56; National Foundation for Infantile Paralysis, Fourteenth Annual Report (1951), 84, 87, 89–94.

22. Turner to Basic O'Connor, Sept. 9, 1955, Turner papers, box 50564, "Mr. Basil O'Connor" folder; JHSPH Advisory Board Minutes, Jan. 28, 1952, p. 49, and Jan. 25, 1954, p. 237.

23. Williams, *Virus Hunters*, 276; Turner, *Heritage of Excellence*, 373; Shonick, *Government and Health Services*, 425; James Shannon, "The Advancement of Medical Research: A Twenty-Year View of the Role of the National Institutes of Health," *Journal of Medical Education* 42 (Feb. 1967), 99–101.

24. JHSPH 1939–40, 1945–46, 1948–49, 1949–50, and 1955–56 Budgets, 3b O.D. Financial, boxes 506104–05; Wilson G. Smillie, "Training of Public Health Personnel in the United States and Canada," *AJPH* 49.4 (1959), 455–62.

25. Report of the Director of the School of Hygiene and Public Health 1946–47; Harry Eagle to Turner, Jan. 16, 1947, Thomas B. Turner papers, box 50564, "Harry Eagle" folder,

AMC; SHPH Advisory Board Minutes, Oct. 28, 1947, p. 166 and Dec. 16, 1947, p. 177; Korstad, *Dreaming of a Time*, 59; John J. Wright and Cecil G. Sheps, "Role of Case Finding in Syphilis Control Today," *AJPH* 40.7 (July 1950) 844–49.

26. Turner to Perrin Long, June 7, 1948, "Miscellaneous" folder, box 50564, Turner papers.

27. Ann Pietrangelo, "Complement Test," healthline.com (published June 4, 2012, accessed Sept. 28, 2015). For examples of the prewar work on complement, see Harry Eagle and George Brewer, "Mechanism of Hemolysis by Complement: I. Complement Fixation as an Essential Preliminary to Hemolysis," *Journal of General Physiology* 12.6 (1929), 845–62, and Harry Eagle's early 1940s articles in the *Journal of Experimental Medicine* on the serology of syphilis.

28. Manfred M. Mayer bio file, AMC; Turner, *Heritage of Excellence*, 546; Thomas Turner, Microbiology 1957–58 Annual Report, "President's Report" folder; "An Account of Activities at The Johns Hopkins University and Hospital Directed Toward a Solution of the Cancer Problem," undated [1953], Joint Committee on Cancer Teaching and Research subject file folder 2, AMC, p. 3; Rose, "America's First Department of Immunology," 240–47.

29. Turner, Microbiology 1957–58 Annual Report; Manfred M. Mayer, Herbert J. Rapp, Bernard Roizman, S. Wayne Klein, Keith M. Cowan, David Lukens, Carlton E. Schwerdt, Frederick L. Schaffer, and Jesse Charney, "The Purification of Poliomyelitis Virus as Studied by Complement Fixation," *Journal of Immunology* 78.6 (June 1957), 435–55; JHU Treasurer's Report, 1952–53 through 1957–58; Bernard Roizman, bio file, AMC.

30. Turner to Ferrell, Oct. 18, 1938; JHU Treasurer's Report, 1946–47, 1947–48, and 1948–49.

31. Shonick, *Government and Health* Services, 35–49; Turner to Alan M. Chesney, Mar. 26, 1952, "Johns Hopkins Medical School" folder, box 50564, Turner to Ernest Stebbins, Apr. 28, 1952, "Advisory Board" folder, box 50562, Turner papers.

32. Turner to Stebbins, Apr. 3, 1950, in JHSPH 1949–50 budget.

33. Lloyd E. Rozeboom to Ernest L. Stebbins, Jan. 4, 1957, Subcommittee to Review the Curriculum binder; Brown, *Rockefeller Medicine Men*, 107–9, quote p. 107; Fee and Rosenkrantz, "Professional Education for Public Health in the United States," 250–51.

34. Allan M. Brandt, "The Syphilis Epidemic and Its Relation to AIDS," *Science* 239.4838 (1988), 375–80; Robert A. Nelson and Manfred A. Mayer, "Immobilization of Treponema pallidum by Antibody Produced in Syphilitic Infection," *Journal of Experimental Medicine* 89 (1949), 369–93; Virgil Scott, Charles R. Rein, Ira L. Schamberg, J. E. Moore, and Harry Eagle, "The Serologic Differentiation of Syphilitic and False Positive Sera," *American Journal of Syphilis, Gonorrhea and Venereal Disease* 29 (1945), 505; J. E. Moore and C. F. Mohr, "Biologically False Positive Tests for Syphilis," *JAMA* 150 (1952), 467–73; A. Mc Gehee Harvey, "AutoImmune Disease and the Chronic Biologic False Positive Test for Syphilis," *JAMA* 182 (1962), 513–18; Ilana Lowy, " 'Scientific Facts' and Their Public: The History of the Diagnosis of Syphilis," *Revue de Synthèse* 116 (1995), 42–44.

35. A. McGehee Harvey, *Adventures in Medical Research*, 248–51; "Names and Addresses" folder and Moore to Carlos Ramirez Corria, Apr. 10, 1950, and Moore to W. W. Peters, Apr. 8, 1950, "Moore, J. E." folder, Turner papers, box 50564; JHSPH Advisory Board Minutes, Jan. 31, 1950, p. 383; M. G. Candau to Lowell J. Reed, July 1, 1955, Records of the Office of the JHU President, "745 (1955)" folder.

36. "Data on TPI Tests," Feb. 10, 1954, Turner papers, box 50563, "TPI Requests" folder; Turner to Basil O'Connor, Sept. 9, 1955, Turner papers, box 50564, "Mr. Basil O'Connor" folder.

37. JHU Board of Trustees minutes, Mar. 4, 1957, p. 4133 and Apr. 1, 1957, p. 4153; Turner, *Heritage of Excellence*, 522; Turner to Stebbins, Jan. 24, 1955, Turner papers, box 50564, "Advisory Board Meeting" folder; Howard A. Howe to Lowell J. Reed, June 7, 1955, Records of the Office of the JHU President, box 185, "745 (1955)" folder; JHU Treasurer's Report, 1939–1960; JHSPH Executive Committee Minutes, May 16, 1957, p. 2, Sept. 26, 1957, p. 3, Nov. 25, 1957, p. 4; "Report of the President," *JHU Circular* (1957–1958), 69, 135; Rose, "America's First Department of Immunology," 244–45.

38. 1956–57 Report of the Dean of the JHSPH, 135, 138; J. E. Moore to C. L. Conley, Apr. 25, 1957, "TPI Laboratory" folder, Turner to Moore, May 20, 1957, and Moore to Turner, May 23, 1957, "Names and Addresses" folder, box 50563, and Moore to Turner, Feb. 12 and 19, 1954, Turner to Moore Feb. 16, 1954, and Turner to Moore, Mar. 1, 1954, "Moore, J. E." folder, Turner papers.

39. Robin Marantz Henig, *The People's Health: A Memoir of Public Health and Its Evolution at Harvard* (Washington, DC: Joseph Henry Press, 1997), 51.

40. Miriam Brailey to Charlotte Silverman and Carol Chandler, Nov. 24, 1958, Miriam Brailey bio file, AMC.

41. Fee, *Disease and Discovery*, 134–36.

42. ASPH minutes, University of Pittsburgh, Apr. 7–8, 1952, 3a D.O. Corresp., box 504579, "Assoc. Schools of Public Health 1952" folder, AMC; 1960 HEW Annual Report, 153–56, 172–77 (total figure for PHS grants to states excludes construction grants).

43. "Annual Report of the President, 1950–51," *JHU Circular* (1951), 71–92, 122–27; National Research Council Committee on Growth, The Research Attack on Cancer 1946, 30–31, suppl. 2, 8; JHU Treasurer's Report 1946–47, p. 66; "Research on the Prevention of Disease," *Rockefeller Foundation Trustees Bulletin,* March 1948, pp. 6–9. After the departments of medicine and psychiatry, preventive medicine was the third largest grant recipient in the School of Medicine in 1946–1947, with 13 grants totaling $169,000, of which $138,000 was from the American Cancer Society. In 1948–1949, it was again third after medicine and surgery.

44. George Rosen, *A History of Public Health* (expanded edition, Johns Hopkins University Press, 1993), 312–19, 462–67; Brandt, *No Magic Bullet*, 176–78; Fee and Rosenkrantz, "Professional Education for Public Health in the United States," 242–53; Elizabeth Fee and Theodore M. Brown, "Preemptive Biopreparedness: Can We Learn Anything from History?" *AJPH* 91 (May 2001), 725; Elizabeth Fee, "Divorce between Theory and Practice: The System of Public Health Training in the United States," *Ciência & Saúde Coletiva* 13 (2008), 846–48; Gary W. Shannon and Gerald F. Pyle, *Disease and Medical Care in the United States: A Medical Atlas of the Twentieth Century* (Macmillan, 1993), 23–73; Starr, *Social Transformation of American Medicine*, 336.

45. Wade Hampton Frost, "The Age Selection of Mortality from Tuberculosis in Successive Decades," *The Milbank Memorial Fund Quarterly* 18.1 (Jan. 1940), 61–66; George Weisz, " Epidemiology and Health Care Reform: The National Health Survey of 1935–1936," *AJPH* 101.3 (2011), 438–47; Gerald M. Oppenheimer, "Becoming the Framingham Study 1947–1950," *AJPH* 95.4 (2005), 602–10.

46. Leonard Scheele, "The Private Physician in the Public Health Program," *Journal of the National Medical Association* 41.4 (Jan. 1949), 9–14; Harvey and Abrams, "For the Wel-

fare of Mankind," 188–92; A. McGehee Harvey, *Adventures in Medical Research*, 251–54; Moore to Turner, Sept. 15, 1953, Turner papers, box 50564, "Moore, J. E." folder; 1953–54 JHSPH Catalog, 63; "Report of the Dean of the JHSPH," *JHU Circular* (1954–1955), 93; "1955–56 Report of the Dean of the JHSPH," *JHU Circular* (1956), 131; 1956–57 JHSPH Catalog, 59; "1956–57 Report of the Dean of the JHSPH," *JHU Circular* (1957), 137–39.

47. Philip Sartwell to Thomas Turner, Oct. 10, 1956, Comments from Staff Members (binder), Committee to Review the Educational Objectives of the School of Hygiene and Public Health, box 50564, Turner papers, AMC.

48. Philip E. Sartwell bio file, AMC; "Philip E. Sartwell, 91, noted Hopkins epidemiologist," *Baltimore Sun*, Dec. 2, 1999.

49. Sartwell and Winston H. Price bio files, AMC; Department of Epidemiology, 3a D.O. Correspondence, box 505348, "President's Report 1958" folder; 1957–58 JHSPH Catalog, 48–49, 137; George W. Corner, *A History of the Rockefeller Institute: 1901–1953, Origins and Growth* (The Rockefeller Institute Press, 1964), 429–33.

50. Philip Sartwell bio file, AMC; P. E. Sartwell, "The Time Factor in Studies of the Outcome of Chronic Disease," *American Review of Tuberculosis* 63 (1951), 608–12; P. E. Sartwell and Margaret Merrell, "Influence of the Dynamic Character of Chronic Disease on the Interpretation of Morbidity Rates," *AJPH* 42 (1952), 579–84; P. E. Sartwell, "Some Approaches to the Epidemiologic Study of Chronic Disease," *AJPH* 45 (1955), 609–14; "On the Methodology of Investigations of Etiologic Factors in Chronic Diseases—Further Comments," *Journal of Chronic Disease* 11 (1960), 61–63.

51. Fee, *Disease and Discovery*; Raymond Pearl, A. C. Sutton, and W. T. Howard, "Experimental Treatment of Cancer with Tuberculin," *Lancet* 216 (1929), 1078–80; Raymond Pearl, "Tobacco Smoking and Longevity," *Science* 87.2253 (1938), 216–17.

52. Morton L. Levin bio file, AMC; M. L. Levin, H. Goldstein, and P. R. Gerhardt, "Cancer and Tobacco Smoking," *JAMA* 143 (May 27, 1950), 336–38; M. L. Levin, "Some Epidemiological Features of Cancer," *Cancer* 1.3 (Sept. 1948), 489–97; *Smoking and Health* (1964), 158, 188; Allan M. Brandt, *The Cigarette Century: The Rise, Fall and Deadly Persistence of the Product That Defined America* (New York: Basic Books, 2007), 134–38.

53. Abraham M. Lilienfeld bio file, AMC; JHSPH Executive Committee minutes, Sept. 25, 1950, p. 158; David Eugene Lilienfeld, "Abe and Yak: The Interactions of Abraham M. Lilienfeld and Jacob Yerushalmy in the Development of Modern Epidemiology (1945–1973)," *Epidemiology* 18.4 (July 2007), 507–14; A. M. Lilienfeld, "National Evaluation of Gamma Globulin," *Public Health Reports* 68 (Oct. 1953), 1001; A. M. Lilienfeld, "Summary of the Report of the National Advisory Committee for Evaluation of Gamma Globulin," *JAMA* 154.13 (1954), 1086–90; Saul Krugman, "The Clinical Use of Gamma Globulin," *New England Journal of Medicine* 269 (July 25, 1963), 195–201.

54. Abraham M. Lilienfeld, "An Overview of the Epidemiology of Cancer," in David L. Levin, ed., *Cancer Epidemiology in the USA and USSR* (GPO, 1980), 4; Commission on Chronic Illness, *Chronic Illness in the United States: Vol. IV, Chronic Illness in a Large City* (Harvard University Press, 1957), 8–20, 366. The PHS conducted local morbidity surveys in Hagerstown, Maryland (1921–1924 and 1941–1944); Cattaraugus County, New York (1929–1932); and Syracuse, New York (1930–1931), and also conducted two national surveys, in cooperation with the Committee on the Costs of Medical Care in 18 states (1928–1931), and the National Health Survey of 2.8 million individuals in 83 cities and 23 rural areas (1935–1936). The US Census Bureau included questions on the prevalence and severity of

disabling illness (but not the cause) in its Current Population Survey (1949–1950), while California conducted the first statewide health survey in 1954–1955.

55. 1953–54 Report of the JHSPH Dean to the President, *JHU Circular* 73 (1954), 99; "Planning for the Chronically Ill: Joint Statement of Recommendations by the American Hospital Association, American Medical Association, American Public Health Association, and American Public Welfare Association," *AJPH* 37 (1947), 1256–66; Morton L. Levin and Dean W. Roberts bio files, AMC.

56. 1953–54 Report of the JHSPH Dean to the President, 99.

57. Commission on Chronic Illness, *Chronic Illness in the United States: Vol. III, Chronic Illness in a Rural Area: The Hunterdon Study* (Harvard University Press, 1959); Jonas N. Muller, review of "Commission on Chronic Illness, *Chronic Illness in the United States, v. 4. Chronic Illness in a Large City: The Baltimore Study*," *AJPH* 48.6 (1958), 813–14; *Smoking and Health: Report of the Advisory Committee to the Surgeon General of the Public Health Service* (PHS publication no. 1103, GPO, 1964), 218–19, 363–67.

58. Margaret Merrell papers, box 505378, "Epid-Stat 1959" folder, and C. A. Smith to Margaret Merrill, Apr. 15, 1955, "Untreated [Sigma] Sample of cases" folder, AMC; William G. Cochran to Ernest Stebbins, Mar. 1, 1950, JHSPH Records, 3b: O.D. Financial, box 506104, "1949–50 Budget" binder.

59. Helen Abbey bio file, AMC; D. P. Murphy and H. Abbey, *Cancer in Families: A Study of the Relations of 200 Breast Cancer Probands* (Harvard University Press, 1959).

60. Brandt, *The Cigarette Century*, 126–27, 150; William G. Rothstein, *Public Health and the Risk Factor: A History of an Uneven Medical Revolution* (University of Rochester Press, 2003); John H. McDonald, *Handbook of Biological Statistics*, 2nd ed. (Sparky House Publishing, 2009), 88–94; William G. Cochran, "Some Methods for Strengthening the Common χ^2 Tests," *Biometrics* 10 (1954), 417–51; N. Mantel and W. Haenszel, "Statistical Aspects of the Analysis of Data from Retrospective Studies of Disease," *Journal of the National Cancer Institute* 22 (1959), 719–48; William G. Cochran, *Experimental Designs* (Wiley, 1950); William G. Cochran, *Sampling Techniques* (Wiley, 1953); James F. Jekel, ed., *Epidemiology, Biostatistics, and Preventive Medicine*, 3rd ed. (Elsevier Health Sciences, 2007), 197.

61. Bernard G. Greenberg, review of *Catalytic Models in Epidemiology* by Hugo Muench, *AJPH* 50 (Feb. 1960), 267; William G. Cochran, review of *Elementary Decision Theory* by Herman Chernoff and Lincoln E. Moses, *AJPH* 50 (Mar. 1960), 417–18; Charles Flagle, Sept. 20, 2010, interview.

62. Annual Letter for 1952 to the ScD Graduates in Parasitology; Ernest Stebbins to Detlev Bronk, Apr. 23, 1953, Records of the Office of the JHU President, box 185, "745 (1953)" folder.

63. Personal communication from Noel Rose, Nov. 15, 2011; Annual Letter for 1952 to the ScD Graduates in Parasitology; Don E. Eyles to Ernest L. Stebbins, Apr. 6, 1953, M. M. Brooke to Detlev W. Bronk, Feb. 25, 1953, Brooke to Bronk, Apr. 20, 1953, William D. Lindquist to Bronk, Apr. 24, 1953, "745 (1953)" folder, box 185, Records of the Office of the JHU President.

64. JHSPH Executive Committee Minutes, Apr. 25, 1955, p. 3; JHSPH Advisory Board Minutes, June 4, 1954, box 501965, AMC; Nicolas Rasmussen, *Picture Control: The Electron Microscope and the Transformation of Biology in America, 1940–1960* (Stanford University Press, 1999), 102–52; F. B. Bang, "The Morphological Approach," in F. M. Burnet and W. M. Stanley, eds., *The Viruses*, vol. 3 (Academic Press, 1959).

65. Philip Bard to Frank R. Ferlaino, Aug. 5, 1953, Joint Committee on Cancer Teaching and Research subject files.

66. F. B. Bang, "Three Dilemmas in the Study of Viruses and Tumor Cells," *Cancer Research* 18.9 (1958), 1004–7 (quote p. 1005); G. O. Gey and F. B. Bang, "Viruses and Cells: A Study in Tissue Culture Applications. II. Effect of Several Viruses on Cell Types and the Amount of Virus Produced," *Transactions of the New York Academy of Science* 14 (1951), 15; 1955–56 JHSPH Catalog, 57.

67. The French biologist A. Borrell, who first advanced the viral theory of cancer causation in 1903, studied the Rous tumor virus. A. Borrell, "Cytologie du sarcome de Peyton Rous et substance specifique," *Comptes Rendus de Société de Biologie* 94 (1926), 500–4.

68. "Annual Report to the American Cancer Society from the Joint Committee on Cancer Teaching and Research of the Johns Hopkins Medical Institutions," 1965, Joint Committee on Cancer Teaching and Research subject files, folder 1, AMC; K. V. Shah, "Neutralizing Antibodies to Simian Virus 40 (SV40) in Human Sera from India," *Proceedings of the Society of Experimental Biology and Medicine* 121 (1966), 303–7; K. V. Shah, "Investigation of Human Malignant Tumors in India for SV40 etiology," *Journal of the National Cancer Institute* 42 (1969), 139–45; K. V. Shah, L. D. Palma, and G.P. Murphy, "The Occurrence of SV40 Neutralizing Antibodies in Sera of Patients with Genitourinary Carcinoma," *Journal of Surgical Oncology* 3 (1971), 443; K. V. Shah, M. Weissman, and G. P. Murphy, "Occurrence of Simian Virus 40 Reacting Antibodies in Sera of Some Patients with Prostatic Cancer," *Journal of Surgical Oncology* 4 (1972), 89–93; L. P. Weiner, R. M. Herndon, O. Narayan, R. T. Johnson, K. V. Shah, L. J. Rubinstein, T. J. Preziosi, and F. K. Conley, "Isolation of Virus Related to SV40 from Patients with Progressive Multifocal Leukoencephalopathy," *New England Journal of Medicine* 286 (1972), 385–90; K. V. Shah, F. B. Bang, and H. Abbey, "Considerations for Epidemiologic Studies to Test the Hypothesis of Viral Causation of Human Breast Cancer," *Journal of the National Cancer Institute* 48 (1972), 1035–38; K. V. Shah, "Does SV40 Infection Contribute to the Development of Human Cancers?" *Reviews in Medical Virology* 10 (2000), 31–43; J. M. M. Walboomers, M. V. Jacobs, M. M. Manos, F. X. Bosch, J. A. Kummer, K. V. Shah, P. J. F. Snijders, J. Peto, C. J. L. M. Meijer, and N. Muñoz, "Human Papillomavirus Is a Necessary Cause of Invasive Cervical Cancer Worldwide," *Journal of Pathology* 189 (1999), 12–19; F. X. Bosch, A. Lorincz, N. Muñoz, C. J. Meijer, and K. V. Shah, "The Causal Relation between Human Papillomavirus and Cervical Cancer," *Journal of Clinical Pathology* 55 (2002), 244–65.

69. "An Account of Activities at The Johns Hopkins University and Hospital Directed Toward a Solution of the Cancer Problem," 3; Frederik Bang, Pathobiology 1957–58 Annual Report, "President's Report" folder; Lowell J. Reed, memo to members of the Joint Committee on Cancer Teaching and Research, Oct. 30, 1951, and "Cancer Research at the Johns Hopkins University," 1957 application for an Institutional Research Grant to the American Cancer Society, p. 11, Joint Committee on Cancer Teaching and Research subject file folder 2, AMC; 1960–61 JHU Treasurer's Report, 82–87.

Chapter 4 · The School and the City

1. Stebbins bio file, AMC; Albert Deutsch, "Dr. Stebbins: Prepared for New York's War Health Problems," *PM*, July 20, 1942; Albert Deutsch, column in *PM*, Mar. 5, 1946; "Dr. Stebbins Leaves," *New York Times*, Oct. 27, 1945; Abel Wolman, faculty reminiscences of Ernest Stebbins, Elizabeth Fee JHSPH History records, "Stebbins" folder.

2. Stebbins bio file; "APHA Past Presidents"; "State to Pioneer Broad-Scale Doctor Course in Public Health," *Wilmington Journal*, Nov. 30, 1950.

3. Huntington Williams and Robert H. Riley bio files, AMC; Elizabeth Fee, "Public Health in Practice: An Early Confrontation with the 'Silent Epidemic' of Childhood Lead Paint Poisoning," *Journal of the History of Medicine and Allied Sciences* 45 (1990), 570–606; "New York State Advances Public Health," *AJPH* 51 (July 1961), 1049–50.

4. Williams bio file; Fee, "Public Health in Practice," quote p. 577.

5. Fee, "Public Health in Practice."

6. "Tuberculosis Called Major Health Problem Not Yet Met," *Baltimore Sun*, Oct. 7, 1941.

7. "Report of the Dean of the School of Hygiene and Public Health," *JHU Circular* (1940–41), 93–104; Kenneth Maxcy, Annual Report of the Department of Epidemiology 1942–43, 3a O. D. Corres., box 502031, Department Reports to the Dean 1942–1943; A. Harvey and Susan L. Abrams, *"For the Welfare of Mankind": The Commonwealth Fund and American Medicine* (Johns Hopkins University Press, 1986), 589; Allen Freeman, Annual Report of the Department of Public Health Administration 1942–43, 3a O. D. Corres., box 502031, "Department Reports to the Dean 1942–1943" folder; "Open Fight on T.B., Syphilis at Forum," *Baltimore Afro-American*, Mar. 27, 1943. For an in-depth discussion of tuberculosis and race in Baltimore, see Samuel Kelton Roberts, *Infectious Fear: Politics, Disease, and the Health Effects of Segregation* (University of North Carolina Press, 2009).

8. Miriam E. Brailey, *Tuberculosis in White and Negro Children: Vol. II. The Epidemiologic Aspects of the Harriet Lane Study* (Commonwealth Fund, 1958).

9. Parran, "The Health of the Nation," 1377; Riley bio file.

10. Arthur J. Viseltear, "Emergence of the Medical Care Section of the American Public Health Association, 1926–1948," *AJPH* 63 (Nov. 1973), 990–91.

11. Parran, "The Health of the Nation," 1377–78; Starr, "The Boundaries of Public Health," chap. 5 in *Social Transformation of American Medicine*, 180–97; Stevens, *In Sickness and in Wealth*, 220–21; Daniel M. Fox, *Health Policies, Health Politics: The British and American Experience, 1911–1965* (Princeton University Press, 1986), 117–31.

12. Viseltear, "Emergence of the Medical Care Section of the American Public Health Association," 992–1004; Derickson, *Health Security for All*, 60, 88–89.

13. Viseltear, "Emergence of the Medical Care Section of the American Public Health Association"; "Health Chief's Zeal Undiminished," *Baltimore Sun*, Aug. 5, 1956.

14. C. Horace Hamilton, "Elements of a State Medical Care Plan" (revised), typescript, Mar. 1945, North Carolina Hospital and Medical Care Study Commission papers, box 1C, North Carolina State Archives, p. 5; Thomas, *Deluxe Jim Crow*, 138–43.

15. "Dr. Freeman Named to Post," *Baltimore Sun*, Sept. 7, 1946; "Dr. Freeman Quits, Ending 50 Years in Public Health," *Baltimore Sun*, Feb. 20, 1954.

16. W. K. Sharp, "PHS District 2 Report, May 1944," June 13, 1944, folder 0243-MD, box 227, Gen. Classified Records: Group III-States, 1936–44, PHS records, RG 90, NA.

17. Committee on Medical Care, Maryland State Planning Commission, *Administering Health Services in Maryland*, 76–77.

18. "1951—Present Budget," Apr. 13, 1951, 3b. O. D. Financial, box 506104, 1951–52 Budget, AMC; Thomas Turner, Memorandum to the CREOSHPH, Sept. 1, 1956, Appendix E: Field Study Areas; JHSPH 1951–52 Budget.

19. Turner, *Heritage of Excellence*, 368.

20. Pietila, *Not in My Neighborhood*, 67–74; Kenneth T. Jackson, *Crabgrass Frontier: The Suburbanization of the United States* (Oxford University Press, 1985), 232–33, 293; Martin V. Melosi, *The Sanitary City: Urban Infrastructure in America from Colonial Times to the Present* (Johns Hopkins University Press, 2000), 224–30, 293–94; Gilbert Sandler, *Jewish Baltimore: A Family Album* (Johns Hopkins University Press, 2000), 24.

21. Thomas Turner to John Ferrell, Feb. 4, 1938, RG 100.1, series 200, box 28, folder 319, RFA; R. A. Vonderlehr to Walter Clarke, Sept. 8, 1941, RG 90: Records of the USPHS, General Classified Records, box 227, 0425 Md (V.D.), National Archives, College Park, MD.

22. Stebbins bio file; *AJPH* 32.8 (Aug. 1942), 933; "Warns of Spread in Venereal Ills," *New York Times*, Mar. 22, 1946.

23. "Survey of Health in City Underway," *Baltimore Sun*, Aug. 4, 1947.

24. "Nurses Claim Dr. Williams 'Browbeater,'" *Baltimore Afro-American*, July 16, 1947; "Nurses Charge Health Survey Deters Work," *Baltimore Evening Sun*, July 21, 1947.

25. Johns Hopkins School of Hygiene and Public Health Department of Biostatistics, "Instructions for Enumerators: Health Survey—Eastern Health District" June 1947, Huntington Williams papers, box 505733, "Eastern Health District—Nurses' Objections to Survey Work" folder, AMC, p. 20.

26. Lowell J. Reed and Huntington Williams, "The Unique Nature of the Eastern Health District Studies and Census Surveys," *Baltimore Health News* 25.9 (Sept. 1948), 57–62, quote p. 60; Postcard to Doctor H. Williams, Aug. 8, 1947, Ant. Romantio to Huntington Williams (undated), East Baltimore Tax Payer to Health Commissioner of Baltimore City, July 26, 1947, Tax Payer to Head Nurse, Health Department, July 21, 1947, Huntington Williams papers, box 505733, "Eastern Health District—Nurses' Objections to Survey Work" folder, AMC.

27. 1947–48 Report of the Dean of the JHSPH, *JHU Circular* 62 (Nov. 1948), 103, 105–6.

28. Hugh H. Smith diary Feb. 25 and July 12, 1948, RG 1.1 Projects, Series 200 United States, box 179, folder 2162 "200 J Johns Hopkins University–Training Area 1945–1949," RFA; Huntington Williams to Mayo L. Emory, Mar. 3, 1949, Huntington Williams papers, box 505733, "Eastern Health District Correspondence 1948–1949" folder; "1948–49 Report of the Dean of the JHSPH," *JHU Circular* 68 (Nov. 1949), 95–96; "1950–51 Report of the Dean of the JHSPH," *JHU Circular* 70 (Nov. 1951), 114–15.

29. JHSPH Advisory Board Minutes, Feb. 28, 1950, p. 390; 1949–50 Report of the Director of the JHSPH, *JHU Circular* 69 (Nov. 1950), 105–6; "School History" (http://www.mailman.hs.columbia.edu/about-us/school-history, accessed May 5, 2010); Ernest L. Stebbins to Huntington Williams, Mar. 5, 1949, box 185, 745 (1949) folder, Records of the Office of the JHU President; Elizabeth Fee, "Partners in Community Health: The Baltimore City Health Department, the Johns Hopkins School of Hygiene and Public Health, and the Eastern Health District, 1932–1992," *Maryland Medical Journal* 42.8 (Aug. 1993), 740–42.

30. Stebbins interview by Fee, Oct. 15, 1979; Huntington Williams to Thomas D'Alesandro Jr., Mar. 8, 1949, "Eastern Health District Correspondence 1948–1949" folder.

31. "Certification of Employee of the City of Baltimore, Subversive Activities Act of 1949," Charlotte Silverman papers, box 505225, "Ober Law" folder, AMC; Park et al., *The Harriet Lane Home: A Model and a Gem*, 198; "Oust Dr. Brailey, Williams Warned," *Baltimore Sun*, Mar. 17, 1950; Charlotte F. Gerczak, "The Courage of Her Convictions: The

Story of Miriam Brailey," unpublished manuscript, July 2001, Miriam Brailey papers, pp. 7–8, AMC; Miriam Brailey to Charlotte Silverman, Aug. 9, 1949, and Carl Bassett, Oct. 12, 1950, letter to opponents of the Ober Law, "Ober Law" folder.

32. Brailey to Silverman, Aug. 9, 1949; "Joseph Sherbow, Powerful Lawyer and Judge, dies," *Baltimore Sun*, Dec. 17, 1979; Ralph W. Ballin, MD, letter to the editor, *Baltimore Sun*, Mar. 17, 1950; "Dr. Brailey Fights Ober-Law Firing," *Baltimore Sun*, Dec. 22, 1950; Gerczak, "The Courage of Her Convictions," 8–9; JHSPH Executive Committee Minutes, Jan. 29, 1951, p. 163; "Report of the Office of the Vice President and Provost," Jan. 1969, "Ober Law" folder.

33. APHA Committee on Professional Education, "Report of the Subcommittee on Field Training of Public Health Personnel," *AJPH* 44 (1954), 673–75; APHA Committee on Administrative Practice, "The State Health Department—Services and Responsibilities," *AJPH* 44 (1954), 235–52.

34. Campbell and Connor, Variations in State Public Health Programs during a Five-Year Period, 6, 12, 39, 110, 126, 128; 1955 HEW Annual Report, 117–18; Ernest L. Stebbins, "Contribution of the Graduate School of Public Health—Plans for the Future," *AJPH* 47 (Dec. 1957), 1509; Wallace F. Janssen, "Introduction," Food and Drug Administration Annual Reports 1950–1974 (1974), xi–xii.

35. "Appendixes: I Trends and Needs for Official Community Health Services—As Seen by Health Officials in 28 States," *AJPH* 47 (1957), 33; Kenneth T. Jackson, *Crabgrass Frontier: The Suburbanization of the United States* (Oxford University Press, 1985), 283–85; SHPH 1951–52 Budget; Baltimore City Health Department, *Guarding the Health of Baltimore* (1961), 13; 1957–58 SHPH Catalog, 35.

36. JHSPH Advisory Board Minutes, June 8, 1951, p. 563; John Black Grant diary, Mar. 29–Apr. 1, 1958, box 187, folder 2237, "200 L Johns Hopkins University–School of Hygiene and Public Health 1958–61," RFA.

37. "Dr. Williams Quizzed on Health Dept.," *Baltimore Sun*, Dec. 6, 1956; "Action Is Seen Revolt against Dr. Williams," *Baltimore Sun*, June 17, 1958; "Dr. Williams Quizzed on Health Dept.," *Baltimore Sun*, Dec. 6, 1956.

38. "1956–57 Report of the SHPH Director," *JHU Circular* 76 (Nov. 1957), 142; "Baltimore Department Reorganized," *AJPH* 47 (June 1957), 793; "Pleas for Dr. Williams, Miss Lazarus Increase," *Baltimore Sun*, July 20, 1956; "Action Is Seen Revolt against Dr. Williams," *Baltimore Sun*, June 17, 1958; Huntington Williams bio file, AMC.

39. Fee and Rosenkrantz, "Professional Education for Public Health in the United States," 240–41.

40. "Accounts of Grant Money Received and Spent," 34–35, 40, 70–73, 80–82, 92, 96–97, 118–19, 124; JHSPH Budgets 1924–67, box 506105, AMC; Winslow, 1949 APHA accreditation report.

41. JHSPH Advisory Board Minutes, vol. 5, Sept. 23, 1947, p. 155, Oct. 28, 1947, p. 165, Nov. 25, 1947, p. 173, Dec. 16, 1947, p. 177; Commission on University Education in Hospital Administration, "Report on the Program in Hospital Administration at Johns Hopkins University," January 1955, Records of the Office of the President, box 185, "745 (1955)" folder, JHU Hamburger University Archives; Stevens, *In Sickness and in Wealth*, 71–75, 156–58.

42. Report on the Program in Hospital Administration at Johns Hopkins University; Charles Flagle interview, Sept. 29, 2010. Crosby served from 1954 to 1972 as executive vice-president and director of the American Hospital Association.

43. JHSPH Executive Committee Minutes, Dec. 18, 1950, p. 162; Paul A. Lembcke, "Medical Auditing by Scientific Methods Illustrated by Major Female Pelvic Surgery," *JAMA* 162 (1956), 646–55; Commission on University Education in Hospital Administration, "Report on the Program in Hospital Administration at Johns Hopkins University."

44. Margaret Merrell, "Report of the Committee on Applications and Curriculum, Sub-Committee on Alumni and their MPH Curriculum Suggestions," Records of the Office of the JHU President, box 185, "745 (1955)" folder, p. 14; "1955–56 Report of the Director of the JHSPH," *JHU Circular* 75 (Nov. 1956), 120; Thomas B. Turner to Ernest L. Stebbins, "Report of the Curriculum Committee," May 18, 1956, "Advisory Board Meeting" folder.

45. "Report of Sub-Committee of Applications and Curriculum Committee on Alumni and Their MPH Curriculum Suggestions," 14, 20.

46. Shonick, *Government and Health Services*, 92; 1950 Federal Security Administration Annual Report; 1968 Health, Education and Welfare Annual Report.

47. Allan Brandt, *No Magic Bullet: A Social History of Venereal Disease in the United States since 1880* (Oxford University Press, 1987), 176–78; Fee and Rosenkrantz, "Professional Education for Public Health in the United States," 236–37, 242–53; Elizabeth Fee and Theodore M. Brown, "Preemptive Biopreparedness: Can We Learn Anything from History?" *AJPH* 91 (May 2001), 725; Elizabeth Fee, "Divorce between Theory and Practice: The System of Public Health Training in the United States," *Ciência & Saúde Coletiva* 13 (2008), 846–48; Shonick, *Government and Health Services*, 94–95; B. S. Sanders, "Local Health Departments: Growth or Illusion?" *Public Health Reports* 74 (1959), 13–20; Milton Terris, "The Changing Face of Public Health," *AJPH* 49 (1959), 1119; Jesse B. Aronson, "The Politics of Public Health—Reactions and Summary," *AJPH* 49 (1959), 311.

48. "News from the Field," *AJPH* 40.7 (July 1950), 1054; *Congress and the Nation 1945– 1964* (Congressional Quarterly, 1965), 1114.

49. Elaine Tyler May, *Homeward Bound: American Families in the Postwar Era*, rev. ed. (Basic Books, 1999), 120; US Department of Health, Education, and Welfare, National Center for Health Statistics, "Fertility Tables for Birth Cohorts by Color: United States, 1917–73," 1976; Keith Wailoo, *Dying in the City of the Blues: Sickle Cell Anemia and the Politics of Race and Health* (University of North Carolina Press, 2001), 92–95, 104–9.

50. Anne Baber Kennedy, " 'Many Hidden Springs': Celebrating 50 Years of Maternal and Child Health Sciences at Johns Hopkins and a Century of Maternal and Child Health in Maryland," 3a D.O. Corresp., box 507939, "Department of Maternal and Child Health" folder, AMC, pp. 16–17; JHSPH Advisory Board minutes, Jan. 28, 1947, p. 102, Feb. 5, 1947, p. 108, and Dec. 16, 1947, p. 178; Edwards Park, John W. Littlefield, Henry M. Seidel, and Lawrence S. Willow, *The Harriet Lane Home: A Model and a Gem* (Department of Pediatrics, School of Medicine, Johns Hopkins University, 2006), 311.

51. Parran–Farrand Report, 34, 38.

52. Park, *The Harriet Lane Home*, 247–56, 260, 311; Harper, Division of Maternal and Child Health 1957–58 Annual Report; Edward Davens to Detlev W. Bronk, July 9, 1951, 3a D.O. correspondence, box 505343, "Appointments, Resignations, 1951–1957, Various and A–J" folder; Josiah Macy Jr. Foundation Study of the Future of the Johns Hopkins School of Hygiene and Public Health (1975), 77.

53. Ruth Benson Freeman bio file, AMC.

54. Paul Lemkau to Ernest Stebbins, Apr. 1, 1950, JHSPH records, 3b: O.D. Financial, box 506104, "1949–50" binder; "Report on the Eastern Health District to the IHD 1943,"

3a D. O. Corres., box 502037, "Rockefeller Foundation" folder; 1946–47 JHSPH Catalog, 36; 1947–48 JHSPH Catalog, 44; 1948–49 JHSPH Catalog, 44; 1951–52 JHSPH Catalog, 57–63; 1952–53 JHSPH Catalog, 59–61; Ruth B. Freeman to Ernest L. Stebbins Apr. 22, 1952, Thomas Turner papers, box 505461, "Development Committee" folder.

55. Fee, *Disease and Discovery*, 201–4, 218; George Rosen, "Public Health and Mental Health: Converging Trends and Emerging Issues," in *Mental Health Teaching in Schools of Public Health* (Association of Schools of Public Health, 1961), 22; Gerald R. Grob, *From Asylum to Community: Mental Health Policy in Modern America* (Princeton University Press, 1991), 102–3.

56. "1956–57 Report of the JHSPH Director," *JHU Circular* 76 (Nov. 1957), 143.

57. William M. Schmidt and Isabelle Valadian, "A Maternal and Child Health Bookshelf," *AJPH* 54 (Apr. 1964), 551–62; Helen M. Wallace, *Health Services for Mothers and Children* (Saunders, 1962); Harold C. Stuart and Dane G. Prugh, eds., *The Healthy Child: His Physical, Psychological and Social Development* (Harvard University Press, 1960).

58. 1955–56 JHSPH Catalog, 13–19.

59. JHSPH Directory of Graduates, 1919–1962.

60. Thomas, *Deluxe Jim Crow*, 85–96; Johanna Schoen, *Choice and Coercion: Birth Control, Sterilization, and Abortion in Public Health and Welfare* (University of North Carolina Press, 2005), 22–23; Justin Lessler, C. Jessica E. Metcalf, Rebecca F. Grais, Francisco J. Luquero, Derek A. T. Cummings, and Bryan T. Grenfell, "Measuring the Performance of Vaccination Programs Using Cross-Sectional Surveys: A Likelihood Framework and Retrospective Analysis," *PLoS Medicine* 8.10 (2011), e1001110; Janet Golden, "The Iconography of Child Public Health: Between Medicine and Reform," in Cheryl Kranick Warsh and Veronica Strong-Boag, eds., *Children's Health Issues in Historical Perspective* (Wilfred Laurier University Press, 2005), 391–407, quote p. 404.

61. Virginia Apgar papers, Profiles in Science, National Library of Medicine (http://profiles.nlm.nih.gov/ps/retrieve/Collection/CID/CP, accessed Sept. 12, 2011).

62. Virginia Apgar to Paul A. Harper Mar. 24, 1958, Virginia Apgar papers; 1968–69 JHSPH Catalog, 84; 1972–73 JHSPH Catalog, 77.

63. Virginia Apgar papers.

64. Lowell Reed, "Annual Report of the Department of Biostatistics 1942–43," 3a O. D. Corres., box 502031, "Department Reports to the Dean 1942–1943" folder, AMC; Fee, *Disease and Discovery*, 192–204, 225; Margaret Merrell, "The Family as a Unit in Public Health Research," *Human Biology* 24.1 (Feb. 1952), 1–11, quote p. 9; "The Work of Selwyn D. Collins," *Public Health Reports* 75.6 (1960), 565–66.

65. W. H. Frost, "The Familial Aggregation of Infectious Diseases," *AJPH* 28.1 (Jan. 1938), 2–13; Frost, "The Importance of Epidemiology as a Function of Health Departments," 113–14 (quote); Merrell, "The Family as a Unit in Public Health Research."

66. Merrell, "The Family as a Unit in Public Health Research."

67. Alan Mason Chesney Medical Archives JHSPH institutional records photograph collection and People at Work Photograph Collection, Public health student nurse photographs by Dennis Stock for Johns Hopkins Magazine, 1964.

68. Starr, *Social Transformation of American Medicine*, 322–26.

69. Martha Rogers, Abraham M. Lilienfeld, and Benjamin Pasamanick, *Prenatal and Paranatal Factors in the Development of Childhood Behavior* (Acta Psychiatric Neurology Supplement No. 102, 1955), 12–18.

70. Abraham M. Lilienfeld bio file, AMC; David Lilienfeld, "Abe and Yak: The Interactions of Abraham M. Lilienfeld and Jacob Yerushalmy in the Development of Modern Epidemiology," 507–14; Halbert L. Dunn, "Record Linkage," *AJPH* 36.12 (Dec. 1946), 1412–16; H. B. Newcombe, J. M. Kennedy, S. J. Axford, and A. P. James, "Automatic Linkage of Vital Records," *Science* 130.3381 (Oct. 1959), 954–59; Abraham M. Lilienfeld and E. Parkhurst, "A study of the Association of Factors of Pregnancy and Parturition with the Development of Cerebral Palsy: A Preliminary Report," *American Journal of Hygiene* 53 (1951), 262–82; JHSPH Executive Committee minutes, Sept. 25, 1950, p. 158. Although Sweden's cerebral palsy registry was initiated in 1954, most countries did not begin tracking population data on cerebral palsy until the 1970s, and the United States still has no central registry. Christine Cans, Geraldine Surman, Vicki McManus, David Coghlan, Owen Hensey, and Ann Johnson, "Cerebral Palsy Registries," *Seminars in Pediatric Neurology* 11.1 (Mar. 2004), 18–23; Nigel Paneth, T. Ting Hong, and Steven Korzeniewski, "The Descriptive Epidemiology of Cerebral Palsy," *Clinics in Perinatology* 33 (2006), 251–67.

71. Abraham M. Lilienfeld, Benjamin Pasamanick, and Martha Rogers, "Relationship between Pregnancy Experience and the Development of Certain Neuropsychiatric Disorders in Childhood," *AJPH* 45 (1955), 637–43.

72. Benjamin Pasamanick bio file, AMC; Benjamin Pasamanick, "A Comparative Study of the Behavioral Development of Negro Infants," *Journal of Genetic Psychology* 69 (1946), 3–44.

73. Lilienfeld, Pasamanick, and Rogers, "Relationship between Pregnancy Experience and the Development of Certain Neuropsychiatric Disorders in Childhood," 638–40, quote p. 640.

74. Benjamin Pasamanick, Hilda Knobloch, and Abraham M. Lilienfeld, "Socioeconomic Status and Some Precursors of Neuropsychiatric Disorder," *American Journal of Orthopsychiatry* 26 (1956), 594–601; Rowland V. Rider, Matthew Tayback, and Hilda Knobloch, "Associations between Premature Birth and Socioeconomic Status," *AJPH* 45.8 (Aug. 1955), 1022–28; J. Katz, A. C. C. Lee, N. Kozuki, J. E. Lawn, S. Cousens, H. Blencowe, et al. and the CHERG Small-for-Gestational-Age-Preterm Birth Working Group, "Mortality Risk in Preterm and Small-for-Gestational-Age Infants in Low-Income and Middle-Income Countries: A Pooled Country Analysis," *Lancet* 382.9890 (2013), 417–25; A. C. C. Lee, J. Katz, H. Blencowe, S. Cousens, N. Kozuki, J. P. Vogel, et al. and the CHERG SGA-Preterm Working Group, "Born Too Small: National and Regional Estimates of Term and Preterm Small-for-Gestational-Age in 138 Low-Middle Income Countries in 2010," *Lancet Global Health* 1 (2013), e26–36.

75. Lilienfeld, Pasamanick, and Rogers, "Relationship between Pregnancy Experience and the Development of Certain Neuropsychiatric Disorders in Childhood"; Joseph Wortis, "Mental Retardation as a Public Health Problem," *AJPH* 45.5 (May 1955), 632–36; 1966 HEW Annual Report, 50.

76. Debora Jackson Perrone, "The Legacy of Paul Harper: Childhood's Man for All Seasons," *Johns Hopkins Public Health* (Spring 1998), 10–13; Paul A. Harper, *Preventive Pediatrics, Child Health and Development* (Appleton-Century-Crofts, 1962).

77. William M. Schmidt and Isabelle Valadian, "A Maternal and Child Health Bookshelf," *AJPH* 54 (Apr. 1964), 551–52; James Colgrove, "Reform and Its Discontents: Public Health in New York City during the Great Society," *Journal of Policy History* 19.1 (2007), 8.

78. Park, *The Harriet Lane Home*, 267; Edward Shorter, *The Kennedy Family and the Story of Mental Retardation* (Temple University Press, 2000), 73–74; A. T. Sigler, B. H. Cohen, A. M. Lilienfeld, J. E. Westlake, and W. H. Hetznecker, "Reproductive and Marital Experience of Parents of Children with Down's Syndrome (Mongolism)," *Journal of Pediatrics* 70 (1967), 608–14; Abraham M. Lilienfeld with Charlotte H. Benesch, *Epidemiology of Mongolism* (Johns Hopkins Press, 1969); B. H. Cohen and A. M. Lilienfeld, "The Epidemiological Study of Mongolism in Baltimore," *Annals of the New York Academy of Science* 171 (1970), 320–27; B. H. Cohen, A. M. Lilienfeld, S. Kramer, and L. C. Hyman, "Parental Factors in Down's Syndrome—Results of the Second Baltimore Case-Control Study," in E. Hook and I. Porter, eds., *Population Cytogenetics Studies in Humans* (Academic Press, 1977).

79. Shorter, *The Kennedy Family*, 7–9.

80. Park, *The Harriet Lane Home*, 270–71; "Planning in Mental Retardation," *AJPH* 47.11 (Nov. 1957), 1482; Paul V. Lemkau, memo on suggestions for collaboration between the School of Hygiene and Kennedy Habilitation Center for Physically and Mentally Handicapped Children Jan. 10, 1967, 3a: D.O. Correspondence, box 504582, "Mental Hygiene" folder; Robert E. Farber to Ernest L. Stebbins, Jan. 22, 1965, 3a: D.O. Correspondence, box 506162, "Eastern Health District 1963–65" folder.

81. Shorter, *The Kennedy Family*, 80–82; Park, *The Harriet Lane Home*, 311–12; Robert E. Cooke to Wilbur J. Cohen, assistant secretary of HEW, Mar. 30 and July 10, 1961, Robert E. Cooke papers, box 14JF, "NICHD: Comprehensive, General (through December 31, 1961)" folder, AMC; "Chronology of Events," *The NIH Almanac*.

82. Park, *The Harriet Lane Home*, 271, 300; Kennedy, "Many Hidden Springs," 18–19.

83. Shonick, *Government and Health Services*, 92.

Chapter 5 · Rethinking the Public Health Curriculum

1. JHSPH Executive Committee Minutes, Mar. 1, 1949, p. 136 and Mar. 29, 1949, p. 141; Ernest L. Stebbins, "Confidential: The Financial Situation of the School of Hygiene and Public Health," March 2, 1951, Ernest L. Stebbins to Lowell J. Reed, May 21, 1951, and Alan M. Chesney, Memorandum re: the Budget of the School of Medicine for 1951–52, May 19, 1951, all in Series 3b O.D. Financial, box 506104, 1951–52 budget, AMC; JHSPH Advisory Board Minutes, Apr. 27, 1953; School of Hygiene budgets from 1951–52 through 1956–57, Series 3b O.D. Financial, box 506104.

2. Perrin H. Long, "Memorandum—A Proposed Plan for Post-War Undergraduate and Graduate Training in the Department of Preventive Medicine in the Johns Hopkins University School of Medicine," Dec. 17, 1945, Series 1.2, box 146, folder 1307, RFA.

3. John J. Phair to Lewis H. Weed, Jan. 2, 1945, and Perrin H. Long to Weed, Jan. 26, 1945, folder 1307; Lewis Weed to Alan Gregg, Feb. 26, 1946, Gregg to Alan M. Chesney, Apr. 3, 1952, and Memorandum, Mar. 14, 1946, RG 1.1 Projects, Series 200 United States, box 95, folder 1141 "200A Johns Hopkins University–Preventive Medicine 1942–52," RFA; National Research Council Committee on Growth, *The Research Attack on Cancer 1946*, 30–31, suppl. 2, 8; JHU Treasurer's Report 1946–47, p. 66; "Research on the Prevention of Disease," *Rockefeller Foundation Trustees Bulletin*, March 1948, 6–9; Turner, *Heritage of Excellence*, 441.

4. School of Medicine Committee on Preventive Medicine, "Report to the Advisory Board," Jan. 16, 1952, Turner papers, box 505461, "Comm. on Teaching of Public Health to Med. Students, Committee on Preventive Med.-J. H. Med. Sch." folder, AMC. The Com-

mittee on Preventive Medicine, chaired by Alan Chesney, dean of the medical school, with A. McGehee Harvey, chair of Medicine; E. Kennerly Marshall Jr., chair of Pharmacology; Francis F. Schwentker, chair of Pediatrics; and Ernest Stebbins.

5. Katharine G. Clark, *Preventive Medicine in Medical Schools*, 41–43; School of Medicine Committee on Preventive Medicine, "Report to the Advisory Board."

6. W. G. Cochran to Members of the Committee on Teaching of Public Health to Medical Students, "Report of the Committee on Teaching Public Health to Medical Students" (Cochran Report), May 27, 1953, "Comm. on Teaching of Public Health to Med. Students, Committee on Preventive Med.-J. H. Med. Sch." folder; Clark, *Preventive Medicine in Medical Schools*, 1–10; Robert H. Riley bio file, AMC; "American Board of Preventive Medicine and Public Health Incorporated," *AJPH* 38 (Sept. 1948), 1348–49.

7. Cochran Report. In 1940, only 9 percent of Americans were covered by hospital insurance; by 1950, fully half were. Stevens, *In Sickness and in Wealth*, 259.

8. Cochran Report.

9. Debora Jackson Perrone, "The Legacy of Paul Harper: Childhood's Man for All Seasons," *Johns Hopkins Public Health*, Spring 1998, 10–13; MPDC Reference Book No. 2, 1953–56 Item No. 60, "Application for Financial Support of Home and Office Care Program During a Five Year Build-Up Period," May 20, 1953, and "Present Status of Home and Office Care Program" (c. 1953), MPDC records, box 507842, AMC.

10. Alexander D. Langmuir, "The Training of the Physician: Education and Training in Preventive Medicine and Public Health," *New England Journal of Medicine* 271 (Oct. 8, 1964), 772–74.

11. Fee, "Partners in Community Health," 742; "Application for Financial Support of Home and Office Care Program during a Five Year Build-Up Period"; Kenneth D. Durr, *Behind the Backlash: White Working-Class Politics in Baltimore, 1940–1980* (University of North Carolina Press, 2003), 102.

12. Cochran Report; A. McGehee Harvey and Susan L. Abrams, *"For the Welfare of Mankind": The Commonwealth Fund and American Medicine* (Johns Hopkins University Press, 1986), 238–42; MPDC Reference Book No. 2, 1953–56 Item No. 60, "Application for Financial Support of Home and Office Care Program during a Five Year Build-Up Period," May 20, 1953, Ernest Stebbins to Lester J. Evans, June 1, 1953, and "Present Status of Home and Office Care Program" (c. 1953), MPDC records, box 507842, AMC.

13. Barry Wood, "Teachers of Medicine," *Journal of Laboratory and Clinical Medicine* 41.6 (1953), 6–10; "Present Status of Home and Office Care Program."

14. 1954–55 SOM Catalog, 124; 1957–58 SOM Catalog, 134; 1958–59 SOM Catalog, 137; 1959–60 SOM Catalog, 95; 1963–64 SOM Catalog, 106; John Black Grant diary, Mar. 29–Apr. 1, 1958, RG 1.1 Projects, Series 200 United States, box 187, folder 2237 "200 L Johns Hopkins University–School of Hygiene and Public Health 1958–61," RAC; "1958–59 Report of the Director of the JHSPH," *JHU Circular* 78 (Nov. 1959), 83.

15. MPDC, "A Report on the Johns Hopkins Medical Institutions" Jan. 1, 1950, p. 41, Alfred Blalock papers, "Correspondence: Medical Planning and Development Committee 1949–1950" folder, AMC; W. W. Cort to Ernest Stebbins Mar. 31, 1950, JHSPH Records, 3b: O.D. Financial, box 506104, "1949–50 Budget" binder.

16. JHSPH Executive Committee Minutes, Nov. 1, 1949, p. 146; "First Report of Committee on the Doctor of Science Program," "Advisory Board Meeting February 1, 1956" folder; Thomas Turner, Memorandum to the CREOSHPH, Sept. 1, 1956.

17. Turner to Stebbins, Dec. 1, 1954, "Advisory Board Meeting" folder; "First Report of Committee on the Doctor of Science Program," "Advisory Board Meeting February 1, 1956" folder; Thomas Turner, Memorandum to the CREOSHPH, Sept. 1, 1956.

18. Roger M. Herriott to Turner Mar. 29, 1954, Turner papers, box 50564, "Miscellaneous" folder.

19. Turner to Herriott Apr. 19, 1954, Turner papers, box 50564, "Miscellaneous" folder.

20. Frederik B. Bang to Thomas B. Turner, Nov. 16, 1956, Paul Lemkau, "Biological Basis of Public Health" (undated, c. Dec. 1956), CREOSHPH Book I binder.

21. Paul Lemkau, Division of Mental Hygiene 1957–58 Annual Report, "President's Report" folder.

22. Manfred Mayer, memo on Proposed Course Entitled "Biology of Populations," Dec. 6, 1956, CREOSHPH Book I binder; Carl Lamanna to Thomas B. Turner, Dec. 6, 1956, CREOSHPH Book I binder.

23. 1957–58 JHSPH Catalog, 53; Thomas B. Turner, "Comment on Dr. Sartwell's Memorandum of Nov. 9, 1956," Nov. 14, 1956, CREOSHPH Comments from Staff Members binder; Carl Lamana to Thomas Turner, Apr. 26, 1956, Turner papers, box 50564, "Misc." folder.

24. Paul V. Lemkau to Thomas Turner, Mar. 9, 1956, Turner papers, box 50564, "Curriculum Committee Background Material" folder.

25. 1936–37 JHSPH Catalog, 28–30; 1948–49 JHSPH Catalog, 37; JHSPH Advisory Board Minutes, June 4, 1954; 1954–55 JHSPH Catalog, 41–43, 75–76; Roger M. Herriott papers finding aid, AMC.

26. JHSPH Advisory Board Minutes, June 4, 1954; Bacon F. Chow to Turner, Jan. 17, 1957, Turner papers, box 50564, CREOSHPH Subcommittee to Review the Curriculum binder; Lemkau to Turner, Mar. 9, 1956.

27. John C. Whitehorn, "Proposed Study of Educational Objectives and Program in the Johns Hopkins Medical Institutions," March 1954, Turner papers, box 50564, "Med. Planning and Develop. Comm.-D. Whitehorn" folder; Committee to Review the Educational Objectives of the School of Hygiene and Public Health, Book I binder, Turner papers, box 50564, AMC. The chair of the Department of Environmental Medicine had remained vacant since Joseph Lilienthal's death in late 1955.

28. "Report of the American Public Health Association Task Force," *AJPH* 47.2 (Feb. 1957), 218–34.

29. Thomas Turner, Memorandum to the CREOSHPH, Sept. 1, 1956, pp. 8, 12–13, and Philip Sartwell to Thomas Turner Oct. 10, 1956, CREOSHPH Book I binder.

30. Turner to O'Connor July 24, 1956, Turner papers, box 50564, Mr. Basil O'Connor folder.

31. "Report of Sub-Committee of Applications and Curriculum Committee on Alumni and their MPH Curriculum Suggestions," 20; Turner, Memorandum to the CREOSHPH, Sept. 1, 1956, pp. 15, 23–33; "Interim Report of the CREOSHPH," Dec. 11, 1956, CREOSHPH Book I.

32. Manfred M. Mayer to Turner, Feb. 6, 1957, CREOSHPH Book I.

33. Margaret Merrill to Thomas Turner, Jan. 28, 1957, and Lloyd E. Rozeboom to Ernest Stebbins, Jan. 4, 1957, CREOSHPH Book I.

34. Ruth B. Freeman to Turner, Jan. 25, 1957, CREOSHPH Subcommittee to Review the Curriculum binder; Paul Harper to CREOSHPH, memo re: Two Proposals in

Dr. Turner's Working Papers, undated (c. Oct. 1956), CREOSHPH Book I; "Report of the Committee on Applications and Curriculum, Sub-Committee on Alumni and their MPH Curriculum Suggestions," 9, 13; Commission on University Education in Hospital Administration, "Report on the Program in Hospital Administration at Johns Hopkins University."

35. E. B. Wilson to Lowell Reed, Dec. 11, 1941, 3a: D.O. Corres., box 502032, "Harv-Hay Feb 1941–Aug 1943" folder, AMC.

36. Commission on University Education in Hospital Administration, "Report on the Program in Hospital Administration at Johns Hopkins University"; Freeman to Turner, Jan. 25, 1957; "Report of the Committee on Applications and Curriculum, Sub-Committee on Alumni and their MPH Curriculum Suggestions," 9, 13; Carl Lamanna to Thomas B. Turner, Dec. 6, 1956, CREOSHPH Book I binder.

37. Whitehorn, "Proposed Study of Educational Objectives and Program in the Johns Hopkins Medical Institutions"; "Interim Report of the CREOSHPH," Dec. 11, 1956; Kenneth L. Zierler to Thomas B. Turner, Feb. 15, 1957, Manfred M. Mayer to T. B. Turner, Feb. 26, 1957, CREOSHPH Book I binder.

38. Stebbins to Turner, "Comments on the Memorandum of September 1st, Entitled 'A Memorandum to the Committee to Review the Educational Objectives of the School of Hygiene,'" Dec. 7, 1956, CREOSHPH Book I binder.

Chapter 6 · *The Postwar Geopolitics of American Public Health*

1. Paul Johnson, *Modern Times: The World from the Twenties to the Nineties*, rev. ed. (Harper Perennial, 1992), 446–52.

2. 1964 HEW Annual Report, 228–29.

3. Pan American Sanitary Bureau, "Proceedings of the Latin American Fellowship Conference," February 12, 1943, 3a D.O. Correspondence, box 502036, "Otto-Proceedings of the Latin American Fellowship Conference" folder.

4. Leroy E. Burney, "Veterans' Preference in Public Health Agencies of the United States," *AJPH* 35 (Mar. 1945), 253–56; Richard W. Steward, ed., *American Military History Volume II: The United States Army in a Global Era, 1917–2008* (US Army Center of Military History, 2010), chap. 9, "The Army of the Cold War: From the 'New Look' to Flexible Response," 255–88.

5. Ernest L. Stebbins, "Current Problems in Postgraduate Education in Public Health," attachment to letter to William McPeak, July 24, 1956, 3a D.O. Corresp., box 506162, "Ford Foundation 1956–66" folder; W. L. Treuting to Silas B. Hays, May 22, 1957, 3a D.O. Corresp., box 504580, "ASPH Exec. Comm. 1961" folder.

6. 1955–56 JHU Treasurer's Report, 68; "JHU School of Hygiene and Public Health Expenditures from Research Grants, Training Grants, and Government Contracts," in JHU Board of Trustees minutes, Oct. 27, 1958, pp. 4562–64.

7. Langmuir, "The Surveillance of Communicable Diseases of National Importance," quote p. 183; Martin D. Young, "In Memoriam: Justin M. Andrews (1902–67)," *Journal of Parsitology* 56.1 (Dec. 1970), 1248–49; JHSPH Executive Committee Minutes, Nov. 1, 1949, p. 145.

8. Langmuir, "The Surveillance of Communicable Diseases of National Importance," 182–84, quote p. 184; Amy L. Fairchild, Ronald Bayer, and James Colgrove, *Searching Eyes:*

Privacy, the State, and Disease Surveillance in America (University of California Press, 2007), xviii, 17, 22, 247.

9. Alexander D. Langmuir, "The Epidemic Intelligence Service of the Center for Disease Control," *Public Health Reports* 95 (Sept.–Oct. 1980), 471–73, quote p. 471.

10. Langmuir, "The Epidemic Intelligence Service of the Center for Disease Control," 471–73; Martin Frobisher bio file, AMC; Donald A. Henderson oral history interview, Jan. 29, 2009.

11. Langmuir, "The Epidemic Intelligence Service of the Center for Disease Control," 473–75; Elizabeth W. Etheridge, *Sentinel for Health: A History of the Centers for Disease Control* (University of California Press, 1992).

12. Campbell and Connor, *Variations in State Public Health Programs during a Five-Year Period*, 6, 12, 39, 110, 126, 128; 1950 FSA Annual Report, 115–16, 127, 129, 163; 1955 HEW Annual Report, 13, 134, 140–41, 190–91; 1960 HEW Annual Report, 174–75, 271–72; 1964 HEW Annual Report, 228–29; Langmuir, "The Epidemic Intelligence Service of the Center for Disease Control," 473.

13. JHSPH Advisory Board Minutes, vol. 5, Mar. 30, 1948, p. 209 and Apr. 30, 1948, pp. 215, 217; "News from the Field," *AJPH* 40.8 (Aug. 1950), 1063.

14. MPDC Reference Book No. 1, 1947–1952, No. 28, "Proposal of a Joint Medical School and School of Hygiene Enterprise in Environmental Medicine," Feb. 3, 1950, box 507841, AMC.

15. Stebbins to Joseph Lilienthal, Oct. 15, 1951, Turner papers, box 505461, "Air Force Students' Curriculum" folder; USAF School of Aerospace Medicine, "The United States Air Force Specialty Training Program in Aviation Medicine," August 1961 and Calvin C. Chapman, "The United States Air Force Aviation Medicine Residence Training Program," Aug. 26, 1964, 3a D.O. Corresp., box 50995, "Aerospace Med. Assoc." folder, AMC; 1956–57 JHSPH Catalog, 21; Ernest L. Stebbins, review of *Human Factors in Air Transportation*, *AJPH* 43.8 (Aug. 1953), 1052; "Airborne Infection in a Space Capsule," presented at National Academy of Science conference, Woods Hole, July 1966, Richard L. Riley bio file.

16. JHSPH Executive Committee minutes, June 5, 1952, p. 187; USAF School of Aerospace Medicine, "The United States Air Force Specialty Training Program in Aviation Medicine," August 1961 and Calvin C. Chapman, "The United States Air Force Aviation Medicine Residence Training Program," Aug. 26, 1964, 3a D.O. Corresp., box 50995, "Aerospace Med. Assoc." folder, AMC; 1956–57 JHSPH Catalog, 21.

17. Grant Action Form, "Johns Hopkins University–School of Hygiene and Public Health—Request to Foundation for Further Support," Mar. 22, 1948, RG 1.1, Series 200L, box 186, folder 2234, RFA; Joseph Lilienthal papers finding aid, AMC; Joseph Lilienthal curriculum vita, c. 1949, Records of the Office of the JHU President, box 185, "745 (1949)" folder; 1955–56 Report of the Dean of the Medical Faculty, 62–63; Joseph L. Lilienthal papers finding aid and bio file, AMC; Joe Lilienthal to W. Horsley Gantt, Nov. 30, 1950 and Sept. 24, 1951, W. Horsley Gantt papers, General Correspondence Series III, "Lilienthal, Joe 1950–1951" folder, AMC.

18. Nancy A. Heaton, *The W. Horsley Gantt Papers* (Johns Hopkins University School of Medicine, 1986).

19. Jos. L. Lilienthal Jr. to Lowell J. Reed, July 31, 1955, and W. F. Hamilton to Reed, Dec. 5, 1955, Records of the Office of the President, JHU, Series 1, box 185, "745 (1955)" folder, Hamburger Archives.

20. Alfred P. Ashton to William D. McCuin, Dec. 4, 1953, Harry R. Walsh to NYOO Contractors, Oct. 31, 1957, Harry Ridgely Warfield to Frederik B. Bang, Mar. 3, 1954, "Institute for Cooperative Research J.H.U. 1957–47" folder.

21. "Ninth and Final Report of Research carried out by the Johns Hopkins University Department of Microbiology under the direction of Dr. Carl Lamanna for the Biological Department, Chemical Corps, Camp Detrick to Sept. 1, 1954," 3a D.O. Corresp., box 504571, "Institute for Cooperative Research J.H.U. 1957–47" folder, pp. 1–2, AMC.

22. "Ninth and Final Report of Research," 3, 12.

23. John C. Reed and Andreas G. Ronhovde, *Arctic Laboratory: A History (1947–1966) of the Naval Arctic Research Laboratory at Point Barrow, Alaska* (Arctic Institute of North America, 1971); JHSPH Records, 5e PHA Problems, box 502119, AMC; Naval Photographic Center, "Operation Deepfreeze No. 54, Ross Sea and Coulman Island, Antarctica, Oct. 15, 1958" (motion picture), RG428: General Records of the Department of the Navy, 1941–2004, "Moving Images Relating to Military Activities," NARA, College Park, MD; Rozeboom, *Medical Zoology at the JHSPH*, 92, 122–25; John Hume to Colin F. Vorder Bruegge, July 17, 1967, Records of the Office of the JHU President, series 9, box 33, "Hygiene-General 1967" folder. The Records of the Office of the President in the JHU Hamburger Archives (box 35) document the ties that Detlev W. Bronk, president of Johns Hopkins and chairman of the National Research Council, fostered beginning in 1949 between Hopkins and the PHS Arctic Health Research Center. John Rodman Paul and George Comstock conducted research on Eskimo health at the center during the 1950s.

24. John B. Hozier, "Responsibilities of the Public Health Service in Civil Defense," *JAMA* 160.14 (Apr. 7, 1956), 1206–8, quote p. 1206.

25. Hozier, "Responsibilities of the Public Health Service in Civil Defense," 1207; US Department of Health, Education and Welfare, *1955 Annual Report*, 13.

26. Hozier, "Responsibilities of the Public Health Service in Civil Defense," 1207.

27. Ibid., 1207; David A. Cook, *A History of Narrative Film* (W. W. Norton and Company, 1981), 437.

28. Socrates Litsios, "John Black Grant: A 20th-Century Public Health Giant," *Perspectives in Biology and Medicine* 54.4 (2011), 532–49; John Farley, *To Cast Out Disease: A History of the International Health Division of the Rockefeller Foundation (1913–1951)* (Oxford University Press, 2004), 15–16.

29. Reed to Ferrell Sept. 9, 1941, and Dec. 19, 1941, 3a O. D. Corres., box 502037, "Rockefeller Foundation Sept 1941–Mar 1942," AMC; Gisela Cramer and Ursula Prutsch, "Nelson A. Rockefeller's Office of Inter-American Affairs (1940–1946) and Record Group 229," *Hispanic American Historical Review* 86.4 (Nov. 2006), 785–806; Pan American Sanitary Bureau, "Proceedings of the Latin American Fellowship Conference," Feb. 12, 1943, 3a O.D. Corres., box 502036, "Otto-Latin American Fellowship Conference" folder; Institute of Inter-American Affairs Health and Sanitation Division, "The Bilateral Cooperative Health Programs of the United States of America and Other Countries of the Americas," 7; M. E. Bustamante, "Public Health Administration in Latin America," *AJPH* 40 (1950), 1067–71; Paulina Pino and Giorgio Solimano, "The School of Public Health at the University of Chile: Origins, Evolution, and Perspectives," *Public Health Reviews* 33.1 (2011), 315–22.

30. *Journey into Medicine*, script, RG 306 US Information Agency records, box 20, Entry 1098, "Movie Scripts 1942–1965," National Archives-College Park, MD; "A Film for Recruitment," *AJPH* 39.8 (Aug. 1949), 1042.

31. *Journey into Medicine*, The Internet Movie Database (www.imdb.com)—the film's evocative black-and-white cinematography was done by Boris Kaufman, who later won an Oscar for *On the Waterfront* (1954); "Medical Motion Pictures," *JAMA* 141.10 (Nov. 5, 1949), 749; K. C. Chaudhury, "An Eye Witness Account of the Fifth International Congress of Pediatrics, New York," *Indian Journal of Pediatrics* 15.1 (Jan. 1948), 9–16.

32. Fee, *Disease and Discovery*, 57–60, 98–111, 151–54; Medical Planning and Development Committee, "A Report on the Johns Hopkins Medical Institutions," Jan. 1, 1950, p. 7; JHSPH Catalogs for 1937–38, 1944–45, 1957–58; John J. Hanlon, *Principles of Public Health Administration* (C. V. Mosby Company, 1950), 295–97; Transcript of the ASPH Advisory Committee meeting on the International Role of the North American schools of public health, Nov. 28–29, 1961, 3a: D.O. Corresp., box 504579, "ASPH-Rosenthal Foundation Project 1961" folder, AMC, p. 7.

33. High Commission for Hygiene and Public Health, Commission for the Study of the Reorganization of the Health Care Services, *Reports of the Consultants*, vol. II (Rome, Italy, 1949).

34. Pan American Sanitary Bureau, *Proceedings of the Latin American Fellowship Conference*, Feb. 12, 1943; Rosenfeld, Gooch, and Levine, *Report on Schools of Public Health in the United States*, 53–54; ASPH minutes, University of Pittsburgh, Apr. 7–8, 1952.

35. Hubert H. Humphrey, "The United States and the World Health Organization," Committee Print for the Senate Committee on Government Operations Subcommittee on Reorganization and International Organizations, 86th Cong. 1st Sess., May 11, 1959, 121–41; Hanlon, *Principles of Public Health Administration*, 3rd ed. (C. V. Mosby Company, 1960), 362–68; Hanlon, *Principles of Public Health Administration*, 5th ed. (C. V. Mosby Company, 1969), 235–40; Maurice Pate, "UNICEF Goals in Maternal and Child Health," *AJPH* 50 (June 1960), 8–12.

36. Transcript of the ASPH Advisory Committee meeting on the International Role of the North American schools of public health, Nov. 28–29, 1961, 3a Director or Dean's Office: Correspondence, box 506164, "ASPH-Rosenthal Foundation Project 1961" folder, AMC, pp. 7–8.

37. Edyth Schoenrich, "Study of Foreign Medical Graduates," Jan. 1983, Abel Wolman papers, series 9, box 3, JHU Hamburger Archives, Table VIII: Degree Recipients; Report of the President 1949–50, *JHU Circular* (1950), 188; Kishore Chandra Patnaik obituary, *Indian Journal of Public Health* 16.2 (1972), 95–97.

38. JHSPH Advisory Board Minutes, vol. 4, June 6, 1944, pp. 174–75; John Hume bio file, AMC; No. 35, Interinstitutional Committee on Venereal Disease Control to Lowell Reed, Dec. 19, 1950, MPDC Reference Book No. 1, 1947–1952, MPDC Records, box 507841, AMC; "International VD Experts Study U.S. Control Programs for WHO," *AJPH* 39.11 (Nov. 1949), 1508–9.

39. Huan-Ying Li interview, May 14, 2012.

40. Ibid.

41. Ibid.

42. Ibid.

43. Amrith, *Decolonizing International Health*, 146; Li interview.

44. Li interview; Huan-Ying Li, "Application of *T. pallidum* Immobilization Test in the Diagnosis of Syphilis," *Chinese Medical Journal* 49.12 (1963), 759–62.

45. Charles D. Flagle, Oct. 16, 1998, interview by Edward Berkowitz, Baltimore, Maryland, National Library of Medicine, transcript, pp. 19–22; Michel Lechat, "Diary: Graham Greene at the Leproserie," *London Review of Books* 29 (Aug. 2, 2007), 34–35; Charles D. Flagle and Michel F. Lechat, "Allocation of Medical and Associated Resources to the Control of Leprosy," *Acta Hospitals* 2 (June 1962); WHO Neglected Tropical Diseases website, "In memoriam: Professeur Michel Lechat, 1927–2014," May 7, 2014 (http://www.who.int/neglected_diseases, accessed Feb. 11, 2016).

46. Ernest M. Allen to Turner, Sept. 20, 1956, Turner papers, box 50564, National Advisory Council on Health Research Facilities folder, AMC; "Laboratory Research Council," AJPH 47 (Jan. 1957), 148.

47. JHSPH Executive Committee Minutes, Dec. 13, 1956, pp. 3–4, Jan. 25, 1957, p. 2.

48. W. Barry Wood to Keith Spalding, Jan. 16, 1957, and Milton S. Eisenhower to William S. Carlson, Jan. 22, 1957, Records of the Office of the JHU President, box 185, "745 (1957)" folder; JHU Trustees minutes, Apr. 1, 1957, p. 4148 and May 6, 1957, pp. 4172–74.

49. JHU Board of Trustees minutes Mar. 4, 1957, p. 4133 and Apr. 1, 1957, p. 4153; Turner, *Heritage of Excellence*, 522; Turner to Stebbins, Jan. 24, 1955, Turner papers, box 50564, "Advisory Board Meeting" folder; Howard A. Howe to Lowell J. Reed, June 7, 1955, Records of the Office of the JHU President, box 185, "745 (1955)" folder; JHU Treasurer's Report, 1939–1960; JHSPH Executive Committee Minutes, May 16, 1957, p. 2, Sept. 26, 1957, p. 3, Nov. 25, 1957, p. 4; "Report of the President," *JHU Circular* (1957–1958), 69, 135; Rose, "America's First Department of Immunology," 244–45; K. Frank Austen, "Manfred Martin Mayer, 1916–1984," *Biographical Memoirs* (National Academy of Sciences, 1990), 257–80.

50. John Black Grant diary, Mar. 29–Apr. 1, 1958; JHU Trustees Executive Committee minutes, June 13, 1960, p. 4727; 1956–57 Report of the Dean of the JHSPH, 135, 138; Margaret Merrell to Ernest L. Stebbins, Nov. 6, 1957, Margaret Merrell papers, box 505378, "Office of the President" folder, AMC; Kenneth Zierler to W. Barry Wood, Jan. 10, 1958, W. Barry Wood to Merrell, Jan. 28, 1958, Wood to Zierler, Jan. 28, 1958, "Office of the Vice-Pres." folder; JHU Trustees minutes, June 1, 1959, p. 4632; JHU Trustees Executive Committee minutes, May 2, 1960, p. 4714 and Dec. 5, 1960, p. 4781.

51. John C. Bugher to Barry Wood, May 14, 1958, and Barry Wood to Lester Evans, June 23, 1958, RG 1.1, series 200, box 187, folder 2237 "200 L Johns Hopkins University–School of Hygiene and Public Health 1958–61," RFA.

52. Fee, *Disease and Discovery*, 217; HHS Diary Note, Sept. 7, 1945, and Grant Action Form, Oct. 26, 1945, R.G. 1.1, series 100, box 41, folder 374, RFA; Alan Gregg to James B. Conant, Oct. 1, 1943, folder 374.

53. Clyde Gunsalus declined the chair of Microbiology (JHU Trustees minutes, Jan. 13, 1958, p. 4357 and Mar. 17, 1958, p. 4396); James Franklin Crow declined the chair of Environmental Medicine (JHU Trustees minutes, Dec. 8, 1958, p. 4573 and Jan. 12, 1959, p. 4578); Victor P. Bond declined a professorship of Radiological Health in Environmental Medicine (JHU Trustees minutes, Mar. 2, 1959, p. 4599); Lincoln E. Moses declined the chair of Biostatistics (JHU Trustees Executive Committee minutes, Mar. 7, 1960, p. 4694); Aaron Klug declined the chair of Biophysics (JHU Trustees Executive Committee minutes, Apr. 7, 1960, p. 4710 and Oct. 3, 1960, p. 4757).

54. Johnson, *Modern Times*, 625–30.

55. Randall M. Packard, "'Roll Back Malaria, Roll in Development'? Reassessing the Economic Burden of Malaria," *Population and Development Review* 35 (Mar. 2009), 53–87; John Sharpless, "Population Science, Private Foundations, and Development Aid: The Transformation of Demographic Knowledge in the United States, 1945–1965," in Frederick Cooper and Randall Packard, eds., *International Development and the Social Sciences: Essays on the History and Politics of Knowledge* (University of California Press, 1997), 176–78; Timothy D. Baker interview, Aug. 31, 2010.

56. Myron E. Wegman, "Introduction," *AJPH* 50 (June 1960 suppl.), 1–2; Myron E. Wegman, "Organization for New Responsibilities in Public Health, Part I: Health Needs and Trends," *AJPH* 52 (May 1962), 766.

57. Hubert H. Humphrey, "The United States and the World Health Organization," Committee Print for the Senate Committee on Government Operations Subcommittee on Reorganization and International Organizations, 86th Cong. 1st Sess., May 11, 1959, 121–41; Oscar Ewing, speech to the Conference of Presidents of Negro Land Grant Colleges, Oct. 18, 1950, box 41, Oscar Ewing papers, Harry S. Truman Presidential Library, Independence, Missouri, 7; Randall Packard, "Visions of Postwar Health and Development and Their Impact on Public Health Interventions in the Developing World," in Frederick Cooper and Randall Packard, eds., *International Development and the Social Sciences: Essays on the History and Politics of Knowledge*, 96–103, quote p. 98; Sunil S. Amrith, *Decolonizing International Health: India and Southeast Asia, 1930–65* (Palgrave McMillan, 2006), 128–33, 146, 173–74.

58. Amrith, *Decolonizing International Health*, 130–35, 150.

59. James N. Giglio and Stephen G. Rabe, *Debating the Kennedy Presidency* (Rowman and Littlefield, 2003), 12–42; William J. Lederer and Eugene Burdick, *The Ugly American* (Random House, 1962); National Research Council Division of Medical Sciences, "Tropical Health: A Report on a Study of Needs and Resources" (1962), ix.

60. JHU Board of Trustees minutes, June 1, 1959, p. 4632; "Senator Humphrey Asks Public Health Training Grants, Scholarships," press release May 2, 1955, Ernest L. Stebbins papers, box 505656, "Assoc. Schools of Public Health 1952" folder; John A. Logan, "Counteracting Communism Through Foreign Assistance Programs in Public Health," *AJPH* 45.8 (Aug. 1955), 1017–21.

61. Malcolm E. Jewell, *Senatorial Politics and Foreign Policy* (University of Kentucky Press, 1962), 133–34; Hubert Humphrey, "U.S. MUST KEEP MANTLE OF PEACE-MAKER, SENATOR HUMPHREY DECLARES," press release Oct. 8, 1959, Speech Text Files, Hubert H. Humphrey papers, Minnesota Historical Society; Humphrey, "The United States and the World Health Organization," 79–80; Hubert Humphrey to Henry Labouisse, June 23, 1961, 3a Director or Dean's Office: Correspondence, box 504580, "ASPH-Legislation S. 1983 1961" folder, AMC; US Senate Committee on Government Operations, Subcommittee on Reorganization and International Organizations, *The U.S. Government and the Future of International Medical Research*, 1961.

62. M. G. Candau, "Problems in Developing International Health Programs," *AJPH* 50 (June 1960), 5–6; National Research Council Division of Medical Sciences, "Tropical Health: A Report on a Study of Needs and Resources" (1962), ix; "International Research," *AJPH* 52 (Jan. 1962), 153; Humphrey, "The United States and the World Health Organization," 81; "The NIH Almanac—Historical Data" (http://nih.gov/about/almanac/historical/chronology_of_events.htm, accessed Nov. 9, 2013); US Senate Committee on Government

Operations, Subcommittee on Reorganization and International Organizations, *The U.S. Government and the Future of International Medical Research*, 1961, Appendix, part II, p. 319; NRC Division of Medical Sciences, "Tropical Health: A Report on a Study of Needs and Resources," ix.

63. JHU Board of Trustees Executive Committee minutes, Sept. 19, 1960, p. 4740.

Chapter 7 · Missionaries and Mercenaries

1. V. Rajagopalan to Abel Wolman, Dec. 25, 1963, Abel Wolman papers, series 5, box 4, "India" folder, JHU Hamburger Archives. Visvanathan Rajagopalan (JHU Engineering 1954) was a sanitary engineer and student of Abel Wolman's who returned to India as professor of public health engineering at the University of Madras. From 1954 to 1964, he directed India's national water supply and sanitation program to expand access to safe drinking water, then available to only 6 percent of the Indian population. The program became the largest in the world and among the most successful. He joined the World Bank as a senior engineering adviser on water projects and became a senior World Bank official, directing the Department of Environment in the late 1980s and early 1990s.

2. William H. Foege, "Foreword," in Michael H. Merson, Robert E. Black, and Anne J. Mills, eds., *Global Health: Diseases, Programs, Systems and Policies*, 3rd ed. (Jones & Bartlett Learning, 2012), xv.

3. Gaylord W. Anderson, "Health Education—A One-World Challenge," *AJPH* 50 (Feb. 1960), 127–33; Kingsley Davis, "Population Policy: Will Current Programs Succeed?" (1963), in Heer, *Kingsley Davis*, 447.

4. Eugene P. Campbell, "Proposal for ICA to Participate in the Development of a Facility or Center of International Health at the Johns Hopkins School of Public Health," Dec. 30, 1960, 3a Dean's or Director's Office Correspondence, 6e Ernest Stebbins, box 505343, "International Health 1961" folder, pp. 1–6, AMC.

5. Ibid., 10–12.

6. Timothy D. Baker, Dec. 15, 2008, and Aug. 31, 2010, interviews; 1960–61 JHSPH Catalog, 45.

7. Campbell, "Proposal for ICA," 7–9; John C. Snyder, "Suggestions for Improving the Health Activities of the International Cooperation Administration," Feb. 14, 1961, 3a Dean's or Director's Office Correspondence, 6e Ernest Stebbins, box 50995, "AID 1960–1965" folder, AMC.

8. Campbell, 1960 ICA proposal for Johns Hopkins Division of International Health, 23; International Cooperation Administration grant contract with Johns Hopkins University, Apr. 7, 1961, and "Summation of Five Years' Activities of the Division of International Health, 1961–1966," Carl Taylor papers, box 21, "Dept. International Health" folder, AMC; 1962–63 JHSPH Catalog, 56.

9. P. Stewart Macaulay to Ernest L. Stebbins, Mar. 27, 1961, and H. Ridgely Warfield to Ernest L. Stebbins, Mar. 23, 1961, "International Health 1961" folder.

10. Amendment No. 1 to Grant by the United States of America to The Trustees of the Johns Hopkins University, June 25, 1962, "International Health 1961" folder; Jacob H. Landes to Timothy D. Baker, May 10, 1962, "International Health 1962" folder.

11. US House Committee on Foreign Affairs, "Hearings on 87 H.R. 7372, International Development and Security Act, Part 3," 87th sess., 1st Cong. (1961), June 26–29, July 6, 1961, p. 920; Carl Taylor, "Memo re Conversation with Dr. Stebbins at Johns Hopkins,"

June 21, 1961, "Department of International Health" folder; Timothy D. Baker to Eugene Campbell, Jan. 15, 1962, 3a: Dean's or Director's Office Correspondence box 505343, "International Health 1962" folder, AMC; Timothy D. Baker interview, Aug. 31, 2010.

12. Timothy D. Baker interview, Aug. 31, 2010; "Edward Hicks Hume," *Biographical Dictionary of Chinese Christianity* (http://www.bdcconline.net/en/stories/h/hume-edward -hicks.php, accessed Oct. 10, 2010).

13. Humphrey, "The United States and the World Health Organization," 91, 140; C. W. Krusé and Abel Wolman, "A Memorandum on the Modern Scope of Environmental Hygiene," Feb. 4, 1957, CREOJHSPH binder.

14. Edyth Schoenrich, "Study of Foreign Medical Graduates, Degree Recipients, and International Health Planners," Jan. 1983, Wolman papers, series 9, box 3, JHU Hamburger Archives, pp. 28–30.

15. Mark H. Haefele, "Walt Rostow's Stages of Economic Growth: Ideas and Action," in David C. Engerman et al., eds., *Staging Growth: Modernization, Development, and the Global Cold War* (University of Massachusetts Press, 2003), 88–95; David C. Engerman, "West Meets East: The Center for International Studies and Indian Economic Development," in Engerman, *Staging Growth*, 7, 81–97, 210–12; Michael E. Latham, *Modernization as Ideology: American Social Science and "Nation Building" in the Kennedy Era* (University of North Carolina Press, 2000), 56–57.

16. "Memorandum for the Record, Summary Record of the President's Meeting with Indian Planning Minister Asoka Mehta, May 4, 1966," in Gabrielle S. Mallon and Louis J. Smith, eds., *Foreign Relations of the United States, 1966–1968 vol. 25, South Asia* (GPO, 2000), 637–39; US Census Bureau, "Table No. 1292, U.S. Foreign Grants and Credits by Type and Country: 1966 to 1999," *Statistical Abstract of the United States: 2011* (US Census Bureau, 2010); "AID 1960–1965" folder.

17. "Trustees Recently Elected" undated, c. 1963, Records of the Office of the JHU President, series 8, box 1, "Trustees Correspondence-General 1960–1963" folder.

18. John Sharpless, "Population Science, Private Foundations, and Development Aid: The Transformation of Demographic Knowledge in the United States, 1945–1965," in Frederick Cooper and Randall Packard, eds., *International Development and the Social Sciences: Essays on the History and Politics of Knowledge*, 176.

19. Reed, "Annual Report of the Department of Biostatistics 1942–43"; Isaiah Bowman to Lowell Reed, Nov. 25, 1940, "Bowman Oct. 1940–Dec. 1940" folder and Reed to Bowman, Mar. 7, 1942, 3a O. D. Corres., box 502029, "Bowman Jan. 1942–Apr. 1942" folder, AMC; Rockefeller Foundation 1951 Annual Report, 18.

20. Chidambara Chandrasekaran, *The Life and Works of a Demographer: An Autobiography* (New Delhi: Tata McGraw-Hill, 1999), 41–44, 87–90; Raymond Pearl, *The Natural History of Population* (Oxford University Press, 1939); Fee, *Disease and Discovery*, 207–9.

21. "Report of Subcommittee to Consider Courses on 'Populations,'" Jan. 23, 1957, Clark P. Read to Turner, Feb. 5, 1957, Subcommittee to Review the Curriculum binder.

22. "Gadabouting in Baltimore with Lula Jones Garrett," *Baltimore Afro-American*, Mar. 20, 1948.

23. Sushila Nayar bio file, AMC; Chandrasekaran, *The Life and Works of a Demographer*, 91–96.

24. Nayar bio file; Paul A. Harper bio file, AMC; Catia Cecilia Confortini, "Doing Feminist Peace: Feminist Critical Methodology, Decolonization and the Women's Inter-

national League for Peace and Freedom (WILPF), 1945–75," *International Feminist Journal of Politics* 13.3 (2011), 349–70; Sushila Nayar, "Preliminary Study of Maternal Mortality in the State of Maryland Exclusive of Baltimore City, January 1947–December 1948," JHSPH DrPH thesis, 1950; UN Department of Public Information, "Fact Sheet on Maternal Mortality," Sept. 2010 (www.un.org/millenniumgoals/pdf/MDG_FS_5_EN_new.pdf, accessed May 21, 2012).

25. *Time*, May 22, 1944.

26. Chandrasekaran, *The Life and Works of a Demographer*, 21; Khan Bahadur M. Yacob and Satya Swaroop, "Longevity in the Punjab," *British Medical Journal* 2.4421 (1945), 433–36, quote p. 36.

27. W. Edwards Deming and Chidambara Chandrasekaran, "On a Method of Estimating Birth and Death Rates and the Extent of Registration," *Journal of the American Statistical Association* 44 (1949), 101–15; Chandrasekaran, *The Life and Works of a Demographer*, 91–96.

28. Chidambara Chandrasekaran bio file, AMC; Chandrasekaran, *The Life and Works of a Demographer*, 44, 106–23; "Chidambara Chandrasekaran 1911–2000," International Union for the Scientific Study of Population website (http://www.iussp.org, accessed Nov. 25, 2011); Chidambara Chandrasekaran, "The Mysore Study," *Population Bulletin of the United Nations* 19/20 (1986), 6–13.

29. United Nations Department of Social Affairs, *The Determinants and Consequences of Population Trends* (United Nations, 1953); George J. Stolnitz, "The Population Commission and Demographic Research: An Overview," *Population Bulletin of the United Nations* 19/20 (1986), 31; Chandrasekaran, *The Life and Works of a Demographer*, 109; Irene B. Taeuber, "The Determinants and Consequences of Population Trends," *Milbank Memorial Fund Quarterly* 33.1 (Jan. 1955), 112–16, quote p. 116.

30. Margaret Bright interview, Aug. 16, 2011; Jean van der Tak, interviews with Irene B. Taeuber and Henry S. Shryock Jr. in *Demographic Destinies: Interviews with Presidents and Secretary-Treasurers of the Population Association of America* (2005) (http://geography.sdsu.edu/Research/Projects/PAA/oralhistory/PAA_Presidents_1947-60.pdf, accessed Oct. 3, 2011), 73, 87, 92.

31. Taylor 2008 interview, transcript pp. 1–2, 7.

32. Taylor 2008 interview.

33. van Zile Hyde, qtd. in Humphrey, "The United States and the World Health Organization," 119.

34. Tim Baker interview, Aug. 31, 2010; Taylor Sept. 30, 2008, video interview; John B. Wyon and John E. Gordon, *The Khanna Study: Population Problems in the Rural Punjab* (Harvard University Press, 1971), 1–3.

35. Turner, *Heritage of Excellence*, 477–78; AJW diary entry, Aug. 4, 1949, folder 374. For positive contemporary reviews of the Khanna Study, see *Economic Development and Cultural Change* 21 (July 1973), 749–51; *Pacific Affairs* 45 (Autumn 1972), 441–43; *Annals of the American Academy of Political and Social Science* 399 (Jan. 1972), 192–93; A. R. Omran, "Population Epidemiology: An Emerging Field of Inquiry for Population and Health Students," *AJPH* 64.7 (July 1974), 674–79.

36. "APHA: Gordon Wyon Awards," APHA website (www.apha.org/membergroups/sections/aphasections/intlhealth/cbphcw/activities/Gordon+Wyon+Awards.htm, accessed Oct. 2, 2010); Connelly, *Fatal Misconception*, 171, 185, 192, 206.

37. Wyon and Gordon, *The Khanna Study*, 1–3; JHSPH Executive Committee Minutes, Jan. 31, 1950, p. 149.

38. Carl E. Taylor, "Hindu Medicine and India's Health," *Atlantic Monthly* 190 (July 1952), 38–42; Carl E. Taylor, "Will India Accept Birth Control?" *Atlantic Monthly* 190 (Sept. 1952), 51–53.

39. C. E. Taylor to J. C. Snyder, "The Possibility of Harvard School of Public Health Engaging in Long-Term Studies of Ecology and Population Dynamics," Sept. 27, 1960, and Carl E. Taylor, "Possible Scope of School's Activities in Research on Population Dynamics," Jan. 27, 1961, Carl Taylor papers, box 21, "Correspondence—Early" folder, AMC; Joe D. Wray, "Population Pressure on Families: Family Size and Child Spacing," in *Rapid Population Growth: Consequences and Policy Implications*, Research Papers, National Academy of Sciences, vol. 2 (Johns Hopkins Press, 1971), 403–61; Nicholas Wright, "Some Estimates of the Potential Reduction in the United States Infant Mortality Rate by Family Planning," *AJPH* 62 (Aug. 1972), 1130–34.

40. Carl E. Taylor interview, Sept. 30, 2008, transcript pp. 4, 7–8; Harvard University School of Public Health, "Draft Proposal to the International Cooperation Administration for Special Training for Teachers of Public Health and Preventive Medicine in ICA Countries," June 26, 1957, Taylor papers; Ernest L. Stebbins to Carl E. Taylor, Dec. 5, 1961, Taylor papers; "Dr. Leavell to India for Two Years," *AJPH* 46 (June 1956), 797; Philip Sartwell to Allyn Kimball July 20, 1961, and Roger Herriott to Allyn Kimball Aug. 16, 1961, "International Health 1961" folder.

41. National Research Council Division of Medical Sciences, *Tropical Health: A Report on a Study of Needs and Resources* (GPO, 1962), 329–31, quote p. 329; Thomas H. Weller, "Tropical Medicine Today," *New England Journal of Medicine* 264 (May 4, 1961), 911–14. James Watt headed the NIH Office of International Health from 1961 to 1967. NIAID was headed by Justin M. Andrews (ScD 1926) from 1957 to 1964 and Dorland J. Davis (MPH 1940) from 1964 to 1975. Joseph Asbury Bell (MPH 1937, DrPH 1948) was medical director of the NIH Laboratory of Infectious Disease. "The NIH Almanac—National Institute of Allergy and Infectious Diseases" (http://www.nih.gov/about/almanac/organization /NIAID.htm, accessed Feb. 21, 2011); Myron Wegman, "In Memoriam: James Watt, 1911–1995," *AJPH* 86 (Oct. 1995), 1488–89; JHSPH Directory of Graduates (1962).

42. "The NIH Almanac—Historical Data, biographical sketches of directors" (http:// www.nih.gov/about/almanac/historical/directors.htm, accessed Feb. 21, 2011); Stephen P. Strickland, *The Story of the NIH Grants Programs* (University Press of America, 1989), 29, 61; NIH Fogarty International Health Center, *Fogarty at 35* (Foundation for the National Institutes of Health, 2003), 10–15.

43. Chamseddine Mofidi bio file, AMC; Akililu Lemma bio file, AMC; "Schistosomiasis Progress Reported by Graduate," *In Brief* SHPH newsletter (Winter–Spring 1975), 2; P. H. Goll, A. Lemma, J. Duncan, and B. Mazengi, "Control of Schistosomiasis in Adwa, Ethiopia, Using the Plant Molluscicide Endod (*Phytolacca dodecandra*)," *Tropical Environmental Medicine and Parasitology* 34.3 (Sept. 1983), 177–83.

44. Lloyd E. Rozeboom, *Medical Zoology at the Johns Hopkins School of Hygiene and Public Health*, 93–94; Elizabeth Fee, unpublished manuscript c. 1990, "The Johns Hopkins Center for Medical Research and Training, Calcutta, India," box 503184, John Hume papers, AMC, 1–4, 9; Timothy D. Baker interview, Aug. 31, 2010.

45. Fred Bang, May 27, 1980, memo to JHSPH Advisory Board, Taylor papers; Rozeboom, *Medical Zoology at the Johns Hopkins School of Hygiene and Public Health*, 94; Carl E. Taylor interview, Sept. 30, 2008.

46. N. Jungalwalla to Frederik B. Bang, June 29, 1963, 3a Dean's or Director's Office Correspondence, box 505343, "J File General 1964–66" folder, AMC; transcript of the ASPH Advisory Committee meeting on the International Role of the North American schools of public health, Nov. 28–29, 1961, 3a Dean's or Director's Office Correspondence, box 504579, "ASPH–Rosenthal Foundation Project 1961" folder, AMC.

47. Fee, "The Johns Hopkins Center for Medical Research and Training, Calcutta, India," 16–18.

48. Ibid., 18–19, 22–24.

49. Ibid., 24–26.

50. Ibid., 26–28; CMRT Executive Committee Minutes, Nov. 13, 1963, R6, box 51, CMRT Committee Minutes, AMC; Frederik Bang to Charles Carpenter, Nov. 19, 1963, R6, box 63, Chronological Correspondence 10-1-63 to 12-31-63, AMC.

51. Fee, "The Johns Hopkins Center for Medical Research and Training, Calcutta, India," pp. 18, 46–52.

52. Ibid., 36–45; J. R. Hughes, S. K. Bose, W. Kloene, D. P. Sinha, and M. R. Cooper, "Acute Lower Respiratory Tract Infections in Calcutta Children: An Etiologic Study," *Indian Pediatrics* 3.6 (1966), 201–11; W. Kloene, F. B. Bang, S. M. Chakraborty, M. R. Cooper, H. Kulemann, K. V. Shah, and M. Ota, "A Two-Year Respiratory Virus Survey in Four Villages in West Bengal, India," *American Journal of Epidemiology* 92.5 (1970), 307–20; W. Kloene, F. B. Bang, M. R. Cooper, H. Kulemann, M. Ota, K. V. Shah, S. M. Chakraborty, and H. G. Pereira, "Isolation of a New Antigenic Type of Influenza B Virus," *Virology* 28.4 (1966), 774–75.

53. N. Jungalwalla to Frederik B. Bang, June 29, 1963, 3a Dean's or Director's Office Correspondence, box 505343, "J File General 1964–66" folder, AMC.

54. Bang to Jungalwalla, July 12, 1963, "J File General 1964–66" folder; Fee, "The Johns Hopkins Center for Medical Research and Training, Calcutta, India," 19–21.

55. Frederik Bang to E. Campbell, Feb. 18, 1963, box 50995, 3a Dean's or Director's Office Correspondence, 6e Ernest Stebbins, "AID 1960–1965" folder, AMC.

56. US Department of State Office of the Historian, "Milestones: 1961–1968: USAID and PL–480, 1961–1969" (https://history.state.gov/milestones/1961-1968/pl-480, accessed Nov. 1, 2015); Godfrey Hodgson, *The Gentleman from New York: Daniel Patrick Moynihan, A Biography* (Houghton Mifflin, 2000), 207–8; Carl Solberg, *Hubert Humphrey: A Biography* (W. W. Norton, 1984), 165; "National Institutes of Health Fiscal Year 1972 Appropriations," HEW 1972 Annual Report, 75; *Report of the JHU Treasurer* for 1960–61, 1965–66, 1970–71, 1974–75.

57. Ernest L. Stebbins to Milton S. Eisenhower, Apr. 21, 1965, Records of the Office of the JHU President, series 6, box 13, "Hygiene-General (1965)" folder; *Congressional Record–Senate*, Feb. 19, 1965, 3120–24; Amalia Vellianitis-Fidas and Eileen Marsar Manfredi, "P.L. 480 Concessional Sales: History, Procedures, Negotiating and Implementing Agreements," Foreign Agricultural Economic Report No. 142 (Foreign Demand and Competition Division, Economic Research Service, US Department of Agriculture, 1977); Carl Taylor interview, Sept. 30, 2008; R. Brad Sack interview, Sept. 28, 2010.

58. Fee, "The Johns Hopkins Center for Medical Research and Training, Calcutta, India," 6–15; Lloyd E. Rozeboom, *Medical Zoology at the Johns Hopkins School of Hygiene and Public Health*, 93–94.

59. William A. Reinke, Jan. 12, 2012, interview. Henry Mosley recalled that the International Centre for Diarrheal Disease Research in Dacca, East Pakistan, had originated as a USAID project that survived on "nearly unlimited soft money" from P.L. 480 grants. W. Henry Mosley interview, Oct. 27, 2010.

60. W. Henry Mosley interview, Oct. 27, 2010, transcript, p. 14.

61. Leslie Corsa Jr., "National Programs to Control Population Growth," USAID working paper, Jan. 1965, cited in "Population Crisis: Hearings on S. 1676," Part 2, pp. 1214–24; Matthew Connelly, *Fatal Misconception: The Struggle to Control World Population* (Belknap Press, 2010), 185. Three members of the Population Council board of trustees had strong Hopkins connections: Eugene R. Black, Detlev W. Bronk, and Thomas Parran. Bernard Berelson, "National Family Planning Programs: A Guide," *Studies in Family Planning* 1 (Dec. 1964), 12.

62. Margaret Bright interview, Aug. 16, 2011.

63. Harper, "Proposal for a New Division of Population Dynamics," 15–16; Paul A. Harper to Oscar Harkavy, July 29, 1965, series 6, box 13, "Hygiene–Financial Reports, Personal Correspondence" folder; 1966–67 JHSPH Catalog, 60.

64. Connelly, *Fatal Misconception*, 162; US Senate Committee on Government Operations, Subcommittee on Foreign Aid Expenditures, "Population Crisis: Hearings on S. 1676," 89th Cong., 2nd sess. (1966), Part 2B, 1159–66.

65. National Research Council Division of Medical Sciences, "Tropical Health: A Report on a Study of Needs and Resources" (1962), x (emphasis added).

66. Packard, "Visions of Postwar Health and Development and Their Impact on Public Health Interventions in the Developing World," in Frederick Cooper and Randall Packard, eds., *International Development and the Social Sciences: Essays on the History and Politics of Knowledge* (University of California Press, 1997), 97–99; John Sharpless, "Population Science, Private Foundations, and Development Aid: The Transformation of Demographic Knowledge in the United States, 1945–1965," in Cooper and Packard, *International Development and the Social Sciences*, 177; May, *Homeward Bound*, 133.

67. Paul Harper, "Proposal for a New Division of Population Dynamics at the Johns Hopkins School of Hygiene and Public Health," Records of the Office of the President, series 6, box 13, "Hygiene-General (1964)" folder, JHU Hamburger Archives, p. 1; "Population Crisis: Hearings on S. 1676," Part 4, p. 878; Paul A. Harper to Milton S. Eisenhower, Feb. 26, 1965, Records of the Office of the JHU President, series 6, box 13, "Hygiene-General (1965)" folder; 3a: Dean's or Director's Office Correspondence, box 505343, "Population Dynamics Conference–AID 1965" folder.

68. Marshall C. Balfour, conference remarks, "Population Dynamics Conference–AID 1965" folder; Corsa, "National Programs to Control Population Growth," 1223.

69. Harper, memo on Development in Physiology of Fertility Regulation at JHSPH, Jan. 27, 1965, "Hygiene–Financial Reports, Personal Correspondence" folder; "Graduate Study in Population Dynamics," brochure undated c. 1970, Population Dynamics subject file, AMC; Larry L. Ewing to John C. Hume, Dec. 9, 1975, 3a D.O. Correspondence, box R111F6, "Public Health Administration" folder.

70. Lyndon B. Johnson, speech for the 20th anniversary of the United Nations, San Francisco, June 25, 1965, qtd. in US Senate Committee on Government Operations, Subcommittee on Foreign Aid Expenditures, "Population Crisis: Hearings on S. 1676," 89th Cong., 2nd sess. (1966), Part 1, Jan. 19, 26, and Feb. 9, 1966, p. 3.

71. Phyllis Piotrow CV (2014); R. T. Ravenholt, P. T. Piotrow, and J. J. Speidel, "Use of Oral Contraceptives: A Decade of Controversy," *International Journal of Gynecology and Obstetrics* 8.6 (1970), 941–56; Phyllis Piotrow, *World Population Crisis: The United States Response* (Praeger Publishers, 1972); P. T. Piotrow, "The United States Commitment to International Family Planning and Population Programs," *International Journal of Health Services* 3.4 (1973), 633–40.

72. Donaldson, *Nature against Us*, 33–42, 56; Leona Baumgartner, "Family Planning and Population Control—Next Steps," *AJPH* 56 (Apr. 1966), 557–60; "Population Crisis: Hearings on S. 1676," 89th Cong., 2nd sess. (1966), Part 1, Jan. 19, 26, and Feb. 9, 1966, pp. 3, 185–200 (1st Johnson quote p. 3, 2nd Johnson quote p. 185). According to the finding aid for the Leona Baumgartner papers (https://collections.countway.harvard.edu/onview /collections/show/16), held at Harvard's Countway Library, Baumgartner played a key role in convincing Lyndon Johnson to embrace population-level family planning as a foreign policy objective.

73. "Letter from the Ambassador to India Chester A. Bowles to President Johnson, May 5, 1966," in Mallon and Smith, *Foreign Relations of the United States, 1966–1968 vol. 25, South Asia*, 641–42; Donaldson, *Nature among Us*, 117.

74. US Department of State, *USAID Country Assistance Program FY 1967, India* (Oct. 1965), part I, V1 to V3 and part II, AB49 to AB68; Timothy D. Baker, "Malaria Eradication in India: A Failure?" *Science* 319 (Mar. 21, 2008), 1616; Connelly, *Fatal Misconception*, 200–1.

75. Joseph M. McDaniel to Milton S. Eisenhower, Apr. 28, 1967, series 6, box 10, "Ford Foundation–Correspondence (1964–1967)" folder, JHU Hamburger Archives; "Summation of Five Years' Activities in the Division of International Health, 1961–1966," 2; *United Nations Yearbook 1970*, 463.

76. Paul A. Harper to Oscar Harkavy, July 29, 1965, and Donald Harting to Paul Harper, Feb. 26, 1965, Records of the Office of the President, series 6, box 13, "Hygiene–Financial Reports, Personal Correspondence" folder; Records of the Office of the President, series 9, box 23, "Ford Foundation 1969–1971" folder; Timothy D. Baker interview, Aug. 31, 2010.

77. S. Seshagiri Rau, "Planning of Public Health Services: Problems in Planning Health Services in India," PHA4/Working Paper No. 3, WHO Expert Committee on Public Health Administration, July 15, 1960, Abel Wolman papers, series 9, box 5, "School of Hygiene International Health" folder, JHU Hamburger Archives, p. 14; *USAID Country Assistance Program FY 1967, India*, Part 2, AB50, AB65–68.

78. Harper, "Proposal for a New Division of Population Dynamics," 11; Corsa, "National Programs to Control Population Growth," 1223; Paul A. Harper to Milton S. Eisenhower, Apr. 18, 1967, Records of the Office of the JHU President, series 6, box 13, "Hygiene-General (1967)" folder; Connelly, *Fatal Misconception*, 204–5; Hugh Leavell, review of Donald J. Bogue, ed., *Progress and Problems of Fertility Control around the World* (Population Association of America, 1968), *AJPH* 60.6 (June 1970), 1168–69.

79. John C. Hume to Ross Jones, Jan. 6, 1964, Records of the Office of the JHU President, series 6, box 13, "Hygiene-General (1964)" folder; "Dr. Norton Reports," *AJPH* 54 (May 1964), 870–71.

80. Connelly, *Fatal Misconception*, 199–215; Warren C. Robinson and John A. Ross, *The Global Family Planning Revolution: Three Decades of Population Policies* (World Bank Publications, 2007), 306–8; USAID Country Assistance Program FY 1967, India, Part 2, AB50, AB65–68.

81. "The Uncertain Trumpet," *Time* 88.27 (Dec. 30, 1966), 22; "Accent on Pragmatics," *Time* 89.12 (Mar. 24, 1967), quote p. 41; "The Loop Way," *Time*, July 23, 1965.

82. Connelly, *Fatal Misconception*, 192, 202.

83. *USAID Country Assistance Program FY 1967, India*, Part 2, AB50, AB65–68; Robinson and Ross, *The Global Family Planning Revolution*, 315–16; figure of 29 million IUDs is from "Memorandum for the Record, Summary Record of the President's Meeting with Indian Planning Minister Asoka Mehta, May 4, 1966," in Gabrielle S. Mallon and Louis J. Smith, eds., *Foreign Relations of the United States, 1966–1968 vol. 25, South Asia* (GPO, 2000), 638; A. deP. Simoes, "India" (paper for International Health Planners course), May 14, 1964, Abel Wolman papers, series 9, box 5, "School of Hygiene International Health" folder, JHU Hamburger Archives, p. 2.

84. *USAID Country Assistance Program FY 1967, India*, Part 2, AB67; Taylor, "Population Planning," 225–26; Connelly, *Fatal Misconception*, 224–27.

85. Connelly, *Fatal Misconception*, 216–30.

86. Envir Adil, testimony before the US Senate Committee on Labor and Public Welfare, Subcommittee on Health, in *Family Planning and Population Research, 1970* (GPO, 1970), 255–57; 1970–71 JHSPH Catalog.

87. Mosley interview, Oct. 27, 2010.

88. W. M. Dobell, "Ayub Khan as President of Pakistan," *Pacific Affairs* 42.3 (Autumn 1969), 294–310, quote p. 297; Mosley interview, Oct. 27, 2010.

89. Donaldson, *Nature against Us*, 110–12; Connelly, *Fatal Misconception*, 234–36.

90. William M. Schmidt to Carl Taylor, Dec. 19, 1960, and Carl E. Taylor, "Possible Scope of School's Activities in Research on Population Dynamics," Jan. 27, 1961, Carl Taylor papers, box 21, "Correspondence—Early" folder, AMC; Carl E. Taylor, "Approval of the Narangwal Population Project by the Government of India," June 6, 1972, Carl Taylor papers, box 21, "Narangwal-General" folder, AMC; Carl Taylor, Sept. 30, 2008, video interview, transcript, p. 10.

91. Taylor 2008 interview, transcript, pp. 9–10; Timothy D. Baker interview, Aug. 31, 2010.

92. US Department of State, *USAID Country Assistance Program FY 1967, India* (Oct. 1965), part I, V1 to V3; Taylor, "Approval of the Narangwal Population Project by the Government of India."

93. Carl Taylor to Timothy Baker, Dec. 12, 1961, Taylor papers; Timothy D. Baker interview, Aug. 31, 2010.

94. Carl E. Taylor, "Economic Triage of the Poor and Population Control," *AJPH* 67.7 (1977), 660–63, quote p. 662.

95. Carl E. Taylor, "Population Planning," chap. 16 in William Reinke, ed., *Topics in Health Planning* (1971), Abel Wolman papers, series 9, box 8, JHU Hamburger Archives,

pp. 223–24; Carl E. Taylor, "Five Stages in a Practical Population Policy," *International Development Review* 10 (1968), 2–7. For a critique of integrating family planning with maternal and child health because it failed to reach out to men, see Vimal Balasubrahmanyan, *Contraception: As If Women Mattered. A Critique of Family Planning* (Centre for Education & Documentation, 1986). Thanks to Rebecca Williams for this reference.

96. Taylor, "Population Planning," 226 (emphasis mine); Connelly, *Fatal Misconception*, Marcolino qtd. 242.

97. J. E. Gordon et al., "The Second Year Death Rate in 27 Less Developed Countries," *American Journal of Medical Science* 254 (1967), 130; C. E. Taylor, "Synergism and Antagonism between Simultaneously Occurring Diseases—General Review of the Ways in Which Diseases Modify Each Other," *Chicago Medical Society Bulletin*, Oct. 4, 1958; C. E. Taylor, N. S. Scrimshaw, and J. E. Gordon, "Interactions of Nutrition and Infection," *American Journal of Medical Science* 237 (Mar. 1959), 367–403; Taylor, "Population Planning," 228 (quotes).

98. Taylor, "Population Planning," 228–30; Donaldson, *Nature against Us*, 60–61, 105–12; "Summation of Five Years' Activities in the Division of International Health, 1961–1966," 4; M-Françoise Hall, "Birth Control in Lima, Peru: Attitudes and Practices," *Milbank Fund Quarterly* 43 (Oct. 1965, Part 1), 409–38; M-Françoise Hall, C. F. Westoff, C. Tietze, and J. M. Stycos, "Family Planning in Lima, Peru," *Milbank Fund Quarterly* 43 (Oct. 1965, Part 2), 100–16.

99. House Committee on Foreign Affairs, *Hearings on the Foreign Assistance Act of 1969* (GPO, 1969), part VII, p. 1484.

100. Freeman, PHS Nursing Faculty Research Development grant narrative; Ruth B. Freeman, "Nursing in the World Health Organization," March 1965, "PHA–Dr. Ruth Freeman 1951–1968" folder.

101. Reinke interview, Jan. 12, 2012.

102. Carl E. Taylor to Timothy D. Baker, Dec. 11, 1968, "Integration of MCH and Family Planning in Rural Health Services" (undated c. 1968), Carl Taylor papers, box 21, "Narangwal-General" folder.

103. Carl E. Taylor to S. Chandrasekhar, Feb. 7, 1969, Carl Taylor papers, box 21, "Narangwal-General" folder, AMC; Robinson and Ross, *The Global Family Planning Revolution*, 315–16.

104. Carl Taylor, "Hearings on H.R. 10042 and H.R. 11136, International Health Agency Act of 1971," p. 162.

105. Nicholas Eberstadt, *Foreign Aid and American Purpose* (American Enterprise Institute for Public Policy Research, 1988), 34–56; JHU Treasurer's Report, "Supporting Schedule A to the Financial Report 1968–1969," 5–18; Vellianitis-Fidas and Manfredi, "P.L. 480 Concessional Sales," 4.

106. US Senate Committee on Foreign Relations, Hearings on S. 489, Nomination of Richard M. Moose as Deputy Under Secretary of State for Management, 95th Cong., 1st sess. (1977), Mar. 8, 1977, pp. 41–42; Carl E. Taylor to D. A. Henderson, Mar. 21, 1977, Carl Taylor papers, box 21, check title folder, AMC.

107. House Committee on Appropriations, Subcommittee on Foreign Operations and Related Agencies, *Foreign Assistance and Related Agencies Appropriations for 1970, Part 2: Economic Assistance* (GPO, 1969), 728.

Chapter 8 · *The Social Sciences, Urban Health, and the Great Society*

1. Margaret Bright interview, Aug. 16, 2011.

2. Bright interview, Aug. 16, 2011; Raymond Forer, "Behavioral Science Activities in a VD Program," *Public Health Reports* 80.11 (Nov. 1965), 1015–20; Alexandra M. Lord, *Condom Nation: The U.S. Government's Sex Education Campaign from World War I to the Internet* (Johns Hopkins University Press, 2010), 113–17.

3. W. Sinclair Harper, Monthly Report–Eastern Health District, Oct. 1960, Mar. 14, 1961, Jan. 9, 1963, Feb. 5, 1963, Oct. 4, 1963, Nov. 1963, Dec. 9, 1963, Feb. 6, 1964, May 25, 1964, JHSPH Dean's Office Correspondence Series 3a, box 506162, "Eastern Health District 1963–1965" folder; Paul V. Lemkau, Report of the Department of Mental Health 1963–64, "Mental Hygiene" folder; DeWitt Bliss, "Abraham Schneidmuhl, Psychiatrist Who Trained Alcoholism Counselors," *Baltimore Sun*, July 20, 1994; Tonya Taliaferro and Rosa Pryor-Trust, *African-American Entertainment in Baltimore* (Arcadia Publishing, 2003), 91–95.

4. Bliss, "Abraham Schneidmuhl"; Mandell interview.

5. Lori Rotskoff, *Love on the Rocks: Men, Women and Alcohol in Post–World War II America* (University of North Carolina Press, 2002), 64–67.

6. Monthly Report–Eastern Health District, June 30, 1964; "Artist's Rendering of New Carling Brewery to Be Built in Baltimore," Cleveland State University Libraries Cleveland Memory Project (www.clevelandmemory.org, accessed Sept. 28, 2011); Brandt, *Cigarette Century*, 332–38.

7. Margaret Bright interview, Aug. 18, 2011; H. D. Chope, "Epidemiology in the Social Sciences," *California Medicine* 91.4 (Oct. 1959), 189–92; F. Stuart Chapin, *Experimental Designs in Sociological Research* (Harper & Brothers, 1947); John E. Gordon and E. Lindemann, "The Biological and Social Sciences in an Epidemiology of Mental Disorders," *American Journal of Medical Science* 223 (July 1954), 316–43; David E. Lilienfeld, "Harold Fred Dorn and the First National Cancer Survey (1937–1939): The Founding of Modern Cancer Epidemiology," *AJPH* 98.12 (Dec. 2008), 2150–58; Rema Lapouse, Mary A. Monk, and Elisabeth Street, "A Method for Use in Epidemiologic Studies of Behavior Disorders in Children," *AJPH* 54.2 (Feb. 1964), 207–22; E. P. Fischer, G. W. Comstock, M. A. Monk, and D. J. Sencer, "Characteristics of Completed Suicides: Implications of Differences among Methods," *Suicide and Life-Threatening Behavior* 23 (1993), 91–100.

8. Margaret Bright interview, Aug. 16, 2011.

9. Ernest L. Stebbins to Thomas Turner, Dec. 7, 1956, Comments from Staff Members binder, and Ruth B. Freeman to Thomas Turner, Jan. 25, 1957, Subcommittee to Review the Curriculum binder, *Committee to Review the Educational Objectives of the School of Hygiene and Public Health.*

10. 1959–60 SHPH Catalog, 43; 1960–61 SHPH catalog, 45; 1962–63 SHPH Catalog, 55–57; 1963–64 SHPH catalog, 35, 55; 1964–65 SHPH Catalog, 56.

11. James S. Coleman to Milton S. Eisenhower, "Proposal for a Program in Sociology and Public Health," Dec. 9, 1964, Records of the Office of the JHU President, series 6, box 13, "Hygiene-General (1964)" folder, JHU Hamburger Archives; "Clyde E. Martin," in Vern L. Bullough and Bonnie Bullough, eds., *Human Sexuality: An Encyclopedia* (Garland Publishing, 1994), quote p. 377.

12. Bright interview, Aug. 16, 2011; Clyde E. Martin, "Epidemiology of Cancer of the Cervix. II. Marital and Coital Factors in Cervical Cancer," *AJPH* 57.5 (May 1967), 803–14; Harold Lamport, letter to the editor, *AJPH* 57.6 (June 1967), 929–30.

13. 1961–62 SHPH Catalog, 45.

14. Paul V. Lemkau, "Community Planning for Mental Health," *Public Health Reports* 76.6 (June 1961), 489–98, quote p. 489; Ernest Gruenberg, "Socially Shared Psychopathology," chap. 7 in A. Leighton, J. A. Clausen, and R. N. Wilson, eds., *Explorations in Social Psychiatry* (Basic Books, 1957); Paul V. Lemkau, "On the Limits of Mental Health," *AJPH* 59.2 (Feb. 1969), 206–7.

15. City of Baltimore 125th Annual Report of the Department of Health, 1939.

16. 1944–45 JHSPH Catalog, 39.

17. JHU Trustees minutes, Mar. 2, 1959, pp. 4600–2 and Sept. 19, 1960, p. 4741; Park, *The Harriet Lane Home*, 248.

18. "Teaching and Research Facilities for the Johns Hopkins University School of Hygiene and Public Health," Dec. 15, 1961, 3a D.O. Correspondence, box 504571, "W. H. Kellogg Found." folder, AMC; Fee, *Disease and Discovery*, 93–95; "A Ten-Year Plan for the School of Hygiene and Public Health," preliminary draft Feb. 1969, 3a D.O. Correspondence, box R111F2.

19. Press release, Dec. 15, 1964, Records of the Office of the President, series 6, box 13, "Hygiene-General (1964)" folder, JHU Hamburger Archives; "Teaching and Research Facilities for the Johns Hopkins University School of Hygiene and Public Health."

20. "A Ten-Year Plan for the School of Hygiene and Public Health," preliminary draft Feb. 1969, JHSPH Dean's Office Correspondence Series 3a, box R111F2; Press release, Dec. 15, 1964, Records of the Office of the JHU President, series 6, box 13, "Hygiene-General (1964)" folder.

21. Guian A. McKee, "Health-Care Policy as Urban Policy: Hospitals and Community Development in the Postindustrial City" (Working Paper 2010-10, Community Development Department of the Federal Reserve Bank of San Francisco, 2010), 5–7, quote p. 6.

22. Ruth B. Freeman to Martha Eliot, Nov. 9, 1961, "PHA–Dr. Ruth Freeman 1951–1968" folder; Jewish Women's Archive, "Public Health Pioneer Margaret Arnstein Appointed Dean of Yale School of Nursing" (http://jwa.org/thisweek/mar/13/1967/margaret-arnstein, accessed Oct. 11, 2015); Ruth B. Freeman, 1957–58 Annual Report of the Division of Public Health Nursing, 3a D.O. Correspondence, box 505348, "President's Report 1958" folder.

23. Timothy D. Baker interview, Nov. 9, 2011; Ernest Stebbins to Ruth B. Freeman, Sept. 14, 1961, 3a D.O. correspondence, box 506168, "PHA–Dr. Ruth Freeman 1951–1968" folder. The Joint Committee on the Study of Education for Public Health was sponsored by the APHA, Association of Schools of Public Health, Association of State and Territorial Health Officers, US Public Health Service, and Canadian Department of National Health.

24. 1961–62 SHPH Catalog, 62, 75, 87; 1964–65 SHPH Catalog, 45; Ruth B. Freeman, 1957–58 Annual Report of the Division of Public Health Nursing; Ruth B. Freeman, grant narrative for PHS Nursing Faculty Research Development grant, June 17, 1964, "PHA–Dr. Ruth Freeman 1951–1968" folder; Mandell interview.

25. "Report on the Teaching of Public Health Nursing in Schools of Public Health to Association of Schools of Public Health," Apr. 9, 1963, and Minutes of the Annual Meeting of the ASPH, Chapel Hill, NC, April 8–9, 1963, 3a Director or Dean's Office: Correspondence, box 504579, "Assoc. of Schools of Public Health 1963" folder, AMC; Ruth Freeman, "Site Visit Nov. 7, 1964 for PHS Nursing Faculty Research Development Program" and Ruth B. Freeman to Don Cornely, Nov. 17, 1966, "PHA–Dr. Ruth Freeman 1951–1968" folder.

26. "Report on the Teaching of Maternal and Child Health," *AJPH* 52.11 (Nov. 1962), 1933; May, *Homeward Bound*, xiv–xvii.

27. "Fertility Tables for Birth Cohorts by Color"; Thomas, *Deluxe Jim Crow*, 80–100; Schoen, *Choice and Coercion*, 23.

28. James T. Patterson, *Freedom Is Not Enough: The Moynihan Report and America's Struggle over Black Family Life from LBJ to Obama* (Basic Books, 2010).

29. August Meier and Elliott Rudwick, *Black History and the Historical Profession, 1915–1980* (University of Illinois Press, 1986), 249–52; Hildrus A. Poindexter, "Handicaps in the Normal Growth and Development of Rural Negro Children," *AJPH* 28.9 (Sept. 1, 1938), 1048; Patterson, *Freedom Is Not Enough*.

30. Patterson, *Freedom Is Not Enough*; Connelly, *Fatal Misconception*, 208, 231; Vance quoted in Robert R. Korstad and James L. Leloudis, *To Right These Wrongs: The North Carolina Fund and the Battle to End Poverty and Inequality in 1960s America* (University of North Carolina Press, 2010), 247–48.

31. Laurie Zabin video interview with Brian Simpson, Sept. 2010.

32. JHSPH scrapbook, AMC; 1957–58 Division of Mental Hygiene Annual Report, 3a D.O. Correspondence, box 505348, "President's Report 1958" folder.

33. Baltimore City Health Department, *Guarding the Health of Baltimore* (1961 Annual Report), 21, 55; Pietila, *Not in My Neighborhood*, 217; Jacques Kelly, "Matthew Tayback, 85, first director of Md. Office on Aging," *Baltimore Sun*, Sept. 22, 2004.

34. Zabin video interview; Department of Gynecology records, box 505158, "Whitridge, John" folder, AMC; Kelly, "Matthew Tayback."

35. Matthew Tayback and Helen Wallace, "Maternal and Child Health Services and Urban Economics," *Public Health Reports* 77.10 (Oct. 1962), 827–34; Application to the Kellogg Foundation for continuation of A Grant for Research in Administration at the Johns Hopkins University School of Hygiene and Public Health," May 17, 1962, "W. H. Kellogg Found." folder. Tayback coauthored one of the earliest articles published on health services research: Frank F. Furstenberg, Matthew Tayback, Harry Goldberg, and J. Wilfrid Davis, "Prescribing, an Index to Quality of Medical Care: A Study of the Baltimore City Medical Care Program," *AJPH* 43.10 (Oct. 1953), 1299–309.

36. Margaret Bright, "Social Indications and Implications for Family Planning Services in Baltimore," 3a D. O. Correspondence, box 504582, "Chronic Disease 1966" folder.

37. Patterson, *Freedom Is Not Enough*.

38. David Lilienfeld, personal communication, Apr. 28, 2012; Bright, "Social Indications and Implications for Family Planning Services in Baltimore"; William Reinke interview, Jan. 27, 2012.

39. Schoen, *Choice and Coercion*, 23–24, 61–63; Julie Fairman, *Making Room in the Clinic: Nurse Practitioners and the Evolution of Modern Health Care* (Rutgers University Press, 2008), 51; Butler A. Stith and Clayton E. Wright, eds., *A Review of the HHS Family Planning Program: Mission, Management, and Measurement of Results*, Institute of Medicine Committee on a Comprehensive Review of the HHS Office of Family Planning Title X Program (National Academies Press, 2009) (http://www.ncbi.nlm.nih.gov/books/NBK215217, accessed Oct. 30, 2015).

40. Reinke interview, Jan. 27, 2012; Connelly, *Fatal Misconception*, 243–44, Notestein qtd. p. 243; Margaret Bright interview, Aug. 16, 2011.

41. JHMI news release, Jan. 31, 1978, and "Department of Population Dynamics" brochure, c. 1978, Population Dynamics subject file.

42. Park, *The Harriet Lane Home*, 202–3; Janet B. Hardy, "The Collaborative Perinatal Project: Lessons and Legacy," *Annals of Epidemiology* 13 (2003), 303–11.

43. Laurie Schwab Zabin interview, May 25, 2012; Stebbins to Virginia H. Patterson, Dec. 9 1963, Stebbins papers, box 504571, "M General 1962–67" folder.

44. Park, *The Harriet Lane Home*, 202–3; Hardy, "The Collaborative Perinatal Project," 310–11; Laurie Zabin interview by Brian Simpson, Aug. 20, 2010.

45. Park, *The Harriet Lane Home*, 202–3; Hardy, "The Collaborative Perinatal Project," 310–11; Laurie Schwab Zabin CV; L. S. Zabin, J. F. Kantner, and M. Zelnik, "The Risk of Adolescent Pregnancy in the First Months of Intercourse," *Family Planning Perspectives* 11.4 (1979), 215–22; L. S. Zabin, "The Effect of Administration Family Planning Policy on Maternal and Child Health," *Journal of Public Health Policy* 4.3 (1983), 268–78; L. S. Zabin, J. D. Hardy, R. Streett, and T. M. King, "A School, Hospital and University-Based Adolescent Pregnancy Prevention Program," *Journal of Reproduction* 29.6 (1984), 421–26; Janet B. Hardy and Laurie Schwab Zabin, *Adolescent Pregnancy in an Urban Environment: Issues, Programs, and Evaluation* (Urban Institute Press, 1991).

46. Ruth B. Freeman, grant narrative for PHS Nursing Faculty Research Development grant, June 17, 1964, and Ruth B. Freeman, "Nursing in the World Health Organization," March 1965, "PHA–Dr. Ruth Freeman 1951–1968" folder.

47. Turner, *Heritage of Excellence*, 260–62; Pietila, *Not in My Neighborhood*, 130; David Lilienfeld, personal communication, July 14, 2015.

48. Charles Flagle interview, Sept. 29, 2010.

49. "1950–51 Report of the Director of the Institute for Cooperative Research," *JHU Circular* 70 (Nov. 1951), 169–70; 1955–56 Report of the JHU Treasurer, 68.

50. Charles D. Flagle bio file, AMC; 1960–61 Report of the JHU Treasurer, 84; Charles D. Flagle, "Some Origins of Operations Research in the Health Services," *Operations Research* 50 (Jan.–Feb. 2002), 53–54.

51. Stevens, *In Sickness and in Wealth*, 175–78, 228; Flagle, "Some Origins of Operations Research in the Health Services," 54–56; Charles D. Flagle, "The Problem of Organization for Hospital Inpatient Care," in C. W. Churchmand and M. Verhulst, eds., *Management Sciences: Models and Techniques*, vol. 2 (Pergamon Press, 1960), 275–87; Charles D. Flagle, H. Lockward, J. H. Moss, and S. Strachan, "The Progressive Patient Care Hospital: Estimating Bed Needs," PHS publication 930-C-2 (1963).

52. Flagle, "Some Origins of Operations Research in the Health Services," 55; "Operations Research in the Health Services," *Operations Research* 10 (1962), 591–603.

53. John Black Grant diary, Mar. 29–Apr. 1, 1958; 1955–56 JHU Graduate Programs Catalog, 155–57. JHSPH faculty who taught in the program included William G. Cochran and Paul Meier in Biostatistics, Abel Wolman in Sanitary Engineering, and Anna Baetjer in Environmental Medicine.

54. Flagle, "Some Origins of Operations Research in the Health Services," 52; Shonick, *Government and Health Services*, 360–61.

55. John E. Wennberg, *Tracking Medicine: A Researcher's Quest to Understand Health Care* (Oxford University Press, 2010), 16; Tayback and Wallace, "Maternal and Child Health Services and Urban Economics," 833.

56. T. J. Bauer, "Appraisal of the Community Health Services and Facilities Act of 1961," *Public Health Reports* 77 (July 1962), 561–62; Public Health Service in HEW 1964 Annual Report, 160; Shonick, *Government and Health Services*, 362; Flagle interview, Sept. 29, 2010.

57. Flagle interview, Sept. 29, 2010.

58. Ibid.

59. Ibid.

60. Donald A. Cornely bio file, AMC.

61. Donald A. Cornely, "Urban Medical Blight," *Journal of Pediatrics* 61.3 (1962), 499–500; *1965–66 Maryland Manual* (Annapolis: State of Maryland, 1966), 78.

62. Park, *The Harriet Lane Home*, 300–1, 312; 1966–67 JHSPH Catalog, 61; 1968–69 JHSPH Catalog, 82.

63. L. Gordis, A. Lilienfeld, and R. Rodriguez, "Studies in the Epidemiology and Preventability of Rheumatic Fever. II. Socioeconomic Factors and the Incidence of Acute Attacks," *Journal of Chronic Diseases* 21 (1969), 655; Leon Gordis, "The Virtual Disappearance of Rheumatic Fever in the United States: Lessons in the Rise and Fall of Disease," *Circulation* 72.6 (1985), 1155–62.

64. Gordis, "The Virtual Disappearance of Rheumatic Fever," 1155–57.

65. *1965–66 Maryland Manual*, 81; *1971–72 Maryland Manual*, 401; Margaret Bright interview, Aug. 16, 2011.

66. Robert D. Wright to Glenn Beall, July 1, 1971, "President's Office 1971–72 Office of Health Care Programs" folder; Fee, *Disease and Discovery*, 52.

67. 1968–69 JHSPH Catalog, 66.

68. Alan Mason Chesney Archives of the Johns Hopkins Medical Institutions, "Johns Hopkins Hospital Institutional Records" (http://medicalarchives.jhmi.edu/hospital.html, accessed Feb. 20, 2016 [quote]); Robert M. Heyssel to Health Care Programs Working Committee, Medical Planning and Development Committee, and Chiefs of Clinical Service, May 22, 1968, Records of the Office of the President, series 9, box 30, "Health Care Programs 1968–69" folder; Guian A. McKee, "Hospitals and Race in the Post-Industrial City: The Johns Hopkins University Hospitals and Inner-City Baltimore," conference paper, Policy History Conference, June 7, 2012, 2–3; "Civilization Here, Savagery There," qtd. in McKee, original source in Sherwood D. Kohn, *Experiment in Planning an Urban High School: The Baltimore Charette* (Educational Facilities Laboratory, 1969), 16–19. McKee notes that "the possibility of JHH leaving East Baltimore appears to have been considered as a standing option in the mid- to late-1960s. For a meeting in which the question was raised directly, see Joint Committee of Trustees of The Johns Hopkins University and Hospital, "Minutes," Apr. 2, 1970, Board of Trustees Book No. 17, Apr. 2, 1970 to Mar. 2, 1971, AMC.

69. John E. Wennberg bio file, AMC; Thomas T. Fenton, "Frustrated Doctor Blocked Drug," *Baltimore Sun*, Feb. 21, 1964; John E. Wennberg, Ronald Okun, Edward J. Hinman, Robert C. Northcutt, Robert J. Griep, and W. Gordon Walker, "Renal Toxicity of Oral Cholecystographic MediaBunamiodyl Sodium and Lopanoic Acid," *JAMA* 186.5 (1963), 461–67; Shannon Brownlee, *Overtreated: Why Too Much Medicine Is Making Us Sicker and Poorer* (Bloomsbury Publishing USA, 2008), 16–18.

70. Willliam J. Perkinson, "Nursing Homes Used as Acute Hospitals, but Lack Adequate Staff and Facilities," *Baltimore Sun*, Mar. 8, 1967.

71. Ibid.

72. McKee, "Hospitals and Race in the Post-Industrial City," 1–2; Centers for Medicare and Medicaid Services, "National Health Expenditure Data—Historical" (https://www.cms.gov/Research-Statistics-Data-and-Systems/Statistics-Trends-and-Reports/NationalHealthExpendData/NationalHealthAccountsHistorical.html, accessed Oct. 1, 2015).

Chapter 9 · Surviving the Seventies

1. Milton S. Eisenhower, Apr. 26, 1965, memorandum to Baker, Herriott, Lemkau, Morgan, and Sartwell, Records of the Office of the JHU President, series 6, box 13, "Hygiene-General (1966)" folder.

2. "Health Dept. in Cabinet Wins Support," *Washington Post*, Mar. 19, 1947; Mike Stobbe, *Surgeon General's Warning: How Politics Crippled the Nation's Doctor* (University of California Press, 2014), 91–92, quote p. 116.

3. Shonick, Government and Health Services, 98–99.

4. Paul V. Lemkau to Milton S. Eisenhower, Dec. 6, 1966, "Confidential Faculty Records" folder.

5. Paul V. Lemkau to members of the Dean Selection Committees and President Milton S. Eisenhower, Dec. 5, 1966, Records of the Office of the JHU President, series 6, box 10, "Confidential Faculty Records" folder.

6. 1968 HEW Annual Report.

7. Alondra Nelson, Body and Soul: The Black Panther Party and the Fight against Medical Discrimination (University of Minnesota Press, 2011), 75–114.

8. Committee on the University's Role in Urban Problems, "The Johns Hopkins University's Role in Urban Affairs," Jan. 5, 1968, Records of the Office of the President, series 9, box 2, "Affirmative Action 1970" folder; Lincoln Gordon, outline for JHSPH faculty talk, Records of the Office of the President, series 9, box 33, "Hygiene–Faculty Coffee 1967" folder, Hamburger Archives. The committee was chaired by John Geyer in Environmental Engineering at Homewood and included JHSPH faculty Paul Lemkau and Cornelius Kruse. At Homewood, JHU administrator Ross Jones led efforts to address the deterioration of the housing around the main liberal arts campus. See Francesca Gamber, " 'Where We Live': Greater Homewood Community Corporation, 1967–1976," in Jessica I. Elfenbein, Thomas L. Hollowak, and Elizabeth M. Nix, eds., *Baltimore '68: Riots and Rebirth in an American City* (Temple University Press, 2011), 208–25.

9. William Bevan to Lincoln Gordon, Oct. 25, 1967, "Hygiene–Faculty Coffee 1967" folder; "The War against Suffering," special issue of *Johns Hopkins Magazine*, summer 1967.

10. Alexander Hollander to William Bevan, Dec. 28, 1967, and Hollander to Lincoln Gordon, Feb. 12, 1968, Records of the Office of the President, series 9, box 30, "Health and Biomedical Planning Institute" folder.

11. Pietila, *Not in My Neighborhood*, 195–96; Peter B. Levy, "The Dream Deferred: The Assassination of Martin Luther King, Jr., and the Holy Week Uprisings of 1968," in Elfenbein, Hollowak, and Nix, *Baltimore '68*, 5–25.

12. Timothy D. Baker interview, Nov. 9, 2011; David M. Paige interview, Aug. 13, 2014.

13. "Freedom School Offers Urban Crisis Courses," *Baltimore Afro-American*, Sept. 23, 1968; "Rats, Rats? Rats!" *Baltimore Afro-American*, November 1968.

14. On the trials and tribulations of Great Society housing and education legislation, see Roger Biles, *The Fate of Cities: Urban America and the Federal Government, 1945–2000* (University of Kansas Press, 2011); on the ways that health policy differed from other aspects of public policy, particularly in its appeal to white middle-class self-interest, see Karen Kruse Thomas, *Deluxe Jim Crow: Civil Rights and American Health Policy* (University of Georgia Press, 2011).

15. Heyssel to Health Care Programs Working Committee, Medical Planning and Development Committee, and Chiefs of Clinical Service, May 22, 1968; "Newark: Negroes Demand and Get Voice in Medical School Plans," *Science* 160.3825 (April 19, 1968), 290–92; Lincoln Gordon, David E. Rogers, Russell A. Nelson, and John C. Hume, Dec. 6, 1968, memo to Faculty of the School of Medicine and School of Hygiene and Public Health and Staff of Hospital, "Health Care Programs 1968–69" folder.

16. Sol Levine bio file, AMC; Margaret Bright interview, Aug. 16, 2011.

17. "Housing Body Welcomes a New Member," *Baltimore Afro-American*, Aug. 2, 1969; Eugene Feinblatt bio file, AMC.

18. David E. Rogers, "The Development of Community Based Health Care Programs by the Johns Hopkins Medical Institutions: A Proposal to the Commonwealth Fund, the Rockefeller Foundation, and the Carnegie Corporation of New York," July 2, 1969, Quigg Newton to Lincoln Gordon, Nov. 14, 1969, Florence Anderson to Gordon, Nov. 19, 1969, Gordon to Newton, Dec. 8, 1969, J. Kellum Smith Jr. to Gordon, Dec. 10, 1969, "Health Care Programs 1969–71" folder.

19. *NBC Evening News*, Feb. 14, 1971, Vanderbilt TV News Archive (http://tvnews.vanderbilt.edu, accessed Apr. 14, 2015).

20. Gordon, Rogers, Nelson, and Hume, Dec. 6, 1968 memo; Rogers, "The Development of Community Based Health Care Programs by the Johns Hopkins Medical Institutions"; Lincoln Gordon to Quigg Newton, Dec. 8, 1969, J. Kellum Smith Jr. to Gordon, Dec. 10, 1969, "Health Care Programs 1969–71" folder.

21. Robert M. Heyssel, "Office of Health Care Programs Progress Report January 1969–December 1969," Dec. 4, 1969, "Health Care Programs 1969–71" folder.

22. "Tayback to Head Aid Programs on Health for Poor," *Baltimore Sun*, June 26, 1969; Frederick P. McGehan, "Health Units Due Changes," *Baltimore Sun*, June 30, 1969.

23. Matthew Tayback, letter to the editor, *Baltimore Sun*, Dec. 4, 1971; Matthew Tayback bio file, AMC.

24. Robert M. Heyssel, "Office of Health Care Programs Progress Report January 1969–December 1969," Dec. 4, 1969, "Health Care Programs 1969–71" folder.

25. Sam Shapiro, "Periodic Screening for Breast Cancer: The HIP Randomized Controlled Trial," *Journal of the National Cancer Institute Monographs* 1997.22 (1997), 27–30; Sam Shapiro, Mar. 6, 1998, oral history interview with Edward Berkowitz, History of Health Services Research Project, National Library of Medicine, pp. 10–15.

26. Fitzhugh Mullan, "Wrestling with Variation: An Interview with Jack Wennberg," web exclusive, posting date: October 7, 2004, *Health Affairs* (http://content.healthaffairs.org/content/early/2004/10/07/hlthaff.var.73.short); John E. Wennberg and Alan M. Gittelsohn, "Small Area Variations in Health Care Delivery: A Population-Based Health Information System Can Guide Planning and Regulatory Decision-Making," *Science* 182.4117 (1973), 1102–8; Wennberg, *Tracking Medicine*, 16–17.

27. *The Dartmouth Atlas of Health Care* (www.dartmouthatlas.org, accessed Apr. 14, 2015); Mullan, Jack Wennberg interview.

28. Margaret Bright interview, Aug. 18, 2011; 1970–71 JHSPH Catalog.

29. 1961–62 SHPH Catalog, 49; Edward Davens obituary, *Baltimore Sun*, Sept. 18, 1992; John Whitridge Jr. to Alan C. Barnes, May 24, 1961, and Sept. 5, 1961, Johns Hopkins School of Medicine, Department of Gynecology records, box 505158, "Whitridge, John" folder, AMC; Arthur Lesser, "The Origin and Development of Maternal and Child Health Programs in the United States," *AJPH* 75.6 (June 1985), 593–94.

30. Fairman, Making Room in the Clinic, 18–19.

31. Donald A. Cornely, "Public Health Nurse–Midwifery Educational Program at Johns Hopkins," Feb. 22, 1977, 3a D.O. Correspondence, box R111F6 (old box 5), "3/14/77 Nurse Midwifery Program Accreditation Site Visit" folder.

32. Cornely, "Public Health Nurse–Midwifery Educational Program at Johns Hopkins"; Bernard Guyer interview, Sept. 26, 2011. The other five master's programs were at Yale, Columbia, Illinois, St. Louis, and Utah.

33. Cornely, "Public Health Nurse–Midwifery Educational Program at Johns Hopkins."

34. Russell Morgan, "Proposal for the Formation of a School of Allied Health Sciences," Nov. 1968, Records of the President, series 9, box 3, "School of Allied Health Sciences—1969" folder, JHU Hamburger Archives.

35. Ibid.

36. Ibid.

37. Allyn W. Kimball to William Bevan, July 2, 1969; William Bevan to Lincoln Gordon, July 18, 1969.

38. Mary Frances Keen, "Tension and Triumph, 1970–1979," in Warren, *Our Shared Legacy*, 164–74.

39. Ibid., 175–78.

40. Robert M. Heyssel and Malcolm L. Peterson to foundation officers, Apr. 14, 1972, "President's Office 1971–72 Office of Health Care Programs" folder.

41. Shapiro interview; Russell H. Morgan to Robert M. Heyssel, May 3, 1972, Records of the Office of the President, series 13, box 9, "President's Office 1971–72 Office of Health Care Programs" folder.

42. Ibid., 179–81.

43. Anna C. Scholl to John C. Hume, Nov. 13, 1975, and Division of Public Health Nursing, Dec. 1975 newsletter, 3a D. O. Correspondence, box R111F6, "Public Health Administration" folder; PHS Notice of Grant Awarded, "An Accelerated Program for the Preparation of Public Health Nursing Supervisors," July 18, 1966, and Ruth B. Freeman to Don Cornely, Nov. 17, 1966, "PHA–Dr. Ruth Freeman 1951–1968" folder.

44. M. Alfred Haynes bio file, AMC; Citizens Board of Inquiry into Hunger and Malnutrition in the United States, *Hunger USA 1968* (The New Community Press, 1968).

45. Hunger and Malnutrition in the United States: Hearings before the Committee on Labor and Public Welfare, Subcommittee on Employment, Manpower, and Poverty, United States Senate 90th Cong. (1968) (statement of M. Alfred Haynes), 16–18.

46. David M. Paige interview July 24, 2013; George G. Graham bio file, AMC; George G. Graham, "Human Copper Deficiency," *New England Journal of Medicine* 285 (1971), 857–58.

47. Ibid.

48. David M. Paige interview, Aug. 14, 2013.

49. Ibid.

50. Ibid.

51. Agriculture, Environmental and Consumer Protection Appropriations, FY72, Part 2: Hearing before the Committee on Appropriations, Subcommittee on Agriculture and Environmental and Consumer Protection Appropriations, United States Senate, 92nd Cong. (1971) (statement of David M. Paige), 1987–2011, quote p. 1988; Victor Oliveira, Elizabeth Racine, Jennifer Olmsted, Linda M. Ghelfi, The WIC Program: Background, Trends, and Issues (U.S. Department of Agriculture, Food Assistance and Nutrition Research Report No. 27, 2002), 7.

52. Improving Nutrition for America's Children in Difficult Economic Times: Hearing Before the Committee on Agriculture, Nutrition and Forestry, United States Senate, 111th Cong. (2009) (statement of David M. Paige), 27–29, quote p. 29.

53. Oliveira et al., *The WIC Program*, 1.

54. Bright interview, Aug. 18, 2011; Margaret Bright bio file, AMC; 1972–73 JHSPH Catalog, 161; 1973–74 JHSPH Catalog, 163–64; "Kay Partridge to Head SHS Nursing Program," The Dome, Sept. 1974; Kay B. Partridge and Paul E. White, "Community and Professional Participation in Decision Making at a Health Center," Health Services Reports 87.4 (Apr. 1972), 336–42.

55. Mandell interview.

56. Philip D. Bonnet, "Mental Hygiene Search Committee," Nov. 6, 1974, "Sch of Hyg Search Committee for Chairman, Department of Mental Hygiene" folder; Wallace Mandell bio file, AMC; Wallace Mandell, Sheldon Blackman, and Clyde E. Sullivan, *Disadvantaged Youth Approaching the World of Work: A Study of Neighborhood Youth Corps Enrollees in New York City* (Wakoff Research Center, Staten Island Mental Health Society, 1969); Bliss, "Abraham Schneidmuhl"; Mandell interview.

57. Caroline Jean Acker, "The Early Years of the PHS Narcotic Hospital at Lexington, Kentucky," *Public Health Reports* 112 (May/June 1997), 245–47; Abraham Wikler, *The Relation of Psychiatry to Pharmacology* (Williams and Wilkins, 1957); Eric C. Schneider, *Smack: Heroin and the American City* (University of Pennsylvania Press, 2008).

58. "Conversation with Jerome H. Jaffe," *Addiction* 94.1 (1999), 13–30, quote p. 20.

59. Stanley F. Yolles, NIMH interview, April 21, 1975.

60. Stanley F. Yolles obituary, *New York Times*, Jan. 21, 2001.

61. NIH Almanac (http://www.nih.gov/about/almanac/historical/chronology_of_events .htm, accessed Sept. 30, 2011); Mandell interview; James Q. Wilson, "The Return of Heroin," *Commentary* Apr. 1975.

62. Mandell bio file; Mandell interview.

63. Ibid.

64. Wallace Mandell to John C. Hume, Oct. 3, 1975, 3a D.O. Correspondence, box R111F6, "Mental Hygiene" folder; 1961–62 JHSPH Catalog, 52; Paul V. Lemkau, Report of the Department of Mental Health 1963–64, "Mental Hygiene" folder; 1973–74 Report of the Dean of the School of Hygiene and Public Health, 6.

65. 3a: D.O. Correspondence, box R111F4, "Sch of Hyg Committee on Ph.D. programs" folder; "Dept. H33 Mental Hygiene Current Grants and Contracts," Dec. 9, 1974, and David E. Price, memo to Steven Muller, Russel H. Morgan, Robert M. Heyssel,

Richard S. Ross, and Harry Woolf, Apr. 7, 1975, 3a D.O. Correspondence, box R111F6, "Sch of Hyg Search Committee for Chairman, Department of Mental Hygiene" folder.

66. Mandell bio file; Mandell to John C. Hume, Oct. 3, 1975.

67. Sol Levine bio file, AMC; Margaret Bright interview, Aug. 16, 2011.

68. Arthur H. Richardson to John C. Hume, Jan. 16, 1973, 3a D. O. Correspondence, box R111F5, "Sch of Hyg Search Committee for Chairman, Dept. of Behavioral Sciences" folder; Kerr L. White to Charles Southwick, July 13, 1972, 3a D.O. Correspondence, box R111F5, "Behavioral Sciences—1972/73 Search Committee" folder; Kerr L. White to Abraham M. Lilienfeld, Oct. 22, 1971, 3a: D.O. Correspondence, box R111F4, "Committee on the Environment" folder; Judith Randal, "A New Look at Schools of Public Health," *Change* 8.9 (Oct. 1976), 52–53.

69. Paul E. White interview, Sept. 9, 2011.

70. Paul E. White interview, Sept. 9, 2011; Charles H. Southwick, Subcommittee Report on Behavioral Sciences Chairman, Jan. 15, 1973, 3a D.O. Correspondence, box R111F5, "Behavioral Sciences" folder; Paul E. White bio file, AMC.

71. "Report of Mental Hygiene Search Committee to Department Chairmen (Advisory Board)," Jan. 7, 1974, and Russell H. Morgan to David E. Price, Apr. 17, 1975, JHSPH Dean's Office Correspondence Series 3a, box R111F6, "Sch of Hyg Search Committee for Chairman, Department of Mental Hygiene" folder; 1974–75 University of North Carolina School of Public Health Catalog, 86.

72. "Report of Mental Hygiene Search Committee to Department Chairmen (Advisory Board)," Jan. 7, 1974, 3a D.O. Correspondence, box R111F6 (old box 5), "Sch of Hyg Search Committee for Chairman, Department of Mental Hygiene" folder.

73. JHSPH Dean's Office Correspondence Series 3a, box R111F6, "Sch of Hyg Search Committee for Chairman, Department of Mental Hygiene" folder; Miller to Eaton, June 12, 2013; Ernest M. Gruenberg CV.

74. 1970–71 JHU Treasurer's Report, 54–55; 1979–80 JHU Long Form Financial Report, 116.

75. Report of the Long Range Planning Committee to the President of the Johns Hopkins University (June 1966), 3a D.O. Correspondence, box R111F2, p. 181.

76. McKee, "Healthcare Policy as Urban Policy," 5.

77. Ann Skinner interview, Mar. 14, 2012.

Chapter 10 · *The Environmental Revolution in Public Health*

1. S. H., "The Fashionable Environment," *Change in Higher Education* 2.2 (Mar.–Apr. 1970), 6–8.

2. Korstad, *Dreaming of a Time*, 111; Norton Nelson, "In Control of Environmental Factors Antithetic to Health," in Bowers and Purcell, *Schools of Public Health: Present and Future*, quote p. 85; Steven Muller to Robert Glaser Jan. 16, 1981, Records of the Office of the President, series 14, box 17, "Office of the President 1972–82 Environmental Health Advisory Council 1980–81" folder, JHU Hamburger Archives.

3. Hiroko Fujita, Kanji Iio and Katsurō Yamamoto, "Brachymesophalangia and Clinodactyly of the Fifth Finger in Japanese Children," *Pediatrics International* 6.1 (June 1964), 26–30; Johannes Abele, "Safety Clicks: The Geiger-Muller Tube and Radiation Protection in Germany, 1928–1960," in Robert Bud, ed., *Manifesting Medicine* (NMSI Trading Ltd., 2004), 79–104; Stan Lee, *Origins of Marvel Comics* (Simon & Schuster, 1974).

4. Ernest L. Stebbins to James Crow, Dec. 1, 1958, Ernest L. Stebbins to Hardin B. Jones, Dec. 1, 1958, Victor P. Bond to Ernest L. Stebbins, Nov. 14, 1958, Ernest L. Stebbins to Victor P. Bond, Dec. 1, 1958, Milton S. Eisenhower to Victor P. Bond, Mar. 5, 1959, 3a Dean's or Director's Office Correspondence, box 505348, "Department of Radiology 1962–1967" folder, AMC. Bond was offered a professorship in 1959 in the Department of Environmental Medicine, but he declined. Other consultants were the University of Wisconsin geneticist James Crow and Hardin B. Jones, professor of medical physics and physiology at the University of California. William B. Looney was involved in the early development of the Radiological Sciences program but left in 1961 to become head of the Radiobiology and Biophysics Laboratory at the University of Virginia Hospital.

5. John Black Grant diary, Mar. 29–Apr. 1, 1958, box 187, folder 2237, "200 L Johns Hopkins University–School of Hygiene and Public Health 1958–61," RFA; National Advisory Committee on Radiation, *Protecting and Improving Health through the Radiological Sciences* (Public Health Service, Department of Health, Education and Welfare, Apr. 1966), 3.

6. Milton S. Eisenhower to Emory W. Morris, July 20, 1960, 3a D.O. Correspondence, box 504571, "W. K. Kellogg Foundation" folder, AMC ; Ernest L. Stebbins to Russell Morgan, Nov. 20, 1963; Russell Morgan, "Institution's Plans," in PHS Research Career Development Program grant application for Shih Yi Wang, "Chemical Studies of Ultraviolet Irradiation Effects on Nucleic Acids and Related Compounds," Aug. 31, 1964, 3a Dean's or Director's Office Correspondence, box 505348, "Radiological Science 1960–1964" folder; "Annual Report to the American Cancer Society from the Joint Committee on Cancer Teaching and Research of the Johns Hopkins Medical Institutions," 1965, Subject files: Joint Committee on Cancer Teaching and Research, folder 1, AMC.

7. Wagner, *A Personal History of Nuclear Medicine*, 111–12, 121–22, 135, 141. PhDs in Radiological Science who later joined the faculty included Bob Dannals, Jonathon Links, Tomas Guilarte, Kwamina Baidoo, James Frost, and Dean Wong; Kanji Iio bio file, AMC.

8. Johns Hopkins Medical Institutions press release, June 7, 1963, "Radiological Science 1960–1964" folder.

9. Kenneth Zierler to W. Barry Wood, Jan. 10, 1958, Margaret Merrell papers, box 505378, "Office of the Vice-Pres." folder, AMC; Joseph November, *Biomedical Computing: Digitizing Life in the United States* (Johns Hopkins University Press, 2012), 19–21, 195.

10. Computer History Museum (http://www.computerhistory.org/atchm/about-the-computer-history-museums-ibm-1401-machines, accessed Nov. 10, 2015); Russel H. Morgan, "Dose Distributions in Diagnostic X-ray Procedures," PHS research R01 grant application, Sept. 10, 1963, "Radiological Science 1960–1964" folder.

11. Morgan, "Dose Distributions in Diagnostic X-ray Procedures."

12. Morgan's publications on diagnostic X-ray exposure included "The Measurement of Radiant Energy Levels in Diagnostic Roentgenology," *Radiology* 76 (1961), 867–76; "Radiation Control in Public Health," *The New Physician* 1 (1961), 430–32; "Radiation Protection Standards," in Joint Committee on Atomic Energy, *Selected Materials on Radiation Protection Criteria and Standards: Their Basis and Use* (May 1960), 63–69; "Radioactive Materials in Man and His Environment: The Character and Magnitude of the Problem," in *Radioactivity in Man*, ed. George R. Meneely (Springfield, IL: Charles C Thomas, 1961), 403–7; "The Dangers of Diagnostic X-ray Exposure," *Post-Graduate Medicine* 29.5 (May 1961), 551–54.

13. Morgan, "Dose Distributions in Diagnostic X-ray Procedures."

14. Ibid.

15. Beers, "Radiobiological Research."

16. Arthur M. Dannenburg Jr., "Enzymes in Pathogenesis of Inflammatory Conditions," PHS R01 research grant, Aug. 25, 1964, Shih Yi Wang, "Chemistry of Nucleic Acids and Related Compounds," PHS R01 research grant application, June 1, 1964, and PHS Research Career Development Program grant application for Shih Yi Wang, "Chemical Studies of Ultraviolet Irradiation Effects on Nucleic Acids and Related Compounds," Aug. 31, 1964, "Radiological Science 1960–1964" folder; Shih Yi Wang, ed., *Photochemistry and Photobiology of Nucleic Acids*, 2 vols. (Elsevier, 1976).

17. 1962–63 Report of the Dean of the JHSPH; Milton S. Eisenhower to Henry T. Heald, July 22, 1963, Records of the Office of the JHU President, series 6, box 10, "Ford Foundation—Grant Application" folder; JHMI Radiological Science, June 7, 1963, press release; Roland F. Beers Jr., "Radiobiological Research," NIH grant application, May 14, 1962, "Radiological Science 1960–1964" folder.

18. Henry Wagner, *A Personal History of Nuclear Medicine* (Springer, 2006), 2–6, 14, 69, 107, 120–21, 135.

19. Wagner, *A Personal History of Nuclear Medicine*, 14, 69, 107, 120–21, 135; John G. McAfee, "Nuclear Instrumentation and Chemistry in Medicine," NIH research grant proposal, Mar. 7, 1962, "Radiological Science 1960–1964" folder.

20. McAfee, "Nuclear Instrumentation and Chemistry in Medicine."

21. Ibid.; Wagner, *A Personal History of Nuclear Medicine*.

22. McAfee, "Nuclear Instrumentation and Chemistry in Medicine."

23. Ibid.

24. Daniel M. Wilner, *Housing Environment and Family Life: A Longitudinal Study of the Effects of Housing on Morbidity and Mental Health* (Johns Hopkins Press, 1962).

25. Daniel Wilner bio file, AMC; Samuel Kelton Roberts, *Infectious Fear*, 202.

26. C. W. Krusé and Abel Wolman, "A Memorandum on the Modern Scope of Environmental Hygiene," Feb. 4, 1957, CREOSHPH binder.

27. Mullan, *Plagues and Politics*, 102, 121; Milazzo, *Unlikely Environmentalists*, 90–99, 108–11.

28. Linda Lear, *Rachel Carson: Witness for Nature* (Henry Holt, 1997).

29. 1960–61 Report of the JHSPH Dean, *JHU Circular* (1962), 92.

30. Cornelius Krusé, "Notes on Reorganization of the Department of Sanitary Engineering, School of Hygiene and Public Health," 1957, "Environmental Health" folder.

31. JHU Trustees minutes, June 5, 1961, 4870–71; 1960–61 Report of the JHSPH Dean, *JHU Circular* (1962), 94; Richard L. Riley, handwritten memo, Sept. 11, 1968, and Cornelius W. Krusé to Aftim Acra, Jan. 10, 1967, "Environmental Health" folder.

32. Syllabus, "Environmental Health 3: Municipal Sanitation," 1967, "Environmental Health" folder; C. W. Krusé, K. Kawata, V. P. Olivieri, and K. E. Longley, "Improvement in Terminal Disinfection of Sewage Effluents," *Water and Sewage Works* 120.6 (1973), 57–64; National Research Council Board on Toxicology and Environmental Health Hazards, *Drinking Water and Health*, vol. 2 (Washington, DC: National Academies Press, 1980).

33. Krusé CV; Kazuyoshi Kawata to Elizabeth Fee, June 11, 1988, Elizabeth Fee papers, "Sanitary Engineering" folder.

34. "pathobiology, n." OED Online, September 2015 (http://www.oed.com/view /Entry/260634, accessed Sept. 27, 2015); Robert D. Cardiff, Jerrold M. Ward, and Stephen W. Barthold, " 'One Medicine—One Pathology': Are Veterinary and Human Pathology Prepared?" *Laboratory Investigation* (2008) 88, 18–26.

35. Arnold Rich to Lewis H. Weed, Feb. 12, 1946, Lewis Weed papers, Correspondence series, Organization and Policy Committee Nov 1945–Jan 1946 folder, AMC.

36. Fee, *Disease and Discovery*, 104–9, 127–29; W. W. Cort, "The Development of the Subject of Helminthology in the SHPH of the Johns Hopkins University," 1939, 3a D.O. Correspondence, box 502103, "Department Reports (Helminthology)" folder.

37. Justin M. Andrews, "A Simple Method for the Devocalization of Dogs," *Science*, New Series, Vol. 64, No. 1664 (Nov. 19, 1926), 502–3; Frances Burman interview, July 31, 2012.

38. Turner, *Heritage of Excellence*, 543; JHSPH Advisory Board Minutes, Oct. 18, 1950, p. 474; "Dog Referendum Battle is Won," *AJPH* 41 (Feb. 1951), 181.

39. For an in-depth look at the Vertebrate Ecology program, see Edmund Ramsden, "Rats, Stress and the Built Environment," *History of the Human Sciences* 25 (2012), 123–47.

40. Paul V. Lemkau to Thomas Turner, Mar. 9, 1956, Turner papers, box 50564, "Curriculum Committee Background Material" folder; Shonick, *Government and Health* Services, 426.

41. Turner, *Heritage of Excellence*, 543; David E. Davis and W. T. Fales, "The Distribution of Rats in Baltimore, Maryland," *American Journal of Hygiene* 49.3 (May 1949), 247–54; Edmund Ramsden and Jon Adams, "Escaping the Laboratory: The Rodent Experiments of John B. Calhoun and Their Cultural Influence," *Journal of Social History* 42.3 (2009), 761–92; Rozeboom, *History of Medical Zoology at JHSPH*, 83–87. Davis served as assistant dean from 1957 until 1960, when he left Hopkins and the Division of Vertebrate Ecology was transferred to Mental Hygiene to become the Division of Animal Behavior.

42. PHS Bureau of State Services, Office of Resource Development (Environmental Health), "Institutes for Environmental Health Studies: A Preliminary Guide to the Development of University-Based and Administered Interdisciplinary Research and Training Activities," April 1964, 1–3 (emphasis added), "Department of Environmental Health" folder.

43. PHS Bureau of State Services, Office of Resource Development (Environmental Health), "Institutes for Environmental Health Studies," 4.

44. Hochschild, Kohn Collection, Maryland Historical Society, box 4, "Penguins" folder; Ethel Poplovski, Aug. 21, 2008, interview; Mark Birkalien, "Remembering Christmastime at the Old Eastpoint Shopping Center," Dec. 18, 2010, Dundalk.Patch.com; JHU Treasurer's Reports, 1960–64, 1970, 1975, 1980; Milazzo, *Unlikely Environmentalists*, 96.

45. William J. L. Sladen to Milton S. Eisenhower, May 13, 1966, Records of the Office of the President, series 6, box 13, "Hygiene-General (1966)" folder, JHU Hamburger Archives; Tom Horton, "Geese's Movie Careers Take Flight: Scientist Dr. William J. L. Sladen Is Director of Environmental Studies at the Airlie Sanctuary in Virginia, Home to Several of the Geese That Star in the Movie 'Fly Away Home,'" *Baltimore Sun*, Sept. 6, 1996.

46. 1971–72 JHSPH Catalog, 35; Rozeboom, *Medical Zoology at the JHSPH*; Charles Rohde interview, Jan. 10, 2012.

47. Charles Rohde interview, Dec. 29, 2011.

48. Rohde interview, Jan. 10, 2012.

49. Russell H. Morgan to Ernest L. Stebbins, May 26, 1964, box 504582, "Department of Environmental Health" folder.

50. Noreen M. Clark, "Population Health and the Environment," in T. J. Goehl, ed., *Essays on the Future of Environmental Health Research: A Tribute to Dr. Kenneth Olden* (Environmental Health Perspectives/National Institute of Environmental Health Sciences, 2005), 142; Bernard D. Goldstein, "NIEHS and Public Health Practice," in Goehl, *Essays on the Future of Environmental Health Research*, 80–89.

51. John C. Snyder, "The Harvard School of Public Health and the Future," 3a: D.O. Correspondence, box 506162, "Harvard Univ. School of Public Health 1959–66" folder, pp. 9, 12.

52. University of North Carolina at Chapel Hill School of Public Health Catalogs, 1959–60 (p. 35) and 1968–69 (pp. 41–42); Korstad, *Dreaming of a Time*, 111; 1970–71 JH-SPH Catalog; B. D. Goldstein, M. Robson, and C. Botnick, "Size Characteristics of Larger Academic Human Environmental Health Programs in the United States," *Environmental Health Perspectives* 106.10 (1998), 615–17.

53. Hollander, *Abel Wolman: His Life and Philosophy*, 206–7; National Research Council Commission on Life Sciences, *Asbestiform Fibers: Nonoccupational Health Risks* (National Academies Press, 1984); J. R. Millette, P. J. Clark, and M. F. Pansing, *Exposure to Asbestos from Drinking Water in the United States* (EPA, 1979).

54. Hollander, *Abel Wolman: His Life and Philosophy*, 206–7; "Andrew J. Rhodes," Canadian Public Health Association CPHA100 (http://cpha100.ca/history/profiles-public-health/rhodes, accessed June 29, 2011); Tulley Long, "The Hybrid Profession: Themes and Tensions in the Development of Sanitary Engineering in the United States, 1850–1970," Aug. 2008, unpublished manuscript; Shonick, *Government and Health Services*, 61–64.

55. Norton Nelson and Morton Lippman, "Organizational Relationships of Schools of Public Health with Schools of Engineering," in John Z. Bowers and Elizabeth F. Purcell, eds., *Schools of Public Health: Present and Future* (Josiah Macy Jr. Foundation, 1974), 24–28; APHA–ASPH Joint Advisory Committee, *Interim Handbook for Accreditation of Schools of Public Health* (Sept. 1972), and Raymond Seltser to Bernard C. Greenberg, Aug. 22, 1977, Records of the University of North Carolina Division of Health Affairs, School of Public Health, Subgroup 1: Administrative Files, Series 2: Office of the Dean, Subseries 1: General Files, box 1:3, "Committees: Core Curriculum Committee Task Force 1974–75" folder, University of North Carolina at Chapel Hill University Archives.

56. C. W. Krusé to E. L. Stebbins, Dec. 10, 1956, Ernest L. Stebbins to Abel Wolman, cc Cornelius Krusé, July 14, 1960, William H. Stewart to Cornelius W. Krusé, July 5, 1962, "Department of Environmental Health" folder; Oscar Sutermeister to Ernest L. Stebbins, Mar. 20, 1963, Anna M. Baetjer to Ernest L. Stebbins, Nov. 18, 1963, box 504582, "Environmental Medicine Anna M. Baetjer" folder.

57. Paul Charles Milazzo, *Unlikely Environmentalists: Congress and Clean Water, 1945–1972* (University Press of Kansas, 2006), 48–50; Hollander, *Abel Wolman: His Life and Philosophy*, 205–10, 310–11, 644; National Research Council Commission on Life Sciences, *Asbestiform Fibers: Nonoccupational Health Risks* (National Academies Press, 1984); J. R. Millette, P. J. Clark, and M. F. Pansing, *Exposure to Asbestos from Drinking Water in the United States* (EPA, 1979).

58. Solbert Permutt, PHS Research Career grant application, Apr. 16, 1963, box 504582, "Environmental Medicine" folder; C. W. Krusé and Abel Wolman, "A Memorandum on the Modern Scope of Environmental Hygiene," Feb. 4, 1957, CREOSHPH binder.

59. Richard L. Riley bio file, AMC; Richard L. Riley, "The Health Effects of Air Pollution," *Transactions of the Studies of the College of Physicians of Philadelphia* 35 (1968), 144–48; Richard L. Riley, "Airborne Infection in a Space Capsule," paper presented at National Academy of Science conference, Woods Hole, July 1966.

60. "Site Visit Air Hygiene Program AP 00424," 22; Richard L. Riley, "Cardiopulmonary Physiology in Bronchial Asthma," PHS R01 grant application, Feb. 1, 1964, "Environmental Medicine" folder.

61. Donald F. Proctor bio file; D. F. Proctor, "Irradiation for the Elimination of Nasopharyngeal Lymphoid Tissue," *Archives of Otolaryngology* 43 (1946), 473–80; W. Willard and D. F. Proctor, "Results and Problems after Four Years of a Conservation of Hearing Program," *AJPH* 38 (1948), 1424–33; D. F. Proctor, L. M. Polovogt, and S. J. Crowe, "Irradiation of Lymphoid Tissue in Diseases of the Upper Respiratory Tract," *Bulletin of the Johns Hopkins Hospital* 83 (1948), 383–428; D. F. Proctor, "Irradiation of the Nasopharynx and the Prevention of Deafness," *Annals of Otolaryngology* 58 (1949), 825–37.

62. James Conant, "Gas Autos Must Go, Says Pollution Expert," *News-American*, Nov. 15, 1967; William J. Perkinson, "Hopkins Professor Says Pollution Poses 4-Prong Threat to Health, Way of Life," *Baltimore Sun*, Nov. 13, 1968; Elaine Stamper, "Asarco Expert Not Worried by Emissions," *El Paso Times*, Jan. 28, 1982.

63. Donald F. Proctor, David L. Swift, Michael Quinlan, Salah Salman, Yasushi Takagi, and Sandra Evering, "The Nose and Man's Atmospheric Environment," *Archives of Environmental Health* 18 (Apr. 1969), 671–80.

64. Richard L. Riley bio file.

65. Goldstein, "NIEHS and Public Health Practice"; Bernard D. Goldstein, "The Need to Restore the Public Health Base for Environmental Control," *AJPH* 85 (1995), 481–83; Baetjer, "Effects of Temperature and Humidity on Respiratory Virus Infections."

66. Anna M. Baetjer, "Body Water and Toxicity of Organic Chemicals," PHS R01 research grant proposal, Oct. 1, 1965, "Environmental Medicine Anna M. Baetjer" folder.

67. Anna M. Baetjer, "Effects of Temperature and Humidity on Respiratory Virus Infections," PHS R01 research grant proposal, Oct. 16, 1962, "Environmental Medicine Anna M. Baetjer" folder; D. F. Swift and D. F. Proctor, "Aerosol Research at the Johns Hopkins School of Hygiene," *Journal of the Air Pollution Control Association* 18 (1968), 675 (abstr.); McAfee, "Nuclear Instrumentation and Chemistry in Medicine."

68. Robert J. Rubin Bio File, AMC.

69. Rudolph J. Jaeger and Robert J. Rubin, "Plasticizers from Plastic Devices: Extraction Metabolism and Accumulation by Biological Systems," *Science* 170 (1970), 460–62; Jaeger and Rubin, "Migration of a Phthalate Ester Plasticizer from Polyvinylchloride Blood Bags into Stored Human Blood and Its Localization in Human Tissues," *New England Journal of Medicine* 287 (1972), 1114–18; Frederick P. McGehan, "Hopkins Researcher Finds A Possible Plastic Danger," *Baltimore Sun*, Feb. 5, 1971; Mary Knudson, "Plastic Blood Storage Bags Too Dangerous to Use, Johns Hopkins Researcher Believes," *Baltimore Sun*, May 28, 1975.

70. W. J. Kozumbo, R. Kroll, and R. J. Rubin, "Assessment of the Mutagenicity of Phthalate Esters," *Environmental Health Perspectives* 45 (1982), 103–9; National Toxicology Program, "National Toxicology Program 1982: Carcinogenesis Bioassay of Di-(2-ethylhexyl)

phthalate (CAS No. 117-81-7) in F344 Rats and B6C3F, Mice (Feed Study)," NTP Technical Reports Series TR No. 217 (NTP, 1982); EPA Integrated Risk Information System (IRIS) entry for DEHP (http://www.epa.gov/iris/subst/0014.htm#carc, accessed June 29, 2011); FDA Center for Devices and Radiological Health, *Safety Assessment of Di(2-ethylhexyl) phthalate (DEHP) Released from PVC Medical Devices* (2009) (http://www.fda.gov/downloads /MedicalDevices/DeviceRegulationandGuidance/GuidanceDocuments/UCM080457.pdf, accessed June 29, 2011), 3, 15, 22; "DEHP in Plastic Medical Devices" (http://www.fda.gov /MedicalDevices/ResourcesforYou/Consumers/ChoosingaMedicalDevice/ucm142643.htm, accessed June 29, 2011).

71. Alan Goldberg interview, Mar. 9, 2012.

72. Alan Goldberg and Ellen K. Silbergeld, Dec. 12, 2014 interview (Silbergeld quotes).

73. Goldberg and Silbergeld interview, Dec. 12, 2014.

74. Goldberg and Silbergeld interview, Dec. 12, 2014 (Silbergeld quote); Goldberg interview, Mar. 9, 2012; E. K. Silbergeld, J. Fales, and A. M. Goldberg, "Lead: Evidence for a Presynaptic Effect on Neuromuscular Function," *Nature* 247 (1974), 49–50; E. K. Silbergeld and A.M. Goldberg, "Hyperactivity: A Lead-Induced Behavior Disorder," *Environmental Health Perspectives* 7 (1974), 227.

75. Ellen K. Silbergeld faculty page (http://www.jhsph.edu/faculty/directory/profile /3806/ellen-silbergeld, accessed Oct. 1, 2015); Goldstein, "NIEHS and Public Health Practice," 82.

76. Ernest M. Gruenberg and J. A. Muir Gray, "The Future of Community Medicine," *The Lancet* 308.7979 (July 31, 1976), 262–63.

77. Bernard D. Goldstein, "NIEHS and Public Health Practice," 82; Bernard D. Goldstein, "The Need to Restore the Public Health Base for Environmental Control," *AJPH* 85 (1995), 481–83.

78. Gareth M. Green to Wolman, Lilienfeld, Billings, Kimball, Goodman, Hume, and Baker, June 28, 1978, Abraham Lilienfeld papers, box 503587, "Correspondence— Appointments to Committees" folder.

Chapter 11 · Chronic Disease Epidemiology

1. JHSPH Catalog 1956–57; Abraham Lilienfeld and George Comstock bio files, AMC.

2. Cook-Deegan and McGeary, "The Jewel in the Federal Crown?" 184; Jack C. Haldeman, memo to division chiefs of the Bureau of State Services, Mar. 27, 1957, "Research in Nursing" folder, box 3, USPHS Records, RG 90, NC3-90-79-1, Selected Files of the Division of Nursing.

3. Bernard L. Harlow, "A Conversation with Henry Blackburn," *Epidemiology* 19 (May 2008), 513–17.

4. Ernest L. Stebbins, "Foreword," in Abraham L. Lilienfeld and Alice J. Gifford, eds., *Chronic Diseases and Public Health* (Johns Hopkins Press, 1966), vii; Brandt, *The Cigarette Century*, 150; Lewis C. Robbins, "The Public Health Service's Program in Cancer Control," *Public Health Reports* 76.4 (Apr. 1961), 341–43.

5. Morgan quoted in "An Account of Activities at The Johns Hopkins University and Hospital Directed toward a Solution of the Cancer Problem," undated c. 1953, Joint Committee on Cancer Teaching and Research subject files, folder 1, AMC, 5; Application to the Kellogg Foundation for continuation of A Grant for Research in Administration at the Johns Hopkins University School of Hygiene and Public Health," May 17, 1962, "W. H.

Kellogg Found." Folder; November, *Biomedical Computing*, 196–97; Nancy Mueller, Alfred Evans, Nancy L. Harris, George W. Comstock, Egil Jellum, Knut Magnus, Norman Orentreich, B. Frank Polk, and Joseph Vogelman, "Hodgkin's Disease and Epstein-Barr Virus," *New England Journal of Medicine* 320 (1989), 689–95.

6. "1958–59 Report of the Director of the JHSPH," *JHU Circular* 78 (Nov. 1959), 83; 1960–61 JHU Treasurer's Report, 84; 1958–59 JHSPH Catalog, 44–45; "Subject-Matter Outline for Chronic Disease Items," revision I, Aug. 1, 1961, 3a D.O. Correspondence, box 504582, "Department of Chronic Diseases 1961–1965" folder, AMC.

7. Jacques Kelly, "Bernice H. Cohen," *Baltimore Sun*, Apr. 18, 2011; Bernice H. Cohen bio file, AMC; Bernice H. Cohen to Milton S. Eisenhower, Jan. 17, 1966, Records of the Office of the President, series 6, box 13, "Hygiene-General (1966)" folder, JHU Hamburger Archives.

8. Department of Biostatistics 1964–65 Annual Report, 1; Bernice H. Cohen, Abraham M. Lilienfeld, and P. C. Huang, eds., *Genetic Issues in Public Health and Medicine* (Springfield, IL: Charles C Thomas, 1978), xiii.

9. David E. Lilienfeld, personal communication, Apr. 28, 2012; A. M. Lilienfeld and E. A. Johnson, "The Age Distribution in Female Breast and Genital Cancers," *Cancer* 8 (1955), 875–82; A. M. Lilienfeld, M. Levin, and G. E. Moore, "The Association of Smoking with Cancer of the Urinary Bladder in Humans," *Archives of Internal Medicine* 98 (1956), 129–35; A. M. Lilienfeld, "Emotional and Other Selected Characteristics of Cigarette Smokers and Nonsmokers as Related to Epidemiological Studies of Lung Cancer and Other Diseases," *Journal of the National Cancer Institute* 22 (1959), 259–82.

10. A. M. Lilienfeld, "Epidemiologic Method of Cancer Research," *Journal of Chronic Diseases* 8 (1958), 649–54; J. Cornfield, W. Haenszel, E. C. Hammond, A. M. Lilienfeld, M. B. Shimkin, and E. L. Wynder, "Smoking and Lung Cancer: Recent Evidence and a Discussion of Some Questions," *Journal of the National Cancer Institute* 22 (1959), 173–203; J. Cornfield and W. Haenszel, "Some Aspects of Retrospective Studies," *Journal of Chronic Diseases* 11 (1960), 523–34; Samuel W. Greenhouse, "Jerome Cornfield's Contributions to Epidemiology," *Biometrics* 38 (1982), 33–45.

11. Leroy E. Burney, "Smoking and Lung Cancer," *JAMA* (Nov. 28, 1959), 1829–37; Dennis L. Breo, "The Unsung Public Health Hero Who Helped Launch the War on Tobacco," *JAMA* 264.12 (1990), 1597–98; *Smoking and Health* (1964); Brandt, *The Cigarette Century*, 150, 226–30; Levin bio file; John C. Hume to N. Franklin, June 4, 1969, records of the Office of the JHU President, series 9, box 32, "Hygiene-Advisory Board 1969" folder; F. A. Stillman et al., "Ending Smoking at the Johns Hopkins Medical Institutions: An Evaluation of Smoking Prevalence and Indoor Air Pollution," *JAMA* 264 (1990), 1565–69.

12. Margaret Bright interview, Aug. 16, 2011; David Celentano interview, August 9, 2011.

13. Bright interview, Aug. 16, 2011; 1961–62 JHSPH Catalog, 73; George D. Miller bio file, AMC; George D. Miller and Lewis H. Kuller, "Trends in Mortality from Stroke in Baltimore, Maryland: 1940–1941 through 1968–1969," *American Journal of Epidemiology* 98.4 (1973), 233–42.

14. Department of Epidemiology 1958 Annual Report, 3a D.O. Correspondence, box 505348, "President's Report 1958" folder.

15. N. E. Aronson, M. Santosham, G. W. Comstock, et al., "Long-Term Efficacy of BCG Vaccine in American Indians and Alaska Natives: A 60-Year Follow-Up Study," *JAMA* 291 (2004), 2086–91.

16. Marie Diener-West interview, Feb. 25, 2013; Frances Burman interview, July 31, 2012.

17. Philip E. Sartwell and George W. Comstock, "Factors Associated with Participation in a Cervical Cytology Screening Program," in "Annual Report to the American Cancer Society from the Joint Committee on Cancer Teaching and Research of the Johns Hopkins Medical Institutions," 1965, Joint Committee on Cancer Teaching and Research subject file, folder 1, AMC.

18. "Nice Guys Finish Last," *Time* 97.3 (Jan. 18, 1971), 63; Knud J. Helsing and Moyses Szklo, "Mortality after Bereavement," *American Journal of Epidemiology* 114 (1981), 41–52; Knud J. Helsing, Moyses Szklo, and George W. Comstock, "Factors Associated with Mortality after Widowhood," *AJPH* 71 (1981), 802–9; Knud J. Helsing, George W. Comstock, and Moyses Szklo, "Causes of Death in a Widowed Population," *American Journal of Epidemiology* 116 (1982), 524–32.

19. Abraham M. Lilienfeld, unpublished manuscript for opening chapter, "An Overview of the Epidemiology of Cancer," in David L. Levin, ed., *Cancer Epidemiology in the USA and USSR* (GPO, 1980), box 503619, "Correspondence—Epidemiology US–USSR Joint Conference" folder, p. 4.

20. "Campaign against Cancer Investigates Hormone Role," JHSPH *In Brief* (Winter–Spring 1975); G. W. Comstock, "Serum 25-Hydroxyvitamin D and Colon Cancer: Eight-Year Prospective Study," *Lancet* 2.8673 (1989), 1176–78; Gina Kolata, "A New Kind of Epidemiology," *Science* 224.4648 (May 4, 1984), 481; A. S. Evans and George W. Comstock, "Presence of Elevated Antibody Titres to Epstein-Barr Virus before Hodgkin's Disease," *Lancet* 1.8231 (1981), 1183–86; Mueller et al., "Hodgkin's Disease and Epstein-Barr Virus."

21. Jacques Kelly, "Philip E. Sartwell, 91, Noted Hopkins Epidemiologist," *Baltimore Sun*, Dec. 2, 1999; FDA Advisory Committee on Obstetrics and Gynecology, "Report on Intrauterine Contraceptive Devices," 1968; FDA Advisory Committee on Obstetrics and Gynecology, "Report on Oral Contraceptives," 1966; P. E. Sartwell, Alfonse T. Masi, Federico G. Arthes, Gerald R. Greene, and Helen E. Smith, "Thromboembolism and Oral Contraceptives: An Epidemiologic Case-Control Study," *American Journal of Epidemiology* 90 (1969), 365–80; Gerald R. Greene and P. E. Sartwell, "Oral Contraceptive Use in Patients with Thromboembolism following Surgery, Trauma, or Infection," *AJPH* 62 (May 1972), 680; *NBC Evening News*, Jan. 20, 1970, broadcast; P. E. Sartwell, "Studies in Iatrogenic Disease," presentation at JHH (undated, c. 1972), Sartwell bio file (quotes).

22. J. Tonascia, L. Gordis, and H. Schmerler, "Retrospective Evidence Favoring Use of Anticoagulants for Myocardial Infarctions," *New England Journal of Medicine* 292 (1975), 1362–66.

23. Moyses Szklo interview, Oct. 19, 2011; Leon Gordis bio file, AMC; JHMI press release, Sept. 1, 1980.

24. Alfonse T. Masi, Philip E. Sartwell, and Lawrence E. Shulman, "The Use of Record Linkage to Determine Familial Occurrence of Disease from Hospital Records (Hashimoto's Disease)," *AJPH* 54.11 (1964) 1887–94; Alfonse T. Masi, "Potential Uses and Limitations

of Hospital Data in Epidemiologic Research," *AJPH* 55.5 (1965), 658–67; Alan M. Gittelsohn bio file, AMC; Alan Gittelsohn, "Tabulation of Vital Records by Computer," *Public Health Reports* 79.10 (1964), 895–904; Alan M. Gittelsohn, "An Information System for Vital Statistics," NIH research grant application, Dec. 23, 1964, 3a Dean's Office correspondence, box 504582, "Biostatistics" folder.

25. November, *Biomedical Computing*, 80–81. Humphrey was influenced by Robert S. Ledley, a former employee at the Johns Hopkins Operations Research Office, who became a leading advocate for computerizing biomedicine, and he may have also interacted with Russell Morgan and Alan Gittelsohn. See Ledley, "Digital Electronic Computers in Biomedical Science," *Science* 130 (Nov. 6, 1959), 1225.

26. Gittelsohn, "An Information System for Vital Statistics."

27. Ibid.

28. Alan M. Gittelsohn, "On the Distribution of Underlying Causes of Death," *AJPH* 72 (1982), 133–40.

29. James Tonascia bio file, AMC; David Celentano interview, August 9, 2011.

30. Celentano interview.

31. Department of Biostatistics Self-Study, Apr. 26, 1978, 3a D.O. Correspondence, box 504582/R111F5, "Committee to Review the Department of Biostatistics" folder, AMC.

32. Paul Brodeur, "Microwaves I," *The New Yorker*, Dec. 13, 1976, 50–110; Paul Brodeur, "Microwaves II," *The New Yorker*, Dec. 20, 1976, 43–83; Statement of William M. Watson to the US House Committee on Appropriations, Subcommittee on State, Justice, Commerce, and Judiciary Appropriations, 95th Cong., 2nd sess. (1978), Hearings on Departments of State, Justice, and Commerce, the Judiciary, and Related Agencies Appropriations for 1979. Part 2: Department of State. Feb. 15, 16, 21, 22, 1978, pp. 432–44; US Senate Committee on Foreign Relations, Hearings on S. 489, Nomination of Richard M. Moose as Deputy Under Secretary of State for Management, 95th Cong., 1st sess. (1977), Mar. 8, 1977, pp. 4–6.

33. "Did Russian Microwaves Harm U.S. Embassy Staff," *SHPH In Brief* newsletter Feb. 1979; *CBS Evening News*, June 27, 1977, and Nov. 20, 1978, broadcasts.

34. Lilienfeld correspondence with Devra Lee Davis in Lilienfeld papers, box 503587, "Correspondence-D Miscellaneous" folder; Christopher Rosen, "Paul Brodeur: I Never Said That Microwaves Take Nutrients Out of Food, Despite 'American Hustle,'" *Huffington Post*, Jan. 7, 2014 (http://www.huffingtonpost.com/2014/01/07/american-hustle-paul -brodeur_n_4555403.html, accessed Nov. 9, 2015); World Health Organization International Agency for Research on Cancer, "IARC Classifies Radiofrequency Electromagnetic Fields as Possibly Carcinogenic to Humans," press release, May 30, 2011 (http://www.iarc .fr/en/media-centre/pr/2011/pdfs/pr208_E.pdf, accessed Nov. 10, 2015); National Cancer Institute, "Cell Phones and Cancer Risk" (http://www.cancer.gov/about-cancer/causes -prevention/risk/radiation/cell-phones-fact-sheet#q5, accessed Nov. 15, 2015).

35. World Health Organization, "What is Ionizing Radiation" (http://www.who.int /ionizing_radiation/about/what_is_ir/en, accessed Nov. 10, 2015); US Nuclear Regulatory Commission website (http://www.nrc.gov/reading-rm/doc-collections/fact-sheets/3mile -isle.html, accessed Nov. 10, 2015); *NBC Evening News*, July 17, 1974, broadcast; Carmel McCoubrey, "Edward Radford, 79, Scholar of the Risks from Radiation," *New York Times*, Oct. 22, 2001, website accessed Nov. 9, 2015.

36. R. Seltser and P. E. Sartwell, "Ionizing Radiation and Longevity of Physicians," *JAMA* 166 (1958), 585–87; R. Seltser and P. E. Sartwell, "The Application of Cohort Analysis to the Study of Ionizing Radiation and Longevity in Physicians," *AJPH* 49 (1959), 1610–20; R. Seltser and P. E. Sartwell, "Mortality and Occupational Exposure to Radiation," *JAMA* 190 (1964), 1046; G. M. Matanoski, R. Seltser, P. E. Sartwell, et al., "The Current Mortality Rates of Radiologists and Other Physician Specialists: Deaths from All Causes and from Cancer," *American Journal of Epidemiology* 101.3 (1975), 188–98; G. M. Matanoski, R. Seltser, P. E. Sartwell, et al., "The Current Mortality Rates of Radiologists and Other Physician Specialists: Specific Causes of Death," *American Journal of Epidemiology* 101.3 (1975), 199–210; Irvin D. J. Bross, "Mindless Use of Technology: Genetic Damage from Low-Level Radiation," 1976, Lilienfeld papers, box 503587, "Correspondence—Bross, Irwin and Dean" folder; Terrell Tannen, "Obituary: Irving D. J. Bross," 364 (October 2, 2004), 1212.

37. November, *Biomedical Computing*, 197; Brandt, "The Syphilis Epidemic and Its Relation to AIDS"; Lilienfeld, "An Overview of the Epidemiology of Cancer," 4.

38. Bross, "Mindless Use of Technology: Genetic Damage from Low-Level Radiation"; Barron Lerner, *The Breast Cancer Wars: Hope, Fear, and the Pursuit of a Cure in Twentieth-Century America* (Oxford University Press, 2003), 244–45; Kevin C. Oeffinger et al., "Breast Cancer Screening for Women at Average Risk: 2015 Guideline Update from the American Cancer Society," *JAMA* 314.15 (Oct. 22, 2015), 1599–614.

39. Abraham M. Lilienfeld, "The Problem of Weak Associations in Epidemiology," draft Aug. 7, 1980, Lilienfeld papers, box 503586, "Correspondence-American Health Foundation" folder; Lilienfeld, "An Overview of the Epidemiology of Cancer," quote pp. 1–2 (emphasis added).

40. Lilienfeld, "An Overview of the Epidemiology of Cancer," 3–7.

41. John R. Wilkins and George W. Comstock, "Source of Drinking Water at Home and Site-Specific Cancer Incidence in Washington County, Maryland," *American Journal of Epidemiology* 14.2 (1981), 178–90.

42. George W. Comstock, "Water Hardness and Cardiovascular Diseases," *American Journal of Epidemiology* 110.4 (Oct. 1979), 375–400 (first quote p. 375, second quote p. 385); Abel Wolman to David A. Hamburg, Abel Wolman papers, Series 5, box 4, "Cardiovascular Diseases–Dr. Comstock" folder, JHU Hamburger Archives.

43. Hollander, *Abel Wolman*, 206–7.

44. Ibid., 206–7; Judith Randal, "New Directions and Dilemmas for NIH," *Change* 9.12 (Dec. 1977), 51–52.

45. Goldstein, "NIEHS and Public Health Practice," 86–87.

46. Ibid., 85.

47. Maryalice Yakutchik, "Two Friends, 40 Years, and One Fresh Cancer Prevention," *Johns Hopkins Public Health Magazine*, Fall 2014; Maryalice Yakutchik, "The Virus That Owns the World," *Johns Hopkins Public Health Magazine*, Spring 2013; Goldstein, "NIEHS and Public Health Practice," 85.

Chapter 12 · Federal Funding and Its Discontents

1. Milton S. Eisenhower, "The Future of Johns Hopkins," *Johns Hopkins Magazine* 8.7 (Apr. 1957), 6–11, first quote p. 11; 1949–50 Report of the JHU Treasurer; 1964–65 Report of the JHU Treasurer, 6–7; and 1965–66 Report of the JHU Treasurer, 24–25; JHU Board of Trustees Executive Committee minutes, Feb. 6, 1961, 4808 (second quote).

2. Thomas L. Hall, Rudolph S. Jackson, and William B. Parsons, *Schools of Public Health: Trends in Graduate Education* (Association of Schools of Public Health, 1980), 29; US Senate Committee on Labor and Human Resources, "Formula Grants to Schools of Public Health," 91st Cong., 1st sess. (1969), 14; Joel D. Howell, "Lowell T. Coggeshall and American Medical Education: 1901–1987," *Academic Medicine* 67 (Nov. 1992), 713–15; Shonick, *Government and Health Services*, 375–402; "Minutes of Annual Meeting, Association of Schools of Public Health, Montreal, Canada," May 8–10, 1967, 3a D.O. Correspondence, box 504579, "ASPH-General—1966–1967" folder, pp. 15, 19, 24; 1967–68 Report of the Dean of the JHSPH, 51.

3. Stephen P. Strickland, *The Story of the NIH Grants Programs* (University Press of America, 1989), 77–80; Shonick, *Government and Health Services*, 99.

4. "A Ten-Year Plan for the School of Hygiene and Public Health," 2.

5. Ibid., draft Feb. 1969; John C. Hume to Paul E. White, July 26, 1976, 3a D.O. Correspondence, box R111F4, "Committee to Reexamine Organization of Research and Teaching of Administration in the School 7/76" folder.

6. National Center for Education Statistics, *Earned Degrees Conferred: Analysis of Trends, 1965–66 through 1974–75* (US Department of Health, Education and Welfare, 1977), 19–21; James L. Troupin, "Graduate Education in Public Health," *JAMA* 214.8 (Nov. 23, 1970), 1536; James L. Troupin, "Graduate Education in Public Health," *JAMA* 210.8 (Nov. 24, 1969), 1529; Troupin, "Graduate Education in Public Health," *JAMA* 238.26 (Dec. 26, 1977), 2826.

7. Smillie, "Training of Public Health Personnel," 455; 1970–71 Report of the Dean of the JHSPH; Johns Hopkins University School of Public Health Registrar's Office; School of Hygiene and Public Health 1983 planning document, 1.

8. Hall, Jackson, and Parsons, *Schools of Public Health: Trends in Graduate Education*, 22–23; Troupin, "Graduate Education in Public Health," *JAMA* (1969), 1531; James L. Troupin, "Graduate Education in Public Health," *JAMA* 234.13 (Dec. 29, 1975), 1398–99; Association of Schools of Public Health, *Schools of Public Health: Educational Data Project 1974–1979* (US Department of Health and Human Services, 1980), 17; Elaine K. Freeman, "Issues of Identity," *Johns Hopkins Magazine*, Fall 2008, 18–19.

9. Hall, Jackson, and Parsons, "Appendix II. Graduate Degrees Awarded by Schools of Public Health by Type of Degree, Sex, and Nationality, 1930–1931 to 1978–1979," *Schools of Public Health: Trends in Graduate Education*, 50; Goldberg and Silbergeld interview, Dec. 12, 2014.

10. US Department of Education, Office of Educational Research and Improvement, *Digest of Education Statistics, 1999* (US Department of Education, 2000), Table 249: Earned Degrees Conferred by Institutions of Higher Education, by Level of Degree and Sex of Student: 1869–70 to 2008–09; Table 294: Earned Degrees in the Health Professions and Related Sciences, by Level of Degree and Sex of Student: 1970–71 to 1996–97; and Table 224: Bachelor's, Master's, and Doctor's Degrees Conferred by Institutions of Higher Education, by Sex of Student and Field of Study: 1987–88.

11. 1953–54 Report of the JHSPH Dean to the President, *JHU Circular* 73 (1954), 94.

12. Fee, *Disease and Discovery*, 63–64; William G. Cochran bio file, AMC; William Reinke interview, Feb. 2012; Alan Goldberg interview, Mar. 9, 2012; Charles Rohde interview, Dec. 29, 2011.

13. Allyn W. Kimball, 1966–67 NIH Division of General Medical Sciences training grant continuation application, 3a D.O. Correspondence, box 504582, "Biostatistics" folder; James Shannon, "The Place of the National Institutes of Health in American Medicine," *New England Journal of Medicine* 269 (1963), 1352–57.

14. Allyn W. Kimball bio file, AMC; Rohde interview, Dec. 29, 2011.

15. Alan Ross to John C. Hume, Sept. 30, 1975, 3a D.O. Correspondence, box 504582/ R111F5, "Allyn W. Kimball" folder; Department of Biostatistics Self-Study.

16. US House Committee on Interstate and Foreign Commerce Subcommittee on Health and the Environment, "Investigation of the National Institutes of Health," 94th Cong., 2nd sess. (GPO, 1976).

17. Frost, "The Importance of Epidemiology as a Function of Health Departments," 113–14; Abraham M. Lilienfeld, "Epidemiology and Health Policy: Some Historical Highlights," *Public Health Reports* 99.3 (1984), 237–41, quote p. 241.

18. W. Henry Mosley CV; "Mosley Heads Hopkins Population Department," *Baltimore Evening Sun*, Aug. 17, 1971; W. Henry Mosley interview, Oct. 27, 2010; Alfred Sommer, Moslemuddin Khan, and Wiley H. Mosley, "Efficacy of Vaccination of Family Contacts of Cholera Cases," *Lancet* (June 12, 1973), 1230–32; Alfred Sommer and Wiley H. Mosley, "Ineffectiveness of Cholera Vaccination as an Epidemic Control Measure," *Lancet* (June 12, 1973), 1232–35, quote p. 1232.

19. Mosley interview, Oct. 27, 2010; Alfred Sommer and Wiley H. Mosley, "East Bengal Cyclone of November 1970: Epidemiological Approach to Disaster Assessment," *Lancet* (May 13, 1972), 1029–36.

20. Alexander Langmuir to Wiley H. Mosley, Feb. 9, 1971, W. Henry Mosley papers, "Ross, Alan, chairman P.D.S.C." folder.

21. Envir Adil, testimony before the US Senate Committee on Labor and Public Welfare, Subcommittee on Health, in *Family Planning and Population Research, 1970* (GPO, 1970), 255–57; William Draper, testimony before the US Senate Committee on Labor and Public Welfare, Subcommittee on Health, in *Family Planning and Population Research, 1970,* 242.

22. R. T. Ravenholt, P. T. Piotrow, and J. J. Speidel, "Use of Oral Contraceptives: A Decade of Controversy," *International Journal of Gynecology and Obstetrics* 8.6 (1970) 2:941–56; Finding aid, Phyllis Piotrow Collection, AMC.

23. Harper, memo on Development in Physiology of Fertility Regulation at JHSPH Jan. 27, 1965, "Hygiene-Financial Reports, Personal Correspondence" folder; "Graduate Study in Population Dynamics," brochure undated c. 1970, Population Dynamics subject file, AMC; Larry L. Ewing to John C. Hume, Dec. 9, 1975, 3a D.O. Correspondence, box R111F6, "Public Health Administration" folder.

24. Quinquennial Report for the Division of Reproductive Biology, Department of Population Dynamics, July 1977–June 1982, Population Dynamics subject file.

25. JHU Board of Trustees Executive Committee minutes, Sept. 19, 1960, p. 4740; JHU Board of Trustees minutes, Oct. 3, 1960, p. 4752; Milton S. Eisenhower to Henry T. Heald, July 22, 1963, and Allocations of Ford Funds, Nov. 10, 1964, Records of the Office of the President, series 6, box 10, "Ford Foundation—Grant Application" folder, JHU Hamburger Archives.

26. George W. Comstock, July 10, 1994, travel diary, London and Belgium, Comstock papers.

27. William Bevan to Milton S. Eisenhower, June 9, 1967, Records of the Office of the President, series 6, box 13, "Hygiene-General (1967)" folder.

28. Alan Ross to John C. Hume, Feb. 18, 1975, and Claude Lenfant to John C. Hume, May 7, 1975, Records of the Office of the President, Series 14, box 17, "Office of the President 1972–82 Environmental Health Sciences 1973–75" folder, JHU Hamburger Archives.

29. Leon Gordis to Steven Muller, Sept. 20, 1976, and Leon Gordis to John Hume, Jan. 27, 1977, Records of the Office of the President, Series 14, box 17, "Office of the President 1972–82 Epidemiology, Dept. of 1973–78" folder, JHU Hamburger Archives.

30. "Current and Pending Research Support by Investigator," Apr. 14, 1980, Abraham Lilienfeld papers, box 503589, "Correspondence—Employee Records" folder, AMC.

31. Hume to Paul E. White, July 26, 1976.

32. Paul White interview, Sept. 8, 2011; Flagle interview, Sept. 29, 2010; "Report to the Policy Committee by the Ad Hoc Committee," May 11, 1976, "Committee to Reexamine Organization of Research and Teaching of Administration in the School 7/76" folder.

33. David E. Rogers to J. Glenn Beall Jr., July 23, 1971, "President's Office 1971–72 Office of Health Care Programs" folder.

34. Ibid.

35. John C. Hume to Harvey Fischman, May 5, 1971, "1975/76 University Affirmative Action Comm." folder and "Additions to the Affirmative Action Program of the Johns Hopkins University," Mar. 23, 1970, "Affirmative Action Program 1970" folder, in Records of the Office of the President, series 9, box 2; Richard T. Smith to W. Henry Mosley, Jan. 16, 1974, 3a D.O. Correspondence, box R111F4, "Affirmative Action" folder.

36. Minutes of the University Affirmative Action Committee, June 12, 1974, in "The Johns Hopkins University Affirmative Action Program Fifth Annual Status Report," Aug. 15, 1974, 3a D.O. Correspondence, box R111F4, "1975/76 University Affirmative Action Comm." folder; John C. Hume to Harvey Fischman, May 5, 1971.

37. "Hygiene General Assembly Notes," *Johns Hopkins Gazette*, Feb. 6, 1975; Barbara Starfield to John C. Hume, Apr. 26, 1974, 3a D.O. Correspondence, box R111F4, "Affirmative Action" folder.

38. Roger M. Herriott to John C. Hume, Jan. 14, 1974, and Barbara Starfield to Paul V. Lemkau, Apr. 26, 1974, "Affirmative Action" folder.

39. Carl Taylor to John Hume, Feb. 1, 1974, "Affirmative Action" folder.

40. Barbara Starfield to John C. Hume, Feb. 18, 1974, Apr. 9, 1974, "Affirmative Action" folder; Minutes of the JHSPH Policy Committee, Jan. 18, 1971, 3a D.O. Correspondence.

41. Lawrence W. Green, "The Johns Hopkins Extended M.P.H. Degree Program in Washington, D.C.," *Health Education Monographs* 3.3 (1975), 281–91.

42. Hall, Jackson, and Parsons, *Schools of Public Health: Trends in Graduate Education*, 29; Edgar E. Roulhac, "Report of Results: Student Opinions and Viewpoints," May 1975, 3a D.O. Correspondence, box R111F2 (old box 1b), "Report of Results—Minority Recruitment Committee" folder; Edgar E. Roulhac bio file, AMC.

43. Betty Addison interview, Sept. 5, 2008.

44. Shonick, *Government and Health Services*, 402; Daniel F. Whiteside, "Training the Nation's Health Manpower: The Next Four Years," *Public Health Reports* 92.2 (Mar.–Apr. 1977), 99–107.

45. US Senate Committee on Labor and Human Resources, "Formula Grants to Schools of Public Health," 20–22; National Center for Education Statistics, *Earned Degrees Conferred: Analysis of Trends, 1965–66 through 1974–75* (US Department of Health, Education and Welfare, 1977), 19–21; Hall, Jackson, and Parsons, *Schools of Public Health: Trends in Graduate Education*, 51.

Chapter 13 · Days of Reckoning and Renewal

1. James Jones, *Bad Blood: The Tuskegee Syphilis Experiment*, rev. ed. (The Free Press, 1993); Jean Heller, "Syphilis Victims in U.S. Study Went Untreated for 40 Years; Syphilis Victims Got No Therapy," *New York Times*, July 26, 1972; Reverby, *Examining Tuskegee*, 96–99, 121, 179, 250.

2. Reverby, "Ethical Failures and History Lessons," 10; Gwatkin, "Political Will and Family Planning"; Jane Lawrence, "The Indian Health Service and the Sterilization of Native American Women," *American Indian Quarterly* 24.3 (2000), 400–19. For another perspective on sterilization in an American context, see Joanna Schoen, *Choice and Coercion: Birth Control, Sterilization, and Abortion in Public Health and Welfare* (University of North Carolina Press, 2005).

3. Mahmood Mamdani, *The Myth of Population Control: Family, Caste, and Class in an Indian Village* (Monthly Review Press, 1972), 13–21, 32–33, 144–53, quote p. 17. Mamdani's book and *The Khanna Study* were reviewed together in several journals, most notably by Burton Benedict, "Other People's Family Planning," *Science* 180 (June 8, 1973), 1045–46. See also P. Visaria's review in *Population Studies* 29.2 (1975), 323–27.

4. Carl E. Taylor, R. S. S. Sarma, Robert L. Parker, William A. Reinke, and Rashid Faruqee, *Child and Maternal Health Services in Rural India: The Narangwal Experiment: Vol. 2. Integrated Family Planning and Health Care* (Johns Hopkins University Press, 1983), Taylor quote p. 12; Connelly, *Fatal Misconception*, 171, 185, 192, 206. For more on how Taylor applied sociology to international health and family planning, see Carl E. Taylor, Charles Leslie, et al., "Asian Medical Systems: A Symposium on the Role of Comparative Sociology in Improving Health Care," *Social Science and Medicine* 7 (1973), 307–18. For a thorough account of critiques of Mamdani, see Rebecca Williams, "Rockefeller Foundation Support to the Khanna Study: Population Policy and the Construction of Demographic Knowledge, 1945–1953," Rockefeller Archive Center Research Reports Online (2011) (http://www.rockarch.org/publications/resrep/, accessed Oct. 1, 2015).

5. Matthew Connelly, "Population Control in India: Prologue to the Emergency Period," *Population and Development Review* 32.4 (2006), 629–667, quote p. 629; Davidson R. Gwatkin, "Political Will and Family Planning: The Implications of India's Emergency Experience," *Population Development Review* 5.1 (1979), 29–59.

6. Tim Baker interview, Aug. 31, 2010; Baker, "Malaria Eradication in India: A Failure?"

7. Amrith, *Decolonizing International Health*, 128–33, 147–50, 173–74.

8. Jonathan B. Tucker, *Scourge: The Once and Future Threat of Smallpox* (Grove Press, 2001), 52–60, quote p. 59; D. A. Henderson interview, Feb. 6, 2009.

9. Randall M. Packard, "'Roll Back Malaria, Roll in Development'? Reassessing the Economic Burden of Malaria," *Population and Development Review* 35 (Mar. 2009), 53–87; Packard, "Visions of Postwar Health and Development and Their Impact on Public Health Interventions in the Developing World," 102–3; Amrith, *Decolonizing International Health*,

128–33, 147–50, 173–74; Mosley interview; Richard Carter and Kamini N. Mendis, "Evolutionary and Historical Aspects of the Burden of Malaria," 582–86.

10. Kerr L. White to Steven Muller, Jan. 16, 1976, Series 13, Office of the President, box 25, "Health Care Organization, Department of 1975–76" folder.

11. D. A. Henderson, *Smallpox: The Death of a Disease* (Prometheus Books, 2009).

12. "Smallpox: Dispelling the Myths: An Interview with Donald Henderson," *Bulletin of the World Health Organization* 86.12 (2008), 917–19.

13. Ibid.

14. D. A. Henderson to JHSPH faculty, March 26, 1978, D. A. Henderson papers.

15. JHSPH 1982–83 Catalog; JHSPH Department of Epidemiology website, "History" (http://www.jhsph.edu/departments/epidemiology/continuing-education/graduate-summer -institute-of-epidemiology-and-biostatistics/about/history.html, accessed Oct. 1, 2015).

16. *NBC Evening News*, Feb. 14, 1971 broadcast; Donald M. Steinwachs interview, Mar. 31, 2013.

17. B. Starfield, B. VandenBerg, D. M. Steinwachs, H. P. Katz, and S. D. Horn, "Variations in Utilization of Health Services by Children," *Pediatrics* 63 (1979) 633–41; Jonathan P. Weiner, Barbara H. Starfield, Donald M. Steinwachs, and L. M. Mumford, "Development and Application of a Population-Oriented Measure of Ambulatory Care Case-Mix," *Medical Care* 29 (1991), 452–72; The Johns Hopkins ACG System website (acg.jhsph.org, accessed Oct. 1, 2015).

18. Steinwachs interview; D. M. Steinwachs and A. Mushlin, "The Johns Hopkins Ambulatory Care Coding Scheme," *Health Services Research* 13 (1978), 36–49.

19. Steinwachs interview.

20. JHSPH catalogs; Steinwachs interview.

21. Steinwachs interview; J. R. Haukin, D. M. Steinwachs, D. Regier, B. Burns, I. Goldberg, and E. Hoeper, "Use of General Medical Care Services by Persons with Mental Disorders," *Archives of General Psychiatry* 39 (1982), 225–31.

22. Gerald N. Grob, "Public Policy and Mental Illnesses: Jimmy Carter's Presidential Commission on Mental Health," *The Milbank Quarterly* 83.3 (2005), 425–56; Ann Skinner interview, Mar. 14, 2012; William W. Eaton interview, Mar. 22, 2012.

23. Carolyn L. Gorman interview, Aug. 21, 2012.

24. Eaton interview, Mar. 22, 2012; A. L. Gross, J. J. Gallo, and W. W. Eaton, "Depression and Cancer Risk: 24 Years of Follow-up of the Baltimore Epidemiologic Catchment Area Sample," *Cancer Causes & Control* 21.2 (2010), 191–99. The Department of Mental Health is currently analyzing the data from four of the five ECA sites and correlating them with the National Death Index to determine the influence of psychopathology on mortality. The outcome will constitute the largest population-based study of mental disorders and mortality ever conducted, with more than 300,000 person-years of observation.

25. Whiteside, "Training the Nation's Health Manpower," 104–5.

26. Abraham Lilienfeld to D. A. Henderson, Feb. 15, 1980, and D. A. Henderson, memo to SHPH Advisory Board, Mar. 25, 1980, Abraham Lilienfeld papers, box 503587, "Correspondence—Appt. as MPH director" folder.

27. JHSPH catalogs.

28. Jones, *Bad Blood*; Susan M. Reverby, *Tuskegee's Truths: Rethinking the Tuskegee Syphilis Study* (University of North Carolina Press, 2000); JHSPH Advisory Board Min-

utes, Jan. 28, 1952, p. 49; Roger M. Herriott bio file, AMC; Faden, *A History and Theory of Informed Consent.*

29. Cecile DeSweemer, "Note on the Rural Health Research Project on Population 1966–73 at Narangwal, Ludhiana District, Punjab, India (March 1975)," Carl Taylor papers, box 21, "Narangwal-General" folder, AMC; Carl E. Taylor to D. N. Chaudhuri, Aug. 3, 1970, Carl Taylor papers, box 21, "Narangwal-General" folder, AMC.

30. Carl Taylor video interview, Sept. 30, 2008, transcript, pp. 10–11; Arnfried A. Kielmann, Carl E. Taylor, et al., *Child and Maternal Health Services in Rural India: The Narangwal Experiment: Vol. 1. Integrated Nutrition and Health Care* (Johns Hopkins University Press, 1983); Daniel Taylor-Ide and Carl E. Taylor, *Just and Lasting Change: When Communities Own Their Futures* (Johns Hopkins University Press, 2002), 126–39; Carl E. Taylor and Cecile DeSweemer, "Lessons from Narangwal about Primary Health Care, Family Planning and Nutrition," in Monica Das Gupta et al., eds., *Prospective Community Studies in Developing Countries* (Clarendon Press, 1997); Brad Sack interview, Sept. 28, 2010.

31. Carl E. Taylor, "Background, Design, and Policy Issues," in Taylor et al., *Child and Maternal Health Services in Rural India*, 2:3–32.

32. John Hume, JHSPH 1973–74 Annual Report, 11; William Reinke interview, Jan. 27, 2012; Carl E. Taylor, "The Future Health Care Delivery Pattern—Lessons from Narangwal," *Indian Journal of Medical Education*, 15.1 (1976), 2–7.

33. Carl E. Taylor, "Ethical Issues Influencing Health for All Beyond the Year 2000," *Infectious Disease Clinics of North America* 9 (June 1995), 223–33, quote p. 232; C. E. Taylor and R. J. Waldman, "Designing Eradication Programs to Strengthen Primary Health Care," in W. R. Dowdle and D. R. Hopkins, eds., *The Eradication of Infectious Diseases* (John Wiley and Sons, 1998), 145–55.

34. Marcos Cueto, "The ORIGINS of Primary Health Care and SELECTIVE Primary Health Care," *AJPH* 94.11 (2004), 1864–74; Theodore M. Brown, Marcos Cueto, and Elizabeth Fee, "The World Health Organization and the Transition from International to Global Health," *AJPH* 96.1 (Jan. 2006), 62–72.

35. John C. Hume to Carl E. Taylor, June 26, 1973, Carl Taylor to Vicente Navarro, Apr. 29, 1977, and Carl Taylor to Vicente Navarro, Apr. 29, 1977, 3a D.O. Correspondence, box R111F6, "International Health" folder.

36. David Sanders and David Werner, *Questioning the Solution: The Politics of Primary Health Care and Child Survival* (HealthWrights, 1997); "Primary Health Care Comes Full Circle: An Interview with Dr Halfdan Mahler," *Bulletin of the World Health Organization* 86.10 (2008), 737–816.

37. Carl E. Taylor and Cecile DeSweemer, "Lessons from Narangwal about Primary Health Care, Family Planning and Nutrition," in Monica Das Gupta et al., eds., *Prospective Community Studies in Developing Countries* (Clarendon Press, 1997); Eberstadt, *Foreign Aid and American Purpose*, 34–56; Martha Finnemore, "Redefining Development at the World Bank," in Cooper and Packard, *International Development and the Social Sciences*, 203–12.

38. R. Brad Sack interview, Sept. 28, 2010; R. B. Sack, "Global View of ORT," *Journal of Diarrheal Disease Research* 5 (1987), 262–64.

39. Mosley interview, Oct. 27, 2010; W. H. Mosley, ed., *Nutrition and Human Reproduction* (New York: Plenum, 1978); W. H. Mosley and L. C. Chen, eds., *Child Survival: Strategies for Research* (Cambridge: Cambridge University Press, 1984).

40. A. Sommer, I. Tarwotjo, G. Hussaini, and D. Susanto, "Increased Mortality in Children with Mild Vitamin A Deficiency," *Lancet* 2 (1983), 585–88; Al Sommer, personal communication, Sept. 19, 2013.

41. Robert E. Black interview, Aug. 2, 2013.

42. Black interview; Cueto, "The ORIGINS of Primary Health Care and SELECTIVE Primary Health Care."

43. Black interview; M. Santosham, A. Chandran, S. Fitzwater, C. Fischer Walker, A. H. Baqui, R. Black, "Progress and Barriers for the control of Diarrheal Disease," *Lancet* 376 (2010), 63–67.

44. John Hume, JHSPH 1973–74 Annual Report, 3.

45. Henderson to JHSPH faculty, March 26, 1978.

46. Gareth M. Green to Wolman, Lilienfeld, Billings, Kimball, Goodman, Hume, and Baker, June 28, 1978, Lilienfeld papers, box 503587, "Correspondence—Appointments to Committees" folder.

47. Richard C. Atkinson and William A. Blanpied, "Research Universities: Core of the US Science and Technology System," *Technology in Society* 30 (2008), 30–48; Michael Yockel, "Rabbit Test," *Warfield's* (May 1986), 40–45; Goldberg and Silbergeld interview, Dec. 12, 2014.

48. Yockel, "Rabbit Test," 40–41.

49. Richard C. Atkinson and William A. Blanpied, "Research Universities: Core of the US Science and Technology System," *Technology in Society* 30 (2008), 30–48; 40–45; Yockel, "Rabbit Test."

50. Ibid., 41–42; Goldberg interview; J. M. Frazier and A. M. Goldberg, "Alternatives to Animals in Toxicity Testing," *Scientific American* 261.2 (1989), 24–30.

51. Yockel, "Rabbit Test," 43–44.

52. Ibid., 45.

53. D. A. Henderson interview, Feb. 21, 2013.

54. Isabel M. Morgan, "Allergic Encephalomyelitis in Monkeys in Response to Injection of Normal Monkey Nervous Tissue," *Journal of Experimental Medicine* 85 (1947), 131–40; Rose, "America's First Department of Immunology"; E. Witebsky, N. R. Rose, K. Terplan, J. R. Paine, and R. W. Egan, "Chronic Thyroiditis and Autoimmunization," *JAMA* 164.13 (1957), 1439–47; Noel R. Rose and Ian R. McKay, eds., *The Autoimmune Diseases* (Academic Press, 1985).

55. Noel R. Rose, "Introduction," in Rozeboom, *Medical Zoology at JHSPH*, iv.

56. Edyth H. Schoenrich to David Paige, Mar. 14, 1975, 3a Dean's or Director's Office Correspondence, box R111F5, "Committee on Residency Training" folder.

Epilogue

1. Council for Education in Public Health, 2013 Annual Report (June 2014), 20; Council for Education in Public Health, 2013 Annual Report (June 2015), 1.

2. David Celentano interview, August 9, 2011.

3. Ibid.

4. Laurie Zabin video interview with Brian Simpson, Aug. 20, 2010.

5. Mandell interview; Celentano interview.

6. Celentano interview.

7. D. Vlahov, J. C. Anthony, A. Munoz, J. Margolick, W. Mandell, K. Nelson, D. Celentano, and B. F. Polk, "A.L.I.V.E.: A Longitudinal Study of Human Immunodeficiency Virus, Type 1 (HIV-1) Infection among Intravenous Drug Users. Description of Methods," *Journal of Drug Issues* 21.4 (Oct. 1991), 759–76; Celentano interview; "Seminal HIV-Injection Drug User Study Marks 20th Anniversary," Nov. 20, 2007, Johns Hopkins School of Public Health News Center (http://www.jhsph.edu/publichealthnews/articles/2007/kirk_ALIVE_anniversary.html, accessed Oct. 15, 2011).

8. Celentano interview; "Seminal HIV-Injection Drug User Study Marks 20th Anniversary"; D. D. Celentano, D. Vlahov, S. Cohn, J. C. Anthony, L. Solomon, and K. E. Nelson, "Risk Factors for Shooting Gallery Use and Cessation among Intravenous Drug Users," *AJPH* 81.10 (Oct. 1991), 1291–95.

9. Lowell J. Reed, Grant Action Form, Mar. 22, 1948, "Johns Hopkins University-School of Hygiene and Public Health-Request to Foundation for Further Support," RG 1.1, series 200, box 186, folder 2234, RFA.

10. Michael Cooper, "Mayor Signs Law to Ban Smoking Soon at Most Bars," *New York Times*, Dec. 12, 2002 (nytimes.com, accessed Oct. 1, 2015).

11. David N. Nabarro and Elizabeth M. Tayler, "The 'Roll Back Malaria' Campaign," *Science* 280.5372 (1998), 2067–68.

12. Marcel Tanner and Don de Savigny, "Malaria Eradication Back on the Table," *Bulletin of the World Health Organization* 86.2 (2008), 82–83; WHO World Malaria Report 2014.